True False 16. Male and female college students are equally likely to wear seatbelts.

True False 17. Alcohol is an important contributor to both intentional and unintentional injuries.

True False 18. "No pain, no gain" is true for receiving health benefits from exercise.

True False 19. The lower a person's cholesterol, the lower his or her risk of dying.

True False 20. Eating a high-protein diet is a healthy choice.

True False 21. Totally eliminating alcohol from one's life is a healthy choice.

True False 22. People who experience chronic pain have underlying psychological disorders that are the real basis of their pain problem.

True False 23. Men are more likely than women to develop heart disease.

True False 24. African Americans are more likely than European Americans to develop and to die of heart disease.

True False 25. Both positive and negative events may produce stress.

True False 26. Psychologists have found that lack of willpower is the primary reason why smokers cannot quit.

True False 27. Sugar pills (placebos) can boost the effectiveness of both psychological and medical treatments.

True False 28. People with a minor illness are about as likely as people with a serious illness to seek medical treatment.

True False 29. People who live with a smoker have about the same risk for cancer and heart disease as do cigarette smokers.

True False 30. Sick people who have a lot of friends usually live longer than sick people who have no close friends.

The answers to these questions appear on the back endpapers. You can also find an answer key on the website for this book: www.cengage.com/psychology/brannon.

HEALTH PSYCHOLOGY

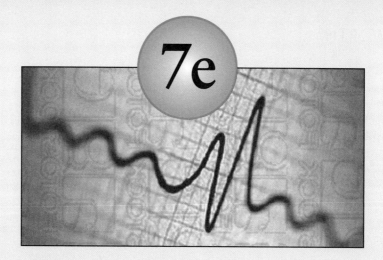

HEALTH PSYCHOLOGY

An Introduction to Behavior and Health

LINDA BRANNON

McNeese State University

JESS FEIST

McNeese State University

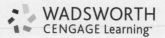

WADSWORTH
CENGAGE Learning

Australia • Brazil • Japan • Korea • Mexico • Singapore • Spain • United Kingdom • United States

WADSWORTH
CENGAGE Learning™

Health Psychology: An Introduction to Behavior and Health, 7th edition
Linda Brannon and Jess Feist

Senior Sponsoring Editor: Jane Potter

Assistant Editor: Paige Leeds

Senior Editorial Assistant: Trina Tom

Associate Media Editor: Rachel Guzman

Marketing Manager: Elisabeth Rhoden

Marketing Coordinator: Molly Felz

Marketing Communications Manager:
Talia Wise

Content Project Manager:
Charlene M. Carpentier

Creative Director: Rob Hugel

Art Director: Vernon Boes

Print Buyer: Paula Vang

Rights Acquisitions Account Manager,
Text: Mardel Glinsky-Schultz

Rights Acquisitions Account Manager,
Image: John Hill

Production Service: Scratchgravel
Publishing Services

Photo Researcher: PrePress PMG

Copy Editor: Margaret C. Tropp

Illustrator: Scratchgravel Publishing
Services

Cover Designer: Larry Didona

Cover Image: Group therapy on lawn,
© Alamy Ltd.; EKG on grid background,
© Age Fotostock; Yoga silhouette, massage
therapy, elderly couple on bikes, vegetables/
fruit, © iStockPhoto; Runner at sunset,
© Shutterstock; Treadmill test, © Masterfile

Compositor: PrePress PMG

For product information and technology assistance, contact us at
Cengage Learning Customer & Sales Support, 1-800-354-9706

For permission to use material from this text or product,
submit all requests online at **www.cengage.com/permissions**
Further permissions questions can be e-mailed to
permissionrequest@cengage.com

Library of Congress Control Number: 2009920060

ISBN-13: 978-0-495-60132-6

ISBN-10: 0-495-60132-2

Wadsworth
10 Davis Drive
Belmont, CA 94002-3098
USA

Cengage Learning is a leading provider of customized learning solutions with
office locations around the globe, including Singapore, the United Kingdom,
Australia, Mexico, Brazil, and Japan. Locate your local office at:
www.cengage.com/global

Cengage Learning products are represented in Canada by
Nelson Education, Ltd.

To learn more about Wadsworth, visit **www.cengage.com/wadsworth**

Purchase any of our products at your local college store or at our preferred
online store **www.ichapters.com**

Printed in the United States of America
1 2 3 4 5 6 7 13 12 11 10 09

Brief Contents

CONTENTS

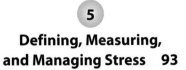
PART 2   Stress, Pain, and Coping

8

Considering Alternative Approaches 188

PART 3 Behavior and Chronic Disease

9

Behavioral Factors in Cardiovascular Disease 221

PART 4 Behavioral Health

12

Smoking Tobacco   307

13

Using Alcohol and Other Drugs   339

PART 5 Looking Toward the Future

16

Future Challenges 437

PREFACE

At the beginning of the 20th century, most serious diseases were caused by contact with viruses and bacteria. People had little individual responsibility for preventing diseases because these microorganisms were nearly impossible to avoid. Today, most serious diseases and disorders occur as the result of individual behaviors—or failures to behave. As health and disease became more closely linked to behavior, psychology—the science of behavior—became involved in many health-related issues. This involvement led to the birth and development of *health psychology*, the scientific study of behaviors that relate to health enhancement, disease prevention, safety, and rehabilitation.

As the profession of health psychology emerged and grew, a need for a comprehensive undergraduate textbook became apparent. Several such books—including the first edition of *Health Psychology: An Introduction to Behavior and Health*—came onto the market. As the field of health psychology developed and expanded, this text evolved to meet the needs of instructors and students who wanted a textbook that included a balance of the science and applications of the field of health psychology. Our purpose in writing the seventh edition of *Health Psychology: An Introduction to Behavior and Health* was to present students with a readable text that will help them keep up to date with the crucial research on behavior and health.

THE SEVENTH EDITION

We have organized the seventh edition of *Health Psychology: An Introduction to Behavior and Health* into five parts. Part 1, which includes the first four chapters, lays a solid foundation in research and theory for understanding

subsequent chapters and approaches the field by considering the overarching issues involved in seeking medical care and adhering to health care regimens. Part 2 deals with stress, pain, and the management of these conditions through conventional and alternative medicine. Part 3 discusses heart disease, cancer, and other chronic diseases. Part 4 includes chapters on tobacco use, drinking alcohol, eating and weight, and physical activity. Part 5 looks toward future challenges in health psychology and addresses how to apply health knowledge to one's life to become healthier.

What's New?

Readers of earlier editions of *Health Psychology: An Introduction to Behavior and Health* will notice a continuation of the concise and accessible writing style and a selective examination of classic and new research studies. The present edition reflects the diversity of health psychology in a number of ways. First, health research has become more international and has come to include more diversity issues, including ethnicity, age, and gender. Second, health research extends into an increasing variety of topics and approaches to health care. The present edition introduces a number of new topics and expands coverage of many more.

Chapter 8, Considering Alternative Approaches, is a new chapter that covers complementary and alternative medicine in detail, including alternative medical systems, alternative practices and products, and mind–body medicine. This chapter also addresses questions of who uses alternative medicine and evaluations of how effective these alternative treatments are, as well as a discussion of the concept of integrative medicine.

The seventh edition also includes some new boxes with presentations of

- The use of technology to enhance adherence
- The stress-relieving potential of biting
- The health risks of watching sports on television
- The health-protective effects of chocolate for heart disease
- The protective effects of a cognitively challenging job
- The importance of adequate sleep for maintaining a healthy weight

Other new or reorganized topics within the chapters include

- An update of several Real-World Profiles and the addition of new ones, including Lindsay Lohan and Norman Cousins
- Placement of information about the training and work of health psychologists in Chapter 1
- A new section in Chapter 16 on using health psychology to improve students' health
- Expanded coverage of the techniques of meta-analysis
- An emphasis on evidence concerning treatment effectiveness based on systematic reviews
- A new organization for Chapters 5 and 7, including material on the management of stress and pain using medical and psychological techniques
- A streamlined and more straightforward presentation of the role of diet in cancer
- Expanded coverage of end-of-life issues in Chapter 11
- Expanded discussions of the role of proinflammatory cytokines in a variety of diseases and psychological disorders
- A streamlined presentation of models for health behaviors in Chapters 3 and 4
- Increased emphasis on the behavioral factors that are important for the development of cardiovascular disease and cancer
- Enlarged coverage of new research on the neurochemical factors in weight regulation

What Has Been Retained?

We have retained the popular features from previous editions, each of which was developed to stimulate critical thinking and to facilitate learning. These features include (1) chapter-opening questions, (2) a "Check Your Health Risks" box in most chapters, (3) a "Would You Believe . . . ?" box in each chapter, and (4) a "Becoming Healthier" feature. The purpose of these features is to actively engage readers in the process of acquiring health-related information that will enhance their personal well-being.

Real-World Profiles A profile of a person in the real world begins each chapter. The purpose of the profile is to illustrate the topics for that chapter, using real people as examples. For the seventh edition, we continue to include well-known people for most real-world profiles. Because these people are familiar to most people, their cases provide intriguing examples, such as Mary-Kate Olsen's eating disorder, Halle Berry's diabetes, Bill Clinton's bypass surgery, Ronald Reagan's Alzheimer's disease, and Lindsay Lohan's problems in coping with her stressful life.

Questions and Answers Each chapter begins with a series of *Questions* that are designed to organize the chapter, preview the material, and enhance active learning. As each chapter unfolds, answers to these questions are revealed through a discussion of relevant research findings. At the end of each major topic, an *In Summary* statement offers a succinct summary of that topic. Then, at the end of the chapter, *Answers* to the chapter-opening questions appear. This *preview, read, and review* method facilitates learning and improves recall.

Check Your Health Risks At the beginning of most chapters, a "Check Your Health Risks" box personalizes material in that chapter. Each box consists of several health-related behaviors or attitudes that readers should check before looking at the rest of the chapter. After checking the items that apply to them and then becoming familiar with the chapter's material, readers can develop a more research-based understanding of their health risks. A special "Check Your Health Risks" appears inside the front cover of the book. Students should complete this exercise before they read the book and look for answers as they proceed through the chapters (or check the website for the answers).

Would You Believe . . . ? Boxes We have kept the popular "Would You Believe . . . ?" boxes, adding six new ones and updating those we retained. Each box begins with the question "Would You Believe . . . ?" and then highlights a particularly intriguing finding in health research. These boxes are designed to explode some preconceived notions and to challenge students to take an objective look at issues that they may have not have evaluated carefully.

Becoming Healthier Embedded in most chapters is a "Becoming Healthier" box with advice on how to use the information in the chapter to enact a healthier lifestyle. Although some people may not agree with all of these recommendations, each is based on the most current research findings. We believe that if you follow these guidelines, you will increase your chances of a long and healthy life.

Other Changes and Additions

We have made a number of subtle changes in this edition that we believe make it an even stronger book than its six predecessors. More specifically, we

- Deleted several hundred old references and exchanged them for more than 800 recent ones
- Reorganized many sections of chapters to improve the flow of information
- Added several new tables and figures to aid students' understanding of difficult concepts
- Highlighted the biopsychosocial approach to health psychology, examining issues and data from a biological, psychological, and social viewpoint
- Drew from the growing body of research from around the world on health to give the book a more international perspective
- Recognized and emphasized gender issues whenever appropriate
- Retained our emphasis on theories and models that strive to explain and predict health-related behaviors

WRITING STYLE

We believe strongly in a readable and engaging writing style, and with each edition we have worked to improve our connection with readers. Although this edition frequently explores complex issues and difficult topics, we use clear, concise, and comprehensible language as well as an informal writing style. The book is designed for upper-division undergraduate students and should be easily understood by those with a minimal background in psychology and biology. Health psychology courses typically draw students from a variety of college majors, necessitating the inclusion of some elementary material that may be repetitive for some students. For other students, this material will fill in the background they need to comprehend the information within the field of health psychology.

Technical terms appear in **boldface type**, and a definition usually appears at that point in the text. These terms also appear in an end-of-book glossary.

INSTRUCTIONAL AIDS

Besides the glossary at the end of the book, we have supplied several other features to help both students and instructors. These include stories of people whose behavior typifies the topic, frequent summaries within each chapter, and annotated suggested readings.

Within-Chapter Summaries

Rather than waiting until the end of each chapter to present a lengthy chapter summary, we have placed shorter summaries at key points within each chapter. In general, these summaries correspond to each major topic in a chapter. We believe these shorter, more frequent summaries keep readers on track and promote a better understanding of the chapter's content.

Annotated Suggested Readings

At the end of each chapter are three or four annotated suggested readings that students may wish to examine. We chose these readings for their capacity to shed additional light on major topics in a chapter. Most of these suggested readings are quite recent, but we have also selected several that have lasting interest. We have included only readings that are intelligible to the average college student and that are accessible in most college and university libraries.

STUDY GUIDE

We have authored the study guide for the seventh edition of *Health Psychology: An Introduction to Behavior and Health* because we feel that a study guide written by the textbook's authors provides students with a more accurate and meaningful account of the contents of the text. Like the textbook, the study guide is divided into 16 chapters. Each chapter of the study guide begins with a set of learning objectives, followed by a challenge to students to "Fill in the Rest of the Story," a feature that should facilitate learning through active participation.

In addition, the study guide contains a variety of *test questions* and a "Let's Get Personal" feature that provides students an opportunity to integrate health information into their personal lives. We believe these features will help students organize their study methods and will also enhance their chances of achieving their best scores on class quizzes.

INSTRUCTOR'S MANUAL WITH TEST BANK

This edition of *Health Psychology: An Introduction to Behavior and Health* is accompanied by a comprehensive instructor's manual. Each chapter begins with a *lecture outline*, designed to assist instructors in preparing lecture material from the text. Many instructors will be able to lecture strictly from these notes; others will be able to use the lecture outline as a framework for organizing their own lecture notes.

A test bank of nearly 1,200 *multiple-choice test items* makes up a large section of each chapter of the instructor's manual. The authors wrote these test items. Some items are factual, some are conceptual, and others ask students to apply what they have learned. These test items will reduce instructors' work in preparing tests. Each item, of course, is marked with the correct answer. The test items are also available electronically on ExamView.

True-false questions and *essay questions* are also included for each chapter. The true-false questions include answers, and each essay question has an outline answer of the critical points.

Each chapter also includes *suggested activities*. These activities vary widely—from video recommendations to student research to classroom debates. We have tried to include more activities than any instructor could feasibly assign during a semester to give instructors a choice of activities.

The growing availability of electronic resources prompted us to include a *Surf the Net* activity. In this section, we suggest online activities, including websites that are relevant to each chapter. This activity expands the electronic resources students may use to explore health-related topics.

INSTRUCTOR'S RESOURCE CD-ROM

Transparencies include art from the text, as well as several physiology video clips and animations in Microsoft® PowerPoint®.

TEXT COMPANION WEBSITE

This website contains practice quizzes, web links, the text's glossary, flashcards, and more for each chapter of the text.

CURRENT PERSPECTIVES: READINGS ON COMPLEMENTARY MEDICINE AND DIVERSITY FROM INFOTRAC® COLLEGE EDITION

Compiled by Erin Strahan of Wilfrid Laurier University, Brantford Campus, this reader contains 15 articles on hot topics in heath psychology. Two or three critical thinking questions for students to answer are posed at the end of each article.

APPLICATIONS IN HEALTH PSYCHOLOGY WORKBOOK

Written by Sussie Eshun of East Stroudsburg University, this guide includes activities that allow students to do basic research and apply investigative skills as they explore such concepts as stress, chronic illness, self-health checks, and more. Each activity includes worksheets and a reflection section called "The Way I See It." The workbook's perforated pages allow students to easily tear out and hand in the worksheets.

ACKNOWLEDGMENTS

Many people have contributed to the completion of this book, and I wish to express my gratitude. I am most grateful to Jess Feist for his participation in the prior six editions of this book. Although he did not participate in the preparation of this edition, his work and words remain as a guide and inspiration for me.

In addition, we would like to thank the people at Cengage Learning for their assistance. Michele Sordi served as editor, beginning with the fifth edition and throughout the preparation of most of this edition. Her skill, diligence, patience, understanding, and support have helped me manage this revision and guided me to produce a better book. Our editors for previous editions, Marianne Taflinger and Ken King, helped shape the book in many ways, and I continue to owe them my thanks. Others who worked on the seventh edition include: Jane Potter, senior sponsoring editor; Paige Leeds, assistant editor; Trina Tom, senior editorial assistant; Rachel Guzman, associate media editor; Elisabeth Rhoden, marketing manager; Molly Felz, marketing coordinator; Talia Wise, marketing communications manager; Charlene M. Carpentier, content project manager; Rob Hugel, creative director; Vernon Boes, art director; Paula Vang, print buyer; Mardel Glinsky-Schultz, John Hill, rights acquisitions account managers; and Anne Draus of Scratchgravel Publishing Services, production service.

I am also indebted to a number of reviewers who read all or parts of the manuscript for this and earlier editions. I am grateful for the valuable comments of the following reviewers:

Soran Susan Dubitsky, Florida International University

Dennis E. Elsenrath, University of Wisconsin, Stevens Point

Sussie Eshun, East Stroudsburg University

Susan K. Johnson, University of North Carolina, Charlotte

Richard Lazarus, University of California, Berkeley

Ralph Paffenbarger, Jr., Stanford School of Medicine

Paul B. Paulus, University of Texas, Arlington

Shirley A. Pavone, Sacred Heart University

Daniel J. Taylor, University of North Texas

Christy Teranishi, Texas A&M International University

Elizabeth Thyrum, Millersville University

Jenny Yi, University of Houston

Authors typically thank their spouses for being understanding, supportive, and sacrificing, and my spouse, Barry Humphus, is no exception. He and Jess's wife, Mary Jo, have given much more than the traditional emotional support. Both have made contributions that have helped to shape the book. In addition to his creative contributions to the book, Barry provided generous, patient, live-in, expert computer consultation and tech support that proved essential in the preparation of the manuscript.

ABOUT THE AUTHORS

Linda Brannon and Jess Feist both spent their careers as Professors in the Department of Psychology at McNeese State University in Lake Charles, Louisiana. Linda joined the faculty at McNeese after receiving her doctorate in human experimental psychology from the University of Texas at Austin, and Jess came to McNeese after receiving his doctorate in counseling from the University of Kansas. Linda and Jess have each been selected to receive the Distinguished Faculty Award from McNeese State University. Jess is currently emeritus Professor of Psychology at McNeese State University.

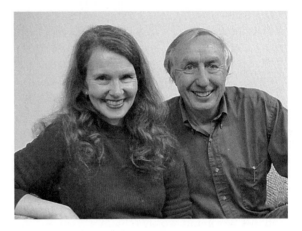

In the early 1980s, Linda and Jess became interested in the developing field of health psychology, which led to their coauthoring the first edition of this book. They have watched the field of health psychology emerge and grow, and the subsequent editions of the book reflect that growth and development.

Their interests converge in the area of health psychology but diverge in other areas of psychology. Jess carries his interest in personality theory to his book *Theories of Personality*, coauthored with his son Greg Feist. Linda's interest in gender and gender issues led her to publish *Gender: Psychological Perspectives*, and she is also coauthor of *Psychology*, an introductory psychology textbook.

Jess now devotes his time to gardening and continues to jog daily. Linda is also a jogger but a more reluctant one than Jess. She enjoys watching movies and practicing tai chi.

HEALTH PSYCHOLOGY

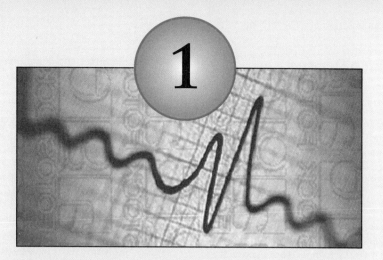

1

INTRODUCING HEALTH PSYCHOLOGY

QUESTIONS

This chapter focuses on three basic questions:

1. How have views of health changed?

2. How did psychology become involved in health care?

3. What type of training do health psychologists receive, and what kinds of work do they do?

Felicia Otchet received her doctoral degree in psychology from the University of Cincinnati in 1996 and took a job in London, Ontario, Canada (Otchet, 1998). Or more accurately, she took several jobs with part-time commitments that equaled a full-time (or more than a full-time) job. Her duties involved providing services to people in a hospital and a community health center, but providing mental health services was not her main duty. Instead, Felicia worked as a clinical health psychologist, acting as part of a multidisciplinary team to provide services to people with chronic pain, HIV, cancer, and other health problems. Her job title was psychologist at the London Health Sciences Centre; she was part of Canada's Behavioural Medicine Service.

Her work at the London Intercommunity Health Centre involved providing services to multicultural clients and consulting with doctors, nurses, social workers, therapists, and community workers to improve adherence to medical advice and manage difficult patients. Another of her jobs was to act as a consultant to a pain management clinic. At the hospital, Felicia acted as part of a team providing consultation and services for female patients with cancers of the reproductive tract. In each of these settings, Felicia supervised students who were receiving training. She also participated in several ongoing research studies and was involved with developing a satisfaction survey for former patients of the hospital.

Felicia's jobs were more varied than those of many health psychologists, but the types of duties and the settings are typical for clinical health psychologists who provide services to patients. Other health psychologists are more involved with research than Felicia was, working in universities or government agencies that conduct research. The training and work settings of health psychologists are part of this introductory chapter. But to introduce health psychology, we must first consider the changing field of health and health care.

THE CHANGING FIELD OF HEALTH

A century ago, most people in the United States saw health as the absence of disease. That view was probably influenced by the diseases that were most common 100 years ago, which differed from the picture of illness today. In the early 1900s, people's diseases were largely the result of contact with impure drinking water, contaminated foods, or sick people. Once they were ill, people were expected to seek medical care to be cured, but medicine had few cures to offer. The duration of most diseases—such as typhoid fever, pneumonia, and diphtheria—was relatively short; a person either died or got well in a matter of weeks. People felt very limited responsibility for contracting a contagious disease because such disease was not controllable. That situation has changed.

During the 20th century, the major challenges to health in the United States shifted from infectious diseases to those related to unhealthy behaviors and lifestyles. Effective treatments were developed to treat and cure many diseases, but these technological developments were expensive. The cost of medical care rose sharply and containing medical costs became a priority, highlighting the importance of educating people about how health-related behaviors could lower (or raise) their risk of becoming ill. As a result of these trends, a new definition of health emerged, one that regarded health as the presence of positive well-being, not merely the absence of disease. This new definition of health led some people in the health care field to advocate a broader perspective on health and disease, questioning the usefulness of the traditional biomedical model.

Patterns of Disease and Death

The 20th century brought about major changes in the patterns of disease and death in the United States, including a shift in the leading causes of death. Infectious diseases such as influenza, pneumonia, tuberculosis, and diphtheria were leading causes of death in 1900, but over the next several decades, chronic diseases such as heart disease, cancer, and stroke became the leading killers. These and other chronic diseases develop and then persist or recur, affecting the person over a long period of time. During the last few years of the 20th century, deaths from chronic diseases—those related to unhealthy lifestyles and behaviors—began to *decrease* while deaths from diseases not closely related to lifestyles and behaviors began to *increase*.

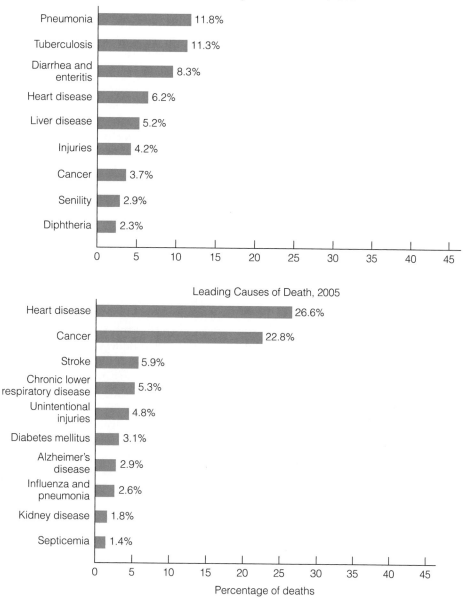

FIGURE 1.1   Leading causes of death, United States, 1900 and 2005.

Sources: "Healthy People, 2010," 2000, by U.S. Department of Health and Human Services, Washington, DC: U.S. Government Printing Office; "Deaths: Final Data for 2005," 2008, by H.-C. Kung, D. L. Hoyert, J. J. Xu, & S. L. Murphy, *National Vital Statistics Reports, 56*(10), Table B.

Causes of Death Chronic diseases are not new, of course, but the proportion of people who die of them has changed dramatically since 1900. Figure 1.1 reveals important differences in the leading causes of death in the United States as recorded in 1900 and 2005. In 1900, the majority of deaths were from diseases that were rooted in public or community health problems, such as pneumonia, tuberculosis, and diarrhea. During the 20th century, most deaths came to be attributable to diseases associated with individual behavior and lifestyle. Heart disease, cancer, stroke, chronic lower respiratory diseases (including emphysema and chronic bronchitis), unintentional injuries, and diabetes have been linked to cigarette smoking, alcohol abuse, unwise eating, stress, and sedentary lifestyle. This change led Robert Sapolsky (1998) to declare: "We are now living well enough and long enough to slowly fall apart" (p. 2).

Recent trends indicate a *decrease* in mortality from several diseases associated largely with individual behavior and lifestyle. Of the top causes of death in the United States, several showed lower mortality rates in 2005 than in 1990. All of these diseases have at least some behavior component. For example, from 1990 to 2005, deaths decreased from heart disease, cancer, and stroke; small increases occurred in violent deaths such as unintentional injuries, suicide, and homicide (Kung, Hoyert, Xu, & Murphy, 2008). Significant increases occurred in Alzheimer's disease, influenza and pneumonia, kidney disease, septicemia (blood infection), and Parkinson's disease. For these causes of death that have recently increased, behavior is a less important component than for those causes that have decreased, but Sapolsky's quote applies—Alzheimer's disease and Parkinson's disease are more likely to affect older individuals, and influenza and pneumonia are more likely to be fatal to them.

Indeed, age is an important factor in mortality. Obviously, older people are more likely to die than younger ones, but the causes of death vary among age groups. Thus, the ranking of causes of death for the entire population may not reflect any specific age group and may lead people to misperceive the risk for some ages. For example, cardiovascular disease (which includes heart disease and stroke) and cancer account for about 60% of all deaths in the United States, but they are not the leading cause of death for young people. For individuals between 1 and 44 years of age, unintentional injuries are the leading cause of death, and violent deaths from suicide and homicide rank high on the list (National Center for Health Statistics [NCHS], 2007). Unintentional injuries account for 28% of the deaths in this age group, suicide for almost 10%, and homicide for

about 8%. As Figure 1.2 reveals, other causes of death account for much smaller percentages of deaths among adolescents and young adults than unintentional injuries, homicide, and suicide.

For adults 45 to 64 years old, the picture is quite different. Cardiovascular disease and cancer become leading causes of death, and unintentional injuries fall to third place. As people age, they become more likely to die, so the causes of death for older people dominate the overall figures for causes of death. However, younger people show very different patterns of mortality.

Ethnicity, Income, and Disease Question 2 from the quiz inside the front cover asks if the United States is among the top 10 nations in the world in terms of life expectancy. It is not; its rank is 14th among industrialized nations (NCHS, 2007) but 45th among all nations (Central Intelligence Agency [CIA], 2008). Within the United States, ethnicity is also a factor in life expectancy, and the leading causes of death show some variation among ethnic groups. Table 1.1 shows the ranking of the 10 leading causes of death for four ethnic groups in the United States. No two groups have identical profiles of causes of death, and some causes do not appear on the list for each group, highlighting the influence of ethnicity on mortality.

If African Americans and European Americans in the United States were considered to be different nations, European America would rank higher in life expectancy than African America—42nd place and 100th place, respectively (CIA, 2008; U.S. Census Bureau [USCB], 2007). Thus, European Americans have a longer life expectancy than African Americans, but neither should expect to live as long as people in Japan, Canada, Iceland, Australia, the United Kingdom, Italy, France, Hong Kong, Israel, and many other countries.

The dramatic life expectancy difference between European and African Americans does not apply as strongly to Hispanic Americans, leading some investigators to proclaim a "Hispanic paradox" for life expectancy. Hispanics have socioeconomic disadvantages similar to those of African Americans (USCB, 2007), including poverty and low educational level. About 10% of European Americans live below the poverty level, whereas

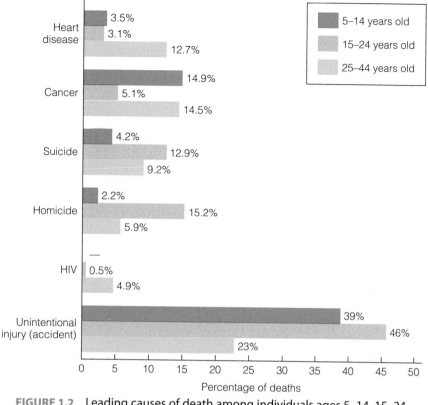

FIGURE 1.2   Leading causes of death among individuals ages 5–14, 15–24, and 55–44, United States, 2004.

Source: Health, United States, 2007, 2007, by National Center for Health Statistics, Table 38.

32% of African Americans and 26% of Hispanic Americans do (USCB, 2007). European Americans also have educational advantages: 86% receive high school diplomas, compared to only 81% of African Americans and 59% of Hispanic Americans. These socioeconomic disadvantages translate into health disadvantages (Crimmins, Ki Kim, Alley, Karlamangla, & Seeman, 2007; Smith & Bradshaw, 2006). That is, poverty and low educational level are related to health problems and lower life expectancy, regardless of ethnicity, so the Hispanic paradox is not so much of a paradox after all.

Access to health insurance and medical care are not the only factors that make poverty a health risk. Indeed, the health risks associated with poverty begin before birth. Even with the expansion of prenatal care by Medicaid, poor mothers, especially teen mothers, are more likely

to deliver low-birth-weight babies, who are more likely than normal-birth-weight infants to die (NCHS, 2007). Also, pregnant women living below the poverty line are more likely than other pregnant women to be physically abused and to deliver babies who suffer the consequences of prenatal child abuse (Zelenko, Lock, Kraemer, & Steiner, 2000).

Income level is strongly related to health, not only at the poverty level but at higher income levels as well. Within any income group, people at higher levels have better health and lower mortality than those at lower levels, which presents a puzzle: Why should very wealthy people be healthier than other wealthy people? One possibility comes from the relation of income to educational level, which, in turn, is related to occupation, social class, and ethnicity. The higher the educational level, the less likely people are to

TABLE 1.1

Ten Leading Causes of Death for Four Ethnic Groups in the United States, 2004

	European Americans	Hispanic Americans	African Americans	Asian Americans
Heart disease	1	1	1	2
Cancer	2	2	2	1
Stroke	3	4	3	3
Chronic lower respiratory disease	4	8	8	7
Unintentional injuries	5	3	5	4
Alzheimer's disease	6	*	*	10
Diabetes	7	5	4	5
Pneumonia & influenza	8	9	*	6
Kidney disease	9	*	7	9
Suicide	10	*	*	8
Septicemia	*	*	10	*
Chronic liver disease	*	6	*	*
Homicide	*	7	6	*
HIV	*	*	9	*
Conditions originating in perinatal period	*	10	*	*

*Not among the 10 leading causes of death for this ethnic group.
Source: "Deaths: Leading causes for 2004," 2007, by M. Heron, *National Vital Statistics Reports*, 56(5), Tables E and F.

engage in unhealthy behaviors such as smoking, eating a high-fat diet, and maintaining a sedentary lifestyle (see Would You Believe . . . ? box). Another possibility is the perception of social status. People's perception of their social standing may differ from their status as indexed by educational, occupational, and income level, and this perception is more strongly related to health status than more objective measures (Operario, Adler, & Williams, 2004). Thus, the possibilities for influence are numerous, and the mechanisms that underlie the relationship of health to income, ethnicity, educational level, and social class require clarification.

Changes in Life Expectancy During the 20th century, life expectancy rose dramatically in the United States and other industrialized nations. In 1900, life expectancy was 47.3 years (USBC, 1975), whereas today it is more than 77 years (USCB, 2007). In other words, infants born today can, on average, expect to live more than a generation longer than their great-great-grandparents born at the beginning of the 20th century.

What factors have accounted for the 30-year increase in life expectancy during the 20th century? Question 3 from the quiz inside the front cover asks if advances in medical care were responsible for this increase. The answer is False; other factors have been more important. The control of many infectious diseases through widespread vaccination and safer drinking water and milk supplies were more important for extending life expectancy. A healthier lifestyle also contributed, as did more efficient disposal of sewage and better nutrition. Medical advances such as antibiotics and new surgical technology, efficient paramedic teams, and more skilled intensive care personnel have played a relatively minor role in increased life expectancy.

Although advances that affect adults' longevity helped extend lives, the single most important contributor to the increase in life expectancy was the lowering of infant mortality. When infants die before their first birthday, these deaths lower the population's average life expectancy much more than do the deaths of middle-aged or older people. Thus, decreasing deaths at a young age can have a

WOULD YOU BELIEVE . . . ?

College Is Good for Your Health

Would you believe that attending college is probably good for your health? Many college students may find it difficult to believe that college improves their health. To the contrary, college seems to add stress, offer opportunities for drug use, and limit the time available for eating a healthy diet, exercising, and sleeping. How could going to college possibly be healthy?

Students may not follow all recommendations for leading a healthy life while they are in college, but people who have been to college have lower death rates than those who have not. This advantage applies to both women and men and to infectious diseases, chronic diseases, and unintentional injuries (NCHS, 2007). On a typical day, better educated people report fewer symptoms and less stress than less educated people (Grzywacz, Almeida, Neupert, & Ettner, 2004). Attending college is not unique in conferring health benefits; education in general provides an overall health advantage.

People who graduate from high school have lower death rates than those who do not, but going to college offers much more protection. For example, people with less than a high school education died at a rate of 667 per 100,000; those who had graduated from high school showed a rate of 477 per 100,000; but people who had attended

college had a death rate of only 208 per 100,000 (NCHS, 2007). That is, people who had attended college showed a death rate less than half that of high school graduates. The benefits of education for health and longevity apply to people around the world. For example, a study of older people in Japan (Fujino et al., 2005) found that low educational level increased the risk of dying. A large-scale study of the Dutch population (Hoeymans, van Lindert, & Westert, 2005) found that education was related to a wide range of health measures and health-related behaviors.

What factors contribute to this health advantage for people with more education? Part of that advantage may be intelligence, which predicts both health and longevity (Gottfredson & Deary, 2004). In addition, people who are well educated tend to live with and around people with similar education, providing an environment with good health-related knowledge and attitudes (Øystein, 2008). Income and occuption may also contribute (Batty et al., 2008); people who attend college, especially those who graduate, have better jobs and higher average incomes than those who do not, and thus are more likely to have better access to health care. In addition, educated people are more likely to be informed consumers of health

care, gathering information on their diseases and potential treatments. Education is also associated with a variety of habits that are positively related to good health and long life. For example, people with a college education are less likely than others to smoke or use illicit drugs (Johnston, O'Malley, Bachman, & Schulenberg, 2007), and they are more likely to eat a low-fat diet and to exercise.

Although separating education and income is almost impossible, a group of Dutch researchers (Schrijvers, Stronks, van de Mheen, & Mackenbach, 1999) examined both financial and behavioral differences related to health. Their analysis indicated that financial factors were a bit more important, but both types of factors contributed independently to health. A longitudinal study of Danish adults (Osler & Prescott, 2003) also showed an advantage for education; this study found that the benefits of education were mediated through income, health behaviors (such as smoking and exercise), and community conditions (such as unemployment and crime). Thus, people who attend college acquire many resources that are reflected in their lower death rate—income potential, health knowledge, more health-conscious spouses and friends, attitudes about the importance of health, and positive health habits.

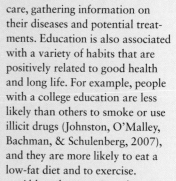

substantial statistical impact. As Figure 1.3 shows, infant death rates declined dramatically between 1900 and 1990, but little decrease has occurred since that time. Unfortunately, this benefit did not apply equally to all ethnic groups. African American infants are more than twice as likely

as European American infants to die in infancy— 13.8 per 1,000 births versus 5.7 (USCB, 2007). The rate among Hispanic Americans is similar to that of European Americans (6.2), despite the disadvantages of lower educational levels, higher rates of poverty, and poorer prenatal care.

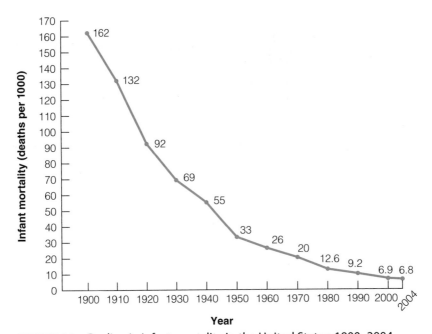

FIGURE 1.3   Decline in infant mortality in the United States, 1900–2004.

Source: Data from *Historical Statistics of the United States: Colonial Times to 1970, 1975*, by U.S. Bureau of the Census, Washington, DC: U.S. Government Printing Office, p. 60; *Statistical Abstract of the United States: 2008* (127th edition), 2007, by U.S. Census Bureau, Washington, DC: U.S. Government Printing Office, Table 108.

Escalating Cost of Medical Care

The second major change within the field of health has been the escalating cost of medical care. These costs, of course, have some relationship to increased life expectancy: As people live to middle and old age, they tend to develop chronic diseases that require extended (and often expensive) medical treatment. About 45% of people in the United States have a chronic condition, and they account for 78% of the dollars spent on health care (Rice & Fineman, 2004). People with chronic conditions account for 88% of prescriptions written, 72% of physician visits, and 76% of hospital stays. Even though today's aging population is experiencing better health than past generations, their increasing numbers will continue to contribute to increasing medical costs.

In the United States, medical costs have increased at a much faster rate than inflation. Between 1960 and 2005, these costs represented a larger and larger proportion of the gross domestic product (GDP). Since 1995, the increases have slowed, but

medical care costs as a percentage of the GDP have crept up to 16% (NCHS, 2007). This percentage is greater than in any other country, although several European countries spend about 10% of their GDP on medical care (USCB, 2007). The total yearly cost of health care in the United States increased from $1,067 per person in 1970 to $6,697 in 2005 (NCHS, 2007), a jump of more than 600% and a much faster annual increase than that reported for the years 1960 to 1980.

Although medical treatment during the 20th century performed nearly miraculous cures for some individuals, the mounting monetary cost of medical miracles militates against the traditional philosophy of health, which emphasizes diagnosis, treatment, and cure. Expensive medical procedures such as heart surgery, hemodialysis, and high-technology imaging techniques contribute to the rising cost of health care in the United States, even though only a relatively small proportion of the population uses such technology.

One strategy for curbing mounting medical costs is to limit services, but another approach requires a

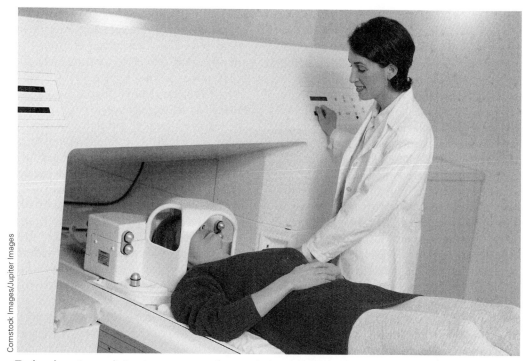

Technology in medicine is one reason for escalating medical costs.

greater emphasis on the early detection of disease and on changes to a healthier lifestyle and to behaviors that help prevent disease. For example, early detection of high blood pressure, high serum cholesterol, and other precursors of heart disease allow these conditions to be controlled, thereby decreasing the risk of serious disease or death. Screening people for risk is preferable to remedial treatment because chronic diseases are quite difficult to cure and living with chronic disease decreases quality of life. Avoiding disease by adopting a healthy lifestyle is even more preferable to treating diseases or screening for risks. Staying healthy is typically less costly than becoming sick and then getting well. Thus, prevention of disease through a healthy lifestyle, early detection of symptoms, and reduction of health risks have all become part of the changing philosophy within the health care field.

What Is Health?

What does it mean to be healthy? Question 1 from the quiz at the beginning of the book asks if health is an absence of disease. But is health more complex? Is health the presence of some positive condition rather than merely the absence of a negative one?

The **biomedical model** is the traditional view of Western medicine, which defines health as the absence of disease (Papas, Belar, & Rozensky, 2004). This view conceptualizes disease exclusively as a biological process that is an almost mechanistic result of exposure to a specific **pathogen,** a disease-causing organism. This view spurred the development of drugs and medical technology oriented toward removing the pathogens and curing disease. The focus is on disease, which is traceable to a specific agent. Removing the pathogen restores health.

The biomedical model of disease is compatible with infectious diseases that were the leading causes of death 100 years ago. Throughout the 20th century, adherence to the biomedical model allowed medicine to conquer or control many of the diseases that once ravaged humanity. When chronic illnesses began to replace infectious diseases as leading causes of death, questions began to arise about the adequacy of the biomedical model (Stone, 1987). While conceding that the biomedical model has been responsible for much progress in the treatment of disease, a few physicians, many psychologists, and some sociologists have expressed dissatisfaction with the biomedical model and have begun to question its usefulness in dealing with the current patterns of disease and death and its definition of health.

An alternative model of health has evolved, one that advocates a holistic approach to medicine. This holistic model considers social, psychological, physiological, and even spiritual aspects of a person's health. An alternative model must have the power of the old model plus the ability to solve problems that the old model has failed to solve. This alternative model is called the **biopsychosocial model,** the approach to health that includes biological, psychological, and social influences. The biopsychosocial model has at least two advantages over the older biomedical model: first, it incorporates not only biological conditions but also psychological and social factors, and second, it views health as a positive condition.

According to the biopsychosocial view, health is much more than the absence of disease. A person who has no disease condition is not sick, but this person may not be healthy either. Because health is multidimensional, all aspects of living—biological, psychological, and social—must be considered. This view diverges from the traditional Western conceptualization, but as Table 1.2 shows, other cultures have held different views.

In 1946, the United Nations established the World Health Organization (WHO) and wrote into the preamble of its constitution a modern, Western definition: "Health is a state of complete physical, mental, and social well-being, and not merely the absence of disease or infirmity." This definition clearly affirms that health is a positive state and not just the absence of pathogens. Feeling good is more than not feeling bad, and research in neuroscience has confirmed the difference (Zautra, 2003). The human brain responds in distinctly different patterns to positive feelings and negative feelings.

Within psychology, a movement that highlights the positive aspects of functioning has become prominent. Proponents of this movement, called *positive psychology*, argue that psychology has emphasized disease and pathology for too much of its history. Psychologists such as Martin Seligman and Mihaly Csikszentmihalyi (2000) have contended that "psychology is not just the study of pathology,

TABLE 1.2
Definitions of Health Held by Various Cultures

Culture	Time Period	Health Is
Prehistoric	10,000 BCE	Endangered by spirits that enter the body from outside
Babylonians and Assyrians	1800–700 BCE	Endangered by the gods, who send disease as a punishment
Ancient Hebrews	1000–300 BCE	A gift from God; disease is a punishment from God
Ancient Greeks	500 BCE	A holistic unity of body and spirit
Ancient China		A state of physical and spiritual harmony with nature
Native Americans	1000 BCE–present	Total harmony with nature and the ability to survive under difficult conditions
Galen in Ancient Rome	130–200 CE	The absence of pathogens, such as bad air or body fluids, that cause disease
Early Christians	300–600 CE	Not as important as disease, which is a sign that one is chosen by God
Descartes in France	1596–1650	A condition of the mechanical body, which is separate from the mind
Western Africans	1600–1800	Harmony achieved through interactions with other people and objects in the world
Virchow in Germany	Late 1800s	Endangered by microscopic organisms that invade cells, producing disease
Freud in Austria	Late 1800s	Influenced by emotions and the mind
World Health Organization	1946	"A state of complete physical, mental, and social well-being"

weakness, and damage; it is also the study of strength and virtue" (p. 7). Thus, positive psychology is compatible with the emerging view of health as a positive state rather than the absence of pathogens. In addition, research in the field of positive psychology extends to health issues, including the impact of optimism on health and life expectancy (Danner, Snowdon, & Friesen, 2001).

IN SUMMARY

Four major trends have changed the field of health care in the past century. One trend is the changing pattern of disease and death in industrialized nations, including the United States. Chronic diseases have replaced infectious diseases as the leading causes of death and disability. These chronic diseases include heart disease, stroke, cancer, emphysema, and adult-onset diabetes, all of which have causes that include individual behavior.

The increase in chronic disease has contributed to a second trend: the escalating cost of medical care. Costs for medical care rose dramatically between 1970 and 2005, but more recent gains have slowed in relation to the gross domestic product. Much of this cost increase is due to a growing elderly population, innovative but expensive medical technology, and inflation.

A third trend is the changing definition of health. Many people continue to view health as the absence of disease, but a growing number of health care professionals view health as a state of positive well-being. To accept this definition of health is to reconsider the biomedical model that has dominated the health care field.

The fourth trend, the emergence of the biopsychosocial model of health, is related to the changing definition of health. Rather than defining disease as the simple presence of pathogens, the biopsychosocial model emphasizes positive health and sees disease, particularly chronic disease, as resulting from the interaction of biological, psychological, and social conditions. An emphasis on positive aspects of health is compatible with positive psychology, which concentrates on people's virtues and strengths.

PSYCHOLOGY'S INVOLVEMENT IN HEALTH

Although chronic diseases have biological causes, individual behavior and lifestyle are strongly implicated in their development. Because behavior is so important for chronic disease, psychology—the science of behavior—has become involved in health care.

Psychology has been involved with people's physical health almost from the beginning of the 20th century. In 1911, the American Psychological Association (APA) convened a panel to discuss the role of psychology in medical education. Psychologists of the time agreed that medical students would profit from instruction in psychology and recommended psychology as part of premedical training or the medical school curriculum. Most medical schools failed to pursue the recommendation.

During the 1940s, medical training typically incorporated the study of psychological factors related to disease, but this limited training was part of the medical specialty of psychiatry, not psychology. A few clinical psychologists provided psychological services, such as testing and psychotherapy for patients with emotional problems, but few were involved in health research (Matarazzo, 1994). Also, psychologists seldom collaborated with medical specialists other than psychiatrists. But psychology's role in medicine began to expand with the creation of new medical schools during the 1960s; the number of psychologists who held academic appointments on medical school faculties nearly tripled from 1969 to 1993 (Matarazzo, 1994). By the beginning of the 21st century, psychologists had made significant progress in their efforts to gain greater acceptance by the medical profession (Pingitore, Scheffler, Haley, Seniell, & Schwalm, 2001).

In 2002, the American Medical Association (AMA) accepted several new categories for health and behavior that permit psychologists to bill for services to patients with physical diseases. Also, Medicare's Graduate Medical Education program now accepts psychology internships, and the APA has worked with the World Health Organization to formulate a new diagnostic system for

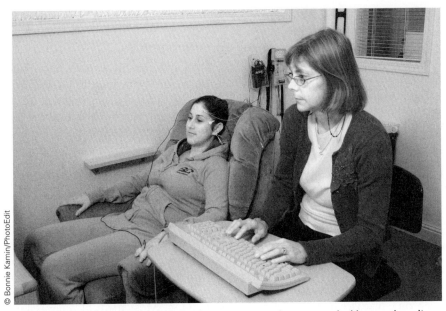

The role of the psychologist in health care settings has expanded beyond traditional mental health problems to include procedures such as biofeedback.

biopsychosocial disorders, the International Classification of Functioning, Disability, and Health (ICF) (Reed & Scheldeman, 2004). Thus, the role of psychologists in medical settings has expanded beyond traditional mental health problems to include procedures and programs to help people stop smoking, eat a healthy diet, exercise, adhere to medical advice, reduce stress, control pain, live with chronic disease, and avoid unintentional injuries.

The Contribution of Psychosomatic Medicine

The notion that psychological and emotional factors can contribute to physical ailments can be traced to the days of Socrates and Hippocrates. Early humans saw disease as spiritual as well as physical, and many cultures include psychological and social factors in their views of health and disease. In the 18th century, a German professor named Gaub anticipated the biopsychosocial approach to disease and health when he wrote, "The reason why a sound body becomes ill or an ailing body recovers very often lies in the mind" (as cited in Fritz, 2000, p. 8).

The notion that emotional factors contribute to illness was compatible with the popular theories of Sigmund Freud, who emphasized the importance of unconscious psychological factors in the development of physical symptoms. Freud's methods relied on clinical experience and intuitive hunches, not research. The search to tie emotional causes to illness drew from Walter Cannon's observation in 1932 that physiological changes accompany emotion (Kimball, 1981). Cannon's research demonstrated that emotion is capable of causing physiological changes that may be related to the development of physical disease; that is, emotion can cause changes, which in turn may cause disease. From this finding, Helen Flanders Dunbar (1943) developed the notion that habitual responses, which people exhibit as part of their personalities, are related to specific diseases. In other words, Dunbar hypothesized a relationship between personality type and disease. A little later, Franz Alexander (1950), a onetime follower of Freud, began to see emotional conflicts as a precursor to certain diseases.

These views led others to begin to see a range of specific illnesses as "psychosomatic." These illnesses included such disorders as peptic ulcer, rheumatoid arthritis, hypertension, asthma, hyperthyroidism, and ulcerative colitis. This belief diverged from the biomedical view, which concentrates on the body and ignores the mind. However, the widespread belief in the separation of mind and body—which can be traced back to Descartes (Papas et al., 2004)—led many laypeople to look at these psychosomatic disorders as not being "real" but merely "all in the head." Thus, psychosomatic medicine exerted a mixed impact, with the positive influence of connecting emotional and physical conditions and the negative influence of belittling the psychological components of illness. Psychosomatic medicine, however, laid the foundation for the transition to the biopsychosocial model of health and disease (Novack et al., 2007). This model holds that many diseases result from some combination of genetics, physiology, social support, personal control, stress, compliance, personality, poverty, ethnic background, and cultural beliefs. We discuss each of these factors in subsequent chapters.

The Emergence of Behavioral Medicine

Two new and interrelated disciplines emerged from the psychosomatic medicine movement: *behavioral medicine* and *health psychology*.

A 1977 conference at Yale University led to the founding of a new field, **behavioral medicine**, defined as "the interdisciplinary field concerned with the development and integration of behavioral and biomedical science knowledge and techniques relevant to health and illness and the application of this knowledge and these techniques to prevention, diagnosis, treatment and rehabilitation" (Schwartz & Weiss, 1978, p. 250). This definition indicates that behavioral medicine is designed to integrate medicine and the various behavioral sciences, especially psychology. The goals of behavioral medicine are similar to those in other areas of health care: improved prevention, diagnosis, treatment, and rehabilitation. Behavioral medicine, then, attempts to use psychology and the behavioral sciences in conjunction with medicine to promote health and treat disease. Chapters 3 through 11 cover topics in behavioral medicine.

The Emergence of Health Psychology

At about the same time that behavioral medicine appeared, a new discipline called *behavioral health* began to emerge. Behavioral health emphasizes the enhancement of health and the prevention of disease in healthy people rather than the diagnosis and treatment of disorders in sick people. Behavioral health includes such concerns as injury prevention, cigarette smoking, alcohol use, diet, and exercise, topics we discuss in Chapters 12 through 15.

Behavioral health has not continued to develop as a strong, formal discipline but has filtered into several fields that use health promotion. Its goals have been incorporated into the field of **health psychology,** the branch of psychology that concerns individual behaviors and lifestyles affecting a person's physical health. Health psychology includes psychology's contributions to the enhancement of health, the prevention and treatment of disease, the identification of health risk factors, the improvement of the health care system, and the shaping of public opinion with regard to health. More specifically, it involves the application of psychological principles to physical health areas such as controlling cholesterol, managing stress, alleviating pain, stopping smoking, and moderating other risky behaviors, as well as encouraging regular exercise, medical and dental checkups, and safer behaviors. In addition, health psychology helps identify conditions that affect health, diagnose and treat certain chronic diseases, and modify the behavioral factors involved in physiological and psychological rehabilitation. As such, health psychology interacts with both biology and sociology to produce health- and disease-related outcomes (see Figure 1.4). Note that neither psychology nor sociology contributes directly to outcomes; only biological factors contribute directly to physical health and disease. Thus, the psychological and sociological factors that affect health must "get under the skin" in some way in order to affect biological processes. One of the goals of health psychology is to identify those ways.

A Brief History of Health Psychology As an identifiable area, health psychology received its first important impetus in 1973, when the Board of Scientific Affairs of the American Psychological Association (APA) appointed a task force to study the potential for psychology's role in health research. Three years later, this task force (APA Task Force, 1976) reported that few psychologists

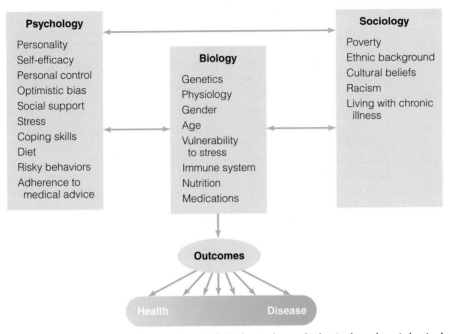

FIGURE 1.4 The biopsychosocial model: Biological, psychological, and sociological factors interact to produce health or disease.

were involved in health research and that research conducted by psychologists in the area of health was not often reported in the psychology journals. However, the report envisioned a future in which health psychology would help in the enhancement of health and prevention of disease.

In 1978, the American Psychological Association established Division 38, Health Psychology, as "a scientific, educational, and professional organization for psychologists interested in (or working in) areas at one or another of the interfaces of medicine and psychology" (Matarazzo, 1994, p. 31). In 1982, the journal *Health Psychology* began publication as the official journal of Division 38. Currently, health psychology is not only a well-established division within the American Psychological Association but is also recognized by the American Psychological Society, another powerful professional organization, which emphasizes research over clinical practice.

Development of Health Psychology In 2001, the APA membership voted to change its bylaws and to include the term "health" in its mission statement. One important objective of the mission

statement is to advance psychology as a science and profession and to promote health and human welfare (Thorn & Saab, 2001). Extending its mission statement to include health signified the impact of the field of health psychology on the profession of psychology.

With its promotion of the biopsychosocial model, health psychology continues to grow. Clinical health psychology continues to gain recognition in providing health care as part of multidisciplinary teams. Health psychology researchers continue to build a knowledge base that will furnish information about the interconnections among psychological, social, and biological factors that relate to health.

IN SUMMARY

Psychology's involvement in health dates back to the beginning of the 20th century, but at that time, few psychologists were involved in medicine. The psychosomatic medicine movement sought to bring psychological factors into the understanding of disease, but that view gave way to the bio-psychosocial approach to health and disease. By the 1970s, psychologists had begun to develop research and treatment aimed at chronic disease and health promotion; this research and treatment led to the founding of two new fields, behavioral medicine and health psychology.

Behavioral medicine is concerned with applying the knowledge and techniques of behavioral research to physical health, including prevention, diagnosis, treatment, and rehabilitation. Health psychology overlaps behavioral medicine, and the two professions have many common goals. However, behavioral medicine is an interdisciplinary field, whereas health psychology is a specialty within the discipline of psychology that is concerned with issues of physical health. Health psychology strives to enhance health, prevent and treat disease, identify risk factors, improve the health care system, and shape public opinion regarding health issues.

THE PROFESSION OF HEALTH PSYCHOLOGY

Health psychology has clearly emerged as a unique profession, having met six criteria for establishing a separate profession. First, it has founded its own national and international associations. Second, it has established a number of professional journals in addition to *Health Psychology*. Third, it has received acknowledgment from professionals in other fields of psychology that its subject matter, methods, and applications are different from theirs. Fourth, health psychology has set up postdoctoral training specific to health psychology and distinct from other fields of psychology. Fifth, it has received recognition from the American Board of Professional Psychology. Sixth, it has been recognized by the American Psychological Association Commission on the Recognition of Specialties and Proficiencies in Professional Psychology (Baum, Perry, & Tarbell, 2004; Thorn & Saab, 2001). In addition, health psychology is becoming recognized within medical schools, schools of public health, universities, and hospitals, and health psychologists

work within all of these settings. However, their training occurs within psychology.

The Training of Health Psychologists

Health psychologists are psychologists first and specialists in health second, but the training in health is extensive because it must prepare clinical health psychologists to practice as part of health care teams. The priority for orienting training around a core in psychology was determined by the landmark Boulder Conference of 1949, which established psychology as both a scientific discipline and a practicing profession. From that time, every doctoral program within a department of psychology has offered nearly the same core of generic course work for psychologists.

Health psychologists usually complete the core courses required of all psychologists and then a program specializing in health psychology. That program may occur during their doctoral training (Baum et al., 2004), but many health psychologists have recommended postdoctoral training, with at least two years of specialized training in health psychology to follow a PhD or PsyD in psychology (Belar, 1997; Matarazzo, 1987). Practicum and internships in health care settings in hospitals and clinics are common components of training (Nicassio, Meyerowitz, & Kerns, 2004).

These standards are consistent with those established by the National Working Conference on Education and Training in Health Psychology of 1983 that defined the core program in psychology for health psychologists. Although this training program was established more than 25 years ago, health psychologists continue to receive a solid core of graduate training in such areas as (1) the biological bases of behavior, health, and disease; (2) the cognitive and affective bases of behavior, health, and disease; (3) the social bases of health and disease, including knowledge of health organizations and health policy; (4) the psychological bases of health and disease, with emphasis on individual differences; (5) advanced research, methodology, and statistics; (6) psychological and health measurement; (7) interdisciplinary collaboration; and (8) ethics and professional issues (Belar, 2008; Belar et al., 2001).

No single discipline in the health care field has the capacity to solve all the problems of health promotion and disease prevention, but the interdisciplinary training of health psychologists equips them to make valuable contributions (Travis, 2001). This interdisciplinary collaboration necessitates skills of cooperation for health psychologists, and their training should prepare them to become part of multidisciplinary teams. Some experts have called for training that equips health psychologists to become primary health care providers in traditional medical settings, including preparation for board certification (McDaniel, Belar, Schroeder, Hargrove, & Freeman, 2002; Tovian, 2004). Thus, training in health psychology is becoming more complex as the work of health psychologists is becoming more varied.

The Work of Health Psychologists

Health psychologists work in a variety of settings, and their work setting varies according to their specialty. Some health psychologists are researchers, who typically work in universities or government agencies that conduct research, such as the Centers for Disease Control and Prevention and the National Institutes of Health. Health psychology research encompasses many topics; it may focus on behaviors related to the development of disease or on evaluation of the effectiveness of new treatments. Clinical health psychologists such as Felicia Otchet are often employed in hospitals, pain clinics, or community clinics. Other settings for clinical health psychologists include health maintenance organizations (HMOs) and private practice.

As Felicia Otchet's work shows, health psychologists may engage in some combination of teaching, conducting research, and providing a variety of services to individuals as well as private and public agencies. Much of their work is collaborative in nature; health psychologists engaged in either research or practice may work with a team of health professionals, including physicians, nurses, physical therapists, and counselors.

The services provided by health psychologists working in clinics and hospitals fit into several categories. One type of service offers alternatives to pharmacological treatment; for example, biofeedback might be an alternative to analgesic drugs for headache patients. Another type of service

was one of Felicia's jobs—the primary treatment of physical disorders that respond favorably to behavioral interventions, such as chronic pain and some gastrointestinal problems. She also provided several other types of services that clinical health psychologists often provide, such as ancillary psychological treatment for patients who are hospitalized with cancer; these patients may also receive stress management training. Felicia also provided another service typical of health psychologists employed in hospitals and clinics—improving the rate of patient compliance with their medical regimens and providing some assessments using psychological and neuropsychological tests. Those who concentrate on prevention and behavior changes are more likely to be employed in health maintenance organizations, school-based prevention programs, or worksite wellness programs. All these organizations use services that trained health psychologists can perform.

Like Felicia Otchet, most health psychologists are engaged in several activities. The combination of teaching and research is common among those in educational settings. Felicia's work in the medical center was typical of that employment setting—she taught medical students, conducted research, and performed clinical services. Those who work exclusively in service delivery settings are much less likely to teach and do research and are more likely to spend the majority of their time providing diagnoses and interventions for people with health problems. Felicia's several jobs allowed her to perform a greater variety of work than many other health psychologists. However, the work of many health psychologists includes more than one of the activities of assessment, research, and provision of services to people in health care settings.

IN SUMMARY

To maximize their contributions to health care, health psychologists must be both broadly trained in the science of psychology and specifically trained in the knowledge and skills of such areas as neurology, endocrinology, immunology, epidemiology, and other medical subspecialties. Health psychologists with a solid background in generic psychology and specialized knowledge in medical fields are currently employed in a variety of settings, including universities, hospitals, clinics, private practice, and health maintenance organizations. They typically collaborate with other health care professionals in providing services for physical disorders rather than for traditional areas of mental health care. Research in health psychology is also likely to be a collaborative effort that may include the professions of medicine, epidemiology, nursing, pharmacology, nutrition, and exercise physiology.

ANSWERS

This chapter has addressed three basic questions:

1. How have views of health changed?

Views of health are changing, both among health care professionals and among the general public. Several trends have prompted these changes, including (1) the changing pattern of disease and death in the United States from infectious diseases to chronic diseases; (2) the increase in medical costs; (3) the growing acceptance of a view of health that includes not only the absence of disease but also the presence of positive well-being; and (4) an emerging new biopsychosocial model of health that departs from the traditional biomedical model and the psychosomatic model by including not only biochemical abnormalities but also psychological and social conditions.

2. How did psychology become involved in health care?

Psychology has been involved in health almost from the beginning of the 20th century. During those early years, however, only a few psychologists worked in medical settings and most were considered adjuncts rather than full partners with physicians. Psychosomatic medicine highlighted psychological explanations of certain somatic diseases, emphasizing the role of emotions in the development of disease. By the early 1970s, psychology and other behavioral sciences were beginning to play a role in the prevention and treatment of chronic diseases and in the promotion of positive health, giving rise to two new fields: behavioral medicine and health psychology.

Behavioral medicine is an interdisciplinary field concerned with applying the knowledge and techniques of behavioral science to the maintenance of physical health and to prevention, diagnosis, treatment, and rehabilitation. Behavioral medicine, which is not a branch of psychology, overlaps with health psychology, a division within the field of psychology. Health psychology uses the science of psychology to enhance health, prevent and treat disease, identify risk factors, improve the health care system, and shape public opinion with regard to health.

3. What type of training do health psychologists receive, and what kinds of work do they do?

Health psychologists receive doctoral-level training in the basic core of psychology, including (1) the biological, cognitive, psychological, and social bases of behavior, health, and disease; (2) advanced research, methodology, and statistics; (3) psychology and health measurement; (4) interdisciplinary collaboration; and (5) ethics and professional issues. In addition, they often receive at least two years of postdoctoral work in a specialized area of health psychology.

Health psychologists are employed in a variety of settings, including universities, hospitals, clinics, private practice, and health maintenance organizations. Clinical health psychologists provide services, often as part of a health care team. Health psychologists who are researchers typically collaborate with others, sometimes as part of a multidisciplinary team, to conduct research on behaviors related to the development of disease or to evaluate the effectiveness of new treatments.

SUGGESTED READINGS

Baum, A., Perry, N. W., Jr., & Tarbell, S. (2004). The development of psychology as a health science. In R. G. Frank, A. Baum, & J. L. Wallander (Eds.), *Handbook of clinical health psychology* (Vol. 3, pp. 9–28). Washington, DC: American Psychological Association. This recent review of the development of health psychology describes the background and current status of the field of health psychology.

Belar, C. D. (2008). Clinical health psychology: A health care specialty in professional psychology. *Professional Psychology: Research and Practice, 39,* 229–233. Clinical health psychology is the applied branch of health psychology. Cynthia Belar traces the development of this field from the beginning, pointing out the widespread influence of health psychology on research and practice in clinical psychology.

Landrine, H., & Klonoff, E. A. (2001). Cultural diversity and health psychology. In A. Baum, T. A. Revenson, & J. E. Singer (Eds.), *Handbook of health psychology* (pp. 851–891). Mahwah, NJ: Erlbaum. In this chapter, Hope Landrine and Elizabeth Klonoff summarize the health beliefs and practices of each of the major ethnic groups in the United States.

Leventhal, H., Musumeci, T., & Leventhal, E. (2006). Psychological approaches to the connection of health and behaviour. *South African Journal of Psychology, 36,* 666–682. This article provides a good introduction to the specifics of the biopsychosocial model by reviewing each of its components and the ways in which health psychologists have related each of them and their interactions to health outcomes.

Schneiderman, N. (2004). Psychosocial, behavioral, and biological aspects of chronic diseases. *Current Directions in Psychological Sciences, 13,* 247–251. This brief article reviews the rise of chronic diseases as leading causes of death, explores the risk factors for these diseases, summarizes the pathways through which these risk factors may cause disease, and evaluates psychosocial interventions.

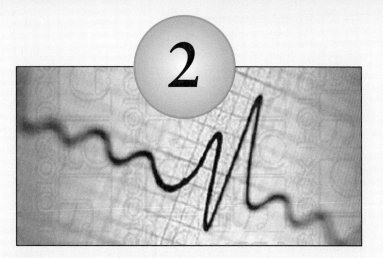

2

CONDUCTING HEALTH RESEARCH

QUESTIONS

This chapter focuses on five basic questions:

1. What are placebos, and how do they affect research and treatment?

2. How does psychology research contribute to health knowledge?

3. How has epidemiology contributed to health knowledge?

4. How can scientists determine if a behavior causes a disease?

5. How do theory and measurement contribute to health psychology?

CHECK YOUR BELIEFS

About Health Research

Check the items that are consistent with your beliefs.

☐ 1. Placebo effects can influence physical as well as psychological problems.

☐ 2. Pain patients who expect a medication to relieve their pain often experience a reduction in pain, even after taking a "sugar pill."

☐ 3. Personal testimonials are a good way to decide about treatment effectiveness.

☐ 4. Newspaper and television reports of scientific research give an accurate picture of the importance of the research.

☐ 5. Information from longitudinal studies is generally more informative than information from the study of one person.

☐ 6. All scientific methods yield equally valuable results, so the research method is not important in determining the validity of results.

☐ 7. In determining important health information, studies with nonhuman subjects can be just as important as those with human participants.

☐ 8. Results from experimental research are more likely than results from observational research to suggest the underlying cause for a disease.

☐ 9. Valuable research is done by people outside the scientific community, but scientists try to discount the importance of such research.

☐ 10. Scientific breakthroughs happen every day.

☐ 11. New reports of health research often contradict previous findings, so there is no way to use this information to make good personal decisions about health.

Items 1, 2, 5, and 8 are consistent with sound scientific information, but each of the other items represents a naïve or unrealistic view of research that can make you an uninformed consumer of health research. Information in this chapter will help you become more sophisticated in your evaluation of and expectations for health research.

REAL-WORLD PROFILE OF SYLVESTER COLLIGAN

Sylvester Colligan was a 76-year-old man who had been having trouble with his right knee for five years (Talbot, 2000). His doctor diagnosed arthritis but had no treatment that would help. However, this physician told Colligan about an experimental study conducted by Dr. J. Bruce Moseley. Colligan talked to Moseley and reported, "I was very impressed with him, especially when I heard he was the team doctor with the [Houston] Rockets. . . . So, sure, I went ahead and signed up for this new thing he was doing" (quoted in Talbot, 2000, p. 36).

Moseley and his colleagues (2002) were conducting a study of the effectiveness of arthroscopic knee surgery. This type of procedure is widely performed but expensive, and Moseley had doubts about its effectiveness (Talbot, 2000). So, Moseley decided to perform an experimental study that included a placebo as well as real arthroscopic surgery. A **placebo** is an inactive substance or condition that has the appearance of an active treatment and that may cause participants to improve or change because of their belief in the placebo's efficacy. Moseley suspected that this type of expectation and not the surgery was producing improvements, so he designed a study in which half the participants received sham knee surgery—they received anesthesia and surgical lesions to the knee, but no further treatment. The other half of the participants received surgical treatment. The participants agreed to be in either group, knowing that they might receive sham surgery. The participants didn't know for several years whether they were in the placebo or the arthroscopic surgery group.

In Moseley's study (Moseley et al., 2002), Sylvester Colligan was in the placebo group, but his knee improved. Two years after the surgery, Colligan reported that his knee hadn't bothered him since the surgery. "It's just like my other knee now. I give a whole lot of credit to Dr. Moseley. Whenever I see him on the TV during a basketball game, I call the wife in and say, 'Hey, there's the doctor that fixed my knee! '" (quoted in Talbot, 2000, p. 36).

Colligan's experience as a patient may be common: Belief in the effectiveness of treatment boosts the treatment's effectiveness. However, this effect presents a problem for researchers like Moseley, who want to determine which effects are due to treatment and which are attributable to expectation. This problem is one of the issues considered in this chapter.

This chapter looks at the way scientists work, emphasizing psychology from the behavioral sciences and epidemiology from the biomedical sciences. These two disciplines share some methods for investigating health-related behaviors, but the two areas also have their own unique contributions to scientific methodology. Before we begin to examine the methods that psychologists and epidemiologists use in their research, we need to consider the situation that Sylvester Colligan experienced—improvement due to the placebo effect.

THE PLACEBO IN TREATMENT AND RESEARCH

Sylvester Colligan knows that his knee is better, and he attributes the improvement to Dr. Moseley and his surgery. Like many people receiving treatment, Colligan benefited from his positive expectations; he improved, even though he received sham surgery. However, these same expectations can become a disadvantage to scientists trying to evaluate the effectiveness of treatments. Thus, the placebo effect may be helpful to individuals who receive treatment but complicate the job of researchers; that is, it can have treatment benefits but research drawbacks.

Treatment and the Placebo

The potency of "sugar pills" has been recognized for years. Henry Beecher (1955) observed the effects of people's beliefs and concluded that the therapeutic effect of the placebo was substantial—about 35% of patients showed improvement. A later review of more than 200 articles dealing with the placebo effect and pain (Turner, Deyo, Loeser, Von Korff, & Fordyce, 1994) revealed that some improvement rates were higher than 35%, but some were lower. For example,

some researchers (Kirsch, Moore, Scoboria, & Nicholls, 2002) have argued that the placebo effect is responsible for up to 80% of the effectiveness of antidepressant drugs. A meta-analysis of migraine headache prevention (Macedo, Baño, & Farré, 2008) indicated a placebo effect of 21%. However, placebos have little effect on broken bones (Kaptchuk, Eisenberg, & Komaroff, 2002).

Both physician and patient expectations can produce reductions in pain, and physicians who appear positive and hopeful about treatment prompt a stronger response in their patients (Moerman, 2003). Placebo responses are also related to other characteristics of the practitioner, such as his or her reputation, attention, interest, and concern (Moerman & Jonas, 2002). The type of treatment is also a factor: Big pills are more effective than little ones; colored pills work better than white tablets; capsules work better than tablets; two doses provoke a larger placebo response than one dose (Shapiro, 1970). An injection is more powerful than a pill, and surgery tends to prompt an even larger placebo response than an injection does.

The underlying cause of the placebo effect has been the subject of intense debate and extensive research. Although improvements due to placebo treatments have been assumed to be psychologically based—"It's in people's heads"—a growing body of research suggests that the effects have a physical as well as a psychological basis (Benedetti, 2006; Scott et al., 2008). For example, placebo analgesic can alter levels of brain activity in ways that are consistent with the activity that occurs during pain relief from analgesic drugs (Wager et al., 2004). Placebo surgery has also demonstrated some effectiveness in alleviating the effects of Parkinson's disease (de la Fuente-Fernández, Schulzer, & Stoessl, 2004; McRae et al., 2004).

Placebos have been found to reduce or cure a remarkable range of disorders and symptoms, including insomnia, low back pain, burn pain, headache, asthma, hypertension, and anxiety (Hróbjartsson & Gøtzsche, 2001, 2004). These findings suggest that the underlying physiological mechanisms for placebo responses are the same as for drug treatments (Finniss & Benedetti, 2005).

In addition, drugs that block the action of analgesic drugs also block the placebo response to analgesic drugs. Placebos can alter neurotransmitters, hormones, and endorphins, potentially producing a variety of perceptual, behavioral, and physical effects.

Placebos are also capable of producing adverse effects, called the **nocebo effect** (Scott et al., 2008; Turner et al., 1994). Nearly 20% of healthy volunteers given a placebo in a double-blind study experienced some negative effect as a result of the nocebo effect. Sometimes, these negative effects appear as side effects to the placebo drugs, which show the same symptoms as other drug side effects, such as headaches, nausea and other digestive problems, dry mouth, and sleep disturbances. The presence of negative effects demonstrates that the placebo effect is not merely improvement but includes any change resulting from receiving a treatment. Recent research (Scott et al., 2008) showed that the nocebo response also activates specific areas of the brain and acts on neurotransmitters, giving additional support to its physical reality.

Expectancy is a major component of the placebo effect (Finniss & Benedetti, 2005; Stewart-Williams, 2004). People act in ways that they *think* they should. Thus, people who are treated without their knowledge do not benefit as much as those who know what to expect. In addition, cultural beliefs about what constitutes effective treatment are important in eliciting a placebo response (Moerman & Jonas, 2002). Learning and conditioning are also factors in the placebo response. Receiving treatment may evoke responses that people have associated with such procedures. That is, through classical and operant conditioning, people associate treatment with getting better, creating situations in which receiving treatment leads to improvements. Thus, both expectancy and learning contribute to the placebo effect.

When patients' positive expectations increase their chances for improvement, the placebo is a valuable adjunct in treatment. *Any* factor that enhances effectiveness is a bonus. Indeed, in most situations involving medical treatment, patients' improvements may result from a combination of treatment plus the placebo effect (Finniss & Benedetti, 2005). Placebo-induced cures are indistinguishable from improvements that occur as a result of other treatments. A cure is a cure, and the method of cure makes no difference to patients' well-being. Placebo effects are a tribute to the ability of humans to heal themselves, and practitioners can enlist this ability to help patients become healthier (Ezekiel & Miller, 2001; Walach & Jonas, 2004). Therefore, the placebo effect may be considered a positive factor in medical and behavioral therapies, as it was for Sylvester Colligan, whose knee improved as a result of sham surgery.

Research and the Placebo

The therapeutic properties of the placebo may be a plus for treatment, but its effects present problems in evaluating treatment effectiveness. For a treatment to be judged effective, it must show a higher rate of effectiveness than that produced by a placebo. This standard calls for researchers to use at least two groups: one that receives the treatment and another that receives a placebo. Both groups must have equal expectations concerning the effectiveness of the treatment. In order to create equal expectancy, not only must the participants be ignorant of who is getting a placebo and who is getting the treatment, but the experimenters who dispense both conditions must also be "blind" as to which group is which. The arrangement in which neither participants nor experimenters know about treatment conditions is called a **double-blind design.** As the Would You Believe . . . ? box points out, this design strategy presents ethical dilemmas.

Psychological treatments such as counseling, hypnosis, biofeedback, relaxation training, massage, and a variety of stress and pain management techniques also produce expectancy effects. That is, the placebo effect also applies to research in psychology, but double-blind designs are not so easy to perform with these treatments. Placebo pills can look the same as pills containing an active ingredient, but this situation is more difficult to arrange for behavioral treatments because the providers always know when they are providing a sham treatment. In these studies, researchers

WOULD YOU BELIEVE . . . ?

Providing Ineffective Treatment May Be Considered Ethical

Would you believe that it is ethical for researchers to treat people with techniques that they know to be bogus? To establish treatment effectiveness, researchers need to arrange conditions that allow them to establish that effectiveness, but the placebo effect complicates this process. In controlling for participants' expectancies, researchers typically use a double-blind design in which neither the participants nor the experimenters know which participants are in the new treatment group and which are in the placebo group. This arrangement places some participants in a group that receives a placebo, which is a treatment known to be ineffective.

Health care providers are supposed to act in the best interest of their patients, yet research with new treatments demands demonstrations of effectiveness, and placebo control designs are a good way to demonstrate such effectiveness. These two goals seem to be contradictory. How do researchers reconcile this ethical difficulty?

Part of the answer to that question lies in the rules governing research with human participants (APA, 2002; World Medical Association, 2004). Providing an ineffective treatment—or any other treatment—may be considered ethical if participants understand the risks fully and still agree to participate in the study. This element of research procedure, known as *informed consent,* stipulates that participants must be informed of factors in the research that may influence their willingness to participate before they consent to participate. Informed consent does not mandate that researchers tell participants exactly what will happen to them, but participants must know about the risks so that they can decide if they want to participate or to withdraw.

When participants in a clinical trial agree to take part in the study, they receive information about the possibility of being assigned to a group that receives a placebo as well as learn about the risks associated with the treatment. Those participants who find the chances of receiving a placebo unacceptable may refuse to participate in the study. Sylvester Colligan, who participated in the study with arthroscopic knee surgery, was told that he might be included in a sham surgery group, and he consented (Talbot, 2000). However, 44% of those interviewed about that study declined to participate (Moseley et al., 2002). Some critics contend that informed consent is not adequate; researchers should also have the ethical obligation to protect participants from exploitation (Resnik, 2008).

The use of placebos in clinical studies is controversial. Despite the value of placebo controls in clinical research, some physicians and medical ethicists consider the use of ineffective treatment to be ethically unacceptable because the welfare of patients is not the primary concern. Rather, clinical studies are oriented toward establishing the effectiveness of treatment, and patient-participants may not receive the accepted standard of care (Kottow, 2007). Critics (Miller & Wager, 2004; Polgar & Ng, 2005) find the use of sham surgery especially unacceptable, citing a series of studies involving sham brain surgery (McRae et al., 2004) in which participants in the control group underwent anesthesia and had holes drilled in their skulls but did not have their brains operated on. Participants in the sham surgery still faced the risks of anesthesia and potential infection but, critics argued, did not have a good chance of benefiting from the procedure. These critics contend that control groups should receive the standard treatment rather than a placebo, and that placebo treatment is acceptable only if no treatment exists for the condition. Thus, opinion regarding the ethical acceptability of placebo treatment is divided, with some finding it acceptable and necessary for research and others objecting to the failure to provide an adequate standard of treatment.

use a **single-blind design** in which the participants do not know if they are receiving the active or inactive treatment, but the providers are not blind to treatment conditions. In single-blind designs, the control for expectancy is not as complete as in double-blind designs, but creating equal expectancies for participants is usually the more important control feature.

A placebo is an inactive substance or condition having the appearance of an active treatment. It may cause participants in an experiment to improve or change behavior because of their belief in the placebo's effectiveness and their prior experiences with receiving effective treatment. Although placebos can have a positive effect from the patient's point of view, they are a continuing problem for the researcher. In general, a placebo's effects are estimated at about 35%; its effects on reducing pain may be higher, whereas its effects on other conditions may be lower. Placebos have been known to influence a wide variety of disorders and diseases.

Experimental designs that measure the efficacy of an intervention, such as a drug, typically use a placebo so that people in the control group (who receive the placebo) have the same expectations for success as do people in the experimental group (who receive the active treatment). Drug studies are usually double-blind designs, meaning that neither the participants nor the people administering the drug know who receives the placebo and who receives the active drug. Researchers in psychological treatment studies are often not "blind" concerning the treatment, but participants are, creating a single-blind design for these studies.

RESEARCH METHODS IN PSYCHOLOGY

Health-related research reports appear daily, but most people have trouble understanding these technical reports (Kertesz, 2003). The reports often contain highly technical terminology and numbers, and many people have no point of reference to interpret these numbers in personally meaningful ways. Indeed, most people do not see these technical reports; rather, they get information about the findings from the media. The news media are in the business of getting people's attention, so the headlines and news coverage of health information may be misleading, because the emphasis is on the most sensational aspects of findings. And, of course, commercial advertisements that champion their product

as a revolutionary new cure for insomnia, an effortless way to eat all you desire and still lose weight, a simple way to stop smoking, or a food that protects you against cancer or heart disease either are not using or are distorting scientific evidence when they make their claims.

Fortunately, scientists have discovered a vast body of health-related information that is relatively objective and free from self-serving claims. This information has been produced by researchers trained in the behavioral and biomedical sciences who typically are associated with universities, research hospitals, and government agencies. Because these women and men use the methods of science in their work, evidence that builds an overall picture usually accumulates gradually over an extended period of time. Dramatic breakthroughs are rare. When scientists are familiar with each other's work, use controlled methods of collecting data, keep personal biases from contaminating results, make claims cautiously, and are able to replicate their studies, evidence is more likely to be evolutionary rather than revolutionary. Claims to the contrary are most often motivated by financial or other personal interests.

How do people separate legitimate research findings from self-serving claims? How do they understand the massive amount of research they hear about in news reports? How do they know which findings should prompt them to make changes in their behavior and which are too tentative? To understand which findings are valid and important, an understanding of research methods used by health researchers is useful. When people know how researchers go about establishing which behaviors are healthy and which are harmful, those people become more knowledgeable in evaluating evidence to make personal health decisions.

Much health-related information comes from studies conducted by behavioral and biomedical scientists using a variety of research methods. The choice of methods depends in large part on what questions the scientists are trying to answer—it is possible to approach any research topic in a variety of ways.

Because of the publicity about overweight and obesity and its growing frequency not only in the United States but also in countries around the world (Rozin, Kabnick, Pete, Fischler, & Shields, 2003), we have chosen to examine this condition to illustrate a variety of research methods. Findings from each method add to an understanding of obesity and its relationship to a variety of behaviors and conditions.

When researchers are interested in what factors predict or are related to either disease or healthy functioning, they use *correlational studies*; when they want to compare people across different age groups, they rely on *cross-sectional studies*; when they desire information on stability or instability of health status or some other characteristic over a period of time, they use *longitudinal studies*; and when they wish to compare one group of participants with another, they use either *experimental designs* or *ex post facto designs*. All these methods from the discipline of psychology have applications in the field of health.

Correlational Studies

Correlational studies yield information about the degree of relationship between two variables, such as body fat and heart disease. Correlational studies *describe* this relationship and are, therefore, a type of *descriptive research* design. Although scientists cannot determine causal relationships through a single descriptive study, the degree of relationship between two factors may be exactly what a researcher wants to know.

To assess the degree of relationship between two variables (such as body mass index [a measure of overweight] and blood pressure), the researcher measures each of these variables in a group of participants and then calculates the **correlation coefficient** between these measures. The computation yields a number that varies between -1.00 and $+1.00$. Positive correlations occur when the two variables increase or decrease together. Negative correlations occur when one of the variables increases as the other decreases. Correlations that are closer to 1.00 (either positive or negative) indicate stronger relationships than do correlations that are closer to 0.00. Small correlations—those less than 0.10—can be *statistically significant* if they are based on a very large number of scores. However, such small correlations, though not random, offer the researcher

very little ability to predict scores on one variable from knowledge of scores on the other variable.

Correlation allowed a group of researchers (Heinrich et al., 2008) to study the relationship between neighborhood factors and overweight. The researchers assessed more than 400 residents of housing developments, measuring physical characteristics of the neighborhood and relating those characteristics to obesity. They found a negative correlation between neighborhood features that supported physical activity and obesity. That is, people who live in housing developments that encourage physical activity were less likely to be obese.

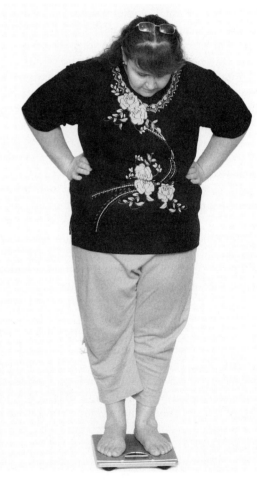

Mikhail Kokhanchikov/istockphoto.com

Blood pressure is a risk factor for cardiovascular disease, which means that people with high blood pressure are at increased risk, but not that high blood pressure causes cardiovascular disease.

Cross-Sectional and Longitudinal Studies

Researchers use two approaches to study developmental issues. **Cross-sectional studies** are those conducted at only one point in time, whereas **longitudinal studies** follow participants over an extended period. In a cross-sectional design, the investigator studies a group of people from at least two different age groups to determine the possible differences between the groups on some measure, such as food preferences, amount of physical activity, number of calories consumed, percent of calories from fat, or other variable.

Longitudinal studies can yield information that cross-sectional studies cannot because they assess the same people over time, which allows researchers to identify developmental trends and patterns. However, longitudinal studies have one obvious drawback: They take time. The time factor usually makes longitudinal studies more costly than cross-sectional studies, and they frequently require a large team of researchers.

Cross-sectional studies have the advantage of speed, but they have a disadvantage as well. Cross-sectional studies compare two or more separate groups of individuals, which makes them incapable of revealing information about changes in individuals over a period of time. For example, a cross-sectional study of obesity in children (Reich et al., 2003) found that obesity was progressively more common among children in the second, fifth, and ninth grades compared to standard weight scores. This apparent trend toward increasing levels of overweight in children is distressing because overweight children also showed increases in factors related to the development of heart disease, such as cholesterol levels and blood pressure. However, only a longitudinal study, looking at the same people over a long period of time, can show the developmental trend in overweight and confirm the relationship to heart disease or other disease conditions.

A longitudinal study of overweight and heart disease risks (Freedman, Khan, Dietz, Srinivasan, & Berenson, 2001) confirmed that overweight children not only showed risk factors for heart disease but also retained these risk factors if they remained overweight as adults.

By comparing measures taken during childhood to the same measures taken 17 years later, this research demonstrated that 77% of overweight children were obese as adults, and they tended to retain the risks for heart disease such as high blood pressure and high cholesterol levels. However, normal weight children who became obese as adults also showed these risks, so being overweight during childhood did not present a special risk—being overweight did.

Experimental Designs

Correlational studies, cross-sectional designs, and longitudinal studies all have important uses in psychology, but none of them can determine causality. Sometimes psychologists want information on the ability of one variable to cause or directly influence another. Such information requires a well-designed experiment.

An experimental design consists of a comparison of at least two groups, often referred to as an experimental group and a control group. The participants in the *experimental group* must receive treatment identical to that of participants in the control group except that those in the experimental group receive one level of the *independent variable*, whereas people in the *control group* receive a different level. The independent variable is the condition of interest, which the experimenter systematically manipulates to observe its influence on a behavior or response—that is, on the *dependent variable*. The manipulation of the independent variable is a critical element of experimental design because this manipulation allows researchers to control the situation by choosing and creating the appropriate levels. In addition, good experimental design requires that experimenters assign participants to the experimental or control group randomly to ensure that the groups are equivalent at the beginning of the study.

Often the experimental condition consists of administering a treatment, whereas the control condition consists of withholding that treatment and perhaps presenting some sort of placebo. If manipulation of the independent variable causes a change in the dependent variable, which can be evaluated by comparing the experimental and control groups, the independent variable has a cause-and-effect relationship with the dependent variable.

For example, an experimental study assessed the effect of a brief intervention to encourage physical activity among obese adults (Bolognesi, Nigg, Massarini, & Lippke, 2006). The participants were obese adults visiting their family physician. The participants were assigned randomly either to the experimental intervention or to a control group for comparison. Physicians delivered a brief counseling concerning physical activity to 48 of the obese patients. A control group of 48 other obese patients received their usual care without any intervention concerning the importance of physical activity. All patients underwent assessments of body mass index (BMI—a measure of obesity) and abdominal girth measurement. The researchers measured how ready the obese adults felt they were to participate in a physical activity program, but these individuals were also assessed 5 to 6 months later for their BMI and abdominal girth. Those who had received the counseling intervention showed lower average BMI and abdominal girth than the control group.

These results suggest that obese people can be influenced by physicians' advice to become more physically active, which in turn can affect their weight. Such an experimental design allows investigators to speak of causation, or at least of probable causes of changes in weight, because the counseling intervention differed between the two groups and other factors were constant. Figure 2.1 shows a typical experimental design comparing an experimental group with a control group, with counseling as the independent variable and BMI as the dependent variable.

Ex Post Facto Designs

Ethical restrictions or practical limitations prevent researchers from manipulating many variables, which means that experiments are not possible, but these limitations do not prevent all research on such variables. When researchers are prevented by either ethical or practical restrictions from manipulating variables in a systematic manner, they sometimes rely on ex post facto designs.

An **ex post facto design,** one of several types of quasi-experimental studies, resembles an experiment in some ways but differs in others. Both types of studies involve contrasting groups to determine differences, but ex post facto designs do not involve the manipulation of independent variables. Instead, researchers choose a variable of interest and select participants who already differ on this variable, called a **subject variable** (or *participant variable*). Both experiments and ex post facto studies involve the measurement of dependent variables. For example, researchers might study degree of obesity (subject variable) and food preference (dependent variable) by selecting a group of participants who are obese and choosing a comparison group of people who are normal weight to determine differences in food choices.

The comparison group in an ex post facto design is not an equivalent control group. These

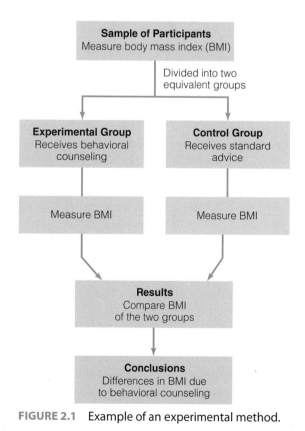

FIGURE 2.1   Example of an experimental method.

participants were not assigned to groups randomly, but rather because of their weight. The groups may also differ on variables other than weight, such as exercise, diet, cholesterol levels, or smoking. The existence of these other differences means that researchers cannot pinpoint the subject variable as the cause of differences in food preferences between the groups. However, findings about differences in level of food preference between the two groups can yield useful information, making this type of study a choice for many investigations.

Ex post facto designs are quite common in health psychology because researchers are often interested in investigating variables they cannot manipulate. For example, a comparison of the eating behavior of obese and normal weight individuals did reveal differences (Laessle, Lehrke, & Dückers, 2007). The researchers measured eating in a laboratory situation for 49 obese and 47 normal weight individuals to determine differences in eating rates and patterns. They found that obese individuals tended to eat faster and to take larger bites, which may relate to their weight.

Ex post facto designs allow comparisons between or among groups, but they do not permit researchers to determine that one variable *causes* changes in another variable. In the study on weight and eating patterns, for example, the researchers could not conclude that eating faster or taking bigger bites caused individuals to be obese, but the study does provide information about differences in eating behaviors for obese versus normal weight individuals.

IN SUMMARY

We have seen that health psychology has contributed to the area of health research through the use of several psychology research methods, including correlational studies, cross-sectional and longitudinal studies, experimental designs, and ex post facto studies. Correlational studies indicate the degree of association between two variables, but they can never show causation. Cross-sectional studies investigate a group of people at one point in time, whereas longitudinal studies follow the participants over an extended period of time. Although longitudinal studies may yield more useful results than cross-sectional studies, they are more time-consuming and more expensive. With experimental designs, researchers manipulate the independent variable so that any resulting differences between experimental and control groups can be attributed to their differential exposure to the independent variable. Experimental studies typically include a placebo given to people in a control group so that they will have the same expectations as people in the experimental group. Ex post facto studies are similar to experimental designs in that researchers compare two or more groups and then record group differences in the dependent variable, but differ in that the independent variable is preexisting rather than manipulated.

RESEARCH METHODS IN EPIDEMIOLOGY

In addition to contributions from psychology methods, the field of health psychology has profited from medical research, especially the research of epidemiologists. **Epidemiology** is a branch of medicine that investigates factors contributing to increased health or the occurrence of a disease in a particular population (Beaglehole, Bonita, & Kjellström, 1993; Tucker, Phillips, Murphy, & Raczynski, 2004). Epidemiology literally means the study of (*logos*) what is among (*epi*) the people (*demos*).

Epidemiology is among the oldest branches of medicine, having its origins in ancient Greece and Babylon when observers first began to compare people who had a particular disease or characteristic to those who did not (Lilienfeld & Lilienfeld, 1980). However, epidemiology did not evolve as a science until the 19th century, when infectious diseases such as cholera, smallpox, and typhoid fever threatened the lives of millions of people. Many of these infectious diseases were controlled or conquered largely through the work of the epidemiologists who gradually and laboriously identified their patterns and mechanisms of transmission, and ultimately, their causes. With the increase in chronic diseases during the 20th century, epidemiologists continued to make fundamental contributions to health by identifying the risk factors for diseases. A **risk factor** is any characteristic or condition that occurs with greater frequency in people with a disease than in people free from that disease. That is, epidemiologists studied those demographic and behavioral factors that were related to heart disease, cancer, and other chronic diseases (Tucker et al., 2004). For example, epidemiology studies were the first to detect a relationship between the behavior of smoking and heart disease.

Two important concepts in epidemiology are prevalence and incidence. **Prevalence** refers to the proportion of the population that has a particular disease or condition at a specific time; **incidence** measures the frequency of *new cases* during a specified period, usually one year (Tucker et al., 2004). With both prevalence and incidence, the number of people in the population at risk is divided into either the number of people with the disorder (prevalence) or the number of new cases in a particular time frame (incidence). The prevalence of a disorder may be quite different from the incidence of that disorder. For example, the prevalence of hypertension is much greater than the incidence because people can live for years after a diagnosis. In a given community, the annual *incidence* of hypertension might be 0.025, meaning that for every 1,000 people of a given age range, ethnic background, and gender, 25 people per year will receive a diagnosis of high blood pressure. But because hypertension is a chronic disorder, the prevalence will accumulate, producing a number much higher than 25 per 1,000. In contrast, for a disease such as influenza with a relatively short duration (due either to the patient's rapid recovery or to quick death), the incidence per year will exceed the prevalence at any specific time during that year.

Research in epidemiology uses three broad methods: (1) observational studies; (2) randomized, controlled trials; and (3) natural experiments. Each method has its own requirements and yields specific information. Although epidemiologists use some of the same methods and procedures employed by psychologists, their terminology is not always the same. Figure 2.2 lists the broad areas of epidemiological study and shows their approximate counterparts in the field of psychology.

Observational Methods

Epidemiologists use observational methods to look at and analyze the occurrence of a specific disease in a given population. These methods do not show causes of the disease, but researchers can draw inferences about possible factors that relate to the disease. Observational methods are similar to correlational studies in psychology; both show an association between two or more conditions, but neither can be used to demonstrate causation.

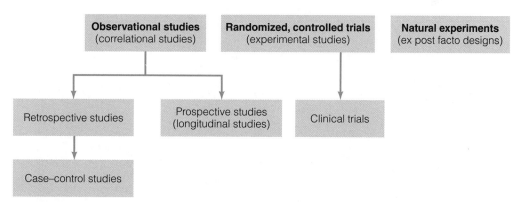

FIGURE 2.2 Research methods in epidemiology, with their psychology counterparts in parentheses.

Two important types of observational methods are prospective studies and retrospective studies. **Prospective studies** begin with a population of disease-free participants and follow them over a period of time to determine whether a given condition, such as cigarette smoking, high blood pressure, or obesity, is related to a later condition, such as heart disease or death. For example, the Japan Public Health Center–Based Study (Chei, Iso, Yamagishi, Inoue, & Tsugane, 2008) followed more than 90,000 Japanese adults between ages 40 and 69 for 11 years to determine the risk of high body mass index and weight gain on the development of heart disease. They found that both having a high body mass index and gaining weight during adulthood increased the risk for heart disease, but only among men. Prospective studies such as this one are longitudinal, making them equivalent to longitudinal studies in psychology: Both provide information about a group of participants over time, and both take a long time to complete.

In contrast, **retrospective studies** use the opposite approach: They begin with a group of people already suffering from a particular disease or disorder and then look backward for characteristics or conditions that marked them as being different from people who do not have that problem.

This approach has an advantage over prospective studies—it need not take as much time or expense. One retrospective study (Nori Janosz et al., 2008) examined groups of people who had participated in a behaviorally based weight management program, all of whom had received a diagnosis of Type 2 diabetes. Some of the individuals had experienced a resolution of their diabetes through an improvement in their regulation of blood glucose, whereas others continued to have problems with blood glucose regulation. Retrospective studies such as this one are also referred to as **case–control studies** because cases (people who had resolved their diabetes) were compared with controls (people who continued to show symptoms of diabetes). In comparing the two groups, the researchers found several differences, including the amount of weight lost. Those individuals whose diabetes had improved lost about twice as much weight as those who continued to have glucose regulation problems.

Randomized, Controlled Trials

A second type of epidemiological studies are randomized, controlled trials, which are equivalent to experiments in psychology. With a randomized, controlled trial, researchers randomly assign

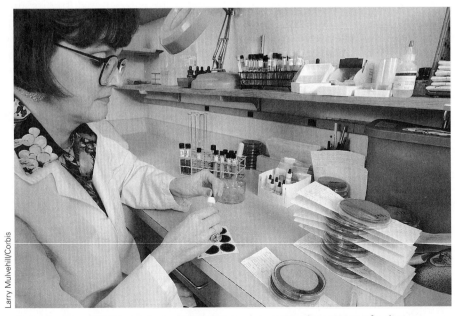

Larry Mulvehill/Corbis

One purpose of epidemiology research is to determine the origins of a disease.

participants to either a study group or a control group, thus making the two groups equal on all pertinent factors except the variable being studied. (In psychology this would be called the independent variable.) Researchers must also control variables other than those being studied to prevent them from affecting the outcome. A randomized, controlled trial, as with the experimental method in psychology, must avoid the problem of **self-selection;** that is, it must not permit participants to choose whether to be placed in the experimental group or the control group, but must assign them to groups randomly.

A test of the effectiveness of a lifestyle intervention for overweight teenagers (Melnyk et al., 2007) assigned participants either to a group that received a 15-week program with nutrition and physical activity components or to a group that received attention but no active intervention for weight control. The random assignment to conditions and the attention placebo make this study an example of a randomized, controlled trial. The results indicated that the teens who received the intervention lost more weight and had lower body mass index scores than those who were in the control condition, who gained weight over the duration of the study. These results suggest the potential effectiveness of this approach for weight loss in overweight adolescents.

A research design that tests the effects of a new drug or medical treatment is called a **clinical trial.** Many clinical trials are randomized, controlled trials that feature random assignment and control of other variables, which allow researchers to determine the effectiveness of the new treatment. The study that assessed the effectiveness of the lifestyle intervention for overweight teenagers (Melnyk et al., 2007) meets the criteria for a clinical trial; this study included random assignment of participants to conditions, a placebo type of control for expectancy and attention, and an assessment of the program's effectiveness.

Clinical trials are more common for establishing the effectiveness of drugs and medical treatments than for behavioral interventions. For example, in a clinical trial to test the efficacy of a weight loss drug (Gadde, Yonish, Foust, & Allison, 2006), obese participants were randomly assigned to one of two groups—the group that received the active drug atomoxetine or a control group that received a placebo pill. Each group received pills for 12 weeks, along with advice to follow a balanced, lower calorie diet. Because the two groups were similar in all other pertinent aspects, any differences between the two groups in subsequent weight loss could be attributed to the differences in treatment. Like most clinical trials, this study was a randomized, placebo-controlled study using the double-blind technique in which neither the participants nor the people who administered the drugs knew which pills contained the active ingredient and which were placebos. All drugs approved by the U.S. Food and Drug Administration (FDA) must first undergo extensive clinical trials of this nature, demonstrating that the drug is effective and has acceptable levels of side effects or other risks. Although the drug atomoxetine had obtained FDA approval for the treatment of attention deficit hyperactivity disorder (ADHD), its use for weight loss required additional clinical trials, the first step of which was successful: Participants showed modest levels of weight loss and minor side effects.

Epidemiologists often regard randomized, placebo-controlled, double-blind trials as the "gold standard" or zenith of research designs (Kertesz, 2003). This design is commonly used to measure the effectiveness of new drugs, and it is also used to assess the efficacy of various psychological and educational interventions. However, John Concato and his colleagues (Concato, Shah, & Horwitz, 2000) presented some evidence that well-designed observational studies are capable of providing the same level of information yielded by randomized, controlled trials. Concato and associates looked at five major medical journals and found 99 studies that evaluated five different treatments. For each treatment, there were several observational studies and several randomized, controlled trials. Results from the observational studies and the randomized, controlled trials were quite similar, indicating that observational studies do not overestimate the size of the treatment effect and can provide the same information as randomized, controlled trials. Moreover, these researchers concluded, observational studies have the advantage of being cheaper and easier to conduct.

Natural Experiments

A third area of epidemiological study is the natural experiment, in which the researcher can only select the independent variable, not manipulate it. Natural experiments are similar to the ex post facto designs used in psychology and involve the study of natural conditions that provide the possibility for comparison.

When two similar groups of people naturally divide themselves into those exposed to a risk or pathogen and those not exposed, natural experiments are possible. Such a situation occurred in 1996 as a result of a change in eligibility for food stamps for immigrants to the United States (Kaushal, 2006). States responded to the change in various ways: Some states enforced the federal ban, resulting in fewer immigrant families' receiving food stamps; other states provided alternative programs to enable immigrant families to continue receiving food stamps. This natural manipulation of conditions allowed a comparison of the body mass index of adult immigrants who continued to receive food stamps versus those who did not to test the hypothesis that receiving food stamps encourages obesity. The results indicated no significant difference in obesity between the two groups, failing to support the hypothesis that food stamps lead to higher rates of obesity.

This natural experiment differs from case–control studies in that it began by examining all the immigrant adults who applied for food stamps, and it differs from randomized, controlled trials in that the researchers selected the participants according to their eligibility rather than manipulating who received assistance and who did not. In a true randomized, controlled trial, researchers would assign participants to nutrition (food stamp) conditions, but of course, ethical considerations prevent researchers from depriving people of assistance to examine the effects on weight.

Meta-analysis

As we have seen, researchers use a variety of approaches to study behavior and health-related outcomes. Unfortunately, research on the same topic may not yield consistent findings, putting researchers (and everyone else) in the position of wondering which outcome is valid. Some studies are larger than others, and when it comes to accepting a result, size matters. But sometimes, even large studies furnish results that seem contradictory. However, the statistical technique of **meta-analysis** allows researchers to evaluate many research studies on the same topic, even if the research methods differed. The results from a meta-analysis include a measure of the overall size of the effect of the variable under study. The ability to offer an estimate of the size of an effect is an advantage. If an effect is statistically significant but small, then people should not be encouraged to change their behavior on the basis of such findings; doing so would provide too few benefits. On the other hand, if an effect is large, then working toward change would be beneficial, even if it is difficult.

For example, a group of researchers (Wang, Chen, Song, Caballero, & Cheskin, 2008) evaluated studies conducted over a period of more than 25 years to determine the relationship between weight and risk for developing kidney disease. These researchers included cross-sectional and case–control designs in their meta-analysis. The results indicated that being overweight raises the risk for kidney disease by about 40%, but being obese almost doubles the risk. Furthermore, the risk is higher for overweight and obese women than for men with comparable body mass indexes. Thus, this meta-analysis allowed researchers to draw conclusions about the impact of weight on this disease.

An Example of Epidemiological Research: The Alameda County Study

Epidemiology provides useful techniques for taking a first look at a health-related problem. A famous example of an epidemiological study is the ongoing Alameda County Study in California, an ongoing prospective study of a single community to identify health practices that may protect against death and disease. As noted earlier, epidemiologists identify risk factors by studying large populations over some period of time and by sifting out behavioral, demographic, or physiological conditions that show a relationship to subsequent disease or death.

The Alameda County Study grew out of the attempt to measure physical, mental, and social aspects of health in accordance with the World Health Organization definition of health (Stallworth & Lennon, 2003). The study identified the health practices and social variables that relate to mortality from all causes. In 1965, epidemiologist Lester Breslow and his colleagues from the Human Population Laboratory of the California State Department of Public Health began a survey of a sample of households in Alameda County (Oakland), California. After determining the number of adults living at these addresses, the researchers sent detailed questionnaires to each resident 20 years of age or older. Usable returns were received from nearly 7,000 people. Among other questions, these participants answered questions about seven basic health practices: (1) getting 7 or 8 hours of sleep daily, (2) eating breakfast almost every day, (3) rarely eating between meals, (4) drinking alcohol in moderation or not at all, (5) not smoking cigarettes, (6) exercising regularly, and (7) maintaining weight near the prescribed ideal.

At the time of the original survey in 1965, only cigarette smoking had been implicated as a health risk. Evidence that any of the other six practices predicted health or mortality was quite tenuous. Because several of these practices require some amount of good health, it was necessary to investigate the possibility that original health status might confound subsequent death rates. To control for these possible confounding effects, the Alameda County investigators asked residents about their physical disabilities, acute and chronic illnesses, physical symptoms, and current levels of energy.

A follow-up 5½ years later (Belloc, 1973) revealed that Alameda County residents who practiced six or seven of the basic health-related behaviors were far less likely to have died than those who practiced zero to three. This decreased mortality risk was independent of their 1965 health status, thus suggesting that healthy behaviors lead to lower rates of death.

In 1974, investigators conducted a major follow-up of living participants and also surveyed a new sample to determine whether the community in general had adopted a healthier lifestyle between 1965 and 1974 (Berkman & Breslow, 1983; Wingard, Berkman, & Brand, 1982). The 9-year follow-up determined the relationship between mortality and the seven health practices, considered individually as well as in combination. Five of the health practices predicted mortality rates independent of participants' use of preventive health services and their physical health in 1965. Cigarette smoking, lack of physical activity, and alcohol consumption were strongly related to mortality, whereas obesity and too much or too little sleep were only weakly associated with increased death rates. As it turned out, skipping breakfast and snacking between meals were not significantly related to mortality.

Men who practiced zero to two health-related behaviors were nearly three times as likely to have died than were those who engaged in four to five of the behaviors. For women, the effect was even more dramatic: When compared to women who practiced four or five of these behaviors, those who engaged in zero to two were more than three times as likely to have died. Moreover, the number of close social relationships also predicted mortality: People with few social contacts were two and a half times more likely to have died than were those with many such contacts (Berkman & Syme, 1979).

If some health practices are inversely related to *mortality*, then a second question concerns how these same factors relate to *morbidity*, or disease. A condition that predicts death need not also predict disease. Many disabilities, chronic illnesses, and illness symptoms do not inevitably lead to death. Therefore, it is important to know whether basic health practices and social contacts predict later physical health. Do health practices merely contribute to survival time, or do they also raise an individual's general level of health?

To answer this question, researchers (Camacho & Wiley, 1983; Wiley & Camacho, 1980) studied a subset of the original sample of Alameda County participants. In addition to the five health practices that related to mortality, this investigation included a Social Network Index that combined marital status, contacts with friends and relatives, and membership in church and other organizations. Each of the five health behaviors as well as the Social Network Index showed a relationship

BECOMING AN INFORMED READER OF HEALTH-RELATED RESEARCH

How can you judge the worth of the abundance of health-related information you read or hear? Several questions serve as criteria for evaluating such information.

1. Is the information based on studies conducted by trained scientists who are affiliated with universities, research hospitals, or government agencies? Useful information does not typically spring from secret sources.

2. Is the information based on testimonials of "satisfied" consumers or from commercial enterprises, with financial gain an obvious motive?

3. Is the information generally consistent with previous research? Dramatic breakthroughs and isolated findings are rare in science.

4. Have the research findings been replicated by other researchers? Valid evidence should emerge from different laboratories.

5. Is the information based on studies using many participants? Information from small studies is usually less reliable than that from large-scale studies.

6. Conversely, is the information based on huge studies involving hundreds of thousands of people? With very large samples, even tiny differences can be statistically significant and can thus appear important even though they have little practical significance or ability to predict health outcomes for a single individual.

7. Are the participants representative of some identified population? If so, the results may be applicable only to similar individuals.

8. Is the information based on correlational or experimental studies? Correlational studies cannot prove causation.

9. If the information comes from an experimental design, did the researchers control for the placebo effect? Did the researchers control for other important variables?

10. Did the researchers use reliable and valid measures of the independent and dependent variables?

11. If the design is prospective or retrospective, did the researchers adequately control for smoking, diet, exercise, and other possible confounding variables?

12. Have the researchers reached conclusions that are consistent with their data?

---

to changes in health. More specifically, (1) both former smokers and nonsmokers had better health than smokers; (2) moderate drinkers were healthier than either heavy drinkers or abstainers; (3) people who slept 7 or 8 hours per night did better than those who got either more or less sleep; (4) both men and women who engaged in high levels of physical activity were healthier than their more sedentary counterparts; (5) normal weight people achieved better health than either overweight participants (30% or more above desirable weight) or underweight individuals (10% or more below desirable weight); and (6) people who scored high on the Social Network Index were healthier than those who received a low rating.

Interestingly, the Social Network Index showed that marriage did not have equal effects on the health of men and women. Among both men and women, individuals who were formerly married—separated, divorced, or widowed—had greater negative changes in health, but women who had never been married were much healthier than men who had never married. Never married men had slightly negative health scores compared with married men, but never married women had considerably higher health scores than either married or formerly married women. Marriage, it seems, provides health benefits to men that do not occur for women.

IN SUMMARY

Epidemiologists conduct research using designs and terminology that differ from those used by psychology researchers. For example, epidemiologists use the concepts of risk factor, prevalence, and incidence. A risk factor is any condition that occurs with greater frequency in people with a disease than it does in people free from that disease. Prevalence refers to the proportion of the population that has a particular disease at a specific time, whereas incidence measures the frequency of new cases of the disease during a specified period of time.

In order to investigate factors that contribute either to health or to the frequency and distribution of a disease, epidemiologists use research methods that are similar to those used by psychologists, but the terminology varies. Among the methods used by epidemiologists are observational studies; randomized, controlled trials; and natural experiments. Observational studies, which are similar to correlational studies, can be either retrospective or prospective. Retrospective studies begin with a group of people already suffering from a disease and then look for characteristics of these people that differ from those of people who do not have the disease; prospective studies are longitudinal designs that follow the forward development of a group of people. Randomized, controlled trials are similar to experimental designs in psychology. Clinical trials, a common type of randomized, controlled trial, are typically used to determine the effectiveness of new drugs, but they can be used in other controlled studies. Natural experiments, which are similar to ex post facto studies, are used when naturally occurring conditions allow for comparisons. The statistical technique of meta-analysis allows researchers to examine a group of studies that have researched the variable of interest and provide an overall estimate of the size of the effect.

DETERMINING CAUSATION

As noted earlier, both prospective and retrospective studies can identify risk factors for a disease, but they do not demonstrate causation. Obesity is a risk for hypertension, heart disease, diabetes, and kidney disease. People who are obese are more likely to develop these conditions than people who are normal weight. However, some people who are not obese—or even overweight—develop heart disease and kidney disease. This section looks at the risk factor

approach as a means of suggesting causation and then examines evidence that cigarette smoking *causes* disease.

The Risk Factor Approach

The risk factor approach was popularized by the Framingham Heart Study (Levy & Brink, 2005), a large-scale epidemiology investigation that began in 1948 and included more than 5,000 men and women in the town of Framingham, Massachusetts. From its early years and continuing to the present, this study has allowed researchers to identify such risk factors for cardiovascular disease (CVD) as serum cholesterol, gender, high blood pressure, cigarette smoking, and obesity. These risk factors do not necessarily cause cardiovascular disease, but they are related to it in some way. Obesity, for example, may not be a direct cause of heart disease, but it is generally associated with hypertension, which is strongly associated with cardiovascular disease. Thus, obesity is a risk factor for CVD.

Two types of expression exist for conveying risk: absolute and relative risk. **Absolute risk** refers to the person's chances of developing a disease or disorder independent of any risk that other people may have for that disease or disorder. These chances tend to be small. For example, a smoker's risk of dying of lung cancer during any one year is about 1 in 1,000. When smokers hear their risk expressed in such terms, they may not be impressed by the hazards of their behavior (Kertesz, 2003).

Relative risk (RR) refers to the ratio of the incidence (or prevalence) of a disease in an exposed group to the incidence (or prevalence) of that disease in the unexposed group. The relative risk of the unexposed group is always 1.00. Thus, an RR of 1.50 indicates that the exposed group is 50% more likely to develop the disease in question than the unexposed group; a relative risk of 0.70 means that the rate of disease in the exposed group is only 70% of the rate in the unexposed group. Expressed in terms of relative risk, smoking seems much more dangerous. For example, male cigarette smokers have a relative risk of about 23.3 for dying of lung cancer and a relative risk of 14.6 for dying of cancer of the larynx (U.S. Department of Health and Human Services

[USDHHS], 2004). This means that, compared with nonsmokers, men who smoke are more than 23 times as likely to die of lung cancer and more than 14 times as likely to die of laryngeal cancer.

The high relative risk for lung cancer among people who have a long history of cigarette smoking may suggest that most smokers will die of lung cancer. However, such is not the case: Most smokers will *not* die of lung cancer. Support for this statement comes largely from two lines of evidence. First, about 39% of male smokers and 40% of female smokers who die of cancer will develop cancer in sites other than the lung (Armour, Woollery, Malarcher, Pechacek, & Husten, 2005). Second, the absolute frequency of death due to heart disease makes a smoker almost as likely to die of heart disease (20% of deaths among smokers) as lung cancer (28% of deaths among smokers). Smokers have a much higher relative risk of dying from lung cancer than cardiovascular disease, but their *absolute risk* of dying from CVD is much more similar.

Cigarettes and Disease: Is There a Causal Relationship?

Although risk factors do not derive from experimental studies, they can determine the *probability* that a person will develop a particular disease. Not all cigarette smokers will develop heart disease, but those who smoke are at least twice as likely to die of cardiovascular disease as those who do not smoke, and some types of people, such as young women, and some smokers, such as those who smoke more than two packs a day, experience much higher risk (USDHHS, 2004). Clearly, smoking cigarettes places one at risk for developing CVD. In a similar fashion, high cholesterol levels, high blood pressure, obesity, and stress are all risk factors for cardiovascular disease, but there is no *experimental* evidence that any of these conditions *cause* coronary heart disease or stroke.

In 1994, representatives from all the major tobacco companies came before the United States Congress House Subcommittee on Health to defend charges that cigarette smoking causes a variety of health problems, including heart disease and lung cancer. The crux of their argument was that no scientific study had ever proven that cigarette smoking causes heart disease or lung cancer in humans. Technically, their contention was correct, because only experimental studies can absolutely demonstrate causation, and no such experimental study has ever been (or ever will be) conducted on humans.

During the past 50 years, however, researchers have used nonexperimental studies to establish a link between cigarette smoking and several diseases, especially cardiovascular disease and lung cancer. Accumulated findings from these studies present an example of how researchers can use those nonexperimental studies to make deductions about a causal relationship. In other words, experimental randomized, placebo-controlled, double-blind studies are not required before scientists can infer a causal link between the independent variable (smoking) and the dependent variables (heart disease and lung cancer). Epidemiologists draw conclusions that a causal relationship exists if certain conditions are met (Susser, 1991; USDHHS, 2004). Using their criteria, does sufficient evidence exist to infer a cause-and-effect relationship between cigarette smoking and heart disease and lung cancer?

The first criterion is that a *dose–response relationship* must exist between a possible cause and changes in the prevalence or incidence of a disease. A **dose–response relationship** is a direct, consistent association between an independent variable, such as a behavior, and a dependent variable, such as a disease; in other words, the higher the dose, the higher the death rate. A body of research evidence (Doll & Hill, 1956; USDHHS, 1990, 2004) has demonstrated a dose–response relationship between both the number of cigarettes smoked per day and the number of years one has smoked and the subsequent incidence of heart disease and lung cancer.

Second, the prevalence or incidence of a *disease should decline with the removal of the possible cause*. Research (USDHHS, 1990, 2004) has consistently demonstrated that quitting cigarette smoking lowers one's risk of cardiovascular disease and decreases one's risk of lung cancer. People who continue to smoke continue to have increased risks of these diseases.

Third, the *cause must precede the disease.* Cigarette smoking almost always precedes incidence of disease. (We have little evidence that people tend to begin cigarette smoking as a means of coping with heart disease or lung cancer.)

Fourth, *a cause-and-effect relationship between the condition and the disease must be plausible;* that is, it must be consistent with other data, and it must make sense from a biological viewpoint. Although scientists are just beginning to understand the exact mechanisms responsible for the effect of cigarette smoking on the cardiovascular system and the lungs (USDHHS, 2004), such a physiological connection is plausible. It is not necessary that the underlying connection between a behavior and a disease be known, but it must be a reasonable possibility.

Fifth, *research findings must be consistent.* For more than 50 years, evidence from ex post facto and correlational studies, as well as from various epidemiological studies, has demonstrated a strong and consistent relationship between cigarette smoking and disease. As early as 1956, British researchers Richard Doll and A. B. Hill noted a straight linear relationship between average number of cigarettes smoked per day and death rates from lung cancer. Although a positive correlation such as this is not sufficient to demonstrate causation, hundreds of additional correlational and ex post facto studies since that time have yielded overwhelming evidence to suggest that cigarette smoking causes disease.

Sixth, the *strength of the association between the condition and the disease must be relatively high.* Again, research has revealed that cigarette smokers have at least a twofold risk for cardiovascular disease and are about 18 times more likely than nonsmokers to die of lung cancer (USDHHS, 2004). Because other studies have found comparable relative risk figures, epidemiologists accept cigarette smoking as a causal agent for both CVD and lung cancer.

The final criterion for inferring causality is the existence of *appropriately designed studies.* Although no experimental designs with human participants have been reported on the relationship between cigarettes and disease, well-designed observational studies can yield the results equivalent

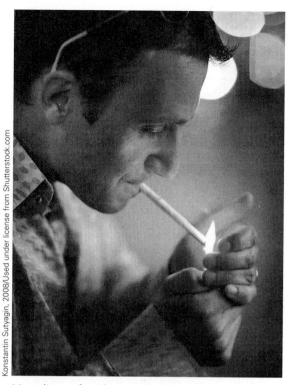

Konstantin Sutyagin, 2008/Used under license from Shutterstock.com

Many lines of evidence point to a causal relationship between smoking and disease.

to experimental studies (USDHHS, 2004), and a large number of these observational studies have consistently revealed a close association between cigarette smoking and both cardiovascular disease and lung cancer.

Because each of these seven criteria is clearly met by the evidence against smoking, epidemiologists are able to discount the argument of tobacco company representatives that cigarette smoking has not been proven to cause disease. When evidence is as overwhelming as it is in this case, scientists infer a causal link between cigarette smoking and a variety of diseases, including heart disease and lung cancer. Criteria for determining causation are summarized in Table 2.1.

IN SUMMARY

A risk factor is any characteristic or condition that occurs with greater frequency in people with a disease than it does in people free from that

TABLE 2.1

Criteria for Determining Causation Between a Condition and a Disease

1. A dose–response relationship exists between the condition and the disease.
2. Removal of the condition reduces the prevalence or incidence of the disease.
3. The condition precedes the disease.
4. A cause-and-effect relationship between the condition and the disease is physiologically plausible.
5. Relevant research data consistently reveal a relationship between the condition and the disease.
6. The strength of the relationship between the condition and the disease is relatively high.
7. Studies revealing a relationship between the condition and the disease are well designed.

disease. Risk may be expressed either in terms of the absolute risk, a person's risk of developing a disease independent of other factors, or the relative risk, the ratio of risk of those exposed to a risk factor compared to those not exposed.

Although the risk factor approach alone cannot determine causation, epidemiologists use several criteria for determining a cause-and-effect relationship between a condition and a disease: (1) A dose–response relationship must exist between the condition and the disease; (2) the removal of the condition must reduce the prevalence or incidence of the disease; (3) the condition must precede the disease; (4) the causal relationship between the condition and the disease must be physiologically plausible; (5) research data must consistently reveal a relationship between the condition and the disease; (6) the strength of the relationship between the condition and the disease must be relatively high; and (7) the relationship between the condition and the disease must be based on well-designed studies. When all seven of these criteria are met, scientists can infer a cause-and-effect relationship between an independent variable (such as smoking) and a dependent variable (such as heart disease or lung cancer).

RESEARCH TOOLS

Psychologists frequently rely on two important tools to conduct research: theoretical models and psychometric instruments. Many, but not all, psychology studies are driven by a theoretical model and are attempts to test hypotheses suggested by

that model. Also, many psychology studies rely on measuring devices to assess behaviors, physiological functions, attitudes, abilities, personality traits, and other variables. This section provides a brief discussion of these two tools.

The Role of Theory in Research

As the scientific study of human behavior, psychology shares the use of scientific methods to investigate natural phenomena with other disciplines. The work of science is not restricted to research methodology; it also involves constructing theoretical models to serve as vehicles for making sense of research findings. Health psychologists have developed a number of models and theories to explain health-related behaviors and conditions, such as stress, pain, smoking, alcohol abuse, and unhealthy eating habits. To the uninitiated, theories may seem impractical and unimportant, but scientists regard them as practical tools that give both direction and meaning to their research.

Scientific **theory** has been defined as "a set of related assumptions that allow scientists to use logical deductive reasoning to formulate testable hypotheses" (Feist & Feist, 2006, p. 4). Theories and scientific observations have an interactive relationship. A theory gives meaning to observations, and observations in turn fit into and alter the theory to explain these observations. Theories, then, are dynamic and become more powerful as they expand to explain more and more relevant observations.

Near the beginning of this cycle, when the theoretical framework is still rudimentary and not yet sufficiently comprehensive to explain a large number of observations, the term **model** is more appropriate than theory. In practice, however, *theory* and *model* are sometimes used interchangeably.

The role of theory in health psychology is basically the same as it is in any other scientific discipline. First, a useful theory should generate research—both descriptive research and hypothesis testing. The goal of descriptive research is to expand the existing theory. This type of research deals with measurement, labeling, and categorization of observations. A useful theory of psychosocial factors in obesity, for example, should generate a multitude of investigations that describe the psychological and social factors related to obesity. On the other hand, hypothesis testing is not specifically carried out to expand the theory but rather to contribute valid data to the body of scientific knowledge. Again, a useful theory of psychosocial factors in obesity should stimulate the formulation of a number of hypotheses that, when tested, produce a greater understanding of the psychological and social conditions that relate to the development and maintenance of obesity. Results of such studies would either support or fail to support the existing theory; they ordinarily do not enlarge or alter it.

Second, a useful theory should organize and explain the observations derived from research and make them intelligible. Unless research data are organized into some meaningful framework, scientists have no clear direction to follow in their pursuit of further knowledge. A useful theory of the psychosocial factors in obesity, for example, should integrate what is currently known about such factors and allow researchers to frame discerning questions that stimulate further research.

Third, a useful theory should serve as a guide to action, permitting the practitioner to predict behavior and to implement strategies to change behavior. A practitioner concerned with helping others change health-related behaviors is greatly aided by a theory of behavior change. For instance, a cognitive therapist will follow a cognitive theory of learning to make decisions about how to help clients and will thus focus on changing the thought processes that affect clients' behaviors. Similarly, psychologists with other theoretical orientations rely on their theories to supply them with solutions to the many questions they confront in their practice.

Theories, then, are useful and necessary tools for the development of any scientific discipline. They generate research that leads to more knowledge, organize and explain observations, and help the practitioner (both the researcher and the clinician) handle a variety of daily problems, such as predicting behavior and helping people change unhealthy practices. Later chapters discuss several theoretical models that are frequently used in health psychology.

The Role of Psychometrics in Research

From the work of Sir Francis Galton (1879, 1883) during the 19th century until the present time, psychology has focused on the measurement of human abilities and behaviors. Indeed, one of psychology's most important contributions to behavioral medicine and behavioral health is its sophistication in assessment techniques. Nearly every important issue in health psychology demands measurement of the phenomenon under investigation. Psychologists have reacted to this demand by constructing a number of instruments to assess such behaviors and conditions as stress, coping, pain, hostility, eating habits, and personal hardiness.

For these or any other measuring instruments to be useful, they must be both *reliable* (consistent) and *valid* (accurate). The problems of establishing reliability and validity are critical to the development of any measurement scale.

Establishing Reliability The **reliability** of a measuring instrument is the extent to which it yields consistent results. In health psychology, reliability is most frequently determined by comparing scores on two or more administrations of the same instrument (*test–retest reliability*) or by comparing ratings obtained from two or more judges observing the same phenomenon (*interrater reliability*).

Reliability is most frequently expressed in terms of either correlation coefficients or percentages. The correlation coefficient, which expresses the degree of correspondence between two sets of scores, is the same statistic used in correlational studies. High reliability coefficients (such as 0.80 to 0.90) indicate that participants have obtained nearly the same scores on two administrations of a test. Percentages can be used to express the degree of agreement between the independent ratings of observers. If the agreement between two or more raters is high (such as 85% to 95%), then the instrument is capable of eliciting nearly the same ratings from two or more interviewers.

Establishing reliability for the numerous assessment instruments used in health psychology is obviously a formidable task, but it is an essential first step in developing useful measuring devices.

Establishing Validity A second step in constructing assessment scales is to establish their validity. **Validity** is the extent to which an instrument measures what it is designed to measure. Measuring scales may be reliable and yet lack validity, or accuracy.

Psychologists determine the validity of a measuring instrument by comparing scores from that instrument with some independent or outside criterion—that is, a standard that has been assessed independently of the instrument being validated. In health psychology, that criterion is often some future event, such as a diagnosis of heart disease or the development of diabetes. An instrument capable of predicting who will receive such a diagnosis and who will remain disease free is said to have *predictive validity*. For example, scales that measure attitudes about body have been used to predict the development of eating disorders. For such a scale to demonstrate predictive validity, it must be administered to participants who are currently free of disease. If people who score high on the scale eventually have higher rates of disease than participants with low scores, then the scale can be said to have predictive validity; that is, it differentiates between participants who will remain disease free and those who will become ill.

IN SUMMARY

The work of scientists is aided by two important tools: useful theories and accurate measurement. Useful theories (1) generate research, (2) predict and explain research data, and (3) help the practitioner solve a variety of problems. Accurate psychometric instruments are both reliable and valid. *Reliability* is the extent to which an assessment device measures consistently, and *validity* is the extent to which an assessment instrument measures what it is supposed to measure.

ANSWERS

This chapter has addressed five basic questions:

1. What are placebos, and how do they affect research and treatment?

A placebo is an inactive substance or condition that has the appearance of an active treatment and that may cause participants to improve or change because of a belief in the placebo's efficacy. In other words, a placebo is any treatment that is effective because patients' expectations based on previous experiences with treatment lead them to believe that it will be effective.

The therapeutic effect of placebos is generally judged to be about 35%, but that rate varies with many conditions, including treatment setting and culture. Placebos, including sham surgery, have been known to be effective in a wide variety of situations, such as decreasing pain, reducing asthma attacks, diminishing anxiety, and decreasing symptoms of Parkinson's disease. Placebos can also produce adverse effects and are then called nocebos.

The positive effects of placebos are usually beneficial to patients, but they create problems for researchers attempting to determine the efficacy of a treatment. Experimental designs that measure the effectiveness of a treatment intervention balance that intervention against a placebo so that people in the control (placebo) group have the same expectations as do people in the experimental (treatment intervention) group. Experimental studies frequently use designs in which the participants do not know which treatment condition they are in (*single-blind* design) or in which neither the participants nor the people administering the treatment know who receives the placebo and who receives the treatment intervention (*double-blind* design).

2. How does psychology research contribute to health knowledge?

Psychology has contributed to health knowledge in at least five important ways. First is its long tradition of techniques to change behavior. Second is an emphasis on health rather than disease. Third is the development of reliable and valid measuring instruments. Fourth is the construction of useful theoretical models to explain health-related research. Fifth are various research methods used in psychology. This chapter is concerned mostly with the fifth contribution.

The variety of research methods used in psychology include (1) correlational studies, (2) cross-sectional studies and longitudinal studies, (3) experimental designs, and (4) ex post facto designs. Each of these makes its own unique contribution to the understanding of behavior and health. Correlational studies indicate the degree of association or correlation between two variables, but by themselves, they cannot determine a cause-and-effect relationship. Cross-sectional studies investigate a group of people at one point in time, whereas longitudinal studies follow the participants over an extended period. In general, longitudinal studies are more likely to yield useful and specific results, but they are more time-consuming and expensive than cross-sectional studies. With experimental designs, researchers manipulate the independent variable so that any resulting differences in the dependent variable between experimental

and control groups can be attributed to their differential exposure to the independent variable. Ex post facto designs are similar to experimental designs in that researchers compare two or more groups and then record group differences on the dependent variable. However, in the ex post facto study, the experimenter merely selects a subject variable on which two or more groups have naturally divided themselves rather than creating differences through manipulation.

3. How has epidemiology contributed to health knowledge?

Epidemiology has contributed the concepts of risk factor, prevalence, and incidence. A risk factor is any characteristic or condition that occurs with greater frequency in people with a disease than it does in people free from that disease. Prevalence is the proportion of the population that has a particular disease at a specific time; incidence measures the frequency of new cases of the disease during a specified time.

Many of the research methods used in epidemiology are quite similar to those used in psychology. Epidemiology uses at least three basic kinds of research methodology: (1) observational studies; (2) randomized, controlled trials; and (3) natural experiments. Observational studies, which parallel the correlation studies used in psychology, are of two types: retrospective and prospective. Retrospective studies are usually *case–control studies* that begin with a group of people already suffering from a disease (the cases) and then look for characteristics of these people that are different from those of people who do not have that disease (the controls). Prospective studies are longitudinal designs that follow the forward development of a population or sample. Randomized, controlled trials are similar to experimental designs in psychology. In these studies, researchers manipulate the independent variable to determine its effect on the dependent variable. Randomized, controlled trials are capable of demonstrating cause-and-effect relationships. The most common type of randomized, controlled trials are clinical trials, which are frequently used to measure the efficacy of medications. Natural experiments, which are similar to ex post facto studies, involve selection rather than manipulation of the independent variable. The statistical technique of meta-analysis allows psychologists and epidemiologists to combine the results of many studies to develop a picture of the size of an effect.

4. How can scientists determine if a behavior causes a disease?

Seven criteria are used for determining a cause-and-effect relationship between a condition and a disease: (1) A dose–response relationship must exist between the condition and the disease; (2) the removal of the condition must reduce the prevalence or incidence of the disease; (3) the condition must precede the disease; (4) the causal relationship between the condition and the disease must be physiologically plausible; (5) research data must consistently reveal a relationship between the condition and the disease; (6) the strength of the relationship between the condition and the disease must be relatively high; and (7) the relationship between the condition and the disease must be based on well-designed studies.

5. How do theory and measurement contribute to health psychology?

Theories are important tools used by scientists to (1) generate research, (2) predict and explain research data, and (3) help the practitioner solve a variety of problems. Health psychologists use a variety of measurement instruments to assess behaviors and theoretical concepts. To be useful, these psychometric instruments must be both reliable and valid.

Reliability is the extent to which an assessment device measures consistently, and validity is the extent to which an assessment instrument measures what it is supposed to measure.

SUGGESTED READINGS

Benedetti, F. (2006). Placebo analgesia. *Neurological Sciences, 27*(Suppl. 2), S100–S102. This short article by one of the leading researchers on the topic of placebo effects describes research on how placebos may work to effect cures.

Kertesz, L. (2003). The numbers behind the news. *Healthplan, 44*(5), 10–14, 16, 18. Louise Kertesz offers a thoughtful analysis of the problems of reporting the findings from health research and gives some tips for understanding findings from research studies, including a definition of some of the terminology used in epidemiology research.

Russo, E. (2004, August 2). New views on mind–body connection. *The Scientist, 18*(15), 28. This short article describes current research on the placebo and how high-tech methods allow the investigation of brain responses to placebos.

Susser, M. (1991). What is a cause and how do we know one? A grammar for pragmatic epidemiology. *American Journal of Epidemiology, 133*, 635–648. Since the 1950s, epidemiologists have developed ways of showing causality in nonexperimental designs; in this practical article, Susser presents criteria for making these causal inferences.

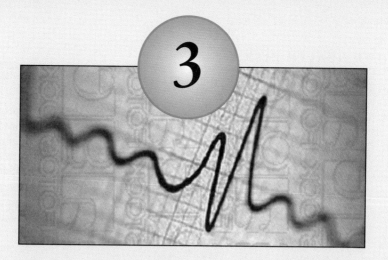

3

SEEKING HEALTH CARE

QUESTIONS

This chapter focuses on three basic questions:

1. Why do people adopt health-related behaviors?

2. What factors are related to seeking medical attention?

3. What problems do people encounter in receiving medical care?

CHECK YOUR HEALTH RISKS

Check the items that apply to you.

☐   1. If I feel well, I believe that I am healthy.

☐   2. I see my dentist twice yearly for regular check-ups.

☐   3. The last time I sought medical care was in a hospital emergency room.

☐   4. If I had a disease that would be a lot of trouble to manage, I would rather not know about it until I was really sick.

☐   5. I try not to allow being sick to slow me down.

☐   6. If I don't understand my physician's recommendations, I ask questions until I understand what I should do.

☐   7. I think it's better to follow medical advice than to ask questions and cause problems, especially in the hospital.

☐   8. When facing a stressful medical experience, I think the best strategy is to try not to think about it and hope that it will be over soon.

☐   9. When I have severe symptoms, I try to find out as much information as possible about my medical condition.

☐ 10. I believe that if people get sick, it is because they were due to get sick, and there was nothing they could have done to prevent their sickness.

☐ 11. I'm a smoker who knows that smoking can cause heart disease and lung cancer, but I believe that other smokers are much more likely to get these diseases than I am.

☐ 12. In order not to frighten patients faced with a difficult medical procedure, it is best to tell them that they won't be hurt, even if they will.

Items 2, 6, and 9 represent healthy attitudes or behaviors, but each of the other items relates to conditions that may present a risk or lead you to less effective health care. As you read this chapter, you will see the advantages of adopting healthy attitudes or behaviors to make more effective use of the health care system.

REAL-WORLD PROFILE OF JEFF WHITE

While playing a game of half-court basketball, Jeff White* jammed his right hand on the backboard and felt an immediate pain. However, he continued playing; he felt that minor injuries were merely "part of the game." For the rest of the day, his hand continued to hurt, and he had difficulty writing, eating, or using the hand for other tasks. The next day, Jeff's hand was somewhat discolored and quite swollen. To reduce the swelling, he wrapped an ice pack around the hand for 20 to 30 minutes two or three times that day. Still, Jeff continued with his daily activities as well as he could, believing that the swelling would soon disappear. On the third day, however, his hand was no better, so he decided to seek advice. But the advice he sought was not from a physician or other health practitioner; rather, it was from two colleagues at his law office, neither of whom had any medical training. Both colleagues advised Jeff to have his hand x-rayed to learn whether it was broken. Still, Jeff hesitated. He feared that taking time to be x-rayed and to see a doctor would be both inconvenient and expensive.

When he finally decided that an X ray was warranted, Jeff went to a local imaging center that specialized in X rays. The person at the imaging center informed Jeff that his hand could not be x-rayed there unless a physician referred him. Indeed, she seemed shocked that anyone would come to the imaging center without a physician's referral. So Jeff, an intelligent attorney with little understanding of how to seek health care in this instance, called his internist and asked her to order an X ray. The internist ordered the X ray and also referred Jeff to an orthopedic specialist, whom he saw the next day. Results of his X ray revealed a broken

*This name has been changed to protect the person's privacy.

metacarpal, a bone in the hand between the wrist and the fingers. The orthopedist placed Jeff's hand in a cast and told him to wait six weeks before playing any more basketball or using his right hand for nearly anything else.

Why was Jeff so reluctant to seek medical care? Why was the pain he experienced not sufficient to prompt him to go to the doctor? Why did he ask the opinion of people with no medical training before getting advice from a trained professional?

ADOPTING HEALTH-RELATED BEHAVIORS

Like Jeff, most people in the world value health and want to avoid disease and disability. Nevertheless, many people behave in ways that work against the goals of maximizing health and minimizing disease and disability. Why do some people, such as Jeff, seem to behave unwisely on issues of personal health? Why do others seek medical treatment when they are not ill? What explains people's reluctance to believe that their own risky behaviors are dangerous and their willingness to believe that those same behaviors place other people in jeopardy? No final answers to these questions are possible at this point, but psychologists have formulated several theories or models in the attempt to predict and to make sense of behaviors related to health. This chapter looks briefly at some of these theories as they relate to health-seeking behavior; Chapter 4 examines theory-driven research about people's adherence to medical advice.

Theories of Health Protective Behaviors

In Chapter 2, we said that useful theories (1) generate research, (2) organize and explain observations, and (3) guide the practitioner in predicting behavior. Health psychologists frequently use theoretical models to meet each of these criteria. These models include the health belief model, which originally grew out of the work of Geoffrey Hochbaum (1958) and his colleagues at the Public Health Service; the theory of reasoned action, developed by Martin Fishbein and Icek Ajzen (Ajzen & Fishbein, 1980; Fishbein & Ajzen, 1975); the concept of planned behavior, which Ajzen developed as an alternative to the theory of reasoned action (Ajzen, 1985, 1991); and Neil Weinstein's (1988) precaution adoption

process model. In Chapter 4, we look at the behavioral model, self-regulation theory, and the transtheoretical model, examining how they apply to adherence to medical advice.

The Health Belief Model Since the early work of Geoffrey Hochbaum (1958), several versions of the *health belief model* (HBM) have appeared. The one that has attracted the most attention and generated the most research is that of Marshall Becker and Irwin Rosenstock (Becker & Rosenstock, 1984).

Like all health belief models, the one developed by Becker and Rosenstock assumes that beliefs are important contributors to health-seeking behavior. This model includes four beliefs that should combine to predict health-related behaviors: (1) perceived *susceptibility* to disease or disability, (2) perceived *severity* of the disease or disability, (3) perceived *benefits* of health-enhancing behaviors, and (4) perceived *barriers* to health-enhancing behaviors, including financial costs.

Each of these factors played a part in Jeff's decision to seek assistance after he hurt his hand. At first, Jeff did not believe that his injury was serious or that he was vulnerable to disability. Thus, he saw little benefit in going to a doctor, an action that would have taken him away from his work as an attorney. After two of his colleagues expressed their belief that his injury might be serious, and after two days of eating, driving, writing, and dressing with his left hand, Jeff changed his beliefs and subsequently sought medical attention. Unlike most people who seek health care, financial cost was not a serious barrier to Jeff, whose most serious obstacle was lack of information about the health care system.

The health belief model corresponds with common sense in many ways. When people perceive that they are susceptible to a severe illness, can benefit from specific behaviors, and can overcome barriers to good health, they should be guided by their own self-interest and actively seek health care. Common sense, however, does not always predict health-related behaviors.

Research on the health belief model has been extensive, but results generally suggest that a model that includes only susceptibility, severity, benefits, and barriers does not predict health-related behaviors as well as more elaborate models. For example, a study that surveyed people from various ethnic groups about choosing to receive an influenza vaccination examined the variables in the health belief model (Chen, Fox, Cantrell, Stockdale, & Kangawa-Singer, 2007). The results indicated that, in general, individuals who believed that they were more susceptible to influenza and that influenza is a serious disease were more likely to obtain a vaccination than those who believed they were less susceptible or that the disease was not so serious. These two variables were much more strongly related to receiving a vaccination for African Americans and European Americans than for Hispanic Americans, for whom barriers were more strongly related than the other factors. These ethnic differences point to the importance of other factors omitted by the health belief model.

The study on influenza vaccination is typical of tests of the health belief model. The components of the model show some relationship to the health-related criterion behavior, but the relationship is weak, and the model seems to be incomplete. Some researchers have dealt with this inadequacy by extending the health belief model, adding factors such as optimism or feelings of personal control (Gillibrand & Stevenson, 2006). Other critics (Armitage & Connor, 2000) have argued that the health belief model emphasizes motivational factors too heavily and behavioral factors too little, and thus will never be a completely adequate model of health behavior. For this reason, some researchers (Poss, 2000) have combined aspects of the health belief model with concepts from other models, including the theory of reasoned action.

The Theory of Reasoned Action The *theory of reasoned action* (Ajzen & Fishbein, 1980; Fishbein &

Ajzen, 1975) assumes that people are generally reasonable and make systematic use of information when deciding how to behave; they think about the outcome of their actions before making a decision to engage or not to engage in a particular behavior (Ajzen, 1985). The theory of reasoned action assumes that behavior is directed toward a goal or outcome and that people freely choose those actions that they believe will move them in the direction of that goal. They can also choose not to act, if they believe that an action would move them away from their goal, as when Jeff decided not to seek immediate medical attention because he believed that a cast on his hand would hamper his regular work routine.

The immediate determinant of behavior is the *intention* to act or not to act. Intentions, in turn, are shaped by two factors. The first is a personal evaluation of the behavior—that is, one's *attitude toward the behavior*. The second is one's perception of the social pressure to perform or not perform the action—that is, one's *subjective norm*. One's attitude toward the behavior is determined by beliefs that the behavior will lead to positively or negatively valued outcomes. One's subjective norm is shaped by one's perception of the evaluation that a particular individual (or group of individuals) places on that behavior and one's *motivation* to comply with the norms set by that individual (or group). In predicting behavior, the theory of reasoned action also considers the relative weight of personal attitudes measured against subjective norms (see Figure 3.1).

In predicting whether Jeff, with a painful, discolored, and swollen hand, will seek medical attention, the theory of reasoned action relies on several pieces of information. First, does Jeff believe that going to the doctor's office is related to his goal of a healthy hand? Second, how strong is his belief that other people expect him to seek medical attention balanced against his need to comply with others' expectations? The answer to the first question reveals Jeff's attitude toward seeking medical assistance, and the answer to the second question suggests the level of social pressure on him to seek assistance. Because Jeff's attitudes and his subjective norms were initially in conflict, his early intention was somewhat mixed,

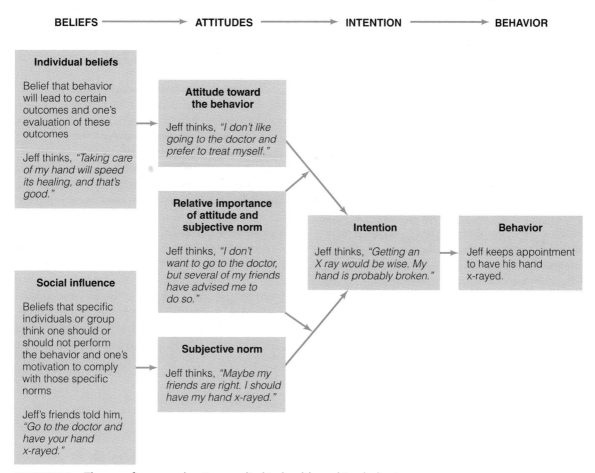

BELIEFS ⟶ ATTITUDES ⟶ INTENTION ⟶ BEHAVIOR

Individual beliefs

Belief that behavior will lead to certain outcomes and one's evaluation of these outcomes

Jeff thinks, *"Taking care of my hand will speed its healing, and that's good."*

Attitude toward the behavior

Jeff thinks, *"I don't like going to the doctor and prefer to treat myself."*

Relative importance of attitude and subjective norm

Jeff thinks, *"I don't want to go to the doctor, but several of my friends have advised me to do so."*

Social influence

Beliefs that specific individuals or group think one should or should not perform the behavior and one's motivation to comply with those specific norms

Jeff's friends told him, *"Go to the doctor and have your hand x-rayed."*

Subjective norm

Jeff thinks, *"Maybe my friends are right. I should have my hand x-rayed."*

Intention

Jeff thinks, *"Getting an X ray would be wise. My hand is probably broken."*

Behavior

Jeff keeps appointment to have his hand x-rayed.

FIGURE 3.1   Theory of reasoned action applied to health-seeking behavior.

Source: Adapted from *Understanding Attitudes and Predicting Social Behavior*, 1st edition, © 1980, p. 8. Adapted by permission of Pearson Education, Inc., Upper Saddle River, NJ.

making prediction of his behavior difficult. Nevertheless, the theory of reasoned action has the potential to make valid predictions when investigators accurately measure both the strength of a person's attitude toward a behavior and the person's need to conform to social norms.

How accurate is the theory of reasoned action in predicting health-seeking behavior? In general, researchers have found the theory to be useful for predicting safe and unsafe health-related behaviors, including use of condoms, exercise, diet, and smoking (Bogart & Delahanty, 2004). In general, the theory of reasoned action fits well with predictions for these behaviors.

Several examples of the success of the theory of reasoned action come from studies on condom use. Two such studies were set in South Africa, where HIV/AIDS has reached pandemic levels and condom use is a pressing health issue. Results of the first study (Chitamun & Finchilescu, 2003) showed that both attitudes and subjective norms predicted South African female students' intention to engage or not to engage in premarital sexual intercourse. In a later investigation of South African students (Mashegoane, Moalusi, Ngoepe, & Peltzer, 2004), researchers interviewed sexually active, unmarried male and female students about their intentions to use condoms. They found that men's attitudes toward condoms predicted their intention to use condoms, but female students' intentions were influenced by additional factors, including **self-efficacy**—the belief that one is capable of performing the behaviors that will produce desired outcomes. The addition of this variable increases the predictive value of the model. Other research on condom use (Beadnell et al., 2008) has confirmed the usefulness of the theory of reasoned action and also the improvement of adding the concept of self-efficacy.

The research evidence that indicates improved prediction as a result of adding self-efficacy may be been as a limitation on the theory of reasoned action. If the theory were adequate, no additions would be necessary. However, the theory of reasoned action is at least as effective as the health belief model in explaining and predicting health-seeking behaviors. Key elements in the theory of reasoned action seem to be attitudes toward the behavior and subjective norms, both of which relate to the intention to perform a behavior.

The Theory of Planned Behavior   One of the originators of the theory of reasoned action decided to add a factor to the model to improve its predictive power. Ajzen has extended the theory of reasoned action to include the concept of perceived behavioral control, an extension he calls the *theory of planned behavior*. The primary difference between the theory of reasoned action and the theory of planned behavior is the latter's inclusion of the *perception of how much control* people have over their behavior (Ajzen, 1985, 1988, 1991). The more resources and opportunities people believe they have, the stronger are their beliefs that they can control their behavior. Figure 3.2 shows that predictions of behavior can be made from knowledge of a person's (1) attitude toward the behavior, (2) subjective norm, and (3) perceived behavioral control. All three components interact to shape the person's intention to behave. Perceived behavioral control is the ease or difficulty one has in achieving desired behavioral outcomes, which reflects both past behaviors and perceived ability to overcome

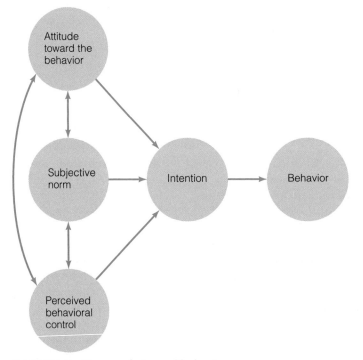

FIGURE 3.2   Theory of planned behavior.

Source: From "The Theory of Planned Behavior," by I. Ajzen, 1991, *Organizational Behavior and Human Decision Processes, 50*, p. 182. Reprinted by permission of Academic Press.

obstacles. The theory assumes that people who believe they can easily perform a behavior are more likely to *intend* to perform that behavior than people who believe they have little control over performing that behavior.

The theory of planned behavior has been used to predict a wide variety of health-related behaviors. An extensive meta-analytic review (Hagger, Chatzisarantis, & Biddle, 2002) included expanded elements of the theories of reasoned action and planned behavior as they apply to participation in a physical activity program, and another meta-analysis (Bogart & Delahanty, 2004) evaluated the theory of planned behavior in relation to condom use. These analyses showed that the theory of planned behavior has some ability to predict these health-related behaviors, but the inclusion of additional variables such as past behavior and self-efficacy improve the model's predictive ability.

A study on the topic of premarital sex among Korean university students (Cha, Doswell, Kim, Charron-Prochownik, & Patrick, 2007) highlights this theory's strengths and weaknesses. These researchers used the theory of planned behavior as a framework to predict premarital sexual behavior. The results indicated that norms were significant predictors for both male and female students, but perceived behavioral control was a factor only for male students. For female students, attitudes were more strongly predictive. Thus, the theory of planned behavior was a good model to explain this behavior, but more so for male students. Female students' behavior was better predicted by the theory of reasoned action.

The theory of planned behavior, then, tends to offer a better model than the theory of reasoned action, but not for all behaviors or all types of participants. In addition, some critics (Armitage & Connor, 2000) have pointed out the limitation of focusing on intentions because intention does not have a straightforward relationship to behavior. To answer this criticism, some researchers have adopted a stage model.

The Precaution Adoption Process Model Neil Weinstein (2000) has criticized other theoretical models for focusing too narrowly on perceived severity of and susceptibility to a disease or disorder and ignoring people's transition from one stage to another in their readiness to adopt health-related behaviors. Weinstein's (1988) *precaution adoption process model* assumes that when people begin new and relatively complex behaviors aimed at protecting themselves from harm, they go through several *stages of belief* about their personal susceptibility. People do not move inevitably from lower to higher stages, and they may even move backward, as when a person who has previously considered stopping smoking subsequently abandons the idea.

Weinstein's precaution adoption process model holds that people move through seven stages in their readiness to adopt a health-related behavior (see Figure 3.3). In stage 1, people have not heard of the hazard and thus are unaware of any personal risk. In stage 2, they are aware of the hazard and believe that others are at risk, but they hold an **optimistic bias** regarding their own level of risk. Stage 3 people acknowledge their personal susceptibility and accept the notion that precaution would be personally effective, but they have not yet decided to take action.

Stages 4 and 5 are critical. In stage 4, people decide to take action, whereas in the parallel stage 5, people decide that action is unnecessary. Some people who branch off to stage 5 may later return to stage 4 and decide to take appropriate action. In stage 6, people have already taken the precautions aimed at reducing risks. Stage 7 involves maintaining the precaution, if needed. Maintenance would not be necessary in the case of polio vaccination (when one dose provides lifetime immunity), but for smoking cessation or dietary changes, maintenance is essential. Before people take action, they must first perceive that the relative benefits of the precaution outweigh its costs.

Although Weinstein's notion of optimistic bias has generated substantial research, his more global concept of the precaution adoption process model has attracted less attention from researchers. In one study, Weinstein and his colleagues (Weinstein, Lyon, Sandman, & Cuite, 2003) hypothesized that barriers to health protective behaviors change from stage to stage. The precaution under investigation was encouraging

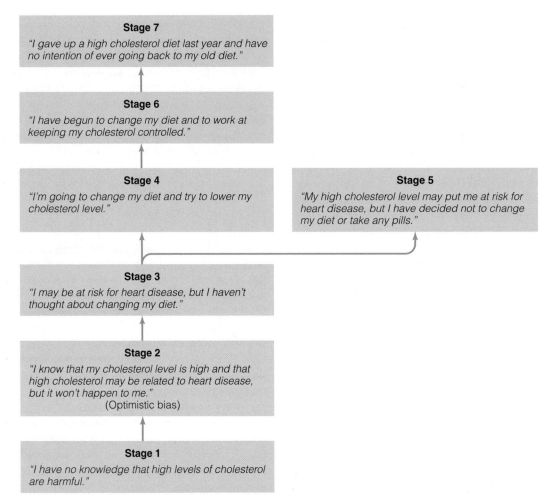

FIGURE 3.3   The seven stages of Weinstein's precaution adoption process model.

homeowners to test their homes for the presence of radon. An education intervention was aimed at getting homeowners in the decided-to-act stage to order a test kit that measured radon level. The study found that interventions that required low effort were more effective in getting decided-to-act people to order test kits than in getting undecided people to decide to test. These findings offer some support for the precaution adoption process model, and some recent research has extended this model to the health-related behaviors of taking calcium supplements (Blalock, 2007), engaging in exercise and taking calcium supplements for protecting against bone loss (Elliott, Seals, & Jacobson, 2007), and parents' following recommended safety procedures for protecting young children (Gielen et al., 2007). Each of these behaviors requires that a person become aware of a hazard and move toward taking appropriate action, and the precaution adoption process model seems to capture the variable nature of these behaviors better than simpler models.

Critique of Health-Related Theories

Chapter 2 suggested that a useful theory should (1) generate significant research, (2) organize and explain observations, and (3) help the practitioner predict and change behaviors. How well do these health-related theories meet these three criteria?

First, both the health belief model and the theory of reasoned action have produced substantial amounts of health-related research, particularly when combined with the concept of self-efficacy. The theory of planned behavior and the precaution adoption process model have prompted less research, but a body of evidence is accumulating for all these models.

Second, do these models organize and explain health-related behaviors? In general, when the theory of reasoned action and the theory of planned behavior are expanded to include self-efficacy, they have some ability to predict perceived behavioral control, subjective norms, attitudes, and intentions. Clearly, all these models are able to do better than chance in explaining and predicting behavior. However, the health belief model, theory of reasoned action, and theory of planned behavior address motivation and attitudes but not actual behavior or behavior change (Armitage & Connor, 2000). Thus, they are only moderately successful in predicting behavior.

Those who seek to build valid models for health-related behaviors face challenges. One challenge is that health-seeking behavior is often determined by factors other than an individual's beliefs or perceptions. Among such factors are poor interpersonal relationships that keep people away from the health care system and public policies (including laws) that affect health-seeking behaviors. In addition, certain health-related behaviors, such as cigarette smoking and dental care, can develop into habits that become so automatic that they are largely outside the personal decision-making process. Other health-producing behaviors, such as dietary changes, may be undertaken for the sake of personal appearance rather than health.

Another type of challenge comes from the necessity of relying on instruments to assess the various components of the models, because such measures are not yet consistent and accurate. The health belief model, for example, might predict health-seeking behavior more accurately if valid measurements existed for each of its components. If a person feels susceptible to a disease, perceives his or her symptoms to be severe, believes that treatment will be effective, and sees few barriers to treatment, then logically that person should seek health care. But each of these four factors is difficult to assess reliably and validly.

These models have been applied to a wide variety of behaviors, including adolescent girls' decision to engage in risky sexual behaviors (Tremblay & Frigon, 2004), cigarette smoking among elementary school children (Swaim, Perrine, & Aloise-Young, 2007) and Chinese adolescents (Guo et al., 2007), behaviors that protect against bone loss among undergraduate women (Blalock, 2007; Sharp & Thombs, 2003), cancer screening procedures (Ross, Kohier, Grimley, & Anderson-Lewis, 2007), alcohol abuse among college students (Codd & Cohen, 2003), and myriad other health-related behaviors. However, a model may have some value for predicting health-seeking behaviors related to one disorder but not to another. Similarly, a theory may relate to health care–seeking behavior but not to prevention behavior or adherence to medical advice, or it may predict the behavior of men but not women. No current theory is comprehensive enough to encompass all these areas.

Finally, most of the models postulate some type of barrier or obstacle to seeking health care, and an almost unlimited number of barriers are possible. Often these barriers are beyond the life experience of researchers. For example, barriers for affluent European Americans may be quite different from those faced by poor Hispanic Americans, Africans living in sub-Saharan Africa, or Hmong immigrants in Canada; thus, the health belief model and the theory of reasoned action may not apply equally to all ethnic and socioeconomic groups (Poss, 2000). Models for health-seeking behavior tend to emphasize the importance of direct and personal control of behavioral choices. Little allowance is made for such barriers as racism and poverty.

IN SUMMARY

Theories of health-seeking behavior, like other theories, should (1) generate research, (2) organize and explain behavior, and (3) help the practitioner solve a variety of problems.

Several theoretical models have been formulated in an effort to meet these three criteria. These models, as well as some to be discussed in Chapter 4, have spurred much research, explained and predicted health behaviors, and aided psychologists and other scientists. Each of these theories has some limitations, however, especially in the ability to predict the health-related behaviors of people who lack the financial resources necessary to pursue medical attention.

If and how people go about seeking medical attention when they feel unwell depends on several factors, many of which are included in one or more of the theories of health-seeking behaviors. Some of these determinants are (1) the characteristics of the symptoms being experienced, (2) the cost of seeking help, (3) the perceived severity of the disease, (4) the person's intention to act, (5) the person's stage of readiness for change, and (6) multiple social and demographic factors.

The health belief model includes the concepts of perceived severity of the disease, personal susceptibility, and perceived benefits of and barriers to health-enhancing behaviors. Research has shown that the health belief model has only limited success in predicting health-related behaviors.

The theory of reasoned action and the theory of planned behavior both include attitudes, subjective norms, and intention in an effort to predict and explain behavior. Research has found that the concepts of intention and perceived behavioral control are powerful predictors of health-seeking behaviors. Weinstein's precaution adoption process model assumes that when people are faced with adopting health protective behaviors, they go through seven possible stages of belief about their personal susceptibility. Among these stages is the necessity of overcoming their *optimistic bias*—that is, their belief that although certain behaviors are dangerous, the danger pertains to other people and not to them.

A limitation of all these models is their inability to accurately measure the many social, ethnic, and demographic factors that also affect people's health-seeking behavior. The balance of this chapter discusses issues involved in seeking medical attention, the problems of health care

that affect patients and their access to care, and the experience of being in the hospital.

⬤ SEEKING MEDICAL ATTENTION

How do people know when to seek medical attention? How do they know whether they are ill or not? When Jeff injured his hand, he experienced pain that persisted for hours, yet he tried several alternatives before he sought medical attention. Those alternatives included home care and consulting nonexperts about his injury. Was Jeff unusually reluctant to seek medical care, or was his behavior typical? Deciding when formal medical care is necessary is a complex problem, compounded by personal, social, and economic factors.

Before we consider these factors, we should define three terms: health, disease, and illness. Although the meaning of these concepts may seem obvious, their definitions have been elusive. Is health the absence of illness, or is it the attainment of some positive state? In the first chapter, we saw that the World Health Organization (WHO) defines health as positive physical, mental, and social well-being, and not merely as the absence of disease or infirmity. Unfortunately, this definition has little practical value for people trying to make decisions about their state of health or illness.

Another difficulty for many people comes from understanding the difference between disease and illness. These terms are often used interchangeably, but most health scientists make a distinction between the two. Disease refers to the process of physical damage within the body, which can exist even in the absence of a label or diagnosis. Illness, on the other hand, refers to the experience of being sick and having been diagnosed as being sick. People can have a disease and not be ill. For example, people with undiagnosed hypertension, HIV infection, or cancer all have a disease, but they may appear quite healthy and be completely unaware of their disease. Although disease and illness are separate conditions, they often overlap—for example, when a person feels ill and has also received a diagnosis of a specific disease.

People frequently experience physical symptoms, but these symptoms may or may not indicate a disease. Symptoms such as a headache, a painful shoulder, sniffles, or sneezing would probably not prompt a person to seek medical care, but an intense and persistent stomach pain probably would. At what point should a person decide to seek health care? Errors in both directions are possible. People who decide to go to the doctor when they are not really sick feel foolish, must pay the bill for an office visit, and lose credibility with people who know about the error, including the physician. If they choose not to seek health care, they may get better, but they may also get worse; trying to ignore their symptoms may make treatment more difficult and seriously endanger their health or increase their risk of death. A prudent action would seem to be to chance the unnecessary visit, but people (for a variety reasons) are often unable or simply reluctant to go to the doctor.

In the United States and other Western countries, people are not "officially" ill until they receive a diagnosis from a physician, making physicians the gatekeepers to further health care. Physicians not only *determine* disease by their diagnoses but also *sanction* it by giving a diagnosis. Hence, the person with symptoms is not the one who officially determines his or her health status. Jeff White's case illustrates this process. He sought a diagnosis by having his hand x-rayed, but the imaging center would not provide this service without a physician's referral. Thus, the gate to medical care was closed without a physician's permission to receive these services.

Dealing with symptoms occurs in two stages, which Stanislav Kasl and Sidney Cobb (1966a, 1966b) called illness behavior and sick role behavior. **Illness behavior** consists of the activities undertaken by people who experience symptoms but who have not yet received a diagnosis. That is, illness behavior occurs *before* diagnosis. These activities are oriented toward determining one's state of health and discovering suitable remedies. Jeff was engaging in illness behavior when he sought the opinion of his colleagues, when he went to the imaging center, and when he called his internist for a referral. All these actions took place before his diagnosis and were oriented toward receiving a diagnosis. In contrast, **sick role behavior** is the term applied to the behavior of people after a diagnosis,

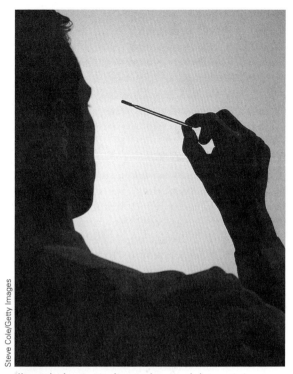

Steve Cole/Getty Images

Illness behavior is directed toward determining health status.

whether from a health care provider or through self-diagnosis. The activities of sick role behavior are oriented toward getting well. Jeff was exhibiting sick role behavior when he got his broken hand put in a cast, kept his appointments to have his hand checked, stopped playing basketball for six weeks, and took care not to reinjure his hand. All of these activities occurred after diagnosis and were oriented toward getting well. A *diagnosis*, then, is the event that separates illness behavior from sick role behavior.

Illness Behavior

Illness behavior, which takes place before an official diagnosis, is directed toward determining health status in the presence of symptoms. People routinely experience symptoms that may signal disease. Symptoms are a critical element in seeking medical care, but the presence of symptoms is not sufficient to prompt a visit to the doctor. Given similar symptoms, some people readily seek help, others do so reluctantly, and still others do not seek help at all. What determines people's decision to seek professional care?

At least six conditions help shape people's response to symptoms: (1) personal factors, (2) gender, (3) age, (4) socioeconomic and ethnic factors, (5) characteristics of the symptoms, and (6) conceptualization of disease.

Personal Factors   Personal factors include people's way of viewing their own body, their level of stress, and their personality traits. An example comes from people who experience irritable bowel syndrome, an intestinal condition characterized by pain, cramping, constipation, and diarrhea. Stress makes this condition worse. Some people with irritable bowel syndrome seek medical services, whereas many others do not. However, the level of symptoms turns out not to be the most important reason for seeking medical care (Ringström, Abrahamsson, Strid, & Simrén, 2007). Instead, seeking medical care is related more strongly to anxiety concerning the condition, coping resources, and level of physical functioning. About half of those who did not seek medical care sought alternative care or the advice of someone with the same condition. Thus, most people with this condition seek help but not necessarily from a physician; those who have adequate resources to cope with the symptoms and feel that the quality of their lives is not too impaired do not seek medical care. These personal factors are more important than the prominence of symptoms in determining who seeks medical care.

Stress is another personal factor in people's readiness to seek care. People who experience a great deal of stress are more likely to seek health care than those under less stress, even with equal symptoms. Those who experience concurrent and prolonged stress are more likely to seek care when the symptoms are ambiguous (Cameron, Leventhal, & Leventhal, 1995; Martin & Brantley, 2004). Ironically, complaining about or being perceived as being under high stress makes it less likely that people will be considered to have a disease. Symptoms that vary along with stress tend to be discounted as not real. This discounting occurs selectively, with women under high stress judged as less likely to have a physical disease than men in the same circumstances (Martin & Lemos, 2002). This tendency to discount symptoms may be a very important factor in the treatment of women who experience symptoms and for the health care providers who hear their reports.

Personality traits may also contribute to illness behavior. In a unique and interesting study headed by Sheldon Cohen (Feldman, Cohen, Gwaltney, Doyle, & Skoner, 1999), investigators inoculated a group of healthy volunteers with a common cold virus to see if participants with different personality traits would report symptoms differently. Participants who scored high on neuroticism—that is, those with strong emotional reactions—generally had high self-reports of illness whether or not objective evidence confirmed their reports. These people also reported more symptoms than other participants, suggesting that people with strong emotional reactions are more likely to complain of an illness. Additional research (Goodwin & Friedman, 2006) has confirmed the role of neuroticism in the readiness to report physical (and mental) symptoms and to seek medical care.

Gender Differences   In addition to personal factors, gender plays a role in the decision to seek treatment, with women more likely than men to use health care (Galdas, Cheater, & Marshall, 2005). The reasons for this difference are somewhat complex. Women tend to report more body symptoms and distress than men (Koopmans & Lamers, 2007). When asked about their symptoms, men tended to report only life-threatening situations, such as heart disease (Benyamini, Leventhal, & Leventhal, 2000). In contrast, women report not only these symptoms but also non-life-threatening symptoms, such as those from joint disease. Given the same level of symptoms, the female gender role allows women to seek many sorts of assistance, whereas the male gender role teaches men to act strong and to deny pain and discomfort. Research on men with prostate disease (Hale, Grogan, & Willott, 2007) confirmed the power of adhering to the male gender role in men's reluctance to seek care. These men were very anxious about their health but were reluctant to seek medical care.

Age Age is yet another factor that influences people's willingness to seek medical care. Young adults show the greatest reluctance to see a health professional, probably because they feel more indestructible.

As people age, they must decide whether their symptoms are due to aging or the result of disease. This distinction is not always easy. In general, people tend to interpret problems with a gradual onset and mild symptoms as resulting from age, whereas they are more ready to see problems with a sudden onset and severe symptoms as being more serious. For example, when older patients with symptoms of acute myocardial infarction are able to attribute these symptoms to age, they tend to delay in seeking medical care. One study (Ryan & Zerwic, 2003) looked at patients who failed to realize that a delay in seeking health care could bring about more severe symptoms as well as increased chance of mortality. Compared with younger and middle-aged patients, these older people were more likely to (1) attribute their symptoms to age, (2) experience more severe and lengthy symptoms, (3) attribute their symptoms to some other disorder, and (4) have had previous experience with cardiac problems. Each of these factors provides information on how older cardiac patients can be treated.

Culture, Ethnicity, and Perception of Illness People from different cultures and ethnic backgrounds have disparate ways of viewing illness. In the United States, people in higher socioeconomic groups experience fewer symptoms and report a higher level of health than people at lower socioeconomic levels (Grzywacz et al., 2004). Yet when higher income people are sick, they are more likely to seek health care. Nevertheless, poor people are overrepresented among the hospitalized, an indication that they are much more likely than middle- and upper-income people to become seriously ill. In addition, people in lower socioeconomic groups tend to wait longer before seeking health care, thus making treatment more difficult and hospitalization more likely. The poor have less access to medical care, have to travel longer to reach health care facilities that will offer them treatment, and must wait longer once they arrive at those facilities.

Ethnic background is another factor in seeking health care, with European Americans being more likely than other groups to report a visit to a physician. Part of the National Health and Nutrition Examination Survey (Harris, 2001) examined some of the reasons behind these ethnic differences, comparing European Americans, African Americans, and Mexican Americans with Type 2 diabetes on access to and use of health care facilities. Ethnic differences appeared in health insurance coverage as well as in common risk factors for diabetes and heart disease.

A study from the United Kingdom confirmed the notion that culture and ethnic background—not lack of knowledge—are primarily responsible for differences in seeking medical care. In this study (Adamson, Ben-Shlomo, Chaturvedi, & Donovan, 2003), researchers sent questionnaires to a large, diverse group of participants. Each questionnaire included two clinical vignettes showing (1) people experiencing signs of chest pain and (2) people discovering a lump in their armpit. The experimenters asked each participant to respond to the chest pain and the lump in terms of needing immediate care. Results indicated that respondents who were black, female, and from lower socioeconomic groups were at least as likely as those who were white, male, and from middle- and upper-class groups to make quick and accurate responses to potential medical problems. These findings suggest that factors other than medical knowledge play an important role in seeking health care. That is, poor black women do not lack information about the potential health hazards of chest pain or a lump in the armpit, but they do lack the resources to respond quickly to these symptoms.

Symptom Characteristics Symptom characteristics also influence when and how people look for help. Symptoms themselves do not inevitably lead people to seek care, but certain characteristics are important in their response to symptoms. David Mechanic (1978) listed four characteristics of the symptoms that determine people's response to disease.

First is the *visibility of the symptom*—that is, how readily apparent the symptom is to the person and to others. A study on intentions to adopt osteoporosis prevention (Klohn & Rogers,

1991) confirmed the importance of the visibility of symptoms. Young women who received messages about osteoporosis as a disfiguring condition were significantly more likely to say that they intended to adopt precautions against osteoporosis than young women who were not alerted to the disfiguring aspects of the disease.

Mechanic's second symptom characteristic was *perceived severity of the symptom*. He contended that symptoms seen as severe would be more likely to prompt action than less severe symptoms. Jeff White did not seek immediate medical care partially because he did not see his symptoms as serious—his hand did not appear to be broken, nor was it discolored until the second day. The perceived severity of the symptom highlights the importance of personal perception and distinguishes between the perceived severity of a symptom and the judgment of severity by medical authorities. Indeed, patients and physicians differ in their perceptions of the severity of a wide variety of symptoms (Peay & Peay, 1998). Symptoms that patients perceived as more serious produced greater concern and a stronger belief that treatment was urgently needed, as a study on women seeking care after experiencing symptoms of heart attack demonstrated (Quinn, 2005). Those women who interpreted their symptoms as indicative of cardiac problems sought care more quickly than women who interpreted their symptoms as some other condition. Thus, perceived severity of symptoms rather than the presence of symptoms is critical in the decision to seek care.

The third symptom characteristic mentioned by Mechanic is the *extent to which the symptom interferes with a person's life*. The more incapacitated the person, the more likely he or she is to seek medical care. The study on irritable bowel syndrome (Ringström et al., 2007) illustrated this principle; those who sought medical care reported a poorer health quality of life than those who did not seek medical care.

Mechanic's fourth hypothesized determinant of illness behavior is the *frequency and persistence of the symptoms*. Conditions that people view as requiring care tend to be those that are both severe and continuous, whereas intermittent symptoms are less likely to generate illness behavior. Severe symptoms prompt people to seek help, but even mild symptoms can motivate people to seek help if those symptoms persist. When ice packs could not reduce the swelling of his hand and when the pain persisted, Jeff decided to take action.

In Mechanic's description and subsequent research, symptom characteristics alone are not sufficient to prompt illness behavior. However, if symptoms persist or are perceived as severe, people are more likely to evaluate them as indicating a need for care. Thus, people are prompted to seek care on the basis of their interpretation of their symptoms, which relates to each person's view of illness.

Conceptualization of Disease Despite a vast amount of knowledge in the fields of physiology and medicine, most people are largely ignorant of how their body works and how disease develops. When people gain information, they integrate it into their existing knowledge structure. If the new information seems incompatible with what they already "know," they may modify this new information to make it fit their preexisting knowledge rather than change their knowledge to conform to the new information. This process may lead to personal conceptualizations of disease that vary substantially from the medical explanation. Both children (Veldtman et al., 2001) and college students (Nemeroff, 1995) showed inaccurate and incomplete conceptualizations of diseases in describing diseases they had and how they became ill.

In exploring how people see various diseases, Howard Leventhal and his colleagues (Benyamini, Leventhal, & Leventhal, 1997, 2000; Leventhal, Leventhal, & Cameron, 2001; Martin & Leventhal, 2004) have looked at five components in the conceptualization process: (1) identity of the disease, (2) time line (the time course of both disease and treatment), (3) cause of the disease, (4) consequences of the disease, and (5) controllability of the disease. Research support exists for all of these components.

The *identity of the disease*, the first component identified by Leventhal and his associates, is very important to illness behavior. People who have identified their symptoms as a "heart attack" should (Martin & Leventhal, 2004) and do (Quinn, 2005) react quite differently from those who label the same symptoms as "heartburn." As we have seen, the presence of symptoms is not sufficient to initiate help seeking, but the labeling that occurs in conjunction with symptoms may be critical in a person's either seeking help or ignoring symptoms.

Labels provide a framework within which symptoms can be interpreted. People experience less emotional arousal when they find a label that indicates a minor problem (heartburn rather than heart attack). Initially, they will probably adopt the least serious label that fits their symptoms. For example, Jeff initially interpreted his broken hand as a bruise. To a large extent, a label carries with it some prediction about the time course of the disease, so if the time course does not correspond to the expectation implicit in the label, the person has to relabel the symptoms. When Jeff's hand failed to respond to the ice packs and the pain continued, he began to doubt the label he had applied. His friends told him he was foolish to ignore the swelling and pain out of a belief that these symptoms would disappear. However, the tendency to interpret symptoms as indicating minor rather than major problems is the source of many optimistic self-diagnoses, of which Jeff's is an example.

The second component in conceptualizing an illness is the *time line*. Even though the time course of a disease is usually implicit within the diagnosis, people's understanding of the time involved is not necessarily accurate. People with a chronic disorder often view their disease as acute and of short duration. For example, patients with heart disease (a chronic disorder) may see their disease as "heartburn," an acute disorder (Martin & Leventhal, 2004). With most acute diseases, patients can expect a temporary disorder with a quick onset of symptoms, followed by treatment, a remission of symptoms, and then a cure. Unfortunately, this scenario does not fit the majority of diseases, such as heart disease and diabetes, which are chronic and persist over a lifetime. However, thinking of chronic diseases as time limited decreases distress; patients who conceptualized their cancer as chronic reported greater distress than those who saw the disease as an acute illness (Rabin, Leventhal, & Goodin, 2004).

The third component of the personal view of illness is the *determination of cause*. For the most part, determining causality is more a facet of the sick role than of illness behavior because it usually occurs after a diagnosis has been made. But the attribution of causality for symptoms is an important factor in illness behavior. For example, if a person can attribute the pain in his hand to a blow received the day before, he will not have to consider the possibility of bone cancer as the cause of the pain.

Attribution of causality, however, is often faulty. People may attribute a cold to "germs" or to the weather, and they may see cancer as caused by microwave ovens or by the will of God. These conceptualizations have important implications for illness behavior. People are less likely to seek professional treatment for conditions they consider as having emotional or spiritual causes. In a study of adults with coronary artery disease (Gump et al., 2001), older patients were more likely than younger ones to believe that age rather than smoking or high cholesterol was the cause of their disease. Culture may also play a role in attributions of causes for diseases. Differences appeared in a study that contrasted White with Pakistani and Indian people with Type 2 diabetes in Great Britain (Lawton, Ahmad, Peel, & Hallowell, 2007). Both groups tried to understand the underlying cause for their disease, but the White Britons were more likely to see their condition as a result of their lifestyle choices, whereas the Pakistani and Indian Britons tended to attribute their disease to external factors and life circumstances. These beliefs may affect how patients care for themselves and manage their disease. Therefore, people's conceptualizations of disease causality can influence their behavior.

The *consequences of a disease* are the fourth component in Leventhal's description of illness. Even though the consequences of a disease are implied by the diagnosis, an incorrect understanding of the consequences can have a profound effect on illness behavior. Many people view a diagnosis of cancer as a death sentence. Some neglect health care because they believe themselves to be in a hopeless situation. Women who find a lump in their breast sometimes delay making an appointment with a doctor, not because they fail to recognize this symptom of cancer but because they fear the possible consequences—surgery and possibly the loss of a breast, chemotherapy, radiation, or some combination of these consequences.

The *controllability* of a disease refers to people's belief that they can control the course of their illness by controlling the treatment or the disease. People who believe that their behaviors will not change the course of a disease are less likely to seek treatment than those who believe that prompt treatment will be effective, but people who are able to control the symptoms of their disease without medical consultation will be less likely to seek professional medical care (Ringström et al., 2007).

The Sick Role

Kasl and Cobb (1966b) defined sick role behavior as the activities engaged in by people who believe themselves ill, for the purpose of getting well. In other words, sick role behavior occurs after a person has been diagnosed. Alexander Segall (1997) modified this concept, proposing that the sick role concept includes three rights or privileges and three duties or responsibilities. The privileges are (1) the right to make decisions concerning health-related issues, (2) the right to be exempt from normal duties, and (3) the right to become dependent on others for assistance. The three responsibilities are (1) the duty to maintain health along with the responsibility to get well, (2) the duty to perform routine health care management and, (3) the duty to use a range of health care resources.

Segall's formulation of rights and duties is meant to be an ideal—not a realistic conception of sick role behavior in the United States. The first right—to make decisions concerning health-related issues—does not extend to children and to many people living in poverty (Bailis, Segall, Mahon, Chipperfield, & Dunn, 2001). The second feature of the sick role is the exemption of the sick person from normal duties. Sick people are usually not expected to go to work, attend school, go to meetings, cook meals, clean house, care for children, do homework, or mow the lawn. However, meeting these expectations is not always possible. Many sick people neither stay home nor go to the hospital, but continue to go to work. People who feel that their jobs are precarious are more likely to go to work when they are sick (Bloor, 2005), but so did those who experienced good working relationships with their colleagues and were dedicated to their jobs (Biron, Brun, Ivers, & Cooper, 2006). Similarly, the third privilege—to be dependent on others—is more of an ideal than a reflection of reality. For example, sick mothers often must continue to be responsible for their children.

Segall's three duties of sick people can all be grouped under the single obligation to do whatever is necessary to get well. However, the goal of getting well applies more to acute than to chronic diseases. People with chronic diseases will never be completely well. This situation presents a conflict for many people with a chronic disease, who have difficulty accepting their condition as one of continuing disability; instead, they erroneously believe that their disease is a temporary state.

IN SUMMARY

No easy distinction exists between health and illness. The World Health Organization sees health as more than the absence of disease; rather, health is the attainment of positive physical, mental, and social well-being. Curiously, the distinction between disease and illness is clearer. Disease refers to the process of physical damage within the body, whether or not the person is aware of this damage. Illness, on the other hand, refers to the experience of being sick; people can feel sick but have no identifiable disease.

At least six factors determine how people respond to illness symptoms: (1) personal factors, such as the way people look upon their own body; (2) gender, with women being more likely than men to seek professional care; (3) age, with older people attributing many ailments to their age; (4) ethnic and cultural factors, with people who cannot afford medical care more likely than affluent people to become ill but less likely to seek health care; (5) characteristics of the symptoms, with symptoms that interfere with daily activities as well as visible, severe, and frequent symptoms most likely to prompt medical attention; and (6) people's conceptualization of disease.

People tend to incorporate five components into their concept of disease: (1) the identity of the disease, (2) the time line of the disease, (3) the cause of the disease, (4) the consequences of the disease, and (5) controllability of the disease. If a disease has been officially identified or diagnosed, then its time course and its consequences are implicit. However, people who know the name of their disease do not always have an accurate concept of its time course and consequence and may wrongly see a chronic disease as having a short time course. People want to know the cause of their illness and to understand how it can be controlled.

Once people's symptoms are diagnosed and they believe they have a disease, they engage in sick role behavior in order to get well. People who are sick should be relieved from normal responsibilities and should have the obligation of trying to get well. However, these rights and duties are difficult and often impossible to fulfill.

RECEIVING HEALTH CARE

From childhood to old age, most people have had some experience of receiving health care. Part of this experience has revolved around the many and varied health care–related problems, including having only limited access to health care, choosing the right practitioner, dealing with managed care, and being in the hospital.

Limited Access to Health Care

The cost of health care prevents many people from receiving proper treatment and care. This limited access to health care is more restricted in the United States than in other industrialized nations (Weitz, 2007). Many countries have developed national health insurance or other plans for universal coverage, but the United States has resisted this strategy. Hospitalization and complex medical treatments are so expensive that most people cannot afford these services. This situation has led to the rise and development of health insurance, which people may purchase as individuals but more often obtain as part of workplace groups that offer coverage to their members.

Individual insurance tends to be expensive and to offer less coverage, especially for people with health problems, but these individuals may be able to get some insurance as part of a workplace group. Thus, employment is an important factor in access to health care in the United States. People who are unemployed or whose jobs do not offer the benefit of health insurance are often uninsured, a situation describing about 17% of people in the United States (NCHS, 2007). However, even people with insurance may face barriers to receiving health care; their policies often fail to cover services such as dental care, mental health services, and eyeglasses, forcing people to pay these expenses out of their own pockets or forego these services. For insured people who experience a catastrophic illness, coverage may be inadequate for many expenses, creating enormous medical costs. Indeed, medical costs are the underlying cause for more than half of all personal bankruptcies in the United States (Hall & Schneider, 2008).

The problem of providing health care for those who cannot afford to pay for these services was a concern throughout the 20th century (Weitz, 2007). In response to these concerns, the U.S. Congress created two programs in 1965—Medicare and Medicaid. Medicare pays hospital expenses for most Americans over the age of 65, and thus few people in this age group are without hospitalization insurance. Medicare also offers medical insurance that those who participate may purchase for a monthly fee, but many expenses are not covered, such as routine dental care. Medicaid provides health care based on low income and physical problems, such as disability or pregnancy. These restrictions make many poor people ineligible; only about 43% of poor people receive coverage through Medicaid (USCB, 2007). Children may be eligible for health insurance, even if their parents are not, through the State Children's Health Insurance Program.

People with low incomes struggle to obtain insurance coverage, but even those with insurance may face barriers such as finding a provider who will accept their plan and the out-of-pocket cost of services (DeVoe et al., 2007). The uninsured face more restrictions. These people are less likely to have a regular physician, more likely to have a

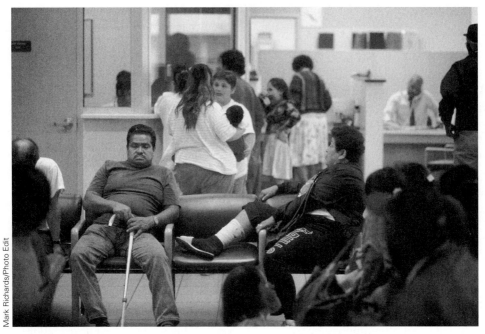

Cost and accessibility of services present barriers to obtaining health care.

chronic health problem, and less willing to seek medical care because of the cost (Pauly & Pagán, 2007). This reluctance has consequences for the management of their diseases. People with chronic diseases and without health insurance have poorly controlled conditions, difficulty in obtaining medications, more health crises, and higher risk of mortality than people with insurance. In addition, a high proportion of people without insurance may create a spillover effect in which those with insurance experience higher costs and poorer quality of care. Thus, health insurance is an important issue in the access to medical care and plays a role in choosing a practitioner.

Choosing a Practitioner

As part of their attempts to get well, sick people usually consult a health care practitioner. Beginning during the 19th century, physicians became the dominant health care providers (Weitz, 2007). Most middle-class wealthy people in industrialized nations seek the services of a physician. Toward the end of the 20th century, however, medical dominance began to decline and other types of health care providers' popularity rose.

For example, midwives, nurses, pharmacists, physical therapists, psychologists, osteopaths, chiropractors, dentists, nutritionists, and herbal healers all provide various types of health care.

Some of these sources of health care are considered "alternative" because they provide alternatives to conventional medical care. Almost a third of U.S. residents who seek conventional health care also use some form of alternative health care, and nearly everyone (96%) who uses alternative health care also uses conventional health care (Weitz, 2007). Some people who consult practitioners such as herbal healers do so because these healers are part of a cultural tradition, such as *curanderos* in Latin American culture. However, the recent growth of alternative medicine has come mainly from well-educated people who are dissatisfied with standard medical care and who hold attitudes that are compatible with the alternative care they seek (Weitz, 2007). Well-educated people are disproportionately represented because they are better able to pay for this care, which is less likely to be covered by insurance than conventional care.

People without health insurance are less likely to have a regular health care provider than are those with insurance (Pauly & Pagán, 2007). Their experience of receiving health care may consist of going to a convenient care clinic or to a hospital emergency room, even for chronic conditions. Convenient care clinics offer basic health care, primarily by physicians' assistants and nurse practitioners (Hanson-Turton, Ryan, Miller, Counts, & Nash, 2007). Seeking care through the emergency room may result in people receiving care only after their condition meets the definition of an emergency. Thus, these patients are sicker than they might have been if they had easier access to care. In addition, seeking care from emergency rooms is more expensive and overburdens these facilities, decreasing their ability to provide care to those with acute conditions.

Access to health care has become increasingly restricted, but attitudes concerning health care have become more consumer oriented. Younger patients are more likely to see their role as that of consumers of health care who, like any consumers, have choices in their selection of services and service providers. Increased access to the Internet has opened a vast source of medical information (and misinformation) to consumers (Wald, Dube, & Anthony, 2007). Patients who go to the web for information become more active in their health care, which is consistent with the consumer philosophy but may decrease physicians' authority and change the nature of the physician–patient relationship. Patients who do not have access to the Internet cannot obtain this information, and without information, people are not in a good position to be effective consumers (Hall & Schneider, 2008).

When people have the freedom to choose their practitioners, they value technical competence but also assume that practitioners will be competent (Bendapudi, Berry, Frey, Parish, & Rayburn, 2006). Other behaviors that differentiate practitioners whom patients rate as providing excellent treatment include being confident, thorough, personable, humane, forthright, respectful, and empathetic. Research indicates that female physicians may be more likely to show these behaviors than male physicians. Two meta-analyses covering nearly 35 years of research (Roter & Hall, 2004) showed that female physicians were more patient centered, spent 10% more time with patients, employed more partnership behaviors, were more positive in their communication, engaged in more psychosocial counseling, asked more questions, and were involved in more emotionally focused talk. Moreover, the patients of female physicians were more likely to disclose more information about their medical symptoms as well as their psychosocial concerns. (Interestingly, male obstetricians and gynecologists had a higher level of emotionally focused talk than their female counterparts.) This research suggests that when choosing a physician, a person may wish to consider the physician's gender.

The Rise of Managed Health Care

Health maintenance organizations (HMOs) originated with the concept that prevention is preferable to treatment. Kaiser Permanente and the Group Health Cooperative of Puget Sound were organized to provide affordable care oriented toward keeping people healthy (Weitz, 2007). HMOs hire health care workers, including physicians, and pay them salaries for their services. This arrangement differs from the fee-for-service payments that most physicians in private or group practice receive. Physicians in HMOs cannot boost their salaries by performing more procedures or seeing more patients. Thus, HMOs came to be seen as a way to contain rising health care costs.

The hope that HMOs could help contain escalating medical care costs led to changes in their operation. Rather than allowing HMO members to choose their services, HMOs began to limit services; that is, they began to manage the amount of health care available to members. A typical arrangement includes a gatekeeper—a primary care physician who is often a general practitioner or family care specialist. Under this arrangement, patients must see a primary care physician when they visit the HMO, and this provider decides if the patient may see specialists or receive additional care. HMOs may pressure their primary care physicians to limit referrals and additional treatment as ways to cut costs (sometimes giving physicians bonuses for limiting these options). This strategy denies access to health care and has led to patient dissatisfaction. This dissatisfaction, in turn, has led to a loss of members for HMOs, with the percentage of the population belonging to an HMO reaching a peak of 30% in 1999 and then dropping to less than 25% in 2006 (NCHS, 2007).

The trends toward managed care and limited access to health care have also affected insurance plan members. Rather than permitting members to seek health care from any practitioner of their choice, many insurance plans now have lists of preferred or exclusive providers whom members may consult and with whom insurance companies have negotiated fixed, discounted prices for services (Hall & Schneider, 2008). Members may choose practitioners who are not on the list, but the financial penalty for this choice is high; insurance companies reimburse a lower percentage of costs, and patients must pay the remainder.

Managed care has not only limited the amount and type of care that individuals receive but has restricted their choice of health care professionals. This situation may prevent people from creating ongoing relationships with health care providers and severely limits the option of seeking alternative health care.

For physicians who provide health care, the practice of medicine has changed. The era of the solo practitioner is coming to an end; most physicians now practice within a multispecialty group of other health care providers or are employed by HMOs. These physicians have less autonomy to make treatment decisions and feel pressure to cut costs, possibly at the risk of their patients' health. The traditional authoritarian role of health care providers is changing; physicians' authority and power have diminished. As a result, health care has become less personal, more difficult to obtain, and more technology oriented. These factors have an impact on all facets of health care, but depersonalization and technology are especially important factors in the experience of being in the hospital.

Being in the Hospital

Over the past 30 years, hospitals and the experience of being in the hospital have both changed. First, many types of surgery and tests that were formerly handled through hospitalization are now performed on an outpatient basis; second, hospital stays have become shorter; third, an expanding array of technology is available for diagnosis and treatment; and fourth, patients feel increasingly free to voice their concerns to their physician (Bell, Kravitz, Thom, Krupat, & Azari, 2001). As a result of these changes, people who are not severely ill are not likely to be hospitalized, and people who are admitted to a hospital are more severely ill than those admitted 30 years ago.

Ironically, although managed care has helped control costs through shorter hospital stays, it has not always been in the interest of the patient. Technological medicine has become more prominent in patient care, and personal treatment by the hospital staff has become less so. These factors can combine to make hospitalization a stressful experience (Weitz, 2007). In addition, understaffing and the challenges of monitoring complex technology and medication regimens have created an alarming number of medical mistakes (see Would You Believe . . . ? box).

The Hospital Patient Role Part of the sick role is to be a patient, and being a patient means conforming to the rules of the health care institution and complying with medical advice. When a person enters the hospital as a patient, that person becomes part of a complex institution and assumes a role within that institution. That role includes some difficult aspects: being treated as a "nonperson," tolerating lack of information, and losing control of daily activities. Patients find incidents such as waits, delays, and communication problems with staff distressing, and such incidents decrease patients' satisfaction (Weingart et al., 2006).

When people are hospitalized, all but their illness becomes invisible, and their status is reduced to that of a "nonperson." Not only are patients' identities ignored, but their comments and questions may also be overlooked. Hospital procedure focuses on the technical aspects of medical care; it usually ignores patients' emotional needs and leaves them less satisfied with their treatment than patients who are treated as persons and informed about their condition (Yarnold, Michelson, Thompson, & Adams, 1998).

The lack of information that patients experience comes from hospital routine rather than from an attempt to keep information from patients. The

WOULD YOU BELIEVE . . . ?

Hospitals May Be a Leading Cause of Death

Would you believe that receiving medical care, especially in an American hospital, can be fatal? Newspaper headlines have painted an alarming picture of the dangers of receiving health care, based on a series of studies. In 1999, a study from the Institute of Medicine made headlines with its findings that at least 44,000—and perhaps as many as 98,000—people die in U.S. hospitals every year as a result of medical errors (Kohn, Corrigan, & Donaldson, 1999). Confirmation of the higher figure (Zhan & Miller, 2003) was followed by another report (HealthGrades, 2004) that contended that 195,000 people die of medical mistakes each year in American hospitals.

These figures created both sensational headlines and immediate controversy. The *New York Times* ("Preventing Fatal Medical Errors," 1999) compared these numbers with fatalities from the Vietnam War, stating that more Americans are killed in U.S. hospitals every 6 months than during the entire war in Vietnam. Although the United States does not recognize medical error as a cause of death, the *Washington Post* (Weiss, 1999) calculated that medical errors are the fifth leading cause of death in the United States.

Unfortunately, medical errors aren't the only cause of unnecessary deaths of patients in U.S. hospitals. Medication, too, can be fatal. An Institute of Medicine study (Aspden, Wolcott, Bootman, & Cronenwett, 2007) estimated that hospitalized patients experience an average of one medication error per patient per day of hospitalization, resulting in morbidity, mortality, and increased cost of hospitalization. A meta-analysis of studies on adverse drug reactions (Lazarou, Pomeranz, & Corey, 1998) found that, even when prescribed and taken *properly*, prescription drugs account for between 76,000 and 137,000 deaths each year. This analysis included patients admitted to a hospital for an adverse drug reaction as well as those already in the hospital who suffered a fatal drug reaction. This meta-analysis also estimated the total number of toxic drug reactions among hospitalized patients at more than 2 million. As with the reports on medical errors, these results created interest in the popular media. *Newsweek* carried an article on the report (Kalb, 1998) and estimated that death from adverse drug reactions is the fourth leading cause of death in the United States, exceeded only by cardiovascular disease, cancer, and stroke. More recent reports (Aspden et al., 2007; HealthGrades, 2004) have suggested that these figures may be underestimates.

Despite widespread publicity and growing concern, little improvement seems to have occurred during the past 10 years. In a report published in the *Journal of the American Medical Association*, Lucian Leape and Donald Berwick (2005) concluded that the medical profession has achieved only limited progress toward solving the problem of medical errors, and a follow-up study (HealthGrades, 2006) indicated that medical errors in hospitals are increasing rather than decreasing.

One barrier to correcting the situation comes from the climate of silence and blame that surrounds errors—health care professionals do not want to admit to errors or report colleagues who have made errors because of the blame involved. Rather than silence and blame, Lucian Leape (Leape & Berwick, 2005) suggested that hospitals should be eager to seek information about errors and that analysis should focus on the systems that allow errors rather than the people who make errors. The practice of medicine will never be free of errors, but creating systems that make errors more difficult to commit will improve patient safety and cut hospitalization costs.

tradition that physicians should decide how much patients ought to know has faded, and most physicians believe that patients should be fully informed about their conditions. However, an open exchange of information between patient and practitioner is difficult to achieve in the hospital, where physicians spend only a brief amount of time talking to patients. In addition, information may be unavailable because patients are undergoing diagnostic tests. The hospital staff may not explain the purpose or results of diagnostic testing, leaving the patient without information and filled with anxiety.

Hospitalized patients are expected to conform submissively to the rules of the hospital and the

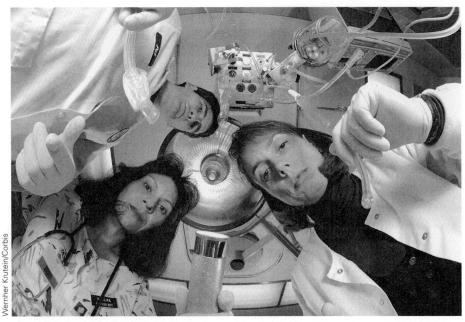

Wernher Krutein/Corbis

Increased use of technology, lack of information, and lack of control contribute to the stress of hospitalization.

orders of their doctor, thus relinquishing much control over their lives. People tend to manifest heightened physiological responses and to react on a physical level to uncontrollable stimulation more strongly than they do when they can exert some control over their condition. Lack of control can decrease people's capacity to concentrate and can increase their tendency to report physical symptoms.

For the efficiency of the organization, uniform treatment and conformity to hospital routine are desirable, even though they deprive patients of information and control. Hospitals have no insidious plot to deprive patients of their freedom, but that is the result when hospitals impose their routine on patients. Restoring control to patients in any significant way would further complicate an already complex organization, but the restoration of small types of control may be effective. For example, most hospitals now allow patients some choice of foods and provide TV remote controls to give patients the power to select a program to watch (or not watch). These aspects of control are small but possibly important, as we discuss in Chapter 5 (Langer & Rodin, 1976; Rodin & Langer, 1977).

Children and Hospitalization Few children negotiate childhood without some injury, disease, or condition that requires hospitalization, and the commonalties of the hospitalization experience are sources of stress and anxiety—separation from parents, an unfamiliar environment, diagnostic tests, administration of anesthesia, immunization "shots," surgery, and postoperative pain. Pediatric hospitals often offer some type of preparation program for children. Training children to cope with their fear of treatment presents special problems to health psychologists. Providing children and parents with information about hospital procedure and equipment can be an effective way to decrease anxiety.

However, reassuring a child is not an effective way to reduce fear in either the child or the parent. In a study with 4- to 6-year-old children who were about to receive preschool immunization shots, researchers (Manimala, Blount, & Cohen, 2000) paired each child with her or his parent and then randomly assigned each dyad to either a distraction group or a reassurance group. Parents of children in the distraction group were asked to distract their child's attention away from the immunization procedure. Parents of children in the reassurance group

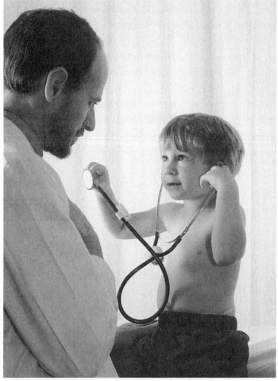

Wernher Krutein/Corbis

Allowing children to become comfortable with medical apparatus can ease their distress.

attempted to reduce their child's anxiety by reassuring them that they had nothing to fear. Results strongly favored the distraction group, with three times as many children in the reassurance group requiring physical restraint. Also, children in the reassurance group showed much more verbal fear then did the other children. An interesting adjunct to these findings involved the training received by parents prior to the immunization process. Those who received training on how to reassure their child expressed a high level of confidence that they would indeed be able to calm their child. Then, after immunization, the reassuring parents not only had problems helping their children, but they rated themselves as being much more distressed than did the other parents. Reassurance, it seems, is not an effective way to reduce stress.

Another strategy for helping children is modeling—that is, seeing another child cope successfully with a similar stressful procedure. A combination of modeling with a cognitive

behavioral intervention and self-talk reduced distress for children who were receiving painful treatments for leukemia (Jay, Elliott, Woody, & Siegel, 1991). Indeed, this intervention was more successful than a drug treatment that included the tranquilizer Valium. A more technological approach involved a virtual reality distraction activity (Gershon, Zimand, Pickering, Rothbaum, & Hodges, 2004) that reduced pain and anxiety for children receiving a painful treatment for cancer. A review of interventions for children (Mitchell, Johnston, & Keppel, 2004) indicated that multicomponent programs were generally more effective than single-component programs; providing information and teaching coping skills are both important for children and their parents when faced with hospitalization.

Cost, not effectiveness, is the main problem with intervention strategies to reduce children's distress resulting from hospitalization for specific medical procedures. The trend is toward cost cutting, and all interventions add to medical care costs. Some of these interventions may be cost-effective if they reduce the need for additional care or decrease other expenses.

IN SUMMARY

The expense of health care has led to restricted access for most U.S. residents. People who have health insurance receive better care and have more choices about their health care than people without insurance. Concerns about health care costs led to the creation of two U.S. government programs: Medicare, which pays for hospitalization for those over age 65; and Medicaid, which pays for care for poor people who are aged, blind, disabled, pregnant, or the parent of a dependent child.

Physicians are primary sources of health care, but alternative sources have become more popular over the past two decades. People without health insurance often have disadvantages and limitations in securing a regular health care practitioner. However, the rise of managed care has affected the health care that most people receive. The drive to cut health care costs has prompted the proliferation of health maintenance organizations and preferred or exclusive provider networks, sometimes at the expense of patient care. Satisfaction with health care in the United States has declined.

Hospitalized patients often experience added stress as a result of being in the hospital. They are typically regarded as "nonpersons," receive inadequate information concerning their illness, and experience some loss of control over their lives. They are expected to conform to hospital routine and to comply with frequent requests of the hospital staff.

Hospitalized children and their parents experience special problems and may receive special training to help them deal with hospitalization. Several types of interventions, including modeling and cognitive behavioral programs, are effective in helping children and their parents cope with this difficult situation.

ANSWERS

This chapter has addressed three basic questions:

1. Why do people adopt health-related behaviors?

Most people value good health and wish to avoid disease, but many fail to seek health care when necessary. Several theories attempt to explain health-related behavior. The health belief model, which was developed specifically to predict and explain health-related behaviors, includes the concepts of perceived severity of the disease, personal susceptibility, and perceived benefits of and barriers to health-enhancing behaviors. Although research has demonstrated some utility for the original health belief model, other studies have introduced new concepts and have had only limited success in predicting health-seeking behavior.

The theory of reasoned action and the theory of planned behavior are general behavior theories that have also been applied to health-related situations. Both theories include attitudes, subjective norms, and intention; in addition, the theory of planned behavior includes the person's perceived behavioral control. These two theories are beginning to produce extensive research, some of which suggests that the concepts of intention and perceived behavioral control add to the predictive ability of theories of reasoned action and planned behavior.

Weinstein's precaution adoption process model assumes that when people are faced with adopting health protective behaviors, they go through seven possible stages of belief about their personal susceptibility. Built into stage 2 is an optimistic bias, a topic that has been heavily researched. Weinstein and his colleagues have conducted the majority of research on the total precaution adoption model, but evidence in support of this model has begun to appear. A limitation of all these models is their inability to accurately predict health-related behaviors, and all omit various social, ethnic, and other demographic factors that also affect people's health-seeking behavior.

2. What factors are related to seeking medical attention?

How people determine their health status when they don't feel well depends not only on social, ethnic, and demographic factors but also on the characteristics of their symptoms and their concept of illness. In deciding whether they are ill, people consider at least four characteristics of their symptoms: (1) the obvious visibility of the symptoms, (2) the perceived severity of the illness, (3) the degree to which the symptoms interfere with their lives, and (4) the frequency and persistence of the symptoms.

Once people are diagnosed as sick, they adopt the sick role that involves relief from normal social and occupational responsibilities and the duty to try to get better.

3. **What problems do people encounter in receiving medical care?**

People encounter problems in paying for medical care, and those without insurance often have limited access to health care. The U.S. government's creation of Medicare and Medicaid has helped people over 65 and some poor people with access to health care, but many people have problems finding a regular practitioner and receiving optimal health care.

The escalating cost of medical care has changed the way many people receive care. The system of private practitioners who provide care has evolved into a system of managed care in which health care is restricted by gatekeepers in health maintenance organizations or by preferred providers specified by insurance companies.

Although hospital stays are shorter than they were 30 years ago, being in the hospital is a difficult experience for both adults and children. As a hospital patient, a person must conform to hospital procedures and policies, which include being treated as a "nonperson," tolerating lack of information, and losing control of daily activities. Children who are hospitalized are placed in an unfamiliar environment, may be separated from parents, and may undergo surgery or other painful medical procedures. Interventions that help children and parents manage this stressful experience may ease the distress, but cost is a factor that limits the availability of these services.

SUGGESTED READINGS

Bogart, L. M., & Delahanty, D. L. (2004). Psychosocial models. In T. J. Boll, R. G. Frank, A. Baum, & J. L. Wallander (Eds.), *Handbook of clinical health psychology: Vol. 3. Models and perspectives in health psychology* (pp. 201–248). Washington, DC: American Psychological Association. This review of models of health-related behaviors critically examines the health belief model and theories of reasoned action and planned behavior. The review is oriented around an evaluation of how well these models predict important health behaviors, including condom use, exercise, smoking, and dieting.

Martin, R., & Leventhal, H. (2004). Symptom perception and health care–seeking behavior. In J. M. Raczynski & L. C. Leviton (Ed.), *Handbook of clinical health psychology* (Vol. 2, pp. 299–328). Washington, DC: American Psychological Association. This article explores the situations and perceptions that underlie seeking health care, including the difficulty of interpreting symptoms and the theories that attempt to explain this behavior.

Weitz, R. (2007). *The sociology of health, illness, and health care: A critical approach* (4th ed.). Belmont, CA: Wadsworth. Weitz critically reviews the health care situation in the United States in this medical sociology book. Chapters 10, 11, and 12 provide a description of health care settings and professions, including many alternatives to traditional health care.

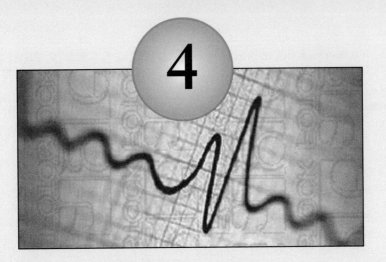

4

ADHERING
TO MEDICAL ADVICE

QUESTIONS

This chapter focuses on four basic questions:

1. What theoretical models have been used to explain adherence?

2. What is adherence, how can it be measured, and how frequently does it occur?

3. What factors predict adherence?

4. How can adherence be improved?

CHECK YOUR HEALTH RISKS

Check the items that apply to you.

☐ 1. I usually stop taking prescription medicine whenever I begin to feel better, even though some of the medication is still left.

☐ 2. If my prescription medicine doesn't seem to be working, I will continue taking it.

☐ 3. I believe that faith will cure disease and heal injuries much more certainly than modern medicine.

☐ 4. I won't have a prescription filled if it costs too much.

☐ 5. I see my dentist twice a year whether or not I have a problem.

☐ 6. Often when I don't feel well, I take medication left over from a previous illness, or I borrow someone else's medication.

☐ 7. I am a woman who doesn't worry about breast cancer because I don't have any symptoms.

☐ 8. I am a man who doesn't worry about testicular cancer because I don't have any symptoms.

☐ 9. I take all my prescribed medications whether or not they seem to be working.

☐ 10. I find prescription labels difficult or confusing to read.

☐ 11. People have advised me to stop smoking, but I have never been able to quit.

☐ 12. I frequently forget to take my medication.

☐ 13. I will take all my prescribed medication even if it makes me feel worse.

☐ 14. The last time I was sick, the doctor gave me advice that I didn't completely understand, but I was too embarrassed to say so.

Items 2, 5, 9, and 13 represent good adherence habits, but each of the other items represents a health risk from failure to follow medical advice. Although it may be nearly impossible to adhere to all good health recommendations (such as not smoking, eating a healthy diet, exercising, and having regular dental and medical checkups), you can improve your health by adhering to sound medical advice. As you read this chapter, you will learn more about the health benefits of adherence.

REAL-WORLD PROFILE OF ALORA GALE

When she was 6 years old, Alora Gale was diagnosed with *human immunodeficiency virus* (HIV), the virus that causes *acquired immune deficiency syndrome* (AIDS) (Folk-Williams, 2002). She was infected with the virus by her mother, who also infected Alora's younger brother Morgan. All three received the diagnosis within the same week. Alora's life has included bouts of sickness, such as pneumonia, as well as regular medical testing and treatment.

When she was 12, Alora began taking a combination of antiviral drugs known as HAART—*highly active antiretroviral therapy* (McCollum, 2003). This regimen required her to take as many as 20 pills a day. Alora commented, "Most people have a medicine cabinet, I have a medicine pantry" (quoted in McCollum, 2003, p. 7). In addition, the timing of the doses was important; she had to take some pills on an empty stomach and others with food. Her father—who has not been diagnosed with HIV—helped by putting out her medicine in paper cups, divided into the correct doses, but when Alora was away from home, she did not always have her medicine or remember to take it.

Like other people who are HIV positive, Alora needs to adhere to this complex medical regimen, because failure to adhere decreases the medication's effectiveness. Alora knows that taking her medication is important: "Yeah, these pills—this fistful of pills—are what's keeping me alive" (quoted in Folk-Williams, 2002). But such a complex regimen makes adherence very difficult. In addition, her drugs produce unpleasant side effects, including nausea, dizziness, sleep problems, and pancreatitis. Alora's brother has not adhered to his medical schedule as well as Alora, which he attributes to the drugs' side effects (Folk-Williams, 2002).

Alora Gale's medical regimen is difficult and demanding, so her "slips" in following it are not surprising. But receiving prescriptions for drugs and instructions for taking them is a common experience, and as with Alora and her brother, failure to comply with medical advice is also common. This chapter explores the factors that affect adherence to medical advice, how common failures are, and how adherence can be improved. The first section frames questions about adherence by examining theories that apply to adherence.

THEORIES THAT APPLY TO ADHERENCE

Why do some people comply with medical advice whereas others fail to comply? Theoretical models to explain adherence include several that apply to behavior in general as well as models specific to health-related behavior. These models include the behavioral model, self-efficacy theory, the theories of reasoned action and planned behavior, and the transtheoretical model.

Behavioral Theory

The *behavioral model* of adherence is based on the principles of operant conditioning proposed by B. F. Skinner (1953). The key to operant conditioning is the immediate *reinforcement* of any response that moves the organism (person) toward the target behavior—in this case, following medical recommendations. Skinner found that reinforcement, either positive or negative, strengthens the behavior it follows. With **positive reinforcement**, a positively valued stimulus is added to the situation, thus increasing the probability that the behavior will recur. An example of positive reinforcement of adherent behavior would be a monetary payment contingent on a patient's keeping a doctor's appointment. With **negative reinforcement**, behavior is strengthened by the removal of an unpleasant or negatively valued stimulus. An example of negative reinforcement would be taking medication to stop one's spouse from nagging about taking one's medication.

Punishment also changes behavior by decreasing the chances that a behavior will be repeated, but psychologists seldom use it to modify noncompliant behaviors. The effects of positive and negative reinforcers are quite predictable: They both strengthen behavior. However, the effects of punishment are limited and sometimes difficult to predict. At best, punishment will inhibit or suppress a behavior, and it can condition strong negative feelings toward any persons or environmental conditions associated with it. Punishment, including threats of harm, is seldom useful in improving a person's adherence to medical advice.

The behavioral model also predicts that adherence will be difficult, because learned behaviors form patterns or habits that are resistant to change. When a person must make changes in habitual behavior patterns to take medication, change diet or physical activity, or take blood glucose readings several times a day, the individual often experiences difficulty in accommodating to a new routine. People need help in establishing such changes, and advocates of the behavioral model use cues, rewards, and contracts to reinforce compliant behaviors. Cues include written reminders of appointments, telephone calls from the practitioner's office, and a variety of self-reminders. Rewards can be extrinsic (money and compliments) or intrinsic (feeling healthier). Contracts can be verbal, but they are more often written agreements between practitioner and patient. Most adherence models recognize the importance of incentives in improving adherence.

Support for the behavioral model has come from studies on children with asthma and on people in substance abuse treatment. An interview study (Penza-Clyve, Mansell, & McQuaid, 2004) explored how children with asthma experience the disorder and how they could be helped to become more compliant. These 9- to 15-year-olds mentioned providing reminders and social support, but the strategy that they endorsed most strongly was rewards for adhering to their medical regimen. Participants in a Veterans Administration substance abuse treatment program were more likely to complete aftercare and to be abstinent from drugs one year later when their program included an aftercare contract, attendance prompts, and reinforcers (Lash et al., 2007).

Self-Efficacy Theory

Albert Bandura (1986, 1997, 2001) has proposed a social cognitive theory that assumes that humans have some capacity to exercise limited control over their lives. That is, they use their cognitive processes for self-regulation. Bandura suggests that human action results from an interaction of behavior, environment, and person factors, especially cognition. Bandura (1986, 2001) referred to this interactive triadic model as **reciprocal determinism.** The concept of reciprocal determinism can be illustrated by a triangle, with behavior, environment, and person factors occupying the three corners of the triangle and each having some influence on the other two (see Figure 4.1). An important component of the person factor is **self-efficacy,** defined by Bandura (2001) as "people's beliefs in their capability to exercise some measure of control over their own functioning and over environmental events" (p. 10).

Self-efficacy is a situation-specific rather than a global concept; that is, it refers to people's confidence that they can perform necessary behaviors to produce desired outcomes in any *particular* situation. Bandura (1986) suggested that self-efficacy can be acquired, enhanced, or decreased in one of four ways: (1) performance, or enacting a behavior; (2) vicarious experience, or seeing another person with similar skills perform a behavior; (3) verbal persuasion, or listening to the encouraging words of a trusted person; and (4) physiological arousal states, such as feelings of anxiety, which ordinarily *decrease* self-efficacy. Bandura believes that the combination of self-efficacy and outcome expectations plays an important role in predicting behavior. According to self-efficacy theory, people's beliefs concerning their ability to initiate difficult behaviors (such as an exercise program) predict their accomplishment of those behaviors.

Self-efficacy theory has been used to predict adherence to a variety of health recommendations, including relapse in a smoking cessation program, maintenance of an exercise regimen, adherence to diabetes management, and compliance with HIV medications. For example, a study on self-efficacy and smoking relapse (Shiffman et al., 2000) found that, after an initial lapse, smokers with high self-efficacy tended to remain abstinent, whereas those with waning self-efficacy were likely to relapse. Self-efficacy was the best predictor of completing versus dropping out of an exercise rehabilitation program (Guillot,

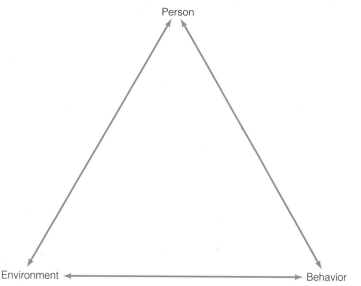

Person

Environment ←——————————————————→ Behavior

FIGURE 4.1 Bandura's concept of reciprocal determinism. Human functioning is a product of the interaction of behavior, environment, and person variables, especially self-efficacy and other cognitive processes.

Source: Adapted from "The Self System in Reciprocal Determinism," by A. Bandura, 1979, *American Psychologist, 33,* p. 345. Adapted by permission of the American Psychological Association and Albert Bandura.

Kilpatrick, Hebert, & Hollander, 2004) and adhering to an exercise program for cardiac rehabilitation (Schwarzer, Luszczynska, Ziegelmann, Scholz, & Lippke, 2008). One team of researchers (Iannotti et al., 2006) studied diabetes management among adolescents and found that self-efficacy was correlated with self-management and with good glycemic control. Research with a group of women with AIDS (Ironson et al., 2005) and women and men with HIV/AIDS (Simoni, Frick, & Huang, 2006) found that self-efficacy was related to adherence to medication and to physical indicators of decreased disease severity. Thus, self-efficacy seems to be a predictor of good adherence and good medical outcomes.

Theories of Reasoned Action and Planned Behavior

The *theory of reasoned action* (Ajzen & Fishbein, 1980; Fishbein & Ajzen, 1975) and the *theory of planned behavior* (Ajzen, 1991) both assume that the immediate determiner of behavior is people's *intention* to perform that behavior. The theory of reasoned action suggests that behavioral intentions, in turn, are (1) a function of people's *attitudes* toward the behavior, which are determined by their beliefs that the behavior will lead to positively or negatively valued outcomes, and (2) their *subjective norms*, which are shaped by their perception of the value that significant others place on that behavior and by their *motivation* to comply with those norms (see Chapter 3, Figure 3.1). The theory of planned behavior includes an additional determinant of intention to act—namely, people's perception of how much *control* they have over their behavior (see Chapter 3, Figure 3.2). Both theories have been used to predict adherence to a number of health-related behaviors, including monitoring of blood glucose levels among adults with diabetes (Shankar, Connor, & Bodansky, 2007), testicular self-examination (McClenahan, Shevlin, Adamson, Bennett, & O'Neill, 2007), and compliance with hypertension treatment (Jeon & Lee, 2007).

A meta-analysis of studies on the usefulness of the theory of reasoned action and the theory of planned behavior (Hausenblas, Carron, & Mack, 1997) found that both theories had value in predicting who will adhere to an exercise program and who will not. More specifically, the analysis revealed a strong connection between attitude toward exercising and intention to exercise and a strong link between intention and exercise behavior. However, the relationship between subjective norms and intention was only moderate. Another meta-analysis on studies using the theory of planned behavior (Armitage & Conner, 2001) also found stronger support for some of the components of the model than for others. Intentions were the strongest predictor and subjective norms the weakest.

Why are these two commonsense theories only moderately successful at predicting adherence to health-related behaviors? A critique of the theories of reasoned action and planned behavior (Ogden, 2003) contended that the constructs of such cognitive models of health behavior are too general to generate hypotheses that are easily testable. The originators of the models (Ajzen & Fishbein, 2004) disputed this contention, but evidence remains that people's past adherence is a better predictor of future adherence than either the theory of reasoned action or the theory of planned behavior (Sutton, McVey, & Glanz, 1999).

The Transtheoretical Model

Another theory that attempts to explain and predict adherence behavior is called the *transtheoretical model* because it cuts across and borrows from other theoretical models; the theory is also called the *stages-of-change model*. The transtheoretical model, developed by James Prochaska, Carrlo DiClemente, and John Norcross (1992, 1994), assumes that people progress as well as regress through five spiraling stages in making changes in behavior: precontemplation, contemplation, preparation, action, and maintenance. An overweight person's progression through these five stages of change in adopting a low-fat diet is illustrated in Figure 4.2.

During the *precontemplation stage*, the person has no intention of altering eating habits. In the *contemplation stage*, the person is aware of the problem, has thoughts about adopting a new diet, but has not yet made an effort to change. The *preparation stage* includes both thoughts (such as intending to adopt a diet within the next month) and action (such as purchasing low-fat food, finding low-fat recipes). During the *action stage*, the person makes overt changes in behavior, such as eliminating fried foods and eating more fruits and vegetables. In

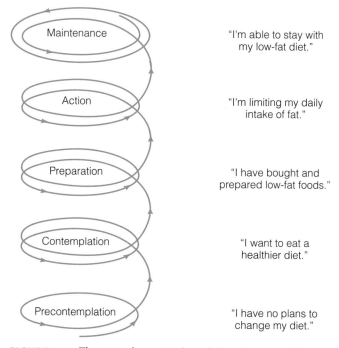

FIGURE 4.2   The transtheoretical model and stages of changing from a high-fat diet to a low-fat diet.

the *maintenance stage*, the person tries to sustain the changes previously made and attempts to resist temptation to relapse back into old eating habits.

Prochaska and his associates maintained that a person moves from one stage to another in a spiral rather than a linear fashion and argue that this model captures the time factor of behavior change better than other models (Velicer & Prochaska, 2008). Relapses propel people back into a previous stage, or perhaps all the way back to the contemplation or precontemplation stages. From that point, the person may progress several times through the stages until completing behavioral change successfully. Thus, relapses are to be expected and can serve as learning experiences that help a person recycle upward through the various stages.

Prochaska and colleagues (1992, 1994) suggested that people in different stages require different types of assistance to make changes successfully. For example, attempts to change people in the precontemplation stage will be unsuccessful because these people do not believe they have a problem. On the other hand, people in the preparation stage will not benefit from messages that they need to

change their behavior—they have passed that stage and need specific suggestions about how to change. People in the maintenance stage need help or information oriented toward preserving their changes. Research tends to supports these contentions. For example, a longitudinal study of adopting a low-fat diet (Armitage, Sheeran, Conner, & Arden, 2004) revealed that people's attitudes and behavior fall into the various stages of the transtheoretical model, and individuals both progress through the stages and regress into earlier stages, much as the model predicts. Furthermore, the interventions that were capable of moving people from one stage to another varied by stage. Unfortunately, these researchers found that moving people from the preparation to the action stage was more difficult than other transitions. A study on mammography adherence (Champion et al., 2007) found that women in all stages except precontemplation benefited from intervention tailored to their stage. Thus, the transitions from one stage to another may not be equally easy to influence.

Does the transtheoretical model apply equally to different problem behaviors? A meta-analysis of 47 studies (Rosen, 2000) attempted to answer this question by looking at the model across several health-related issues, including smoking, substance abuse, exercise, diet, and psychotherapy. The results showed that the transtheoretical model works better with some behaviors than with others. For example, in the case of smoking cessation, cognitive processes were more frequently used in deciding to quit, whereas behavioral techniques were more effective during abstinence. The transtheoretical model is not as successful in predicting adherence to special diets, exercise, or condom use (Bogart & Delahanty, 2004). Craig Rosen (2000) summed up the situation by saying that people who look to the transtheoretical model for "a one-size-fits-all blueprint for interventions are likely to be disappointed" (p. 602).

IN SUMMARY

Several theoretical models attempt to predict and explain adherent and nonadherent behavior. The behavioral model explains adherence in terms of reinforcement and habits that must be changed to adhere to a medical regimen. Bandura's self-efficacy theory emphasizes people's beliefs about illness and about their ability to control their own health. Ajzen and Fishbein's theory of reasoned action assumes that intentions, attitudes, subjective norms, and motivation predict adherence, and Ajzen's theory of planned behavior adds people's subjective belief that they can control their adherence to health-related behaviors. Prochaska's transtheoretical model assumes that people spiral through five stages in making changes in behavior: precontemplation, contemplation, preparation, action, and maintenance. Relapse should be expected, but after relapse, people can move forward again through the various stages.

Research on the effectiveness of these models suggests that people's belief that they can perform healthy behaviors (self-efficacy) combined with their intention to enact these behaviors can contribute to a better understanding of reasons for adherence and nonadherence. However, none of these models provides a comprehensive, accurate prediction of who will adhere and who will not.

ISSUES IN ADHERENCE

For medical advice to benefit a patient's health, two requirements must be met. First, the advice must be valid. Second, the patient must follow this good advice. Both conditions are essential. Ill-founded advice that patients strictly follow may produce new health problems that lead to disastrous outcomes for the compliant patient. On the other hand, excellent advice is essentially worthless if patients do not follow it. As many as 125,000 people in the United States may die each year because they fail to adhere to medical advice, especially by failing to take prescribed medications (Cutting Edge Information, 2004). Two meta-analyses of treatment studies (DiMatteo, Giordani, Lepper, & Croghan, 2002; Simpson et al., 2006) indicated a large difference in the medical outcomes for adherent versus nonadherent patients. These analyses showed that adherence can make a big difference in improvement.

In this section we look at three questions regarding adherence: What is adherence? How is adherence measured? How frequently do people fail to adhere?

What Is Adherence?

Traditionally, people in the medical profession have used the term *compliance* to refer to patient behaviors that conform to physicians' orders (Jaret, 2001). But because the term *compliance* implies reluctant obedience, many health psychologists and some physicians advocate the use of other words, especially *adherence*. However, the terms *cooperation, collaboration,* and *concordance* have also been suggested as substitutes for compliance. Perhaps the most accurate term to describe the *ideal* relationship between physician and patient would be *cooperation* or even *self-management* (Costantini, 2006), terms that suggest active involvement of the patient in restoring health. However, because cooperation is neither a common practice nor an accepted label for this relationship, the terms *compliance* and *adherence* are still the most frequently used words, and we employ these two words interchangeably.

What does it mean to be adherent? We define **adherence** as a person's ability and willingness to follow recommended health practices. R. Brian Haynes (1979) has suggested a broader definition of the term, defining adherence as "the extent to which a person's behavior (in terms of taking medications, following diets, or executing lifestyle changes) coincides with medical or health advice" (pp. 1–2). This definition expands the concept of compliance beyond merely taking medications to include maintaining healthy lifestyle practices, such as eating properly, getting sufficient exercise, avoiding undue stress, abstaining from smoking cigarettes, and not abusing alcohol. In addition, adherence includes making and keeping periodic medical and dental appointments, using seatbelts, and engaging in other behaviors that coincide with the best health advice available. Adherence is a complex concept, with people being compliant in one situation and noncompliant in another (Ogedegbe et al., 2007).

How Is Adherence Measured?

How do researchers know the percentage of patients who fail to comply with practitioners' recommendations? What methods do they use to identify those who fail to adhere? The answer to the first question is that compliance rates are not known with certainty, but the techniques used by researchers have yielded a great deal of information about noncompliance. At least six basic means of measuring patient compliance are available: (1) ask the practitioner, (2) ask the patient, (3) ask other people, (4) monitor medication usage, (5) examine biochemical evidence, and (6) use a combination of these procedures.

The first of these methods, asking the practitioner, is usually the poorest choice. Physicians generally overestimate their patients' compliance rates, and even when their guesses are not overly optimistic, they are usually wrong (Miller et al., 2002). In general, practitioners' accuracy is only slightly better than chance (Parker et al., 2007).

Asking patients themselves is a slightly more valid procedure, but it is fraught with many difficulties. Self-reports are inaccurate for at least two reasons. First, patients tend to report behaviors that make them appear at least a bit better than they are, lying to make their behavior appear more compliant than it is. Second, they may simply not know their own rate of compliance. Interviews are more

prone to these types of errors than asking patients to keep records or diaries of their behavior (Garber, 2004). Because self-report measures have questionable validity, they are often supplemented by other assessment techniques (Parker et al., 2007).

Another technique is to ask hospital personnel and family members to monitor the patient, but this procedure also has at least two inherent problems. First, constant observation may be physically impossible, especially with regard to such regimens as diet and alcohol consumption. Second, persistent monitoring creates an artificial situation and frequently results in higher rates of compliance than would otherwise occur. This outcome is desirable, of course, but as a means of assessing compliance, it contains a built-in error that makes observation by others inaccurate.

A fourth method of assessing compliance is to monitor medicine usage, such as counting pills or assessing whether patients obtain prescriptions or refills (Balkrishnan & Jayawant, 2007). These procedures seem to be more objective, because very few errors are likely to be made in counting the number of pills absent from a bottle or the number of patients who have their prescriptions filled. Even if the required number of pills are gone or the prescriptions filled, however, the patient may not have taken the medication or may have taken it in a manner other than the one prescribed.

The development of electronic technology has made possible more sophisticated methods to determine whether patients take their medication at the prescribed time (Kehr, 2004). Systems such as the Medication Event Monitoring System include a microprocessor in the pill cap that records the date and time of every bottle opening and closing, thus yielding a record of usage (assuming that opening the bottle equals using the medication). In addition, this system includes an Internet link that uploads the data stored in the device so that adherence can be monitored on a daily or weekly basis. This type of assessment does not show high consistency with self-reports (Balkrishnan & Jayawant, 2007; Garber, 2004).

Examination of biochemical evidence is a fifth method of measuring compliance. This procedure looks at the outcome of compliant behavior to find some biochemical evidence, such as analysis of blood or urine samples, to determine whether the patient has behaved in a compliant fashion. Some research (Liu et al., 2001) used biochemical evidence in HIV patients and found that a combination of adherence measures was related to a decrease in the virus that may lead to AIDS. However, problems can arise with the use of biochemical evidence as a means of assessing compliance because individuals vary in their biochemical response to drugs. In addition, this approach requires frequent medical monitoring that may be intrusive and expensive.

Finally, clinicians can use a combination of these methods to assess compliance. Several studies (Liu et al., 2001; Velligan et al., 2007) have used a variety of methods to assess adherence, including interviewing patients, counting pills, electronic monitoring, and measuring biochemical evidence, as well as a combination of all these methods. The results indicate good agreement among pill counts, electronic monitoring, and measuring biochemical evidence but poor agreement between these objective measures and patients' or clinicians' reports. A weakness of using multiple methods of measuring adherence is the cost.

How Frequent Is Nonadherence?

How common are failures of adherence? The answer to this question depends in part on how adherence is defined, the nature of the illness under consideration, the demographic features of the population, and the methods used to assess compliance. When interest in these questions developed in the late 1970s, David Sackett and John C. Snow (1979) reviewed more than 500 studies that dealt with the frequency of compliance and noncompliance. Their findings included higher rates for patients' keeping appointments when patients initiated the appointments (75%) than when appointments were scheduled for them (50%). As expected, compliance rates were higher when treatment was to cure than when it was to prevent a disease. However, adherence was lower for medication taken for a chronic condition over a long period; compliance was around 50% for either prevention or cure.

More recent reviews have confirmed the problem of nonadherence. Robin DiMatteo (2004b) reported on a meta-analysis of more than 500 compliance studies covering a 50-year span; her results indicated that the average rate of nonadherence was 24.8%. The adherence rates tended to be higher in more recent studies than in older ones, but many of the factors identified in Sackett and Snow's (1979) review continued to be significant predictors of adherence. Medication treatments yielded higher compliance rates than recommendations for exercise, diet, or other types of health-related behavior change. However, DiMatteo's analysis revealed that not all chronic conditions yielded equally low compliance rates. Some chronic conditions, such as HIV, arthritis, gastrointestinal disorders, and cancer, showed high adherences rates, whereas diabetes and pulmonary disease showed lower compliance. This analysis also found that compliance rates have improved for some disorders, such as hypertension. Nevertheless, failure to adhere to medical advice is widespread and constitutes a factor in all types of medical treatments.

IN SUMMARY

Adherence is the extent to which a person is able and willing to follow medical and health advice. In order for people to profit from adherence, first, the advice must be valid, and second, patients must follow that advice. Inability or unwillingness to adhere to health-related behaviors increases people's chances of serious health problems or even death.

At least six ways of measuring patient adherence have been suggested: (1) ask the physician, (2) ask the patient, (3) ask other people, (4) monitor medical usage, (5) examine biochemical evidence, and (6) use a combination of these procedures. No one of these procedures is both reliable and valid. However, with the exception of clinician judgment, most have some validity and usefulness. When accuracy is crucial, using two or more of these methods for assessing patient adherence yields greater accuracy than reliance on a single assessment technique.

The frequency of nonadherence depends on the nature of the illness. People are more likely to adhere to a medication regimen than to a program that changes health-related behaviors such as diet or exercise. The average rate of failure to comply is slightly less than 25%.

WHAT FACTORS PREDICT ADHERENCE?

What factors determine who will be compliant and who will not? If we assume that people always act in their own best interests, failures of adherence seem puzzling. Why should people seek medical treatment and then fail to heed the advice? This question leads to another: What are the factors that succeed or fail in predicting compliance? Possible predictors can be divided into five groups: severity of the disease; treatment characteristics, including side effects and complexity of the treatment; personal characteristics, such as age, gender, and personal beliefs; cultural norms; and characteristics of the relationship between the health care provider and the patient, including verbal communication and the personal characteristics of the health care practitioner.

Severity of the Disease

Common wisdom suggests that people with severe, potentially crippling or life-threatening illnesses will be highly motivated to adhere to regimens that protect them against such outcomes. However, little evidence supports this reasonable hypothesis. In general, people with a serious disease are no more likely than people with a less serious problem to seek medical treatment or to comply with medical advice. Indeed, people sometimes seek health care not because they believe they have a serious medical problem but because of appearance or inconvenience. For example, Robin DiMatteo and Dante DiNicola (1982) reported the case of a woman who had been hit by a baseball bat and had suffered some loss of vision in her left eye. The loss of vision, however, did not prompt her to go to a doctor. She sought treatment only after a friend casually commented that her eyelid drooped! If she had been in pain, the woman would have been more likely to seek medical care; pain associated with the illness not only pushes people toward medical care but also increases their level of adherence (Becker, 1979).

A comprehensive review (DiMatteo, 2004b) found that disease severity was not significantly related to compliance. However, a meta-analysis showed that patients' *perception* of the severity of the disease was strongly related to compliance (DiMatteo, Haskard, & Williams, 2007). That is, the objective severity of a disease is less closely related to adherence to medical recommendations concerning treatment or prevention than the threat that people experience from a disease.

Treatment Characteristics

Characteristics of the treatment, such as side effects of the medication and the complexity of the treatment, present potential problems for adherence.

Side Effects of the Medication Early research (Masur, 1981) found little evidence to suggest that unpleasant side effects are a major reason for discontinuing a drug or dropping out of a treatment program. However, more recent research with the complex regimen of drugs for HIV (Gellaitry et al., 2005; Herrmann et al., 2008) indicated that, especially among younger patients, those who experience severe side effects are less likely to take their medications than those with minor side effects. Alora Gale's brother agreed; he listed side effects as the main reason that he failed to comply with his drug regimen.

Complexity of the Treatment Are people less likely to comply as treatment procedures become increasingly complex? In general, the greater the number of doses or variety of medications people must take, the greater is the likelihood that they will not take pills in the prescribed manner (Piette, Heisler, Horne, & Caleb Alexander, 2006). For example, people who need to take one pill per day comply fairly well (as high as 90%), and increasing the dosage to two per day produces little decrease (Claxton, Cramer, & Pierce, 2001). When people must take four doses of medication a day, however, adherence plummets to below 40%. The reason seems to be related to fitting medications into daily routines. For example, pills prescribed once a day can be cued to routine activities, such as taken first thing in the morning; those prescribed twice a day can be cued to early morning and late night; and those prescribed three times a day can be cued to meals. Schedules calling for medication to be taken four or more times a day, or requirements for two or more medications a day, create difficulties and lower compliance rates.

In summary, the more complex the treatment, the lower is the rate of compliance. After looking at the evidence, Philip Ley, who has studied adherence for more than 30 years, concluded that "the simpler the treatment schedule, and the shorter its duration, the greater is compliance" (Ley, 1997, p. 282).

Personal Factors

Researchers have investigated many personal and demographic factors related to compliance. In general, demographic factors such as age and gender show some relationship to adherence, but any of these factors alone is too small to be a good predictor of who will adhere and who will not (DiMatteo, 2004b). Personality was one of the first factors to be considered in relation to compliance, and other personal factors such as emotional factors and personal beliefs have appeared as contributors to adherence.

Age Although age is not a major determinant of adherence, the relationship between the two factors is not a simple one. Indeed, assessing adherence among children is a difficult research endeavor in which the person whose adherence is important is actually the parent and not the child (De Civita & Dobkin, 2005). As children grow into adolescents, they become more responsible for adhering to medical regimens, and this situation continues throughout adulthood. However, older people may face situations that make compliance difficult, such as memory problems, poor health, and regimens that include many medications (Gans & McPhillips, 2003). These varying life situations suggest a complex relationship between age and compliance. One study (Thomas et al., 1995) found a curvilinear relationship between age and compliance with colorectal cancer screening. That is, those who complied best were around 70 years old, with older and younger participants doing worse. Those who are 70 years

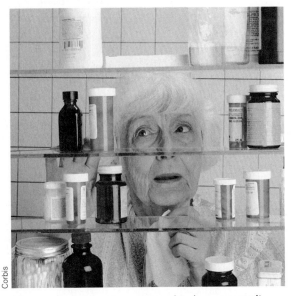

Corbis

More complex treatments tend to lower compliance rates.

old may not be the best at adhering to all medical advice, but this result suggests that both older and younger adults, plus children and adolescents, experience more problems with adherence. Other research confirms the problems with these age groups.

Even with caregivers to assist them, children with asthma (Penza-Clyve et al., 2004), diabetes (Cramer, 2004), and HIV infection (Farley et al., 2004) often fail to adhere to their medical regimens. As they grow into adolescence and exert more control over their own health care, adherence problems become even more prominent (DiMatteo, 2004b). Several studies (Miller & Drotar, 2003; Olsen & Sutton, 1998) have shown that as diabetic children become adolescents, their compliance with recommended exercise and insulin regimens decreases, and conflicts with parents over diabetes management increase. Young adults with these diseases also experience adherence problems (Ellis et al., 2007; Herrmann et al., 2008). Thus, age shows a small but complex relationship with adherence.

Gender With regard to gender, researchers have found few differences in the overall adherence rates of women and men, but some differences exist in following specific recommendations. In general, men and women are about equal in adhering to taking medication (Andersson, Melander, Svensson, Lind, & Nilsson, 2005), controlling diabetes (Hartz et al., 2006), or keeping an appointment for a medical test (Sola-Vera et al., 2008). Women may be better at adhering to healthy diets, such as sodium-restricted diets (Chung et al., 2006) and diets with lots of vegetables (Laforge, Greene, & Prochaska, 1994). However, the overall effect of gender is small and not significant in most cases (DiMatteo, 2004b).

Personality Patterns When the problem of compliance failures became obvious, researchers initially considered the concept of a noncompliant personality. According to this concept, people with certain personality patterns would have low compliance rates. If this concept is accurate, then the same people should be noncompliant in a variety of situations. However, little evidence exists to support this conclusion. On the contrary, some research indicates that noncompliance is specific to the situation (Lutz, Silbret, & Olshan, 1983) and that adherence to one treatment program is independent of adherence to others (Ogedegbe, Schoenthaler, & Fernandez, 2007). Thus, the evidence suggests that noncompliance is not a global personality trait but is specific to a given situation (Haynes, 2001).

Emotional Factors Do emotional factors such as stress and anxiety relate to adherence? Some evidence suggests a positive answer to this question. A study that investigated the effects of stressful life events on subsequent exercise adherence (Oman & King, 2000) found that people who experience several stressful events are likely to drop out of an exercise program. Another study found that individuals taking antiretroviral medication for HIV infection who reported high levels of stress were less adherent (Bottonari, Roberts, Ciesla, & Hewitt, 2005).

Can anxiety and depression reduce adherence rates? A review of studies on the relationship between noncompliance and anxiety and depression (DiMatteo, Lepper, & Croghan, 2000) indicated that the effects of anxiety on adherence are small

but that depression is a large, significant factor in failure to comply. The risk of nonadherence was three times greater in depressed patients than in those who were not depressed.

Emotional factors clearly present risks, but do some personality characteristics relate to better adherence and improved health? Patients who express optimism and positive states of mind are more likely to adhere to their medical regimens (Gonzalez et al., 2004). Furthermore, the factor of conscientiousness, one of the factors in the Five Factor Model of personality (McCrae & Costa, 2003), shows a reliable relationship to adherence and improved health. For example, conscientiousness is related to adherence to an overall healthy lifestyle (Goodwin & Friedman, 2006) as well as good control of diabetes symptoms (Vollrath, Landolt, Gnehm, Laimbacher, & Sennhauser, 2007) and slower progression of HIV infection (O'Cleirigh, Ironson, Weiss, & Costa, 2007). Thus, emotional factors may present either a risk or an advantage for adherence.

Personal Beliefs Some evidence suggests that patients' personal beliefs are related to compliance. We have seen that the theory of reasoned action has some ability both to predict and to explain adherence and nonadherence and that perceived self-efficacy is an even better predictor. People who believe in their personal ability to perform the behaviors necessary to adhere to their medical regimen are more likely to do so. In general, patients' beliefs are an important factor in adherence (Gans & McPhillips, 2003).

Beliefs that affect adherence include a belief in the effectiveness of the treatment. Patients who believe that the recommended course of treatment (Gellaitry et al., 2005) or medications (Menckeberg et al., 2008) will be effective are more likely to comply with the prescribed regimen. Beliefs that treatment will be ineffective or even harmful are related to low adherence. This result appeared in studies with Japanese hospital patients (Iihara et al., 2004), African Americans with hypertension (Lukoschek, 2003), Swedish pharmacy customers (Mårdby, Åkerlind, & Jörgensen, 2007), and individuals taking medication for osteoporosis (McHorney, Schousboe, Cline, & Weiss, 2007).

People who believe that they can take control of their health are more likely to adhere. For example, studies with HIV-positive men (Westerfelt, 2004) and older people (Chia, Schlenk, & Dunbar-Jacob, 2007) revealed that feelings of control over one's health related to adherence. The HIV-positive men reported that they experienced difficulties in complying with their complex drug regimens, but they also felt that compliance was very important and that they were responsible for their health. Indeed, these men felt that the most important piece of advice they could give to someone starting such a regimen was to take responsibility for adhering to it.

Environmental Factors

Although some personal factors are important for adherence, environmental factors exert an even larger influence. These factors include differences in situations and circumstances that may facilitate or pose barriers to adherence. Included in this group of environmental factors are economic factors, social support, and cultural norms.

Economic Factors Economic factors, including income, have a major impact on adherence, health status, and access to health care (DiMatteo, 2004b). Moreover, income is related to educational level and ethnicity in complex ways that are difficult to disentangle (Schnittker, 2004). For example, one study (Gallegos-Macias, Macias, Kaufman, Skipper, & Kalishman, 2003) found a lower rate of compliance with a medical regimen for diabetes among Hispanic American children and adolescents, but this difference disappeared after controlling for income differences. Regardless of which of these factors is the underlying cause, economic factors show a relationship to health; one avenue is through access to health care, and another is through the ability to pay for prescription medications.

In the United States, people without insurance experience difficulties in obtaining access to health care and in follow-up care such as filling prescriptions (Gans & McPhillips, 2003). Many of the people who experience cost concerns have chronic diseases, which often require daily medications over long periods of time (Piette et al.,

2006). In a study of Medicare beneficiaries over age 65 (Gellad, Haas, & Safran, 2007), cost concerns predicted nonadherence, and such concerns were more common for African Americans and Hispanic Americans than for European Americans. People who had been admitted to the hospital for heart disease were more likely to adhere to their medications to reduce cholesterol level during the next year if their insurance plan paid more of the cost of the prescription (Ye, Gross, Schommer, Cline, & St. Peter, 2007). Therefore, how much people must pay for their treatment affects not only access to medical care but also the likelihood that they will adhere to the treatment regimen. These limitations and concerns about costs affect older people and those from ethnic minorities more often than others.

Social Support **Social support** is a broad concept that refers to both tangible and intangible help a person receives from family members and from friends. The introduction to this chapter presented the case of Alora Gale, the young woman who is HIV positive. She has received extensive social support from her father and brother but has often felt isolated from her peers (Folk-Williams, 2002). However, she has benefited from relationships

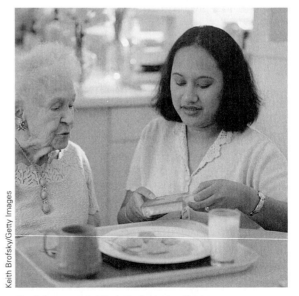

Keith Brofsky/Getty Images

Social support tends to boost adherence.

with other teens who are HIV positive. Her story highlights the importance of the support from family and friends.

Alora's experience is similar to that of other adolescents with chronic diseases, such as asthma and diabetes; a social support network is important for dealing with a chronic disease and for adhering to the required medical regimen (Kyngäs, 2004). Social support networks for adolescents include parents, peers (both those with and without similar conditions), people at school, health care providers, and even pets. In addition, adolescents use technology such as cell phones and computers to contact others and obtain support.

The level of social support one receives from friends and family is a strong predictor of adherence. In general, people who are isolated from others are likely to be noncompliant; those whose lives are filled with close interpersonal relationships are more likely to follow medical advice. A review of 50 years of research (DiMatteo, 2004a) confirmed the importance of social support for adherence.

Social support can be analyzed in terms of the variety and function of relationships that people have and the types of support that they receive from these relationships (DiMatteo, 2004a). For example, living with someone is a significant contributor to adherence; people who are married and those who live with families are more compliant than those who live alone. However, living with someone is not sufficient—family conflict is a negative factor for adherence. Thus, the living situation itself is not the important factor; rather, the support a person receives is the critical issue (DiMatteo, 2004a). Social support may consist of either practical or emotional support. Practical support includes reminders and physical assistance in adhering. Emotional support includes nurturance and empathy. Both types of support are positively related to adherence, but practical support may be more important. In a study of parental support for adolescents with diabetes (Ellis et al., 2007), general support and monitoring were not as effective in boosting adherence as monitoring that was specific to diabetes. Thus, social support is an important factor in compliance, and those who lack a support network have more trouble adhering to a medical regimen.

Cultural Norms

Cultural beliefs and norms have a powerful effect not only on rates of compliance but even on what constitutes compliance. For example, if one's family or tribal traditions include strong beliefs in the efficacy of tribal healers, it seems reasonable that the individual's compliance with modern medical recommendations might be low. A study of diabetic and hypertensive patients in Zimbabwe (Zyazema, 1984) found a large number of people who were not adhering to their recommended therapies. As might be expected, many of these patients believed in traditional healers and had little faith in Western medical procedures. Thus, the extent to which people accept a medical practice has a large impact on adherence to that practice, resulting in poorer adherence for individuals who are less acculturated to Western medicine, such as immigrants or people who retain strong ties to another culture (Barron, Hunter, Mayo, & Willoughby, 2004).

Failures to comply with Western, technological medicine do not necessarily indicate a failure to comply with some other medical tradition. People who maintain a cultural tradition may also retain its healers. For example, a study of Native Americans (Novins, Beals, Moore, Spicer, & Manson, 2004) revealed that many sick people sought the services of traditional healers, sometimes in combination with biomedical services. This strategy of combining treatments might be considered noncompliant by both types of healers.

People who accept a different healing tradition should not necessarily be considered nonadherent when their illness calls for a complex biomedical regimen. Native Hawaiians have a poor record of adherence (Ka'opua & Mueller, 2004), partly because their cultural beliefs are more holistic and spiritual, and their traditions emphasize family support and cohesion. These cultural values are not compatible with those that form the basis of Western medicine. Thus, Native Hawaiians have more trouble than other ethnic groups in Hawaii in adhering to medical regimens to control diabetes and risks for heart disease. The health-related beliefs of Native Hawaiians with heart failure lead them to prefer native healers over physicians (Kaholokula, Saito, Mau, Latimer, & Seto, 2008). However, no differences appear in their rates of compliance with the complex regimen of antiretroviral therapy that helps to control HIV infection, and their cultural value of family support may be a positive factor (Ka'opua & Mueller, 2004).

Cultural beliefs can also increase adherence. For example, older Japanese patients are typically more adherent than similar patients from the United States or Europe (Chia et al., 2006). The Japanese health care system provides care for all citizens through a variety of services, which creates trust in the health care system. This trust extends to physicians; Japanese patients accept their physicians' authority, preferring to allow physicians to make health care decisions rather than making those decisions themselves. Consistent with this attitude, patients tend to respect the advice they receive from physicians and to follow their orders carefully.

Culture and ethnicity also influence adherence through the treatment that people from different cultures and ethnic groups receive when seeking medical care. Physicians and other health care providers are influenced by their patients' ethnic background and socioeconomic status, and this influence relates to patient compliance. Physicians tend to have stereotypical and negative attitudes toward African American and low- and middle-income patients (van Ryn & Burke, 2000), including pessimistic beliefs about their rates of adherence. Perceived discrimination and disrespect appeared as significant factors in a study on ethnic differences in following physicians' recommendations and keeping appointments (Blanchard & Lurie, 2004). African Americans (14.1%), Asian Americans (20.2%), and Hispanic Americans (19.4%) reported that they felt discriminated against or treated with a lack of respect by a physician from whom they had received care within the past two years. In contrast, only about 9% of European American patients felt that they had been treated with disrespect by their physician. In this study, patients' perception of disrespect was related to lower compliance and more missed medical appointments.

These findings have important implications for physicians and other health care providers whose clientele consists largely of people from different cultural backgrounds. In addition, these findings highlight the importance of interactions between patient and practitioner in adhering to medical advice.

Practitioner–Patient Interaction

In addition to looking at disease characteristics and personal factors, researchers have studied patient–practitioner interaction and its relation to adherence and nonadherence. Practitioners who are successful in forming a working alliance with their patients are more likely to have patients who are satisfied and who follow their recommendations (Fuertes et al., 2007). Important factors in building successful practitioner–patient alliances include verbal communication and the practitioner's personal characteristics.

Verbal Communication Perhaps the most crucial factor in patient noncompliance is poor verbal communication between the practitioner and the patient (Cutting Edge Information, 2004). When patients believe that physicians understand their reasons for seeking treatment and that both agree about treatment, adherence increases (Kerse et al., 2004), but problems in communication present barriers to this understanding.

Miscommunication can start when physicians ask patients to report on their symptoms and fail to listen to patients' concerns, interrupting their stories within seconds (Galland, 2005). What constitutes a concern for the patient may not be essential to the diagnostic process, and the practitioner may simply be trying to elicit information relevant to making a diagnosis. However, patients may misinterpret the physician's behavior as a lack of personal concern or as overlooking what patients consider important symptoms. After practitioners have made a diagnosis, they typically tell patients about that diagnosis. If the diagnosis is minor, patients may be relieved and not highly motivated to adhere to (or even listen to) any instructions that may follow. If the verdict is serious, patients may become anxious or frightened, and these feelings may then interfere with their concentration on subsequent medical advice. The patient–practitioner interaction is especially important at this juncture: When patients fail to receive information that they have requested, they feel less satisfied with their physician and are less likely to comply with the advice they receive (Bell, Kravitz, Thom, Krupat, & Azari, 2002).

For a variety of reasons, physicians and patients frequently do not speak the same language. First, physicians operate in familiar territory. They know the subject matter, are comfortable with the physical surroundings, and are ordinarily calm and relaxed with procedures that have become routine to them. Patients, in contrast, may be unfamiliar with medical terminology (Castro, Wilson, Wang, & Schillinger, 2007); distracted by the strange environs; and distressed by anxiety, fear, or pain (Charlee, Goldsmith, Chambers, & Haynes, 1996). In some cases, practitioners and patients do not speak the same language— literally. Differences in native language present a major barrier to communication (Blanchard & Lurie, 2004; Flores, 2006). Even with interpreters, substantial miscommunication may occur (Rosenberg, Leanza, & Seller, 2007). As a result, patients either fail to understand or to remember significant portions of the information their doctors give them, which decreases compliance.

The Practitioner's Personal Characteristics A second aspect of the practitioner–patient interaction is the perceived personal characteristics of the physician. As might be expected, patients' compliance improves as confidence in their physician's technical ability increases (Gilbar, 1989), but patients have difficulty assessing technical competence and tend to assume that their physicians are competent (Bendapudi et al., 2006). In addition, several physician personality variables—as perceived by the patient—are related to compliance. Early research (DiNicola & DiMatteo, 1984) showed that people were more likely to follow the advice of doctors they saw as warm, caring, friendly, and interested in the welfare of patients. Alternatively, when patients believe that physicians look down on them or treat them with disrespect, patients are less likely to follow physicians' advice or keep medical appointments (Blanchard & Lurie, 2004). More recent research (Bendapudi et al., 2006) has confirmed that physicians' personal characteristics are important to patients; patients appreciate physicians who are

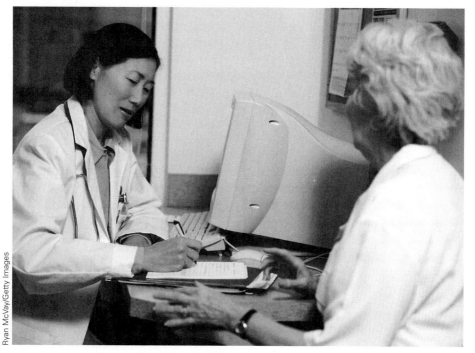

Ryan McVay/Getty Images

Communication is important for compliance, and female physicians tend to encourage interaction and communication.

confident, empathetic, humane, personal, forthright, and respectful.

The physician's gender may also play a role in the exchange of information between doctor and patient. A review of studies of communication during patient visits (Roter & Hall, 2004) found that female physicians spend more time with patients, make more partnership statements, engage in more patient-centered talk, and ask more questions than do male physicians. In addition, patients talk to female physicians more than they do to male physicians. As a result, female physicians have an advantage in establishing the type of relationships that lead to higher adherence rates.

Interaction of Factors

Researchers have identified dozens of factors, each of which shows some relation to adherence. However, many of these factors account for a very small amount of the variation in adhering to medical advice. Some of these factors are statistically significant, but when considered individually, they are poor predictors of who will and who will not adhere (Rietveld & Koomen, 2002). To gain a fuller understanding of adherence, researchers must study the mutual influence of factors that affect adherence. For example, patients' beliefs about the disease are related to compliance, but those beliefs are affected by interactions with physicians, another factor that has been identified as influential for adherence. Thus, the factors are not independent. Many of the factors identified as being related to adherence overlap with and influence other factors in complex ways. Therefore, both researchers and practitioners will benefit from developing an appreciation for and understanding of the interactions among the many factors that affect adherence. This understanding will help in the development of interventions to improve adherence.

IN SUMMARY

Several conditions predict poor adherence: (1) side effects of the medication; (2) long and complicated treatment regimens; (3) personal factors such as old or young age; (4) emotional factors such as conscientiousness and emotional problems such as stress and depression; (5) personal beliefs that the treatment is ineffective or a lack of self-efficacy for performing the medical regimen; (6) economic barriers to obtaining treatment or paying for prescriptions; (7) lack of social support; (8) patients' cultural beliefs that the medical regimen is ineffective; (9) poor patient–practitioner communication, including problems in verbal communication and patients' perceptions of uncaring, incompetent, or disrespectful physicians. Researchers and practitioners need to understand that the factors identified as influencing adherence interact in complex ways. Table 4.1 summarizes the research on what factors predict and fail to predict adherence.

TABLE 4.1
Predictors of Patient Adherence

	Findings	Studies
I. Disease Characteristics		
A. *Severity of illness*		
Illness interferes with appearance	Increases compliance	DiMatteo & DiNicola, 1982
Review of many disorders	No relationship	DiMatteo, 2004b
Patients' perception of severity	Strongly related to compliance	DiMatteo et al., 2007
Pain with the illness	Increases compliance	Becker, 1979
B. *Side effects of medication*		
Unpleasant side effects with HIV drugs	Decreases compliance	Gellaitry et al., 2005; Herrmann et al., 2008
C. *Complex treatment procedures*		
Increasing number of doses	Decreases compliance	Claxton et al., 2001; Piette et al., 2006

TABLE 4.1 Predictors of Patient Adherence—*Continued*

	Findings	Studies
II. Personal Factors		
A. *Increasing age*		
Adults		
Aging	Curvilinear relationship	Thomas et al., 1995
Older ages	Decreases compliance	Gans & McPhillips, 2003
Adolescents		
Growing older	Decreases compliance	DiMatteo, 2004b; Ellis et al., 2008; Herrmann et al., 2008; Miller & Drotar, 2003; Olsen & Sutton, 1998
B. *Gender*		
Keeping medical appointments	Men and women equal	Sola-Vera et al., 2008
Taking medication	Men and women equal	Anderson et al., 2005
Eating a healthy diet	Women more compliant	Chung et al., 2006; Laforge et al., 1994
C. *Personality patterns*		
Noncompliant personality	Situation, not personality, influences adherence	Haynes, 2001; Lutz et al., 1983; Ogedegbe et al., 2007
D. *Emotional factors*		
Stressful life events	Decrease compliance	Bottonari et al., 2005; Oman & King, 2000
Conscientiousness	Increases compliance	Goodwin & Friedman, 2006; O'Cleirigh et al., 2007; Vollrath et al., 2007
Depression	Decreases compliance	DiMatteo et al., 2000
Optimism	Increases compliance	Gonzalez et al., 2004
E. *Personal beliefs*		
Self-efficacy	Increases compliance	Gans & McPhillips, 2003
Belief in treatment effectiveness	Increases compliance	Gellaitry et al., 2005; Menckeberg et al., 2008
No confidence in treatment	Decreases compliance	Iihara et al., 2004; Lukoschek, 2003; Mårdby et al., 2007; McHorney et al., 2007
Feelings of control	Increases compliance	Westerfelt, 2004
III. Environmental Factors		
A. *Economic factors*		
Low income	Decreases compliance	Gallegos-Macias et al., 2003
Insurance fails to cover all prescription costs	Decreases prescription filling and refilling	Gans & McPhillips, 2003; Gellad et al., 2007; Ye et al., 2007
B. *Social support*		
Low social support among adolescents	Decreases compliance	Kyngäs, 2004
Living alone	Decreases compliance	DiMatteo, 2004b
Support for specific health behaviors	Increases compliance	Ellis et al., 2007
C. *Cultural norms*		
Belief in traditional healers	Decreases compliance	Kaholokula et al., 2008; Zyazema, 1984

(Continued)

TABLE 4.1 Predictors of Patient Adherence—*Continued*

	Findings	Studies
Acculturation to Western culture	Increases compliance	Barron et al., 2004; Novins et al., 2004
Culture places trust in physicians	Increases compliance	Chia et al., 2006
Physician's stereotype of African Americans and low-income patients	Decreases compliance	van Ryn & Burke, 2000
Physician disrespect of African Americans, Hispanic Americans, and Asian Americans	Decreases compliance	Blanchard & Lurie, 2004
IV. Practitioner/Patient Interaction		
A. Verbal communication		
Poor verbal communication	Decreases compliance	Cutting Edge Information, 2004
Interrupting patients	Decreases compliance	Galland, 2005
Agreement about treatment	Increases compliance	Kerse et al., 2004
Failing to receive expected information	Decreases compliance	Bell et al., 2002
Problems with language or terminology	Decreases compliance	Blanchard & Lurie, 2004; Castro et al., 2007; Charlee et al., 1996; Flores, 2006; Rosenberg et al., 2007
B. Practitioner's personal qualities		
Patient's confidence in physician's competence	Increases compliance	Bendapudi et al., 2006; Gilbar, 1989
Friendliness	Increases compliance	Bendapudi et al., 2006; DiNicola & DiMatteo, 1984
Practitioner disrespect	Decreases compliance	Blanchard & Lurie, 2004
Gender	Female doctors provide more information	Roter & Hall, 2004

IMPROVING ADHERENCE

We have surveyed several issues related to adherence, including theoretical models that might explain or predict compliance, techniques for measuring compliance, the frequency of compliance, and factors that do or do not relate to compliance. This information, along with knowledge of why some people fail to adhere, can help answer an important question of this chapter: How can adherence be improved?

What Are the Barriers to Adherence?

Like most people taking antiretroviral therapy, Alora Gale has encountered many barriers that make adherence difficult (Folk-Williams, 2002).

In addition to the complexity of the medication regimen and her experience of unpleasant side effects, Alora encountered problems in remembering to take her medication when she deviated from her normal daily routine. She also felt somewhat uncomfortable about taking a handful of pills in public. These barriers are sufficiently serious to prevent Alora from being completely compliant, but many other patients face additional barriers—some of them even more serious than those Alora experienced.

One category of reasons for nonadherence includes all those problems inherent in hearing and heeding physicians' advice. Patients may have financial or practical problems in making and keeping appointments and in filling, taking, and refilling prescriptions. Patients may reject the prescribed regimen as being too difficult, time-consuming, or expensive, or not adequately effective. Or they may just forget. Patients tend to pick and choose among the elements of the regimen their practitioners offer, treating this information as advice rather than orders (Vermeire, Hearnshaw, Van Royen, & Denekens, 2001). These patients may stop taking their medication because adherence is simply too much trouble or does not fit into the routine of their daily lives. Such patients fail to adhere to the prescribed regimen in some ways and so are considered noncompliant.

Patients may stop taking their medication when their symptoms disappear. Paradoxically, others stop because they fail to feel better or begin to feel worse, leading them to believe that the medication is useless. Still others, in squirrel-like fashion, save a few pills for the next time they get sick.

Some patients may make irrational choices about adherence because they have an **optimistic bias**—a belief that they will be spared the negative consequences of nonadherence that afflict other people (Weinstein, 1980, 2001). Other patients may be noncompliant because prescription labels are too difficult to read. Visual handicaps that are common among older patients form one barrier. However, even college students may find prescription labels difficult to understand; fewer than half of college students were able to correctly understand prescription labels that had been randomly selected from a pharmacist's records (Mustard & Harris, 1989).

Another set of reasons for high rates of nonadherence is that the current definition of adherence demands lifestyle choices that are difficult to attain. At the beginning of the 20th century, when the leading causes of death and disease were infectious diseases, compliance was simpler. Patients were compliant when they followed the doctor's advice with regard to medication, rest, and so on. Adherence is no longer a matter of taking the proper pills and following short-term advice. The three leading causes of death in the United States—cardiovascular disease, cancer, and chronic obstructive lung disease—are all affected by unhealthy lifestyles. Thus compliance, broadly defined, currently includes adherence to healthy and safe behaviors as part of an ongoing lifestyle. To be compliant, people must now avoid cigarette smoking, use alcohol wisely or not at all, eat properly, and exercise regularly. In addition, of course, they must also make and keep medical and dental appointments, listen with understanding to the advice of health care providers, and finally, follow that advice. These conditions present a complex array of requirements that are difficult for anyone to fulfill completely. Table 4.2 summarizes some of the reasons patients give for not complying with medical advice.

How Can Adherence Be Improved?

Knowing the barriers to adherence provides hints for improving patient compliance. Methods for improving compliance can be divided into (1) educational and (2) behavioral strategies. Educational procedures are those that impart information, sometimes in an emotion-arousing manner designed to frighten the noncompliant patient into becoming compliant. Included with educational strategies are such procedures as health education messages, individual patient counseling with various professional health care providers, programmed instruction, lectures, demonstrations, and individual counseling accompanied by written instructions. Haynes (1976) reported that strategies that relied on education and threats of disastrous consequences for nonadherence were only marginally effective in bringing about a meaningful change in patients' behaviors; more recent reviews (Harrington, Noble, & Newman, 2004; Schroeder, Fahey, & Ebrahim, 2007) have come to similar conclusions of marginal or no effectiveness. Educational methods may increase patients' knowledge, but behavioral approaches offer a more effective way of enhancing adherence. People, it seems, do not misbehave because they do not know better but because adherent behavior, for a variety of reasons, is less appealing.

Behavioral strategies focus more directly on changing the behaviors involved in compliance. They include a wide variety of techniques, such as notifying patients of upcoming appointments, simplifying medical schedules, providing cues to prompt taking medication, monitoring and rewarding patients' compliant behaviors, and shaping people toward self-monitoring and self-care. Behavioral techniques have been found to be more effective than educational strategies in improving patient compliance.

TABLE 4.2

Reasons Given by Patients for Not Complying With Medical Advice

"It's too much trouble."
"I just didn't get the prescription filled."
"The medication was too expensive, so I took fewer pills to make them last."
"The medication didn't work very well. I was still sick, so I stopped taking it."
"The medication worked after only one week, so I stopped taking it."
"I have too many pills to take."
"I won't get sick. God will save me."
"I forgot."
"I don't want to become addicted to pills."
"If one pill is good, then two pills should be twice as good."
"I saved some pills for the next time I get sick."
"I gave some of my pills to my husband so he won't get sick."
"They're trying to poison me."
"This doctor doesn't know as much as my other doctor."
"The medication makes me sick."
"I don't like the way that doctor treats me, and I'm not going back."
"I feel fine. I don't see any reason to take something to prevent illness."
"My doctor prescribes too many pills. I can't afford all of them."
"I don't like my doctor. He looks down on people without insurance."
"I didn't understand my doctor's instructions and was too embarrassed to ask her to repeat them."
"I don't like the taste of nicotine chewing gum."
"I didn't understand the directions on the label."

Adherence researchers Robin DiMatteo and Dante DiNicola (1982) recommended four categories of behavioral strategies for improving adherence, and their categories are still a valid way to approach the topic. First, various *prompts* can be used to remind patients to initiate health-enhancing behaviors. These prompts may be cued by regular events in the patient's life, such as taking medication before each meal, or they may take the form of telephone calls from a clinic to remind the person to keep an appointment or to refill a prescription. Another type of prompt comes in the form of reminder packaging, which presents information about the date or time that the medication should be taken on the packaging for the medication (Heneghan, Glasziou, & Perera, 2007). In addition, electronic technology can be useful in providing prompts (see Would You Believe...? box).

A second behavioral strategy proposed by DiMatteo and DiNicola is *tailoring the regimen*, which involves fitting the treatment to habits and routines in the patient's daily life. Pill organizers work toward this goal by making medication more compatible with the person's life, and some drug companies are creating medication

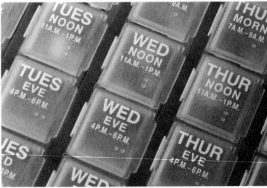

Don Farrall/Getty Images

Finding effective prompts helps patients fit medication into their schedules.

Texting May Improve Your Health

4get ur pills?

If so, you may be able to enlist the aid of your cell phone to text message a reminder (Zimmerman, 2006). Intelecare Compliance Solutions sells a reminder service that customers may receive through voice mail, e-mail, or text messages. These messages can be tailored to the person's medical regimen and daily schedule to boost adherence.

Competition comes from SIMpill, a company that also offers a reminder service (SIMpill, 2008). This service uses wireless technology to supply a special pill bottle that pharmacists can program with a time schedule. Opening the bottle or failing to open the bottle within a specified time span sends a signal to a central server. Forgetting to take a pill results in a message to do so that can come in the form

of a text message. Ignoring the reminder can result in a message to a family member or physician, whose reminder may be more difficult to ignore.

Other types of aids for adherence offer less automation but wider possibilities for health information. The Medication Event Monitoring System (MEMS) offers a recording device embedded in the cap of a pill bottle that makes a record of bottle openings, stores the information, and transmits it through the Internet (Kehr, 2004). That information can be used to formulate e-mails that offer patients the opportunity to consult a health care professional or prompt them to take medication. Another electronic possibility comes from using personal digital assistants (PDAs) to deliver an audiovisual presentation of health information

(Brock & Smith, 2007). This type of patient education showed more promise of changing behavior than most educational approaches, possibly because of its mode of transmission.

However, electronic monitoring is not essential; e-mail reminders and prompts to refill prescriptions can be issued by pharmacists based on records of when medication should be completely used (Cutting Edge Information, 2004). Such reminders can also be mailed, telephoned, faxed, or sent by text message. More low-tech reminders are also possible, such as medication charts to remind patients to use their medication at specific times or alarms that remind patients of the time. Thus, both high-tech and low-tech prompts may remind u 2 take ur meds.

---

packaging, called compliance packaging, that is similar to pill organizers in providing a tailored regimen (Gans & McPhillips, 2003). Another approach that fits within this category is simplifying the medication schedule; a review of adherence studies (Schroeder et al., 2007) indicated that this approach was among the most successful in increasing adherence.

Another way to tailor the regimen involves assessing patients' stages of change as depicted in the transtheoretical model and then orienting change-related messages to a patient's current stage (Gans & McPhillips, 2003). For example, a person in the contemplation stage is aware of the problem but has not yet decided to adopt a behavior (see Figure 4.2). This person might benefit from an intervention that includes information or counseling, whereas a person in the maintenance stage would not. Instead, people in the maintenance stage might benefit from

monitoring devices or prompts that remind them to take their medication or to exercise. Applying this approach to the problem of preventing the complications that accompany heart disease, a group of researchers (Turpin et al., 2004) concluded that tailoring adherence programs to patients' previous levels of adherence was critical; patients who are mostly adherent differ from those who are partially adherent or nonadherent. Similar success occurred with a program to help people adhere to lipid-lowering drugs (Johnson et al., 2006). These successes suggest that differences in stage of readiness to change require different types of assistance to achieve adherence.

A similar way to tailor the regimen involves helping clients resolve the problems that prevent them from changing their behavior. **Motivational interviewing** is a therapeutic approach that originated within substance abuse treatment (Miller & Rollnick, 2002) but has been applied to

BECOMING HEALTHIER

You can improve your health by following sound health-related advice. Here are some things you can do to make adherence pay off.

1. Adopt an overall healthy lifestyle—one that includes not smoking, using alcohol in moderation or not at all, eating a diet high in fiber and low in saturated fats, getting an optimum amount of regular physical activity, and incorporating safety into your life. Procedures for adopting each of these health habits are discussed in *Becoming Healthier* boxes in Chapters 12 through 15.

2. Establish a working alliance with your physician that is based on cooperation and not obedience. You and your doctor are the two most important people involved in your health, and the two of you should cooperate in designing your health practices.

3. Another important person interested in your health is your spouse, parent, friend, or sibling. Enlist the support of a significant person or persons in your life. Research shows that high levels of social support improve one's rate of adherence.

4. Before visiting a health care provider, jot down some questions you would like to have answered; ask the questions, and write down the answers during the visit. If you receive a prescription, ask the doctor about possible side effects—you don't want an unanticipated unpleasant side effect to be an excuse to stop taking the medication. Also, be sure you know how long you must take the medication—some chronic diseases require a lifetime of treatment.

5. If your physician gives you complex medical information

that you don't comprehend, ask for clarification in language that you can understand. Enlist the cooperation of your pharmacist, who can be another valuable health care provider.

6. Remember that some recommendations (such as beginning a regular exercise program) should be adopted gradually. (If you do too much the first day, you won't feel like exercising again the next day.)

7. Find a practitioner who understands and appreciates your cultural beliefs, ethnic background, language, and religious beliefs.

8. Reward yourself for following your good health practices. If you faithfully followed your diet for a day or a week, do something nice for yourself.

health-related behaviors, including adherence (Resnicow et al., 2002). This technique attempts to change a client's motivation and prepares the client to enact changes in behavior. The procedure includes an interview in which the practitioner attempts to show empathy with the client's situation, discusses and clarifies the client's goals and contrasts them with the client's current, unacceptable behavior, and helps the client formulate ways to change behavior. Motivational interviewing has been used with patients with a variety of diseases, and a review of studies (Knight, McGowan, Dickens, & Bundy, 2006) indicated that the technique is effective.

Third, DiMatteo and DiNicola suggested a *graduated regimen implementation* that reinforces successive approximations to the desired behavior.

Such shaping procedures would be appropriate for exercise, diet, and possibly smoking cessation programs, but not for taking medications.

The final behavioral strategy listed by DiMatteo and DiNicola is a *contingency contract* (or behavioral contract)—an agreement, usually written, between patients and health care professionals that provides for some kind of reward to patients contingent on their achieving compliance. These contracts may also involve penalties for noncompliance (Gans & McPhillips, 2003). Contingency contracts are most effective when they are enacted at the beginning of therapy and when the provisions are negotiated and agreed upon by patients and providers. Even with these provisions, contracts have not been demonstrated to boost adherence by a great deal (Bosch-Capblanch, Abba, Prictor, & Garner, 2007).

The ultimate goal of each of these approaches is self-regulation. However, before reaching this goal, patients often need help from others. This outside help, whether from family members or from professionals, is ordinarily given extensively at first and then gradually withdrawn as patients begin to acquire more control over their health-related behaviors.

Despite these suggestions, many health care providers put little effort into improving adherence, and adherence rates have improved little over the past 50 years (DiMatteo, 2004a). Evidence indicates that clear instructions about taking medications are the best strategy to boost adherence for short-term regimens (Haynes, McDonald, & Garg, 2002); the instructions work better if they are both verbal and in writing (Johnson, Sandford, & Tyndall, 2007). For long-term regimens, many strategies show some effectiveness, but none offers dramatic improvement (Haynes et al., 2007). Furthermore, the interventions that dem-

onstrate greater effectiveness tend to be complex and costly. Therefore, adherence remains a costly problem, both in terms of the cost in lives and ill health of failures and in terms of the added costs of even marginally effective interventions.

IN SUMMARY

To improve adherence, many health care professionals first look at the barriers to adherence. These barriers include the difficulty of altering lifestyles of long duration, inadequate practitioner–patient communication, and erroneous beliefs as to what advice patients should follow. Effective programs to improve compliance rates frequently include cues to signal the time for taking medication, clearly written instructions, simplified medication regimens, prescriptions tailored to the patient's daily schedule, and rewards for compliant behavior.

ANSWERS

This chapter has addressed four basic questions:

1. **What theoretical models have been used to explain adherence?**

   Several theoretical models attempt to predict and explain compliant and noncompliant behavior. These include the behavioral model, which explains noncompliance in terms of difficulties in changing long-standing behaviors and advocates reinforcement for compliant behaviors; the self-efficacy model, which holds that people's beliefs that they can perform certain behaviors strongly predict what behaviors they will enact; the theories of reasoned action and planned behavior, both of which posit that intentions, attitudes, subjective norms, and motivation predict adherence; and the transtheoretical model, which proposes that people progress in spiral fashion through five stages in making changes in behavior—precontemplation, contemplation, preparation, action, and maintenance. Each of these models has some

use in predicting and explaining compliance and noncompliance.

2. **What is adherence, how can it be measured, and how frequently does it occur?**

   Adherence is the extent to which a person's behavior coincides with appropriate medical and health advice. For people to profit from medical advice, first, the advice must be accurate and, second, patients must follow the advice. When people do not adhere to sound health behaviors, they may risk serious health problems or even death. As many as 125,000 people in the United States die each year because of adherence failures.

   Patient adherence can be measured in at least six different ways: (1) ask the practitioner, (2) ask the patient, (3) ask other people, (4) monitor use of medicine, (5) examine biochemical evidence, and (6) use a combination of these procedures. Of these, physician judgment is the least valid, but each of the others also has serious flaws; a combination of procedures may provide a better assessment.

These different methods of assessment complicate the determination of the frequency of nonadherence. However, an analysis of more than 500 studies revealed that the average rate of nonadherence is around 25%, with people on medication regimens more compliant than those who must change health-related behaviors.

3. What factors predict adherence?

Researchers have found little evidence that the severity of a disease is an accurate predictor of adherence, but unpleasant or painful side effects of medication tend to lower adherence. Some personal factors relate to compliance, but the noncompliant personality does not exist. Age shows a curvilinear relationship, with older adults and children and adolescents experiencing problems in complying with medication regimens, but gender shows little overall effect. Emotional factors such as stress, anxiety, and depression lower adherence, but conscientiousness improves compliance. Personal beliefs are a significant factor, with beliefs in a regimen's ineffectiveness lowering adherence and self-efficacy beliefs increasing compliance.

A person's life situation also affects compliance. Lower income endangers compliance; people are not able to pay for treatment or medications. Higher income levels and greater social support generally increase adherence. Individuals with a cultural background that fails to accept Western medicine are less likely to comply with such a medical regimen. Ethnicity may also affect the treatment that patients receive from practitioners, and people who feel discriminated against comply at lower rates. Other aspects of the practitioner–patient interaction are important to adherence, especially verbal communication. No one factor accounts for adherence, so researchers must consider a combination of factors.

4. How can adherence be improved?

Knowing the barriers to adherence may help health care professionals detect methods of improving compliance. Strategies for enhancing adherence fall into four approaches: (1) providing prompts, (2) tailoring the regimen, (3) implementing the regimen gradually, and (4) making a contingency contract. Effective programs frequently include clearly written as well as clear verbal instructions, simple medication schedules, follow-up calls for missed appointments, prescriptions tailored to the patient's daily schedule, rewards for compliant behavior, and cues to signal the time for taking medication.

SUGGESTED READINGS

De Civita, M., & Dobkin, P. L. (2005). Pediatric adherence: Conceptual and methodological considerations. *Children's Health Care, 34,* 19–34. Although this article is oriented toward problems for pediatric adherence, the issues of measurement and discussion of the barriers to adherence apply to any age group.

DiMatteo, M. R. (2004). Variations in patients' adherence to medical recommendations: A quantitative review of 50 years of research. *Medical Care, 42,* 200–209. DiMatteo analyzes more than 500 studies published over a span of 50 years to determine factors that relate to failures in adherence. Her concise summary of these results reveals the relative contribution of demographic factors as well as illness characteristics.

Rietveld, S., & Koomen, J. M. (2002). A complex system perspective on medication compliance: Information for healthcare providers. *Disease Management and Health Outcomes, 10,* 621–630. Rietveld and Koomen review models of compliance and factors that affect compliance, integrate this information using a systems perspective, and offer suggestions for improving adherence.

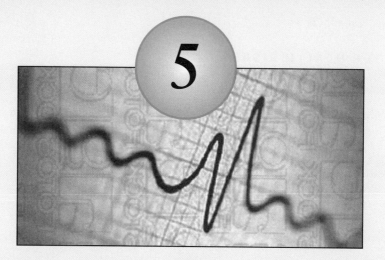

5

DEFINING, MEASURING, AND MANAGING STRESS

QUESTIONS

This chapter focuses on six basic questions:

1. What is the physiology of stress?

2. What theories explain stress?

3. How has stress been measured?

4. What sources produce stress?

5. What factors influence coping, and what strategies are effective?

6. What behavioral techniques are effective for stress management?

CHECK YOUR HEALTH RISKS

Undergraduate Stress Questionnaire

Has this stressful event happened to you at any time during the last two weeks? If it has, please check the box next to it. If it has not, then please leave it blank.

- ☐ Death (of a family member or friend)
- ☐ Death of a pet
- ☐ Working while in school
- ☐ Parents getting a divorce
- ☐ Registration for classes
- ☐ Trying to decide on a major
- ☐ Talked with a professor
- ☐ Trying to get into college
- ☐ Had a class presentation
- ☐ Had projects, research papers due
- ☐ Had a lot of tests
- ☐ It's finals week
- ☐ Applying to graduate school
- ☐ You have a hard upcoming week
- ☐ Lots of deadlines to meet
- ☐ Missed your period and waiting
- ☐ Had an interview
- ☐ Applying for a job
- ☐ Sat through a boring class
- ☐ Can't understand your professor
- ☐ Did badly on a test
- ☐ Went into a test unprepared
- ☐ Crammed for a test
- ☐ Used a fake ID
- ☐ Breaking up with boy-/girlfriend
- ☐ Holiday
- ☐ Bad haircut today

- ☐ Victim of a crime
- ☐ Can't concentrate
- ☐ Coping with addictions
- ☐ Found out boy-/girlfriend cheated on you
- ☐ Did worse than expected on a test
- ☐ Stayed up late writing a paper
- ☐ Problems with your computer
- ☐ Favorite sporting team lost
- ☐ Problems with printing things out
- ☐ Change of environment (new doctor, dentist, etc.)
- ☐ Bothered by having no social support of family
- ☐ Arguments, conflict of value with friends
- ☐ Visit from relatives and entertaining them
- ☐ Noise disturbed you while trying to study
- ☐ Maintaining a long-distance boy-/girlfriend
- ☐ Assignments in all classes due the same time
- ☐ Dealt with incompetence at the registrar's office
- ☐ Someone borrowed something without your permission
- ☐ Exposed to upsetting TV show, book, or movie
- ☐ Problem getting home from bar when drunk
- ☐ Had confrontation with an authority figure
- ☐ Got to class late
- ☐ Parents controlling with money

- ☐ Feel isolated
- ☐ Decision to have sex on your mind
- ☐ No sex in a while
- ☐ Living with boy-/girlfriend
- ☐ Felt some peer pressure
- ☐ Felt need for transportation
- ☐ Couldn't find a parking space
- ☐ Property stolen
- ☐ Car/bike broke down, flat tire, etc.
- ☐ Got a traffic ticket
- ☐ No time to eat
- ☐ Having roommate conflicts
- ☐ Had to ask for money
- ☐ Lack of money
- ☐ Checkbook didn't balance
- ☐ You have a hangover
- ☐ Someone you expected to call did not
- ☐ Lost something (especially wallet)
- ☐ Erratic schedule
- ☐ Thoughts about future
- ☐ Dependent on other people
- ☐ No sleep
- ☐ Sick, injured
- ☐ Fought with boy-/girlfriend
- ☐ Performed poorly at a task
- ☐ Heard bad news
- ☐ Thought about unfinished work
- ☐ Feel unorganized
- ☐ Someone cut ahead of you in line
- ☐ Job requirements changed
- ☐ Someone broke a promise

CHECK YOUR HEALTH RISKS

REAL-WORLD PROFILE OF LINDSAY LOHAN

By age 21, Lindsay Lohan had starred in movies that grossed millions of dollars and recorded hit records ("Celebrity Central," 2008). She had also been through treatment for alcohol and drug abuse twice, as well as being arrested for driving under the influence of alcohol and for possession of cocaine. She later blamed stress and family problems for her behavior: "I hadn't seen my dad; I had a lot of work stress 'cause I was constantly working and never took time to stop" (Silverman, 2008). Lindsay had worked since she was 3 years old, beginning as a child model and becoming a child actor, then a teen movie star and singer. She worked a great deal, but she also partied a lot, using alcohol and drugs. Those behaviors may have also been related to stress.

Although most people find it difficult to accept that people who are wealthy and famous experience stress, research indicates otherwise (Loftus, 1995). Being a celebrity involves stresses that most people do not experience, but those situations are stressful nonetheless. For example, the relentless press coverage that Lindsay Lohan experienced was the type of situation that celebrities rate as stressful. A survey of celebrities found that press coverage was the number one stressor (Loftus, 1995). The type of misbehavior that Lindsay Lohan exhibited is not an unusual reaction to her situation. Indeed, drinking and taking drugs are coping strategies to help manage emotions. Granted, these strategies are neither healthy nor effective, but many people—celebrities and others—have behaved similarly.

This chapter looks at what stress is, how it can be measured, some of the effective and ineffective strategies that people use to cope, and some behavioral management techniques that can help people cope more effectively. Chapter 6 examines the question of whether stress, such as Lindsay Lohan experienced, can cause illness and even death. But first we look at the physiological bases for stress.

THE NERVOUS SYSTEM AND THE PHYSIOLOGY OF STRESS

The basic function of the nervous system is to integrate all of the body's other systems. Small, simple organisms do not need (nor do they have) nervous systems. In larger and more complex organisms, nervous systems provide internal communication and relay information to and from the environment.

The human nervous system contains billions of individual cells called **neurons**, which function electrochemically. Within each neuron, electrically charged ions hold the potential for an electrical discharge. The discharge of this potential produces a minute electrical current, which travels the length of the neuron. The electrical charge leads to the release of chemicals called **neurotransmitters** that are manufactured within each neuron and stored in vesicles at the ends of the neurons. The released neurotransmitters diffuse across the **synaptic cleft,** the space between neurons.

The nervous system is made up of billions of neurons, organized in a hierarchy with major divisions and subdivisions. The two major divisions of the nervous system are the **central nervous system (CNS)** and the **peripheral nervous system (PNS)**. The CNS consists of the brain and the spinal cord, and the PNS comprises all other neurons. The divisions and subdivisions of the nervous system are illustrated in Figure 5.1.

The Peripheral Nervous System

The peripheral nervous system, that part of the nervous system lying outside the brain and spinal cord, is divided into two parts: the **somatic nervous system** and the **autonomic nervous system (ANS)**. The somatic nervous system primarily serves the skin and the voluntary muscles. The autonomic nervous system primarily serves internal organs and is thus involved in responses to stress.

The ANS allows for a variety of responses through its two divisions: the **sympathetic nervous system** and the **parasympathetic nervous system**. These two subdivisions differ anatomically as well as functionally. They, along with their target organs, appear in Figure 5.2.

The sympathetic division of the ANS mobilizes the body's resources in emergency, stressful, and emotional situations. The reactions include an increase in the rate and strength of cardiac contraction, constriction of blood vessels in the skin, a decrease of gastrointestinal activity, an increase in respiration, stimulation of the sweat glands, and dilation of the pupils in the eyes.

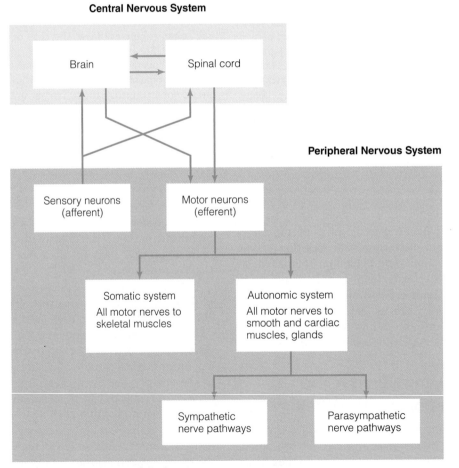

FIGURE 5.1   Divisions of the human nervous system.

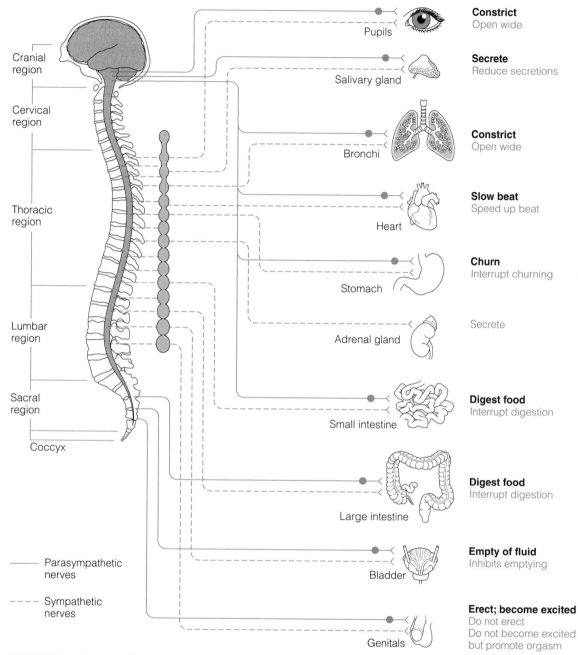

FIGURE 5.2 Autonomic nervous system and target organs. Solid lines and bold type represent the parasympathetic system, whereas dashed lines and lighter type represent the sympathetic system.

The parasympathetic division of the ANS, on the other hand, promotes relaxation and functions under normal, nonstressful conditions. The parasympathetic and sympathetic nervous systems serve the same target organs, but they tend to function reciprocally, with the activation of one increasing as the other decreases. For example, the activation of the sympathetic division reduces the secretion of saliva, producing the sensation of a dry mouth, whereas activation of the parasympathetic division promotes secretion of saliva.

Neurons in the ANS are activated by neurotransmitters, principally **acetylcholine** and **norepinephrine.** These neurotransmitters have complex effects; each has different effects in different organ systems because the organs contain different neurochemical receptors. In addition, the balance between these two main neurotransmitters, as well as their absolute quantity, is important. Therefore, even though there are only two major ANS neurotransmitters, they produce a wide variety of responses.

The Neuroendocrine System

The **endocrine system** consists of ductless glands distributed throughout the body (see Figure 5.3). The **neuroendocrine system** consists of those endocrine glands that are controlled by and interact with the nervous system. Glands of the endocrine and neuroendocrine systems secrete chemicals known as **hormones,** which move into the bloodstream to be carried to different parts of the body. Specialized receptors on target tissues or organs allow hormones to have specific effects, even though the hormones circulate throughout the body. At the target, hormones may have a direct effect, or they may cause the secretion of another hormone.

The endocrine and nervous systems can work closely together because they have several similarities, but they also differ in important ways. Both systems share, synthesize, and release chemicals. In the nervous system, these chemicals are called neurotransmitters; in the endocrine system, they are called hormones. The activation of neurons is usually rapid, and the effect is short term; the endocrine system responds more slowly, and its action persists longer. In the nervous system, neurotransmitters are

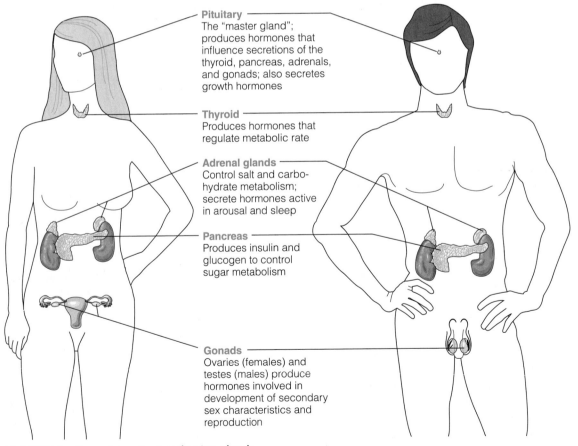

Pituitary
The "master gland"; produces hormones that influence secretions of the thyroid, pancreas, adrenals, and gonads; also secretes growth hormones

Thyroid
Produces hormones that regulate metabolic rate

Adrenal glands
Control salt and carbohydrate metabolism; secrete hormones active in arousal and sleep

Pancreas
Produces insulin and glucogen to control sugar metabolism

Gonads
Ovaries (females) and testes (males) produce hormones involved in development of secondary sex characteristics and reproduction

FIGURE 5.3   Some important endocrine glands.

released by stimulation of neural impulses, flow across the synaptic cleft, and are immediately either reabsorbed or inactivated. In the endocrine system, hormones are synthesized by the endocrine cells, are released into the blood, reach their targets in minutes or even hours, and exert prolonged effects. The endocrine and nervous systems both have communication and control functions, and both work toward integrated, adaptive behaviors. The two systems are related in function and interact in neuroendocrine responses.

The Pituitary Gland Located within the brain, the **pituitary gland** is an excellent example of the intricate relationship between the nervous and endocrine systems. The pituitary is connected to the hypothalamus, a structure in the forebrain. These two structures work together to regulate and produce hormones. The pituitary has been referred to as the "master gland" because it produces a number of hormones that affect other glands and prompt the production of other hormones.

Of the seven hormones produced by the anterior portion of the pituitary gland, **adrenocorticotropic hormone (ACTH)** plays an essential role in the stress response. When stimulated by the hypothalamus, the pituitary releases ACTH, which in turn acts on the **adrenal glands.**

The Adrenal Glands The adrenal glands are endocrine glands located on top of each kidney. Each gland is composed of an outer covering, the **adrenal cortex**, and an inner part, the **adrenal medulla.** Both secrete hormones that are important in the response to stress. The **adrenocortical response** occurs when ACTH from the pituitary stimulates the adrenal cortex to release glucocorticoids, one type of hormone. **Cortisol**, the most important of these hormones, exerts a wide range of effects on major organs in the body (Kemeny, 2003). This hormone is so closely associated with stress that the level of cortisol circulating in the blood can be used as an index of stress. Its peak levels appear 20 to 40 minutes after a stressor, allowing time for measurement of this stress hormone.

The **adrenomedullary response** occurs when the sympathetic nervous system actives the adrenal medulla. This action prompts secretion of **catecholamines**, a class of chemicals containing **epinephrine** and norepinephrine. Epinephrine (sometimes referred to as adrenaline) is produced exclusively by the adrenal medulla and accounts for about 80% of the hormone production of the adrenal glands. Norepinephrine is not only a hormone; it is also a neurotransmitter produced in many places in the body besides the adrenal medulla. Neurotransmitters work at the synapse, whereas hormones circulate through the blood. Norepinephrine has both actions and is produced at many places in the body, not exclusively in the adrenal medulla.

Epinephrine, on the other hand, is produced exclusively in the adrenal medulla. It is so closely and uniquely associated with the adrenomedullary stress response that it is sometimes used as an index of stress. The amount of epinephrine secreted can be determined by assaying a person's urine, thus measuring stress by tapping into the physiology of the stress response. Such an index can be helpful because it does not rely on personal perceptions of stress, and its use as a measure of stress can provide an alternative perspective. Like other hormones, epinephrine and norepinephrine circulate through the bloodstream, and their action is both slower and more prolonged than the action of neurotransmitters.

Physiology of the Stress Response

The physiological reactions to stress begin with the perception of stress. That perception results in activation of the sympathetic division of the autonomic nervous system, which mobilizes the body's resources to react in emotional, stressful, and emergency situations. Walter Cannon (1932) termed this configuration of responses the "fight or flight" reaction because this array of responses prepares the body for either option. Sympathetic activation prepares the body for intense motor activity, the sort necessary for attack, defense, or escape. This mobilization occurs through two routes and affects all parts of the body.

One route is through direct activation of the sympathetic division of the ANS (called the adrenomedullary system), which activates the adrenal medulla to secrete epinephrine and norepinephrine (Kemeny, 2003). The effects occur throughout the body, affecting the cardiovascular, digestive, and respiratory systems.

The other route is through the hypothalamic-pituitary-adrenal axis, which involves all of these structures. The action begins with perception of a threatening situation, which prompts action in the hypothalamus. The hypothalamic response is the release of corticotropin-releasing hormone, which stimulates the anterior pituitary (the part of the pituitary gland at the base of the brain) to secrete adrenocorticotropic hormone (ACTH). This hormone stimulates the adrenal cortex to secrete glucocorticoids, including cortisol. The secretion of cortisol mobilizes the body's energy resources, raising the level of blood sugar to provide energy for the cells. Cortisol also has an anti-inflammatory effect, giving the body a natural defense against swelling from injuries that might be sustained during a fight or a flight. Figure 5.4 shows these two routes of activation.

The point of the physiological reaction to stress is to furnish a variety of responses that allow adaptation to a threatening situation. Maintaining an appropriate level of activation under

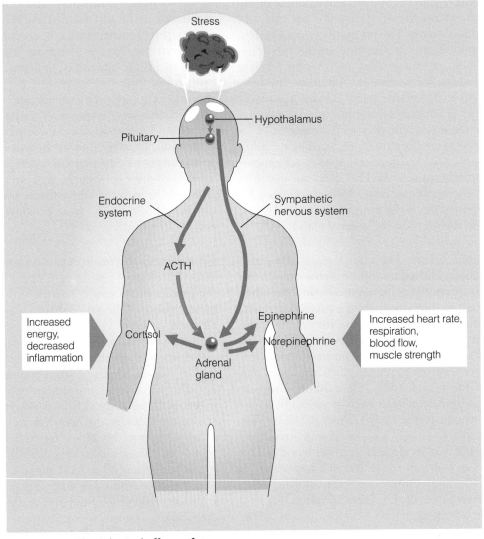

FIGURE 5.4   Physiological effects of stress.

changing circumstances is referred to as **allostasis,** and the wide range of circumstances that people encounter requires different levels of physiological activation (McEwen, 2005). Activation of the sympathetic nervous system is the body's attempt to meet the needs of the situation during emergencies. At its optimum in maintaining allostasis, the autonomic nervous system adapts smoothly, adjusting to normal demands by parasympathetic activation and rapidly mobilizing resources for threatening or stressful situations by sympathetic activation. However, prolonged activation of the responses of the sympathetic nervous system creates *allostatic load,* which can overcome the body's ability to adapt. Thus, allostatic load may be the source of problems (Gunnar & Quevedo, 2007).

Shelly Taylor and her colleagues (Taylor, 2002, 2006; Taylor et al., 2000) raised objections to the traditional conceptualization of the stress response, questioning the basic notion that it is a fight-or-flight response. These theorists contended that research and theory on stress responses have been biased by concentrating on men, for whom fight-or-flight is a more valid model than for women. Although they acknowledged that men's and women's nervous system responses to stress are virtually identical, they argued that women exhibit neuroendocrine responses to stress that differ from men's reactions, and that these differences lay the biological foundation for gender differences in behavioral responses to stress. They proposed that the stress response in women is better characterized as "tend and befriend" than "fight or flight." That is, women tend to respond to stressful situations with nurturing responses and by seeking and giving social support, rather than by either fighting or fleeing.

Taylor and her colleagues argued that this pattern of responses arose in women during human evolutionary history and is more consistent with the biological and behavioral evidence than the fight-or-flight conceptualization of stress responses. This view has been the target of criticism (Geary & Flinn, 2002), but a limited amount of human research is consistent with its contentions (Taylor, 2006). For example, the patterns of hormone secretion during competition differ for women and men (Kivlinghan, Granger, & Booth, 2005). In a study of children's responses to mothers

whose behavior was frightening, girls tended to seek the company of mothers who were behaving in a frightening way, whereas boys tended to avoid the frightening mother (David & Lyons-Ruth, 2005). This finding is consistent with the hypothesis that females tend to affiliate under conditions of stress, whereas males tend to flee.

IN SUMMARY

The physiology of the stress response is complex. When a person perceives stress, the sympathetic division of the autonomic nervous system rouses the person from a resting state in two ways: by stimulating the sympathetic nervous system and by producing hormones. The ANS activation is rapid, as is all neural transmission, whereas the action of the neuroendocrine system is slower but longer lasting. The pituitary releases ACTH, which in turn affects the adrenal cortex. Glucocorticoid release prepares the body to resist the stress and even to cope with injury by the release of cortisol. Together the two systems form the physiological basis for allostasis, adaptive responses under conditions of change.

An understanding of the physiology of stress does not completely clarify the meaning of stress. Thus, several models have been constructed in an attempt to better define and explain stress.

THEORIES OF STRESS

Despite a great deal of scientific research on the subject and the widespread use of the term in everyday conversation, *stress* has no simple definition (McEwen, 2005). Indeed, it has been defined in three different ways: as a stimulus, as a response, and as an interaction. When some people talk about stress, they are referring to an environmental *stimulus,* as in "I have a high-stress job." Others consider stress a physical *response,* as in "My heart races when I feel a lot of stress." Still others consider stress to result from the *interaction* between environmental stimuli and the person, as in "I feel stressed when I have to make financial decisions at work, but other types of decisions do not stress me."

These three views of stress also appear in the different theories of stress. The view of stress as an external event was the first approach taken by stress researchers, the most prominent of whom was Hans Selye. During the course of his research, Selye changed to a more response-based view of stress, concentrating on the biological aspects of the stress response.

The most influential view of stress among psychologists has been the interactionist approach, proposed by Richard Lazarus. The next two sections discuss the views of Selye and Lazarus.

Selye's View

Beginning in the 1930s and continuing until his death in 1982, Hans Selye (1956, 1976, 1982) researched and popularized the concept of stress, making a strong case for its relationship to physical illness and bringing the importance of stress to the attention of the public. Although he did not originate the concept of stress, he researched the effects of stress on physiological responses and tried to connect these reactions to the development of illness.

Selye first conceptualized stress as a stimulus and focused his attention on the environmental conditions that produce stress. In the 1950s, he shifted his focus to stress as a response that the organism makes. To distinguish the two, Selye started using the term *stressor* to refer to the stimulus and *stress* to mean the response.

Selye's contributions to stress research included a model for how the body defends itself in stressful situations. Selye conceptualized stress as a nonspecific response, repeatedly insisting that stress is a general physical response caused by any of a number of environmental stressors. He believed that a wide variety of different situations could prompt the stress response, but the response would always be the same.

The General Adaptation Syndrome The body's generalized attempt to defend itself against noxious agents became known as the **general adaptation syndrome (GAS)**. This syndrome is divided into three stages, the first of which is the **alarm reaction.** During alarm, the body's defenses against a stressor are mobilized through activation of

the sympathetic nervous system. This division activates body systems to maximize strength and prepares them for the fight-or-flight response. Adrenaline (epinephrine) is released, heart rate and blood pressure increase, respiration becomes faster, blood is diverted away from the internal organs toward the skeletal muscles, sweat glands are activated, and the gastrointestinal system decreases its activity. As a short-term response to an emergency situation, these physical reactions are adaptive, but many modern stress situations involve prolonged exposure to stress and do not require physical action.

Selye called the second phase of the GAS the **resistance stage.** In this stage, the organism adapts to the stressor. How long this stage lasts depends on the severity of the stressor and the adaptive capacity of the organism. If the organism can adapt, the resistance stage will continue for a long time. During this stage, the person gives the outward appearance of normality, but physiologically the body's internal functioning is not normal. Continuing stress will cause continued neurological and hormonal changes. Selye believed that these demands take a toll, setting the stage for what he described as *diseases of adaptation*— diseases related to continued, persistent stress. Figure 5.5 illustrates these stages and the point in the process at which diseases develop.

Among the diseases Selye considered to be the result of prolonged resistance to stress are peptic ulcers and ulcerative colitis, hypertension and cardiovascular disease, hyperthyroidism, and bronchial asthma. In addition, Selye hypothesized that resistance to stress would cause changes in the immune system, making infection more likely.

The capacity to resist stress is finite, and the final stage of the GAS is the **exhaustion stage.** At the end, the organism's ability to resist is depleted, and a breakdown results. This stage is characterized by activation of the parasympathetic division of the autonomic nervous system. Under normal circumstances, parasympathetic activation keeps the body functioning in a balanced state. In the exhaustion stage, however, parasympathetic functioning is at an abnormally low level, causing a person to become exhausted.

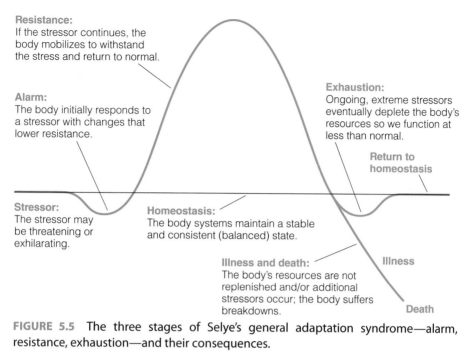

Resistance:
If the stressor continues, the body mobilizes to withstand the stress and return to normal.

Alarm:
The body initially responds to a stressor with changes that lower resistance.

Exhaustion:
Ongoing, extreme stressors eventually deplete the body's resources so we function at less than normal.

Return to homeostasis

Stressor:
The stressor may be threatening or exhilarating.

Homeostasis:
The body systems maintain a stable and consistent (balanced) state.

Illness and death:
The body's resources are not replenished and/or additional stressors occur; the body suffers breakdowns.

Illness

Death

FIGURE 5.5 The three stages of Selye's general adaptation syndrome—alarm, resistance, exhaustion—and their consequences.

Source: An Invitation to Health (7th ed., p. 40) by D. Hales, 1997, Pacific Grove, CA: Brooks/Cole. Copyright 1997 by Brooks/Cole Publishing Company. Reprinted by permission.

Selye believed that exhaustion frequently results in depression and sometimes even death.

Evaluation of Selye's View Selye's early concept of stress as a stimulus and his later concentration on the physical aspects of stress have both been influential in researching and measuring stress. The stimulus-based view of stress prompted researchers to investigate the various environmental conditions that cause people to experience stress and also led to the construction of stress inventories, such as the Undergraduate Stress Questionnaire that introduces this chapter. These inventories ask people to check or list the events they have experienced in the recent past and measure the amount of stress by totaling these events.

Selye's view of the physiology of stress was probably too simplistic (McEwen, 2005). He considered the stress response to all events to be similar, a contention that research has not confirmed. He also believed that the physiological responses to stress were oriented toward maintaining functioning within a narrow range of the optimal level. That view has been replaced by the concepts of

allostasis and *allostatic load*, which emphasize the processes of adaptation and change rather than narrow regulation. Allostatic load occurs when many changes are required by the persistence of a stressor or the presence of many stressors. Thus, allostatic load can become overload, resulting in damage and disease. This view of stress is similar to Selye's but shows subtle differences that are more compatible with modern research.

Selye largely ignored the situational and psychological factors that contribute to stress, including the emotional component and the individual interpretation of stressful events (Mason, 1971, 1975), which makes his view of stress incomplete in the view of most psychologists. Although Selye's view has had great influence on the popular conception of stress, an alternative model formulated by psychologist Richard Lazarus has had a greater impact among psychologists.

Lazarus's View

In Lazarus's view, the interpretation of stressful events is more important than the events themselves.

Neither the environmental event nor the person's response defines stress; rather, the individual's *perception* of the psychological situation is the critical factor. This perception includes potential harms, threats, and challenges as well as the individual's perceived ability to cope with them.

Psychological Factors Lazarus's emphasis on interpretation and perception differs from that of Selye. This emphasis necessitated another difference: Lazarus worked largely with humans rather than nonhuman animals. The ability of people to think about and evaluate future events makes them vulnerable in ways that other animals are not. Humans encounter stresses because they have high-level cognitive abilities that other animals lack.

According to Lazarus (1984, 1993), the effect that stress has on a person is based more on that person's feelings of threat, vulnerability, and ability to cope than on the stressful event itself. For example, losing a job may be extremely stressful for someone who has no money saved or who believes that finding another job will be very difficult. In Lazarus's view, a life event is not what produces stress; rather, it is one's view of the situation that causes an event to become stressful. For example, Lindsay Lohan, who was introduced at the beginning of this chapter, apparently perceived her work demands as stressful. Other actors may have experienced her level of employment as a positive event; many actors find unemployment more stressful than working (Loftus, 1995). Indeed, Lohan's problems led to decreased demand for her services, which she reported as distressing (Silverman, 2008).

Lazarus and Susan Folkman defined psychological stress as a "particular relationship between the person and the environment that is appraised by the person as taxing or exceeding his or her resources and endangering his or her well-being" (1984, p. 19). This definition has several important points. First, Lazarus and Folkman's theory takes an interactional or *transactional* position, holding that stress refers to a relationship between person and environment. Second, this theory holds that the key to that transaction is the person's appraisal of the psychological situation. Third, the situation must be seen as threatening, challenging, or harmful.

Appraisal Lazarus and Folkman (1984) recognized that people use three kinds of appraisal to assess situations: primary appraisal, secondary appraisal, and reappraisal. **Primary appraisal** is not necessarily first in importance, but it is first in time. When people first encounter an event, such as an offer of a job promotion, they appraise the offer in terms of its effect on their well-being. They may view the event as irrelevant, benign-positive, or stressful. It is unlikely that an offer of a job promotion would be seen as irrelevant, but many environmental events, such as a snowstorm in another state, have no implications for a person's well-being. A benign-positive appraisal means that the event is seen as having good implications. A stressful appraisal can mean that the event is seen as harmful, threatening, or challenging. Each of these three—harm, threat, and challenge—is likely to generate an emotion. Lazarus (1993) defined *harm* as damage that has already been done, such as an illness or injury; *threat* as the anticipation of harm; and *challenge* as a person's confidence in overcoming difficult demands. An appraisal of harm may produce anger, disgust, disappointment, or sadness; an appraisal of threat is likely to generate worry, anxiety, or fear; an appraisal of challenge may be followed by excitement or anticipation. These emotions do not produce stress; instead, they are generated by the individual's appraisal of an event. Research indicates that the perception of threat or challenge makes a difference for performance; perception of challenge led to better performance than perception of threat (Gildea, Schneider, & Shebilske, 2007).

After their initial appraisal of an event, people form an impression of their ability to control or cope with harm, threat, or challenge, an impression called **secondary appraisal.** People typically ask three questions in making secondary appraisals. The first is "What options are available to me?" The second is "What is the likelihood that I can successfully apply the necessary strategies to reduce this stress?" The third is "Will this procedure work—that is, will it alleviate my stress?"

When people believe they can do something that will make a difference—when they believe they can successfully change a situation to achieve a positive outcome—stress is reduced. Lindsay Lohan did not have that confidence. She had not found any successful strategy for balancing her work demands with the other aspects of her life. Her father had been convicted of driving under the influence of alcohol and sentenced to prison. Many celebrities anchor their lives around their families, and without that possibility, Lindsay had difficulty finding effective coping strategies.

The third type of appraisal is **reappraisal.** Appraisals change constantly as new information becomes available. Reappraisal does not always result in more stress; sometimes it decreases stress.

Vulnerability Stress is most likely to be aroused when people are vulnerable—when they lack resources in a situation of some personal importance. These resources may be either physical or social, but their importance is determined by psychological factors, such as perception and evaluation of the situation. An arthritic knee, for example, would produce physical vulnerability in a professional athlete but might be a minor inconvenience to the professional life of someone who works behind a desk.

Lazarus and Folkman (1984) insisted that physical or social deficits alone are not sufficient to produce vulnerability. What matters is whether people consider the situation personally important. Vulnerability differs from threat in that it represents only the *potential* for threat. Threat exists when people perceive that their self-esteem is in jeopardy; vulnerability exists when people's lack of resources creates a potentially threatening or harmful situation. Celebrities remain popular by pleasing people, so their continued fame is always uncertain (Loftus, 1995). Many feel that they are undeserving of their success and consequently fear its loss. These situations provide good examples of threat and vulnerability.

Coping An important ingredient in Lazarus's theory of stress is the ability or inability to cope with a stressful situation. Lazarus and Folkman defined coping as "constantly changing cognitive and behavioral efforts to manage specific external and/or internal demands that are appraised as taxing or exceeding the resources of the person" (1984, p. 141). This definition spells out several important features of coping. First, coping is a process, constantly changing as one's efforts are evaluated as more or less successful. Second, coping is not automatic; it is a learned pattern of responding to stressful situations. A response that is automatic (such as closing one's eyes to block out intense light) or that becomes automatic through experience (such as shifting one's weight while riding a bicycle) would not be considered coping. Third, coping requires effort. People need not be completely aware of their coping response, and the outcome may or may not be successful, but effort must have been expended. Fourth, coping is an effort to *manage* the situation; control and mastery are not necessary. For example, most of us make an effort to manage our physical environment by striving for a comfortable air temperature. Thus, we cope with our environment even though complete mastery of the climate is impossible. How well people are able to cope depends on the resources they have available and the strategies they use.

IN SUMMARY

Two leading theories of stress are those of Hans Selye and Richard Lazarus. Selye, the first researcher to look closely at stress, first saw stress as a stimulus but later viewed it as a response. Whenever animals (including humans) encounter a threatening stimulus, they mobilize themselves in a generalized attempt to adapt to that stimulus. This mobilization, called the general adaptation syndrome (GAS), has three stages—alarm, resistance, and exhaustion—and the potential for trauma or illness exists at all three stages.

In contrast, Lazarus held a cognitively oriented, transactional view of stress and coping. Stressful encounters are dynamic and complex, constantly changing and unfolding, so that the outcomes of one stressful event alter subsequent appraisals of new events. Individual differences in coping strategies and in the appraisal of stressful events are crucial to a person's experience of stress; therefore, the likelihood of developing any stress-related disorder varies with the individual. The relationship between stressful events and subsequent health is complex, and any attempt to measure stress and people's attempts to cope with it must also be complex.

MEASUREMENT OF STRESS

Measuring stress is an important part of health psychology. In order to understand the sources of stress and the effect of stress on disease, researchers must first measure stress. This section discusses some of the more widely used methods and addresses the problems involved in determining their reliability and validity.

Methods of Measurement

Researchers have used a variety of approaches to measure stress, but most fall into two broad categories: physiological measures and self-reports. Physiological measures assume that stress is a biological response that can be measured much as any other biological response. Self-reports are often used to measure either **life events** or **daily hassles.** Both approaches hold some potential for investigating the effects of stress on illness and health.

Physiological Measures   One method of measuring stress uses various physiological and biochemical measures, including blood pressure, heart rate, galvanic skin response, respiration rate, and increased secretion of stress hormones such as cortisol and epinephrine. The physiological indexes of blood pressure, heart rate, galvanic skin response, and respiration rate all change with activation of the sympathetic division of the autonomic nervous system. Therefore, stress and emotion produce changes in these responses. Indeed, these measures are the ones used in polygraphs, and their relationship with emotion is the basis for use of polygraphs as "lie detectors." This use is controversial (National Research Council, 2003), but these physiological indexes show some relationship to stress.

A more common approach to the physiological measurement of stress is through its association with the release of hormones. Epinephrine and norepinephrine are produced in the adrenal medulla in association with the experience of stress. Measurement of these two hormones, in either blood or urine samples, can provide an index of stress (Eller, Netterstrøm, & Hansen, 2006; Krantz, Forsman, & Lundberg, 2004). The levels of these hormones circulating in the blood decrease within a few minutes after the stressful experience, so measurement must be quick to capture the changes. The levels of hormones persist longer in the urine, but factors other than stress contribute to urinary levels of these hormones. In addition, taking these measurements may itself be a stressful experience, contaminating the assessment. The stress hormone cortisol persists for at least 20 minutes, and measurement of salivary cortisol provides an index of the changes in this hormone.

The advantage of these physiological measures of stress is that they are direct, highly reliable, and easily quantified. A disadvantage is that the mechanical and electrical hardware and clinical settings that are frequently used may themselves produce stress. Thus, this approach to measuring stress is useful but not the most widely used method. Self-report measures are far more common.

Life Events Scales   Since the late 1950s and early 1960s, researchers have developed a number of self-report instruments to measure stress. The earliest and best known of these self-report procedures is the Social Readjustment Rating Scale (SRRS), developed by Thomas H. Holmes and Richard Rahe in 1967. The scale is simply a list of 43 life events arranged in rank order from most to least stressful. Each event carries an assigned value, ranging from 100 points for death of a spouse to 11 points for minor violations of the law. Respondents check the items they have experienced during a recent period, usually the previous 6 to 24 months. Adding each item's point value and totaling scores yields a stress score for each person. These scores can then be correlated with future events, such as incidence of illness, to determine the relationship between this measure of stress and the occurrence of physical illness.

Life events scales like the SRRS have sometimes appeared in the popular press with the

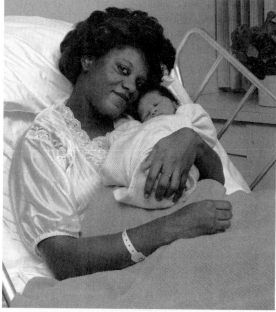

Life events scales also include positive events because such events also require adjustment.

(2) major events, and (3) changes in coping resources. Respondents answer *never, almost never, sometimes, fairly often,* or *very often* to items that ask about their stressful situations during the past month. Researchers have used the PSS in a variety of situations, such as assessing stress during final exams for undergraduate college students (Pollard & Bates, 2004), determining the effectiveness of a relaxation program for elementary teachers (Nassiri, 2005), and predicting symptoms such as headache, sore throat, and fatigue in graduate students (Lacey et al., 2000). Its brevity combined with good reliability and validity have led to use of this scale in a variety of research projects.

More recent life events scales include the Weekly Stress Inventory (Brantley et al., 2007; Brantley, Jones, Boudreaux, & Gatz, 1997), which assesses stress over a few weeks or months; the Stress in General Scale (Stanton, Balzer, Smith, Parra, & Ironson, 2001), designed to measure general work stress; the Life Events Inventory (Sharpley, Tanti, Stone, & Lothian, 2004), which considers the likelihood that some people will view many negative events as positive and some positive events as negative; and the Stress Symptom Checklist (Schlebuisch, 2004), a South African scale that looks at the participant's level of stress rather than the stimuli precipitating the stress.

implication that people should count their stress points and use care to avoid additional stress that might put them beyond some critical total, usually 300 points on the SRRS. This advice ignores the fact that many people accumulate far more than 300 points in a year and never become ill.

Other stress inventories exist, including the Undergraduate Stress Questionnaire (USQ) (Crandall, Preisler, & Aussprung, 1992), the assessment that appears as Check Your Health Risks at the beginning of this chapter. This stress inventory is similar to the SRRS in providing a list of sources of stress and asking people to check the ones that have happened to them during the past two weeks. College students who check more stress situations tend to use health services more than students who check fewer events.

The Perceived Stress Scale (PSS) (Cohen, Kamarck, & Mermelstein, 1983) emphasizes perception of events. The PSS is a 14-item scale that attempts to measure the degree to which situations in people's lives are appraised as "unpredictable, uncontrollable, and overloading" (Cohen et al., 1983, p. 387). The scale assesses three components of stress: (1) daily hassles,

Everyday Hassles Scales Richard Lazarus and his associates pioneered an approach to stress measurement that looks at daily hassles rather than life events. Daily hassles are "experiences and conditions of daily living that have been appraised as salient and harmful or threatening to the endorser's well-being" (Lazarus, 1984, p. 376). Recall from the discussion of theories of stress that Lazarus views stress as a transactional, dynamic complex shaped by people's *appraisal* of the environmental situation and their *perceived capabilities to cope* with this situation. Consistent with this view, Lazarus and his associates insisted that measurement instruments must not conceptualize stress as an objective environmental stimulus but instead must allow for subjective elements such as personal appraisal, beliefs, goals, and commitments (Lazarus, 2000; Lazarus, DeLongis, Folkman, & Gruen, 1985).

Robert Marien/Corbis

As a consequence, Lazarus and his associates (Kanner, Coyne, Schaefer, & Lazarus, 1981) developed the original Hassles Scale, which consisted of 117 items of annoying, irritating, or frustrating ways in which people may *feel* hassled. A companion inventory, the Uplifts Scale, contained 138 items that might make a person feel good. In addition to checking hassles or uplifts that occurred during the past month, respondents rated the degree of each on a 3-point scale. This second rating was consistent with Lazarus's belief that an individual's *perception* of stress is more crucial than the objective event itself.

Research on the Hassles Scale (Kanner et al., 1981) indicated only a modest correlation between hassles and life events, which suggests that these two types of stress are not the same thing. In addition, the Hassles Scale was a more accurate predictor of psychological health than the life events scale (Lazarus, 1984). This finding suggests that the Hassles Scale supplements life events scales as a measure of stress and that the life events scale added little to the predictive value of the Hassles Scale.

Later, Anita DeLongis, Susan Folkman, and Lazarus (1988) published a completely revised Hassles and Uplifts Scale. The revised scale asks participants to think of how much of a hassle or uplift each of 53 items was to them that day.

Respondents rate such items as "Your spouse" or "The weather" on a 4-point scale, ranging from *none* to *a great deal*. The revised Hassles and Uplifts Scale has the advantage of being much shorter than the 255 items on the original scales. In addition, the revised scale showed better predictive power than the Social Readjustment Rating Scale in predicting both the frequency and intensity of headaches (Fernandez & Sheffield, 1996) and episodes of inflammatory bowel disease (Searle & Bennett, 2001), indicating its success in predicting disease.

Using the concept of assessing stress by measuring hassles has also been extended to specific situations. For example, the Urban Hassles Index (Miller & Townsend, 2005) and the Family Daily Hassles Inventory (Rollins & Garrison, 2002) target specific groups and situations. Table 5.1 lists some of the many self-report inventories developed to measure stress. Some of these instruments have been translated into different languages and have used different norms.

Reliability and Validity of Stress Measures

The usefulness of stress measures rests on their ability to predict some established criterion and to do so consistently. For health psychology, the criterion is usually illness or some risk factor

TABLE 5.1

Examples of Self-Report Stress Scales

Scale Name	Author(s)	Goal	Number of Items and Scoring
Computer Hassles Scale	Richard A. Hudiburg	To define a measure for a specific type of stress	37 items rated on a 4-point scale of severity ranging from *not at all* to *extremely*
Daily Stress Inventory	Phillip J. Brantley Sheryl L. Catz Edwin Boudreaux	To determine the occurrence of daily stressors and the experience of symptoms	58 items rated on a 7-point scale ranging from *not stressful* to *caused panic*
Illness Effects Questionnaire	Glen D. Greenberg Rolf A. Peterson	To capture patients' illness experience and the impairment of daily function	20 items rated on an 8-point scale ranging from *agree to disagree*

TABLE 5.1 Examples of Self-Report Stress Scales—*Continued*

Scale Name	Author(s)	Goal	Number of Items and Scoring
Index of Teaching Stress	Richard R. Abidin Ross W. Greene	To measure the presence of teaching stress and the potential for problems with students	90 items rated on a 5-point scale ranging from *never stressful* to *very often stressful*
Mental Health Professionals Stress Scale	Delia Cushway Patrick A. Tyler Peter Nolan	To identify sources of stress for mental health professionals	42 items with 7 subscales
Nurse Stress Index	Stephen Williams Cary L. Cooper	To locate the main sources of stress in the daily work of nurses	30 items with 6 subscales
Occupational Stress Indicator	Stephen Williams Cary L. Cooper	To provide a comprehensive set of measurements for mental and physical health, sources of pressure, locus of control, and coping strategies	167 items rated on a 6-point scale, divided into 28 subscales
Parenting Stress Index	Richard R. Abidin	To measure the characteristics of parenting stress associated with the child, parent, and situation	120 items rated on a 5-point scale and yes/no format; a 36-item short form exists
Stress Schedule	Edmond Hallberg Kaylene Hallberg Loren Sauer	To provide a comprehensive measure of stress so that people with high stress get an "early warning"	60 items rated on a 5-point agree/disagree scale
Weekly Stress Inventory	Phillip J. Brantley Glen N. Jones Edwin Boudreaux	To assess minor stressors ("hassles") for the time span of a week	87 items rated on 7-point scale ranging from *not stressful* to *extremely stressful*

Source: Evaluating Stress: A Book of Resources, edited by C. P. Zalaquett & R. J. Wood, 1997, Lanhan, MD: Scarecrow Press.

for disease. To predict future stress-related illness, these inventories must be both reliable and valid. Reliability is the consistency with which an instrument measures whatever it measures, and validity is the extent to which it measures what it is supposed to measure.

The *reliability* of self-report inventories is most frequently determined by either the paired-associate method or the test–retest technique. In the paired-associate method, close associates (usually a spouse) fill out the inventory, answering as if the item applied to their associate. The degree of agreement between the two associates is usually quite high for moderately or severely stressful events (Slater & Depue, 1981) but lower for less stressful experiences (Zimmerman, 1983).

The second approach to determining reliability is the test–retest technique, in which the same person completes the stress inventory at two different times. Inaccuracies in memory are the main reason for less than perfect agreement, and a review of test–retest reliability (Turner & Wheaton, 1995) indicated that the relationship is far from perfect. Techniques to improve memory such as cues and question wording to prompt recall can increase reliability scores for important events to a very high level for both the associate method and the individual test–retest approach.

To consider the *validity* of self-report inventories, we must begin with the question "What are these instruments supposed to measure?" At least three approaches to answering this question are possible. First, the scales should accurately represent all of the life events experienced by the respondents. Second, because these scales are designed to measure stress, scores on self-report inventories should correlate with some other measure of stress, such as judgments of a spouse or close associate or physical measurements of stress. Third, as they are most frequently used, self-report inventories are supposed to measure or predict the incidence of future illness. Let's consider these three approaches in more detail.

First, do self-report inventories accurately represent all experiences of stressful life events? Some investigators (Turner & Wheaton, 1995) have suggested that many people tend to underreport (omit) life events, whereas other critics contended that sick people overreport life events, providing a kind of justification for their illness. Other critics (Gorin & Stone, 2001) have argued that memory distortion and the biases of recall prevent self-reports from being valid indicators of past events. Either overreporting or underreporting decreases the validity of life events measures. Research (Turner & Avison, 2003) has indicated that life events scales tend to underestimate the stress that African Americans experience.

The second approach asks how one can determine the degree to which a person is accurately reporting stressful events. One method is to compare reports from a spouse or close associate. But the result generally yields significant levels of disagreement between partners, especially when mildly distressful events are included.

The third and most useful type of validity for stress inventories is the extent to which they predict future illnesses or disorders. If self-report scales can demonstrate predictive validity, then they will play a valuable role in determining who may be at risk for stress-related illnesses. One problem in measuring the relationship between stress inventories and illness is the confounding of items on the major life events scales with the presence of physical disorders. Being ill can be stressful, of course, but it can also lead to answers that have been included in the Social Readjustment Rating Scale, such as sex difficulties, revision of personal habits, change in sleeping habits, and change in eating habits. Therefore, a high score on the SRRS or other similarly constructed life events scale may be a consequence rather than a cause of illness. However, an analysis of 30 years of research on the SRRS (Scully, Tosi, & Banning, 2000) concluded that the SSRS predicts occurrence of stress-related symptoms, making it a useful tool.

IN SUMMARY

Stress can be measured by several methods, including physiological and biochemical measures and self-reports of stressful events. The most popular life events scale is the Social Readjustment Rating Scale, which emphasizes change in life events. Despite its popularity, the SRRS is not a good predictor of subsequent illness. Lazarus and his associates pioneered the measurement of stress as daily hassles and uplifts. These inventories emphasize the perceived severity and importance of daily events. In general, the revised Hassles and Uplifts Scale is more accurate than the SRRS in predicting future illness.

The prediction of future illness is one measure of validity, or how accurate stress inventories are in their assessment. Another important characteristic of stress measurement is reliability, which is how consistent the measures are.

Self-report inventories of stress have only moderate levels of reliability and low levels of validity, and even hassles scales have limited validity for predicting illness.

SOURCES OF STRESS

Stress can flow from myriad sources—cataclysmic events with natural or human causes, change in an individual's life history, and ongoing hassles of daily life. In organizing sources of stress, we have followed the model set forth by Richard Lazarus and Judith Cohen (1977), but as these two researchers emphasized, an individual's perception of a stressful event is more crucial than the event itself.

Cataclysmic Events

Lazarus and Cohen defined cataclysmic events as "sudden, unique, and powerful single life-events requiring major adaptive responses from population groups sharing the experience" (p. 91). A number of cataclysmic events, both intentional and unintentional, strike unpredictably in areas around

the world. Unintentional major events include such natural disasters as hurricanes, typhoons, fires, tornadoes, floods, earthquakes, and other cataclysmic events that kill large numbers of people and create stress, grief, and fear among survivors. Some of these events, such as hurricanes, typhoons, and floods are unique and powerful but not necessarily sudden.

Occasionally, stressful events are so powerful that they affect nearly the entire globe, such as the great tsunami in the Indian Ocean in late December 2004 and hurricane Katrina and its aftermath, which destroyed New Orleans and other cities on the Gulf of Mexico in late August 2005, followed by hurricane Rita, which devastated southeast Texas and southwest Louisiana about a month later. The physical damage of these natural events was astronomical. More than 200,000 people were killed or missing and countless others left injured, sick, and homeless. Survivors of the tsunami (Dewaraja & Kawamura, 2006) and residents in the New Orleans area (Weems et al., 2007) experienced symptoms of depression and **posttraumatic stress disorder (PTSD)**. For the

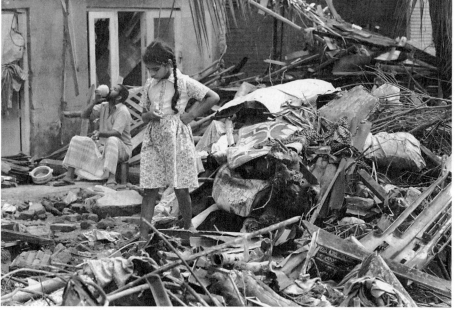

Cataclysmic events require major adaptive responses from large groups of people.

U.S. Gulf Coast residents, their symptoms were moderated or exacerbated by feelings of support from others, discrimination, and their proximity to the destruction.

Natural disasters can be devastating to huge numbers of people, but they cannot be blamed on any single person or group of persons. In contrast, the assassination of President John Kennedy, the 1995 bombing of the Murrah Federal Building in Oklahoma City, and the attack on the World Trade Center and the Pentagon on September 11, 2001, were all *intentional* acts. Each was sudden, unique, and powerful, and each required adaptive responses from large numbers of people. The aftermath of these cataclysmic events was brought into millions of homes by the media, resulting in multitudes of people having similar stress-related experiences.

Several factors contribute to how much stress an event creates, including physical proximity to the event, time elapsed since the event, and the intention of the perpetrators. The September 11 attack on the World Trade Center included all three factors for those living in New York City, creating lingering trauma for people close to the site (Hasin, Keyes, Hatzenbuehler, Aharonovich, & Alderson, 2007). For those not in New York City, stress associated with the attacks began to dissipate within weeks (Schlenger et al., 2002), but some evidence (Richman, Cloninger, & Rospenda, 2008) suggests that individuals in the midwestern United States continued to experience negative effects several years later. The intentional nature of the attacks added to the stress, making these violent events more traumatic than natural disasters.

Both adults and children reacted to the September 11 attacks with concern, distress, and worry. A national survey 3 to 5 days after the event (Schuster et al., 2001) reported that 90% of Americans experienced some stress as a result of the attacks. In addition, 35% of the adults said that they had children who showed signs of stress. People living closest to the attack were three times more likely to have experienced severe stress than those living farther away (Galea et al., 2002). Those individuals who were most severely affected were also more likely to experience effects a year later (Adams & Boscarino, 2005). People living in the Washington, D.C.,

area reported lower levels of stress than people in other metropolitan areas (Schlenger et al., 2002), possibly because the Pentagon building is somewhat isolated and only part of the structure was damaged, or possibly because people regard the Pentagon as part of the military and saw the attack as an act of war rather than terrorism.

Intentional acts seem to produce more widespread stress than do natural disasters. For example, more than one-third of the survivors of the Oklahoma City blast suffered from posttraumatic stress disorder (PTSD) six months after the bombing (North et al., 1999), whereas 24% of the survivors of an earthquake in Iceland were identified as having PTSD three months after the event (Bödvarsdóttir & Elklit, 2004). In addition, intentional violence driven by political motives is a widespread experience, whereas the effects of natural disasters are more confined to those who lived through the event (Norris, Byrne, Diaz, & Kaniasty, 2001).

In summary, cataclysmic events can be either intentional or unintentional, with different effects on stress. Such events strike suddenly, without warning, and people who survive them as well as those who help with the aftermath often see their experience as life altering. Despite the power of cataclysmic events to affect people, however, they have received less attention than life events as sources of stress (Richman et al., 2008).

Life Events

The second type of stress involves life events that affect us all. Experiencing the death of a spouse, getting a divorce, being fired from your job, or moving to a different country are major sources of stress, but minor life events can also be stressful. Some of the items on the Undergraduate Stress Questionnaire at the beginning of this chapter are life events, and the popular Holmes and Rahe (1967) Social Readjustment Rating Scale described earlier in this chapter consists of life events.

Life events differ from cataclysmic events in three important ways. Life events and life event scales emphasize the importance of *change*. When people are required to make some sort of change or readjustment, they feel stressed. Positive events such as getting married, becoming a parent, and starting a new job all require some adjustment, but negative events such as losing a job, the death of a family member, or being a victim of a violent crime also require adaptation. Unlike cataclysmic events that affect huge numbers of people, stressful life events affect a few people or perhaps only one. Divorce that happens to you can be more profound in changing your life than an earthquake in a far-off location that affects thousands. Lindsay Lohan mentioned her father's arrest and her separation from him as stresses in her life that affected her problem behavior and drug use (Silverman, 2008).

Cataclysmic events occur suddenly, but life events usually evolve more slowly. Divorce does not happen in a single day, and being dismissed from one's job is ordinarily preceded by a period of interpersonal friction. Crime victimization, however, is often sudden and unexpected. All of these life events produce stress, and subsequent problems are common. For example, divorce may decrease stress between the divorcing partners (Amato & Hohmann-Marriott, 2007) but more often creates short-term and sometimes long-term problems not only for the adults but also for their children (Michael, Torres, & Seemann, 2007). Losing a job may or may not be a major stressor, depending on the person's resources. When losing a job results in long-term unemployment, this situation creates a cascade of stressors, including financial problems and family conflict (Howe, Levy, & Caplan, 2004). Being the victim of a violent crime "transforms people into victims and changes their lives forever" (Koss, 1990, p. 374). Crime victims tend to lose their sense of invulnerability, and their risk of PTSD increases (Koss, Bailey, Yuan, Herrera, & Lichter, 2003). This risk applies to a variety of types of victimization, and the risk of PTSD has been established for children (Sebre et al., 2004) as well as for adults. Even exposure to community violence increases risks for children (Rosario, Salzinger, Feldman, & Ng-Mak, 2008).

Daily Hassles

Unlike life events that call for people to make adjustments in their lives, daily hassles are part of everyday life. Although some hassles are rare or occasional (such as misplacing one's car keys), others are repetitive, chronic, and often beyond personal control. Living in poverty, fearing crime, arguing with one's spouse, balancing work with family life, living in crowded and polluted conditions, and fighting a long daily commute to work are examples of daily hassles. The stress brought on by daily hassles can originate from both the physical and the psychosocial environment.

Daily Hassles and the Physical Environment Many people associate environmental sources of stress with urban life. They think of noise, pollution, crowding, fear of crime, and personal alienation as being associated with city living. Although these environmental sources of stress may be more concentrated in urban settings, rural life can also be noisy, polluted, hot, cold, humid, or even crowded, with many people living together in a one- or two-room dwelling. Air and water pollution originating in urban or industrial settings may disperse to other, nonurban settings. Nonetheless, the crowding, noise, pollution, fear of crime, and personal alienation more typical of urban living combine to produce what Eric Graig (1993) termed **urban press.** The results from one study (Christenfeld, Glynn, Phillips, & Shrira, 1999) suggested that the combined sources of stress affecting residents of New York City are factors in that city's higher heart attack death rate. Living in a polluted, noisy, and crowded environment creates chronic daily hassles that not only make life unpleasant but may also affect behavior and performance (Evans & Stecker, 2004) and pose a risk to health (Schell & Denham, 2003). Access to a garden or park can diminish this stress; individuals whose living situations included such access reported lower stress (Nielsen & Hansen, 2007).

People tend to deal with problems produced by *pollution* in one of two ways—by ignoring the threat or by concentrating on the impact the pollution will have on them personally (Hatfield & Job, 2001). When neither of these strategies is possible, people may feel threats from environmental pollution, producing stress. For example, a study that examined residents who lived in an area contaminated by industrial pollution showed that these people exhibited significantly

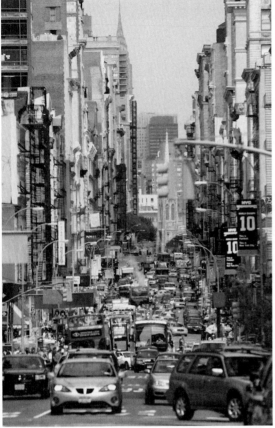

Crowding, noise, and pollution increase the stress of urban life.

more physical and psychological symptoms of stress than did people who lived in an uncontaminated area (Matthies, Hoeger, & Guski, 2000).

Noise is considered a type of pollution because it is a noxious, unwanted stimulus that intrudes into a person's environment, but it is quite difficult to define in any objective way. Definitions are invariably subjective because noise is a sound that a person does not want to hear. One person's music is another person's noise. The importance of subjective attitude toward noise was illustrated by a study (Nivision & Endresen, 1993) that asked residents living beside a busy street about their health, sleep, anxiety level, and attitude toward noise. The level of noise was not a factor, but the residents' subjective view of noise showed a strong relationship to the number of their health complaints. Similarly, workers who were more

sensitive to noise (Waye et al., 2002) showed a higher cortisol level and rated a low-frequency noise as more annoying than workers who were less sensitive. Other research demonstrated that noise and vibration affected performance on a cognitive task (Ljungberg & Neely, 2007). However, the most likely health effects of noise are probably hearing loss from the direct influence of exceedingly loud noise rather than an indirect effect produced by increased stress.

Another source of hassles is *crowding*. A series of classic experiments with rats living in crowded conditions (Calhoun, 1956, 1962) showed that crowding produced changes in social and sexual behavior that included increases in territoriality, aggression, and infant mortality and decreases in levels of social integration. These results suggest that crowding is a source of stress that affects behavior, but studies with humans are complicated by several factors, including a definition of crowding.

A distinction between the concepts of population density and crowding helps in understanding the effects of crowding on humans. In 1972, Daniel Stokols defined **population density** as a *physical* condition in which a large population occupies a limited space. **Crowding**, however, is a *psychological* condition that arises from a person's perception of the high-density environment in which that person is confined. Thus, density is necessary for crowding but does not automatically produce the feeling of being crowded. The crush of people in the lobby of a theater during intermission of a popular play may not be experienced as crowding, despite the extremely high population density. The distinction between density and crowding means that personal perceptions, such as a feeling of control, are critical in the definition of crowding. Crowding in both neighborhoods and residences plays a role in how stressed a person will be (Regoeczi, 2003).

Pollution, noise, and crowding often co-occur in "the environment of poverty" (Ulrich, 2002, p. 16). The environment of poverty may also include violence or the threat of violence and discrimination. On a daily basis, wealthier people experience fewer stressors than poor people (Grzywacz et al., 2004), but even wealthy people are not exempt.

Michalnapa.../Dreamstime.com

The threat of violence and fear of crime have become a part of the stress of modern life. Some evidence suggests that community violence is especially stressful for children and adolescents (Ozer, 2005; Rosario et al., 2008). However, the fear of crime is more widespread than is victimization: People who have never been victims are still afraid. This fear is exacerbated by media coverage that creates the impression that violence is more common than it is, cultivating fear (Van Den Buick, 2004). For example, many people are surprised to learn that violent crime has actually decreased over the past 50 years in the United States (USCB, 2007). The fear experienced over the possibility of victimization can isolate people from their neighbors, worsening the community climate and even affecting individual health (Stafford, Chandola, & Marmot, 2007).

In the United States, poverty is more common among ethnic minorities than among European Americans (USCB, 2007), and discrimination is another type of daily hassle that is often associated with the environment of poverty. However, discrimination is part of the psychosocial environment.

Daily Hassles and the Psychosocial Environment
People's psychosocial environment can be fertile ground for creating daily hassles. These stressors originate in the everyday social environment from sources such as community, workplace, and family interactions.

Discrimination is a stressor that occurs with alarming regularity in a variety of social situations in the community and workplace for African Americans in the United States (Landrine & Klonoff, 1996), but other ethnic groups (Edwards & Romero, 2008), women, and gay and bisexual men (Huebner & Davis, 2007) also face discrimination. Unfair treatment creates disadvantage for the individuals discriminated against and also creates a stigma that is stressful (Major & O'Brien, 2005). Discrimination is a source of stress that may increase the risk for cardiovascular disease (Troxel, Matthews, Bromberger, & Sutton-Tyrrell, 2003). Indeed, discrimination may be a factor in a variety of health problems (McKenzie, 2003).

Discrimination is not the only stressor that occurs in the workplace—some jobs are more stressful than others. Contrary to some people's

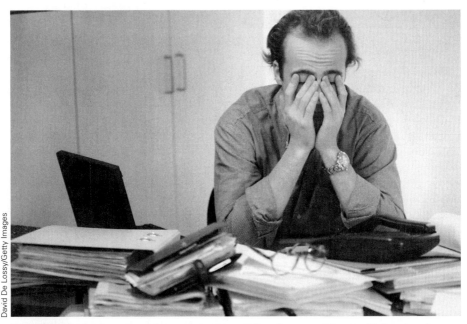

High job demands can produce stress, especially when combined with low levels of control.

assumption, business executives who must make many decisions every day have *less* job-related stress than their employees who merely carry out those decisions. Most executives have jobs in which the demands are high but so is their level of control, and research indicates that lack of control is more stressful than the burden of making decisions. Lower level occupations are actually more stressful than executive jobs (Wamala, Mittleman, Horsten, Schenck-Gustafsson, & Orth-Gomér, 2000). Using stress-related illness as a criterion, the jobs of construction worker, secretary, laboratory technician, waiter or waitress, machine operator, farmworker, and painter are among the most stressful. These jobs all share a high level of demand combined with a low level of control, status, and compensation. Middle-level managers such as foremen and supervisors also have highly stressful jobs. They must meet demands from two directions: their bosses and their workers. Thus, they have more than their share of stress (and stress-related illness).

Although it may seem ironic, celebrities such as Lindsay Lohan may experience job stress (Loftus, 1995). They are rarely in control of their careers and experience frequent periods of unemployment, creating stress.

High demands and low control combine to produce stress in a variety of work situations for both men and women (Wang, Lesage, Schmitz, & Drapeau, 2008). Men were also affected by lack of job security, whereas creating a balance between work and family life was more stressful for women. High demands and low control also combine with other workplace conditions to increase on-the-job stress. A situation such as working in a noisy environment may not be sufficient to produce stress, but when it is combined with other workplace factors such as rotating shift work (Cottington & House, 1987), signs of stress appear in both blood pressure and stress hormone production.

Stress from trying to balance the roles of worker and family member affects men as well as women. Half of all workers are married to someone who is also employed, creating multiple roles for both women and men (Moen & Yu, 2000). Problems may arise from work stress spilling over into the family or from family conflicts intruding into the

workplace (Ilies et al., 2007). The differences in men's and women's roles and expectations within the family mean that family and work conflicts influence women and men in different ways. Women often encounter stress because of the increased burden of doing the work associated with their multiple roles as employee, wife, and mother, but overall, these multiple roles offer health benefits (Barnett & Hyde, 2001; Schnittker, 2007).

The positive or negative effects of work and family roles depend on the resources people have available. Both men and women are affected by partner and family support, but women's health is more strongly affected by their absence (Walen & Lachman, 2000). Women with children and no partner are especially burdened and, therefore, stressed (Livermore & Powers, 2006). Thus, filling

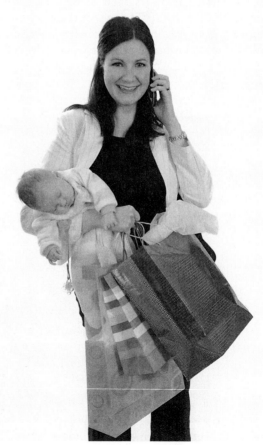

carebott/istock photo

Multiple roles can be a source of stress.

multiple obligations is not necessarily stressful for women, but low control and poor support for multiple roles can produce stress for both men and women. Partners perceive a lack of support as stressful (Dehle, Larsen, & Landers, 2001). Despite the possibilities for conflict and stress, families are a major source of social support, a resource that is important for coping with stress. Celebrities mention the importance of family as anchoring forces in their lives that can decrease their stress (Loftus, 1995). Lindsay Lohan's lack of family support may have contributed to her problems.

IN SUMMARY

Stress has a number of sources, which can be classified according to the magnitude of the event: cataclysmic events, life events, and daily hassles. Cataclysmic events include natural disasters such as floods and earthquakes and intentional violence such as terrorist attacks. Intentional violence tends to produce more distress, including an increased risk for post-traumatic stress disorder (PTSD).

Life events are events that produce changes in people's lives that require adaptation. Life events may be either negative or positive. Negative life events such as divorce, death of a family member, or crime victimization can produce severe and long-lasting stress.

Daily hassles are everyday events that create repetitive, chronic distress. Some hassles arise from the physical environment; others come from the psychosocial environment. Stress from pollution, noise, crowding, and violence combine in urban settings with commuting hassles to create a situation described as urban press. Each of these sources of stress may also be considered individually. Noise and crowding are annoyances, but there is some evidence that even low levels of these stressors can prompt stress responses, which suggests that long-term exposure may have negative health consequences. The combination of community stressors such as crowding, noise, and threat of violence is common in poor neighborhoods, creating an environment of poverty.

Daily hassles in the psychosocial environment occur within the situations of the everyday social environment, including community, workplace, and family. Within the community, racism and sexism produce stress for the targets of these types of discrimination. Within the workplace, jobs with high demands and little control create stress, and poor support adds to the stress. Within the family, relationships such as spouse and parent present possibilities for conflict and stress as well as support. In addition, the conflict between family and work demands is a source of stress for many people.

COPING WITH STRESS

People constantly attempt to manage the problems and stresses of their lives, and most of these attempts fit into the category of coping. However, the term **coping** is usually applied to strategies that individuals use to manage the distressing problems and emotions in their lives. The term first appeared in psychology research in the 1960s; the 1970s were a time of explosive growth on the topic (Folkman & Moskowitz, 2004; Martin & Brantley, 2004). Researchers have conducted thousands of studies on coping, exploring the personal and situational characteristics that affect coping efforts as well as the effectiveness of various coping strategies.

Personal Resources That Influence Coping

Lazarus and Folkman (1984) listed *health and energy* as one important coping resource. Healthy, robust individuals are better able to manage external and internal demands than are frail, sick, tired people. A second resource is a *positive belief*: the ability to cope with stress is enhanced when people believe they can successfully bring about desired consequences. This ability is related to a third resource: *problem-solving skills*. Knowledge of anatomy and physiology, for example, can be an important source of coping when receiving information about one's own health from a physician who is speaking in technical terms. *Material resources* are another important means of coping. Having the money to get one's car repaired decreases the stress of having a transmission problem. A fifth coping resource is *social skills*. Confidence in one's ability to get other people to cooperate can be an important source of stress management. Closely allied to this resource is *social support*, listed by Lazarus and Folkman as a sixth coping resource. During the 1980s, evidence began to emerge suggesting that people who receive support from friends, family members, and health care providers tend to live longer and healthier lives than people who lack support.

Social Support **Social support** refers to a variety of material and emotional supports a person receives from others. The related concepts of **social contacts** and **social network** are sometimes used interchangeably; both refer to the number and types of people with whom one associates. The opposite of social contacts is **social isolation**, which refers to an absence of specific, meaning-

ful interpersonal relations. People with a high level of social support ordinarily have a broad social network and many social contacts; socially isolated people have neither.

The Alameda County Study (Berkman & Syme, 1979) was the first to establish a strong link between social support and longevity. This study indicated that lack of social support was as strongly linked to mortality as cigarette smoking and a sedentary lifestyle. Figure 5.6 shows that women in all age groups had lower mortality rates than men (as indicated by the height of the bar in the graph). However, for both men and women, as the number of social ties decreased, the death rate increased. In general, participants with the fewest social ties were two to four times more likely to die than participants with the most social ties. The effects were not uniform for all age groups, but the benefits of social support apply to many age groups, including college students (Hale, Hannum,

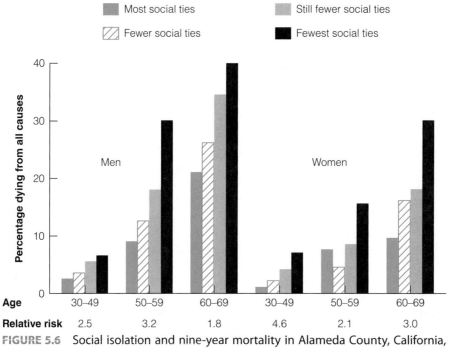

FIGURE 5.6 Social isolation and nine-year mortality in Alameda County, California, 1965–1974.

Source: From "Social Networks, Host Resistance, and Mortality: A Nine-Year Follow-up of Alameda County Residents," by L. F. Berkman & S. L. Syme, 1979, *American Journal of Epidemiology, 109,* p. 190. Copyright © 1979 by the Johns Hopkins University School of Hygiene and Public Health. Reprinted by permission of Oxford University Press.

& Espelage, 2005). Social support was related to better perceptions of health for college women and fewer physical symptoms for college men.

Social support may influence stress in several ways. For example, stressed individuals may benefit from a support network with members who encourage them to adopt healthier habits, such as stopping smoking, beginning an exercise program, or keeping doctor's appointments. Social support may also help people gain confidence in their ability to handle stressful situations; thus, when they experience stress, they may appraise the stressor as less threatening than do people who have fewer coping resources (Wills, 1998). Another possibility is that social support may alter the physiological responses to stress (DeVries, Glasper, & Detillion, 2003; Kiecolt-Glaser & Newton, 2001). This view, referred to as the *stress-buffering hypothesis*, suggests that social support lessens or eliminates the harmful effects of stress and therefore protects against disease and death. A longitudinal study of Canadians (Shields, 2004) provided limited support for this view. For adults who experienced little stress, social support was not very important in their feelings of distress; for those who experienced more stress, emotional support exerted a buffering effect for women but not for men. However, emotional support provided only short-term psychological buffering effects, not long-term benefits in terms of physical symptoms. Thus, the benefits of social support probably operate indirectly through psychosocial channels to benefit health.

The positive effects of social support for health are well established (Martin & Brantley, 2004), but some individuals benefit more than others. For example, marriage (or at least happy marriage) would seem to provide excellent social support for both partners, but the benefits of marriage are not equal for women and men—being married benefits men's health more than women's (Kiecolt-Glaser & Newton, 2001). The reason for men's advantage is not clear, but one possibility is that women's role as caregivers puts them in the position of providing more care than they receive. Providing companionship is a positive factor for the caregiver as well as the recipient, but providing help comes at a cost to the helper (Strazdins & Broom, 2007). This situation may describe women's more than men's caregiving and thus the gender difference.

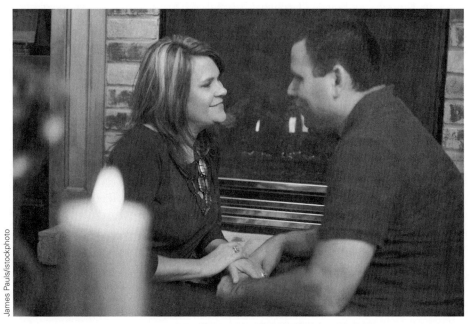

James Pauls/istockphoto

Emotional support and companionship are both beneficial to health.

Social support is a significant factor in predicting both the development of disease and the course of chronic disease (Martin & Brantley, 2004). Its benefits are entwined with another factor that influences coping: perceptions of personal control.

Personal Control   A second factor that may affect people's ability to cope with stressful life events is a feeling of **personal control**—that is, confidence that they have some control over the events that shape their lives. Both classic and current research confirms the benefits of a sense of control. One classic approach is Julian Rotter's (1966) concept of locus of control, a continuum that captures the extent to which people believe they are in control of the important events in their lives. According to Rotter, people who believe that they control their own lives have an *internal locus of control*, whereas those who believe that luck, fate, or the acts of others determine their lives score high on *external locus of control*. The value of an internal locus of control appeared in a study of people with chronic illness (Livneh, Lott, & Antonak, 2004); those who had adapted well showed a higher sense of control than those who had adapted poorly. Unfortunately, a longitudinal analysis of college students in the United States (Twenge, Liqing, & Im, 2004) showed a movement toward external locus of control over the past 40 years, which may be a danger signal for health.

Another classic example of the effects of personal control was reported by Ellen Langer and Judith Rodin (1976), who studied older nursing home residents. This research project encouraged some residents to assume more responsibility for and control over their daily lives, whereas others had decisions made for them. The areas of control were fairly minor, such as rearranging furniture, choosing when and with whom to visit in the home, and deciding what leisure activities to pursue. In addition, residents were offered a small growing plant, which they were free to accept or reject and to care for as they wished. A comparison group of residents received information that emphasized the responsibility of the nursing staff, and each of them also received a live plant. Although equal in

most other ways, the amount of control made a substantial difference in health. Residents in the responsibility-induced group were happier, more active, and more alert, with a higher level of general well-being. In just three weeks, most of the comparison group (71%) had become more debilitated, whereas nearly all the responsibility-induced group (93%) showed some overall mental and physical improvement. An 18-month follow-up of these same residents (Rodin & Langer, 1977) showed that residents in the original responsibility-induced group retained their advantage, and their mortality rate was lower than that of the comparison group.

These studies suggest that even a minimal amount of control can be beneficial to health, and an analysis of the components of control (Montpetit & Bergeman, 2007) suggests that self-efficacy is an important factor in the sense of control. However, the benefits of control may be bound to Western cultures that emphasize individual autonomy and effort. In a comparison of stress and coping among people from Japan and Great Britain (O'Connor & Shimizu, 2002), the Japanese participants reported a lower sense of personal control, but only the British reported that loss of control produced stress. Thus, the results concerning the benefits of personal control may be restricted to people in Western societies.

Personal Hardiness   In 1977, Suzanne Kobasa and her mentor Salvatore Maddi proposed the notion of the hardy personality as an explanation for why some people are resilient to stress and others are not. Kobasa and Maddi (1977) hypothesized that hardiness buffers the harmful effects of stress and thus protects the hardy personality from stress-related illness. A longitudinal test of this model on business executives (Kobasa, 1979) revealed a difference between executives who were able to withstand stress and those who were not in terms of (1) a sense of *commitment* to self, (2) *control* over their lives, and (3) a view of necessary readjustments as *challenges* rather than stress. These three factors—commitment, control, and challenge—separated the hardy executives from those who became sick, even though both groups experienced equal amounts of stress.

The notion that some people possess personal traits that help protect them against the harmful effects of stress is an appealing one, and a great deal of research has been conducted in this area. With its origins embedded in existential philosophy and psychology, the concept of hardiness is probably not applicable to all people (Klag & Bradley, 2004; Turnipseed, 2003). However, hardiness is one of the concepts that contributes to an explanation of why some people are more resilient to stress than others (Bonanno, 2004) and represents one of the "pathways to resilience" (Maddi, 2005, p. 261). Another approach to understanding differences in stress focuses on coping strategies.

Personal Coping Strategies

Coping strategies can be categorized in many ways, but Folkman and Lazarus's (1980) conceptualization of coping strategies as emotion focused or problem focused has been influential. **Problem-focused coping** is aimed at changing the source of the stress, whereas **emotion-focused coping** is oriented toward managing the emotions that accompany the perception of stress. Both approaches can be effective in making the stressed individual feel better, but the two approaches may not be equally effective in managing the stressful situation.

Several different strategies fall within the emotion-focused and problem-focused categories. For example, taking action to try to get rid of the problem is a problem-focused strategy, but so is making a plan of the steps to take or asking someone to help you in solving the problem. Getting upset and venting emotions is clearly emotion focused, but seeking the company of friends or family for comfort and reassurance and refusing to accept the situation are also strategies oriented toward managing the negative emotions associated with stress.

If an upcoming exam is a source of stress, a problem-focused strategy might be making (and following) a schedule for studying. Calling up a friend and complaining about the test or going out to a movie might help manage the distress, but these strategies are almost certainly not the most effective ways of dealing with the upcoming

test. The problem-focused strategy clearly sounds like a better choice in this case, but emotion-focused coping can be effective in some situations (Folkman & Moskowitz, 2004). In situations in which the stress is unavoidable, finding a way to feel better may be the best option. For example, a person has few options for problem-focused coping while undergoing an unpleasant dental procedure, and distancing oneself from unpleasant feelings may be the best way to cope during the procedure (although avoiding having a necessary procedure would *not* be a wise coping strategy). For an unusual coping strategy, see the Would You Believe...? box.

Additional categories have been considered to label coping strategies (Folkman & Moskowitz, 2004). These possibilities include *social coping*, such as seeking support from others, and *meaning-focused coping*, in which the person concentrates on deriving meaning from the stressful experience. For example, people who have experienced a trauma such as loss of a loved one or a diagnosis of a serious disease often attempt to understand the personal (and often spiritual) meaning within the situation. People who take this approach often succeed (Folkman & Moskowitz, 2000), and in doing so experience positive well-being (Helgeson, Reynolds, & Tomich, 2006). All of these coping strategies involve reactions to existing stressors, but people may also act to avoid stress.

Anticipating a problem and taking steps to avoid it is known as **proactive coping** (Aspinwall & Taylor, 1997). The process includes accumulating resources that will be useful, recognizing upcoming problems, and appraising the situation before attempting preliminary coping. This process may sound ideal because it allows a person to avoid stress, but proactive coping has the disadvantage of expending effort in preparation for an event that may not occur or may not be as stressful as anticipated.

A meta-analysis of the effects of coping strategies on psychological and physical health (Penley, Tomaka, & Wiebe, 2002) revealed benefits for some coping strategies but risks for some others. The relationships between coping strategies and health outcomes were mediated by the type of

WOULD YOU BELIEVE . . . ?

You May Be Able to Take a Bite Out of Stress

As unlikely as it may seem, the act of biting may reduce stress. This finding appeared in a study with rats (Okada et al., 2007) in which researchers exposed rats to stress by restraining them for an hour. Half of the rats were allowed to bite a wooden stick during the restraint, and the other half were not. Measurements of blood pressure, body core temperature, and immune system function indicated that biting moderated the stress response. Chewing may play a role in coping with stress.

Do these results apply to humans? Other research suggests that they do. In a study conducted with human participants in a laboratory stress experiment, the participants who chewed gum experienced lower levels of stress than those who did not (Scholey, Robertson, Haskell, Milne, & Kennedy, 2008). The participants rated their stress and anxiety, but researchers also measured cortisol in saliva samples. The results indicated that the laboratory stressor was successful in inducing stress, and chewing

gum was helpful in reducing stress. This effect appeared both in the self-ratings and in the physiological measurement of salivary cortisol.

These findings may explain why some people bite their fingernails, chew their lips, pencils, or gum, or eat when they are stressed. The act of chewing may be an effective coping strategy, helping people take a bite out of stress.

---

stressor and whether the impact was on psychological or physical health. In general, problem-focused coping showed positive associations with good health, whereas emotion-focused coping strategies tended to show negative associations. For example, people who used avoidance-oriented coping, such as eating more, drinking, sleeping, or using drugs, reported poorer overall health. Results from another meta-analysis on studies available through a database in Taiwan (Yu, Chiu, Lin, Wang, & Chin, 2007) offered support for some of these findings, including the complex relationship between stress and coping strategies and differences in the use of coping strategies. For example, individuals who are stressed are less likely to use problem-focused and more likely to use emotion-focused coping strategies, although those who use problem-focused approaches tend to report less stress.

Problem-focused strategies typically show advantages over emotion-focused approaches because problem-focused coping has the potential to change the situation. One study (Park & Adler, 2003) found that students who used both were healthier; another study (Sasaki & Yamasaki, 2007) showed health benefits for students who used

problem-solving strategies but poorer outcomes for those whose use of emotional expression increased. Ideally, the process of coping would allow people to manage their distress in the short term and change the stressor in the long term.

Culture exerts a powerful influence on coping, and gender also shows some effects. One might imagine that people who live in cultures that emphasize social harmony would be more likely to use social coping strategies, but such is not the case (S. E. Taylor et al., 2004). Indeed, Koreans and Asian Americans reported that, when experiencing stress, they would be less likely than European Americans to seek assistance from their families. However, another study (Lincoln, Chatters, & Taylor, 2003) found that African Americans were more likely than European Americans to seek social support from their families.

Some studies have found cross-cultural similarities in coping strategies, and those studies tend to study people in similar situations. For example, a study of adolescents in seven European nations (Gelhaar et al., 2007) found similarities among coping strategies for adolescents in all of the nations, especially in job-related situations. Research on gender differences in coping has also tended to find small differences between women's and men's coping strategies when studying individuals in similar situations (Adams, Aranda, Kemp, & Takagi, 2002; Ronan, Dreer, Dollard, & Ronan, 2004; Sigmon, Stanton, & Snyder, 1995) but larger gender differences when studies fail to control for situation (Matud, 2004). Because gender roles vary among cultures, gender and culture may interact to create different situational demands for coping by men and women in various cultures.

IN SUMMARY

Humans have a natural tendency toward health and away from distress, disease, and pain, and both personal resources and a variety of coping strategies allow people to cope in order to avoid or minimize distress. Social support, defined as the emotional quality of one's social contacts, is inversely related to disease and death. In general, people with high levels of social support experience health advantages and lower mortality. People with adequate social support probably receive more encouragement and advice regarding good health practices and may react less strongly to stress, which may buffer them against the harmful effects of stress more than people who are socially isolated.

Adequate feelings of personal control also seem to enable people to cope better with stress and illness. People who believe that their lives are controlled by fate or outside forces have greater difficulty changing health-related behaviors than do those who believe that the locus of control resides with themselves. The classic studies of nursing home residents demonstrated that when people are allowed to assume even small amounts of personal control and responsibility, they seem to live longer and healthier lives.

People who have high personal hardiness are probably better able to cope with stress than are people with low hardiness scores. Research on the concept of hardiness has yielded mixed results, but hardiness is one of the factors in resilience.

Coping strategies may be classified in many ways, but the distinction between problem-focused coping, which is oriented toward solving the problem, and emotion-focused coping, which is oriented toward managing distress associated with stress, has been useful. In addition, meaning-focused coping helps people find underlying meaning in negative experiences, and proactive coping can even prevent stress. In general, problem-focused coping is more effective than other types, but all types of coping strategies may be effective in some situations. The key to successful coping is flexibility, leading to the use of an appropriate strategy for the situation.

BEHAVIORAL INTERVENTIONS FOR MANAGING STRESS

Psychologists have been prominent in devising techniques that teach people how to manage stress. Some authorities consider these behavioral techniques to be part of mind–body medicine and thus part of alternative medicine (Barnes et al., 2004), which is explored in Chapter 8. Other authorities consider that approaches such as relaxation training, biofeedback, and cognitive behavioral therapy have demonstrated sufficient effectiveness to be part of conventional medicine (Bassman & Uellendahl, 2003). Psychologists tend to focus on the behavioral aspects of these techniques and to consider them part of psychology. Health psychologists employ these techniques in the interventions they use to help people with stress-related problems.

Relaxation Training

Relaxation training is perhaps the simplest and easiest to use of all psychological interventions, and relaxation may be the key ingredient in other types of therapeutic interventions for managing stress.

What Is Relaxation Training? During the 1930s, Edmond Jacobson (1938) discussed a type of relaxation he called *progressive muscle relaxation*. With this procedure, patients first receive the explanation that their present tension is mostly a physical state resulting from tense muscles.

BECOMING HEALTHIER

Progressive muscle relaxation is a technique that you may be able to use to cope with stress and pain. Although some people may need the help of a trained therapist to master this approach, others are able to train themselves. To learn progressive muscle relaxation, recline in a comfortable chair in a room with no distractions. You may wish to remove your shoes and either dim the lights or close your eyes to enhance relaxation. Next, breathe deeply and exhale slowly. Repeat this deep breathing exercise several times until you begin to feel your body becoming more and more relaxed.

The next step is to select a muscle group (for example, your left hand) and deliberately tense that group of muscles. If you begin with your hand, make a fist and squeeze the fingers into your hand as hard as you can. Hold that tension for about 10 seconds and then slowly release the tension, concentrating on the relaxing, soothing sensations in your hand as the tension gradually drains away. Once the left hand is relaxed, shift to the right hand and repeat the procedure, while keeping your left hand as relaxed as possible. After both hands are relaxed, go through the same

tensing and relaxing sequence progressively with other muscle groups, including the arms, shoulders, neck, mouth, tongue, forehead, eyes, toes, feet, calves, thighs, back, and stomach. Then repeat the deep breathing exercises until you achieve a complete feeling of relaxation. Focus on the enjoyable sensation of relaxation, restricting your attention to the pleasant internal events and away from irritating external sources of pain or stress. You will probably need to practice this procedure several times to learn to quickly place your body into a state of deep relaxation.

While reclining in a comfortable chair, often with eyes closed and with no distracting lights or sounds, patients first breathe deeply and exhale slowly. After this, the series of deep muscle relaxation exercises begins, a process described in the Becoming Healthier box. Once patients learn the relaxation technique, they may practice independently or with prerecorded audiotapes at home. Length of relaxation training programs varies, but six to eight weeks and about 10 sessions with an instructor are usually sufficient to allow patients to easily and independently enter a state of deep relaxation (Blanchard & Andrasik, 1985).

Autogenics training is another approach to relaxation. Pioneered by Johannes Schultz during the 1920s and 1930s in Germany, the technique was refined by Wolfgang Luthe (Naylor & Marshall, 2007). Autogenics training consists of a series of exercises designed to reduce muscle tension, change the way people think, and change the content of people's thoughts. The process begins with a mental check of the body

and proceeds with suggestions for relaxation and warmth throughout the body. Advocates contend that practicing autogenics for 10 minutes at least twice a day reduces stress and thus improves health.

How Effective Is Relaxation Training? Like other psychological interventions, relaxation can be regarded as effective only if it proves more powerful than a control situation, or placebo. Research generally indicates that relaxation techniques meet this criterion (Jacobs, 2001). Indeed, relaxation may be an essential part of other interventions such as biofeedback and hypnotic therapies (see Chapter 8).

Relaxation techniques have been quite successful in treating stress. Relaxation training was a component in a successful stress management program for college students (Iglesias et al., 2005), and children were able to learn and to benefit from relaxation training (Lohaus & Klein-Hessling, 2003). Progressive muscle relaxation has been a component in effective treatment programs for

TABLE 5.2

Effectiveness of Relaxation Techniques

Problem	Findings	Studies
1. Stress management for college students	Relaxation is a component in successful stress management.	Iglesias et al., 2005
2. Hypertension, insomnia, stress of cancer treatment	Progressive muscle relaxation is an effective component in programs to manage these disorders.	McCallie et al., 2006
3. Laboratory stress	Progressive muscle relaxation produces changes in heart rate, skin conductance, and skin temperature in children.	Lohaus & Klein-Hessling, 2003

such stress-related disorders as depression, hypertension, insomnia, and the stressful effects of cancer treatment (McCallie, Blum, & Hood, 2006).

Cognitive Behavioral Therapy

Health psychologists use the same types of interventions for managing stress that they use for other behavior problems, including *cognitive behavioral therapy*. This approach is a combination of *behavior modification*, which arose from the laboratory research on operant conditioning, and *cognitive therapy*, which can be traced to research on mental processes. Cognitive behavioral therapy has demonstrated greater effectiveness than any other approach for stress management.

What Is Cognitive Behavioral Therapy? **Cognitive behavioral therapy** (CBT) is a type of therapy that aims to develop beliefs, attitudes, thoughts, and skills to make positive changes in behavior. Like cognitive therapy, CBT assumes that thoughts and feelings are the basis of behavior, so CBT begins with changing attitudes. Like behavior modification, CBT focuses on modifying environmental contingencies and building skills to change observable behavior.

An example of CBT for stress management is the stress inoculation program developed by Donald Meichenbaum and Roy Cameron (1983; Meichenbaum, 2007). The procedure works in a manner analogous to vaccination. By introducing a weakened dose of a pathogen (in this case, the pathogen is stress), the therapist attempts to build some immunity against high levels of stress. Stress inoculation includes three stages: conceptualization, skills acquisition and rehearsal, and follow-through or application. The *conceptualization* stage is a cognitive intervention in which the therapist works with clients to identify and clarify their problems. During this overtly educational stage, patients learn about stress inoculation and how this technique can reduce their stress. The *skills acquisition and rehearsal* stage involves both educational and behavioral components to enhance patients' repertoire of coping skills. At this time, patients learn and practice new ways of coping with stress. One of the goals of this stage is to improve self-instruction by changing cognitions, a process that includes monitoring one's internal monologue—that is, self-talk. During the *application and follow-through* stage, patients put into practice the cognitive changes they have achieved in the two previous stages.

Another CBT approach to stress is cognitive behavioral stress management (CBSM; Antoni, Ironson, & Scheiderman, 2007), a 10-week group intervention that shares many features with stress inoculation training. CBSM also works toward changing cognitions concerning stress, enlarging clients' repertoire of coping skills, and guiding clients to apply these skills in effective ways. Other researchers have also used variations of CBT to investigate the effectiveness of this approach to stress management.

How Effective Is Cognitive Behavioral Therapy? Research on the efficacy of CBT indicates that it is effective for both prevention and management of stress and stress-related disorders. Furthermore, CBT has been effective with a wide variety of clients.

An early meta-analysis (Saunders, Driskell, Johnston, & Sales, 1996) of nearly 40 studies found that stress inoculation training was effective in decreasing anxiety and raising performance under stress. Stress inoculation training is effective for a range of stressors. For example, one program (Sheehy & Horan, 2004) tested the benefits of stress inoculation training for first-year law students to determine if the training helped these students alleviate some of their anxiety and stress. The results indicated that the program was successful in meeting those goals and also in raising grades.

Stress inoculation can also be effective in helping victims of trauma manage their severe distress (Cahill & Foa, 2007). For example, stress inoculation is helpful for crime victims who experience posttraumatic stress disorder (Hembree & Foa, 2003). A version of stress inoculation has been adapted for use on the Internet, making this therapy available to a larger number of people (Litz, Williams, Wang, Bryant, & Engel, 2004).

Other varieties of cognitive behavioral therapy are effective for stress management, including cognitive behavioral stress management. This intervention may even help counteract the negative effects of stress by moderating the increased cortisol production that accompanies the stress response (Gaab et al., 2003; Gaab, Sonderegger, Scherrer, & Ehlert, 2007), an accomplishment that few techniques have achieved (see Chapter 6). However, these effects may not include dramatic improvement in immune functioning. A meta-analysis of cognitive behavioral interventions for people who are HIV positive (Crepaz et al., 2008) revealed significant positive effects for reductions in stress, depression, anxiety, and anger, but immune functioning was less improved.

Cognitive behavioral stress management has also been successful in helping those with substance abuse problems manage stress-induced cravings, which could give a significant boost to substance abuse treatment (Back, Gentilin, & Brady, 2007). Group cognitive behavioral therapy and trauma-focused cognitive behavioral therapy are also among the most effective interventions for posttraumatic stress disorder (Bisson & Andrew, 2007). Cognitive behavioral techniques have been applied to workplace stress management, and this approach has demonstrated consistently larger effects than other programs (Richardson & Rothstein, 2008). Furthermore, cognitive behavioral stress techniques can help students improve their performance; a cognitive behavioral stress intervention improved students' motivations and scores on standardized exams (Keogh, Bond, & Flaxman, 2006).

In summary, many studies show that cognitive behavioral therapy interventions can be effective for stress management for people with a variety of stress-related problems. These techniques are among the most effective types of behavioral management strategies. Table 5.3 summarizes the effectiveness of cognitive behavioral therapy for stress-related problems.

Emotional Disclosure

Research by James Pennebaker and colleagues (Pennebaker, Barger, & Tiebout, 1989) provided evidence that emotional self-disclosure improves both psychological and physical health. Prompted by this finding, other researchers have discovered that the positive effects of emotional disclosure extend to a variety of people, in myriad settings, and among diverse cultures.

What Is Emotional Disclosure? **Emotional disclosure** is a therapeutic technique in which people express their strong emotions by talking or writing about negative events that precipitated those emotions. For centuries, confession of sinful deeds has been part of personal healing in many religious rituals. Then, during the late 19th century, Joseph Breuer and Sigmund Freud (1895/1955) recognized the value of the "talking cure," and **catharsis**—the verbal expression of emotions—became an important part of psychotherapy. Pennebaker took the notion of catharsis beyond Breuer and Freud and has been able to demonstrate the health benefits of talking or writing about traumatic life events.

The general pattern of Pennebaker's research is to ask people to write or talk about traumatic events for 15 to 20 minutes, three or four times a week. Emotional disclosure should be distinguished from emotional expression. The latter term simply

TABLE 5.3

Effectiveness of Cognitive Behavioral Therapy

Problem	Findings	Studies
1. Performance anxiety	Inoculation training reduces performance anxiety and boosts performance under stress.	Saunders et al., 1996
2. Stress of law school	Stress inoculation training decreases stress and increases grades.	Sheehy & Horan, 2004
3. Posttraumatic stress disorder	Inoculation procedures lessen negative effects of posttraumatic stress disorder.	Cahill & Foa, 2007; Hembree & Foa, 2003; Litz et al., 2004
4. Hormonal stress responses affect immune system functioning	Cognitive behavioral stress management moderates cortisol production during stress response.	Gaab et al., 2003; Gaab et al., 2007
5. Stress, anxiety, depression in people with HIV	Cognitive behavioral therapy improves these symptoms of HIV.	Crepaz et al., 2008
6. Stress-related cravings	Cognitive behavioral stress management decreased cravings.	Back et al., 2007
7. Posttraumatic stress disorder	Cognitive behavioral therapy is among the most effective treatments.	Bisson & Andrew, 2007
8. Workplace stress	Cognitive behavioral therapy is effective.	Richardson & Rothstein, 2008
9. School-related stress	Cognitive behavioral therapy boosts motivation and test performance.	Keogh et al., 2006

refers to emotional outbursts or emotional venting, such as crying, laughing, yelling, or throwing objects. Emotional disclosure, in contrast, involves the transfer of emotions into language and thus requires a measure of self-reflection. Emotional outbursts are often unhealthy and may add more stress to an already unpleasant situation.

In one of their early studies on emotional disclosure, Pennebaker and colleagues (Pennebaker et al., 1989) asked survivors of the Holocaust to talk for one to two hours about their war experiences. Those survivors who disclosed the most personally traumatic experiences had better subsequent health than survivors who expressed less painful experiences. Since then, Pennebaker and his colleagues have investigated other forms of emotional disclosure, such as asking people to talk into a tape recorder or speak to a therapist about highly stressful events. With each of these techniques, the key ingredient is language—the emotions must be expressed through language.

The physical and psychological changes in people who use emotional disclosure are typically compared with those of a control group, who are asked to write or talk about superficial events. This relatively simple procedure seems to be responsible for such physiological changes as fewer physician visits, improved immune functioning, and lower rates of asthma, arthritis, cancer, and heart disease. In addition, disclosure has produced psychological and behavioral changes, such as better grades among college students, increased ability to find new jobs, and an enhanced sense of well-being (Pennebaker & Graybeal, 2001).

How Effective Is Emotional Disclosure? A substantial number of studies by Pennebaker's team as well as by other researchers have demonstrated the effectiveness of disclosure in reducing a variety of illnesses. One early study (Pennebaker, Colder, & Sharp, 1990) showed that students who disclosed feelings about entering college had fewer illnesses than those who merely wrote about superficial topics. However, some people may benefit from writing about stresses more than others. One study indicated that both gender and initial level of distress moderated the effectiveness of emotional disclosure (Manier & Olivares, 2005).

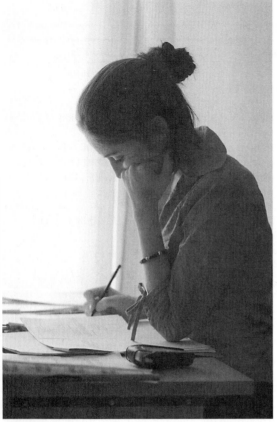

Writing about traumatic or highly stressful events produces physical as well as emotional benefits.

were asked to write about ways in which a traumatic life event had contributed to their personal growth, they received health benefits comparable to those who wrote about a traumatic experience without including episodes of personal growth (King & Miner, 2000). In another study, when participants were led to a less negative interpretation of a traumatic event, they experienced greater benefits than did those whose negative interpretations were validated (Lepore, Fernandez-Berrocal, Ragan, & Ramos, 2004). Other research (Lestideau & Levallee, 2007) suggested that when writing about a stressful situation, developing a plan for dealing with the situation boosted the benefits of expressive writing. These findings extend Pennebaker's research on disclosure by suggesting that people who concentrate on the positive aspects of a traumatic experience or develop a plan to deal with the stressful situation can receive health benefits equal or superior to those who simply write about a traumatic life event.

Pennebaker's research has added an effective and easily accessible tool to the arsenal of strategies for managing stress. Indeed, benefits can occur through a program of writing by e-mail (Sheese, Brown, & Graziano, 2004). See Table 5.4 for a summary of the effectiveness of self-disclosure through writing or talking.

The benefits of writing about stressful experiences extend to specific health problems as well as feelings of distress. Despite its emotional basis, a meta-analysis of studies on emotional disclosure (Frisina, Borod, & Lepore, 2004) indicated that this approach was more effective in helping people with physical than psychological problems. Emotional disclosure may reduce symptoms in patients with asthma and arthritis (Smyth, Stone, Hurewitz, & Kaell, 1999) and buffer some of the problems associated with cancer (Zakowski, Ramati, Morton, & Flanigan, 2004).

Must the emotional disclosure focus on trauma? Some evidence indicates that when people focus on finding some positive aspect of a traumatic experience, they may accrue even more benefits than when they focus on the negative aspects of the experience. When college students

IN SUMMARY

Health psychologists help people cope with stress by using relaxation training, cognitive behavioral therapy, and emotional disclosure. Relaxation techniques include progressive muscle relaxation and autogenics training. Relaxation approaches have demonstrated some success in helping patients manage stress and anxiety. Relaxation is generally more effective than a placebo.

Cognitive behavioral therapy draws upon operant conditioning and behavior modification as well as cognitive therapy, which strives to change behavior through changing attitudes and beliefs. Cognitive behavioral therapists attempt to get patients to think differently about their stress experiences and teach strategies that lead to more effective self-management.

TABLE 5.4
Effectiveness of Emotional Disclosure

Problem	Findings	Studies
1. General health problems	Holocaust survivors who talked most about their experience had fewer health problems 14 months later.	Pennebaker et al., 1989
2. Anxiety about entering college	Students who disclosed had fewer illnesses.	Pennebaker et al., 1990
3. Asthma, rheumatoid arthritis, and living with cancer	Keeping a journal of stressful events reduces symptoms and improves functioning.	Smyth et al., 1999; Zakowski et al., 2004
4. Visits to a health center for illness	Writing about the positive aspects of traumatic events is as effective as writing only about negative aspects of traumatic events.	King & Miner, 2000
5. Emotional and physical symptoms	Focusing on less traumatic aspects of situation produced greater benefits than focusing on negative.	Lepore et al., 2004
6. Emotional and physical symptoms	Focusing on developing a plan produced greater benefits than focusing only on emotions.	Lestideau & Levallee, 2007
7. Problems in mental and physical health	E-mail writing about traumatic events showed benefits.	Sheese et al., 2004

Stress inoculation and cognitive behavioral stress management are types of cognitive behavioral therapy interventions. Stress inoculation introduces low levels of stress and then teaches skills for coping and application of those skills. Stress inoculation and cognitive behavioral stress management have been successful interventions for preventing stress and in treating a wide variety of stress problems, including anxiety and depression in people with HIV, stress-cravings in people with substance use disorders, posttraumatic stress disorder, workplace stress, and school-related stress.

Emotional disclosure calls for patients to disclose strong negative emotions, most often through writing. People using this technique write about traumatic life events for 15 to 20 minutes, three or four times a week. Emotional disclosure generally enhances health, relieves anxiety, and reduces visits to health care providers, and may reduce the symptoms of asthma, rheumatoid arthritis, and cancer.

ANSWERS

This chapter has addressed six basic questions:

1. What is the physiology of stress?

The nervous system plays a central role in the physiology of stress. When a person perceives stress, the sympathetic division of the autonomic nervous system stimulates the adrenal medulla, producing catecholamines and arousing the person from a resting state. The perception of stress also prompts a second route of response through the pituitary gland, which releases adrenocorticotropic hormone (ACTH). This hormone, in turn, affects the adrenal cortex, which produces glucocorticoids. These hormones prepare the body to resist stress.

2. What theories explain stress?

Hans Selye and Richard Lazarus both proposed theories of stress. During his career, Selye defined stress first as a stimulus and then as a response. Whenever the body encounters a disruptive stimulus, it mobilizes itself in a generalized attempt to adapt to that stimulus. Selye called this mobilization the general adaptation syndrome. The GAS has three stages—alarm, resistance, and exhaustion—and the potential for trauma or illness exists at all three stages. Lazarus insisted that a person's perception of a situation is the most significant component of stress. To Lazarus, stress depends on one's appraisal of an event rather than on the event itself. Whether or not stress produces illness is closely tied to one's vulnerability as well as to one's perceived ability to cope with the situation.

3. How has stress been measured?

Stress has been assessed by several methods, including physiological and biochemical measures and self-reports of stressful events. Most life events scales are patterned after Holmes and Rahe's Social Readjustment Rating Scale. Some of these instruments include only undesirable events, but the SRRS and other self-report inventories are based on the premise that any major change is stressful. Lazarus and his associates have pioneered scales that measure daily hassles and uplifts. These scales, which generally have better validity than the SRRS, emphasize the severity of the event as perceived by the person.

Physiological and biochemical measures have the advantage of good reliability, whereas self-report inventories pose more problems in demonstrating reliability and validity. Although most self-report inventories have acceptable reliability, their ability to predict illness remains to be established. For these stress inventories to predict illness, two conditions must be met: first, they must be valid measures of stress; second, stress must be related to illness. Chapter 6 takes up the question of whether stress causes illness.

4. What sources produce stress?

Sources of stress can be categorized as cataclysmic events, life events, and daily hassles. Cataclysmic events include sudden, unexpected events that produce major demands for adaptation. Such events include natural disasters such as earthquakes and hurricanes and intentional events such as terrorist attacks. Posttraumatic stress disorder is a possibility in the aftermath of such events.

Life events such as divorce, criminal victimization, or death of a family member also produce major life changes and require adaptation, but life events are usually not as sudden and dramatic as cataclysmic events. Daily hassles are even smaller and more common, but produce distress. Such daily events may arise from the community, as with noise, crowding, and pollution; from workplace conditions, such as work with high demands and little control; or from conflicts in relationships.

5. What factors influence coping, and what strategies are effective?

Factors that influence coping include social support, personal control, and personal hardiness. Social support, defined as the emotional quality of one's social contacts, is important to a person's ability to cope and to one's health. People with social support receive more encouragement and advice to seek medical care, and social support may provide a buffer against the physical effects of stress. Second, people's beliefs that they have control over the events of their life seem to have a positive impact on health. Even a sense of control over small matters may improve health and prolong life. The factor of personal hardiness includes components of commitment, control, and interpreting events as challenges rather than as stressors.

People use a variety of strategies to cope with stress, all of which may be successful. Problem-focused coping is often a better choice than emotion-focused efforts because problem-focused coping can change the source of the problem, eliminating the stress-producing situation. Emotion-focused coping is oriented toward managing the distress that accompanies stress. Proactive coping involves anticipating future stress and finding ways to prevent it. Research indicates that most people use a variety of coping strategies, often in combination, and this flexibility is important for effective coping.

6. What behavioral techniques are effective for stress management?

Three types of interventions are available to health psychologists in helping people cope with stress. First, relaxation training can help people cope with a variety of stress problems. Second, cognitive behavioral therapy—including stress inoculation and cognitive behavioral stress management—is effective in reducing both stress and stress-related disorders such as posttraumatic stress disorder. Third, emotional disclosure—including writing about traumatic events—can help people recover from traumatic experiences and experience better psychological and physical health.

SUGGESTED READINGS

Kemeny, M. E. (2003). The psychobiology of stress. *Current Directions in Psychological Science, 12*, 124–129. This concise review furnishes a summary of the physiology of stress, how stress can "get under the skin" to influence disease, and some psychosocial factors that moderate this process.

Lazarus, R. S., & Folkman, S. (1984). *Stress, appraisal, and coping*. New York: Springer. In this classic book, Richard Lazarus and Susan Folkman present a comprehensive treatment of Lazarus's views of stress, cognitive appraisal, and coping. This book also discusses the relevant literature up to that time.

McEwen, B. S. (2005). Stressed or stressed out: What is the difference? *Journal of Psychiatry and Neuroscience, 30*, 315–318. This brief, readable article summarizes the evolution of the concept of stress, including Selye's work and changes to that framework.

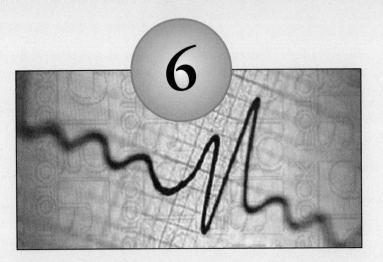

UNDERSTANDING STRESS
AND DISEASE

QUESTIONS

This chapter focuses on three basic questions:

1. How does the immune system function?

2. How does the field of psychoneuro-immunology relate behavior to disease?

3. Does stress cause disease?

This chapter reviews the evidence relating to stress as a possible cause of disease and follows Lindsay Lohan to see whether her stress and conflict place her at an elevated risk for disease or death. If stress, a psychological factor, can influence physical disease, some mechanism must exist to allow this interaction. We begin with a discussion of the immune system, which protects the body against stress-related diseases and could provide the mechanism for stress to cause disease.

PHYSIOLOGY OF THE IMMUNE SYSTEM

The immune system consists of tissues, organs, and processes that protect the body from invasion by foreign material, such as bacteria, viruses, and fungi (Schindler, Kerrigan, & Kelly, 2002). In addition, the immune system performs house-keeping functions by removing worn-out or damaged cells and patrolling for mutant cells. Once the invaders and renegades are located, the immune system activates processes to eliminate them.

Organs of the Immune System

Rather than being a centralized system, the immune system is spread throughout the body in the form of the **lymphatic system**. The tissue of the lymphatic system is **lymph**; it consists of the tissue components of blood other than red cells and platelets. In the process of vascular circulation, fluid and *leukocytes* (white blood cells) leak from the capillaries, escaping the circulatory system. Body cells also secrete white blood cells. This tissue fluid is referred to as lymph when it

enters the lymph vessels, which circulate lymph and eventually return it to the bloodstream.

Lymph circulates by entering the lymphatic system and then reentering the bloodstream rather than staying exclusively in the lymphatic system. The structure of the lymphatic system (see Figure 6.1) roughly parallels the circulatory system for blood. In its circulation, all lymph travels through at least one **lymph node**. The lymph nodes are round or oval capsules spaced throughout the lymphatic system that help clean lymph of cellular debris, bacteria, and even dust that has entered the body.

Lymphocytes are a type of white blood cell found in lymph. There are several types of lymphocytes, the most fully understood of which are T-lymphocytes, or **T-cells**; B-lymphocytes, or **B-cells**; and **natural killer (NK) cells**. Lymphocytes arise in the bone marrow, but they mature and differentiate in other structures of the immune system. In addition to lymphocytes, two other types of leukocytes are granulocytes and monocytes/macrophages. These leukocytes are involved in the nonspecific and specific immune system responses (discussed more fully later).

The **thymus**, which has endocrine functions, secretes a hormone called **thymosin**, which seems to be involved in the maturation and differentiation of the T-cells. Interestingly, the thymus is largest during infancy and childhood and then atrophies during adulthood. Its function is not entirely understood, but the thymus is clearly important in the immune system because its removal impairs immune function. Its atrophy also suggests that the immune system's production of T-cells is more efficient during childhood and that aging is related to lowered immune efficiency; research confirms this prediction (Briones, 2007).

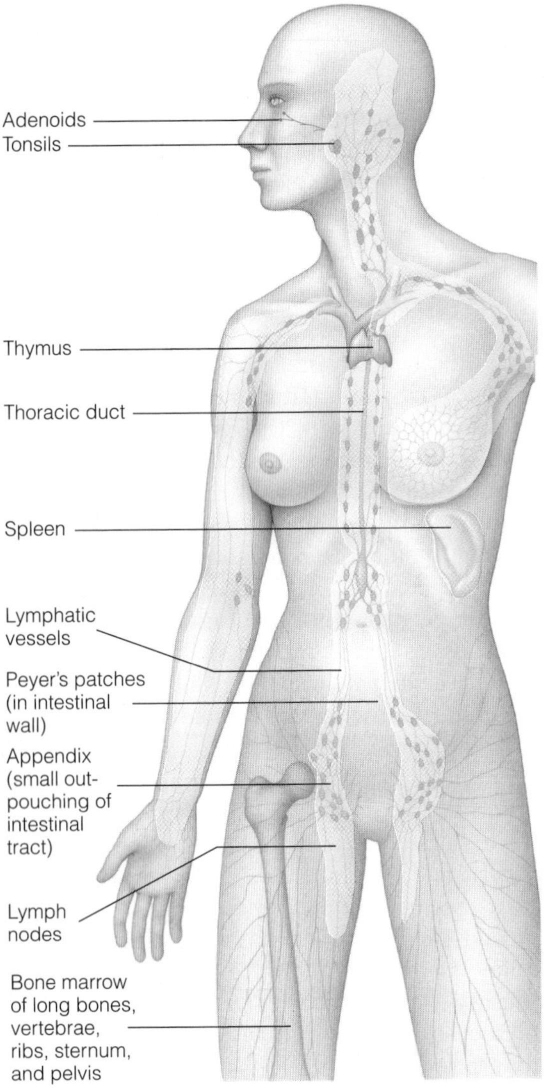

Adenoids
Tonsils

Thymus

Thoracic duct

Spleen

Lymphatic
vessels

Peyer's patches
(in intestinal
wall)

Appendix
(small out-
pouching of
intestinal
tract)

Lymph
nodes

Bone marrow
of long bones,
vertebrae,
ribs, sternum,
and pelvis

FIGURE 6.1 Lymphatic system.

Source: Introduction to Microbiology (p. 407), by J. L. Ingraham &
C. A. Ingraham, 1995, Belmont, CA: Wadsworth. Copyright 1995 by
Wadsworth Publishing Company. Reprinted by permission.

The **tonsils** are masses of lymphatic tissue located
in the throat. Their function seems to be similar
to that of the lymph nodes: trapping and killing
invading cells and particles. The **spleen**, an organ
near the stomach in the abdominal cavity, is one
site of lymphocyte maturation. In addition, it
serves as a holding station for lymphocytes as
well as a disposal site for worn-out blood cells.

The surveillance and protection that the immune system offers is not limited to the lymph
nodes but takes place in other tissues of the body
that contain lymphocytes. Thus, although the organs of the immune system may be considered to
be all those structures that manufacture, differentiate, store, and circulate lymph, immune function relies on more than these structures and is
not confined to the lymphatic system. To protect
the entire body, immune function must occur in
all parts of the body.

Function of the Immune System

The immune system's function is generally to
protect against injury and specifically to maintain vigilance against foreign substances that the
body encounters. The immune system must be
extraordinarily effective to prevent 100% of the
invading bacteria, viruses, and fungi from damaging our bodies. Few other body functions must
operate at 100% efficiency, but when this system
performs at some lesser capacity, the person (or
animal) becomes vulnerable.

Invading organisms have many ways to enter
the body, and the immune system has means to
combat each mode of entry. In general, immune
system responses to invading foreign substances
are of two types: general (nonspecific) and specific responses. Both may be involved in fighting
an invader.

Nonspecific Immune System Responses Intact skin
and mucous membranes are the first line of
defense against foreign substances, but some invaders regularly bypass them and enter the body.
Those that manage to do so face two general
(nonspecific) mechanisms. One is **phagocytosis**,
the attacking of foreign particles by cells of the
immune system. Two types of leukocytes perform this function. **Granulocytes** contain gran-
ules filled with chemicals. When these cells come
into contact with invaders, they release their
chemicals, which attack the invaders. **Macrophages** perform a variety of immune functions,
including scavenging for worn-out cells and debris, assisting in the initiation of specific immune
responses, and secreting a variety of chemicals
involved in breaking down the cell membranes

of invaders. Thus, phagocytosis, which is part of the nonspecific immune system response, involves several mechanisms that can quickly result in the destruction of invading bacteria, viruses, and fungi. However, some invaders escape this nonspecific action.

A second type of nonspecific immune system response is **inflammation**, which works to restore tissues that have been damaged by invaders. When an injury occurs, blood vessels in the area of injury contract temporarily. Later they dilate, increasing blood flow to the tissues and causing the warmth and redness that accompany inflammation. The damaged cells release enzymes that help destroy invading microorganisms; these enzymes can also aid in their own digestion, should the cells die. Both granulocytes and macrophages migrate to the site of injury to battle the invaders. Finally, tissue repair begins. Figure 6.2 illustrates the process of inflammation.

Specific Immune Systems Responses Two types of lymphocytes, T-cells and B-cells, carry out specific immune responses—that is, an immune response that is specific to one invader. When a lymphocyte encounters a foreign substance for the first time, both the general response and a specific response occur. Invading microorganisms are killed and eaten by macrophages, which present fragments of these invaders to T-cells that have moved to the area of inflammation. This contact sensitizes the T-cells, and they acquire specific receptors on their surfaces that enable them to recognize the invader. An army of *cytotoxic T-cells* forms through this process, and it soon mobilizes a direct attack on the invaders. This process is referred to as *cell-mediated immunity* because it occurs at the level of the body cells rather than in the bloodstream. Cell-mediated immunity is especially effective against fungi, viruses that have already entered the cells, parasites, and mutations of body cells.

The other variety of lymphocyte, the B-cells, mobilizes an indirect attack on invading microorganisms. With the help of one variety of T-cell (the *helper T-cell*), B-cells differentiate into **plasma cells** and secrete **antibodies**. Each antibody is specifically manufactured in response to a specific invader. Foreign substances that provoke antibody

manufacture are called **antigens** (for *anti*body *gen*erator). Antibodies circulate, find their antigens, bind to them, and mark them for later destruction. Figure 6.3 shows the differentiation of T-cells and B-cells.

The specific reactions of the immune system constitute the *primary immune response*. Figure 6.4 shows the development of the primary immune response and depicts how subsequent exposure activates the *secondary immune response*. During initial exposure to an invader, some of the sensitized T-cells and B-cells replicate and, rather than going into action, are held in reserve. These *memory lymphocytes* form the basis for a rapid immune response on second exposure to the same invader. Memory lymphocytes can persist for years but will not be activated unless the antigen invader reappears. If it does, then the memory lymphocytes initiate the same sort of direct and indirect attacks that occurred at the first exposure, but much more rapidly. This specifically tailored rapid response to foreign microorganisms that occurs with repeated exposure is what most people consider **immunity**.

This system of immune response through B-cell recognition of antigens and their manufacture of antibodies is called **humoral immunity**, because it happens in the bloodstream. The process is especially effective in fighting viruses that have already entered the cells, parasites, and mutations of body cells.

Creating Immunity One widely used method to induce immunity is **vaccination**. In vaccination, a weakened form of a virus or bacterium is introduced into the body, stimulating the production of antibodies. These antibodies then confer immunity for an extended period. Smallpox, which once killed thousands of people each year, was eradicated through the use of vaccination. As a result, people are no longer vaccinated against this disease. Concerns about smallpox as a biological weapon are based on this lack of immunity.

Other vaccines exist for a variety of diseases. They are especially useful in the prevention of viral infections. However, immunity must be created for each specific virus, and thousands of viruses exist. Even viral diseases that produce similar symptoms, such as the common cold, may be caused by

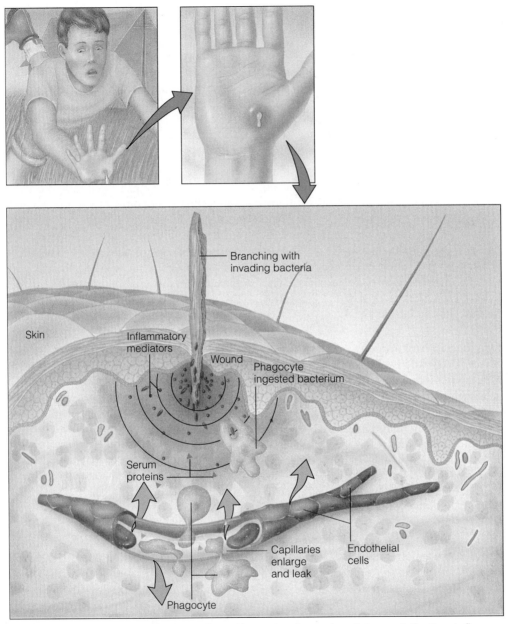

FIGURE 6.2 Acute inflammation is initiated by a stimulus such as injury or infection. Inflammatory mediators, produced at the site of the stimulus, cause blood vessels to dilate and increase their permeability; they also attract phagocytes to the site of inflammation and activate them.

Source: Introduction to Microbiology (p. 386), by J. L. Ingraham & C. A. Ingraham, 1995, Belmont, CA: Wadsworth. Copyright 1995 by Wadsworth Publishing Company. Reprinted by permission.

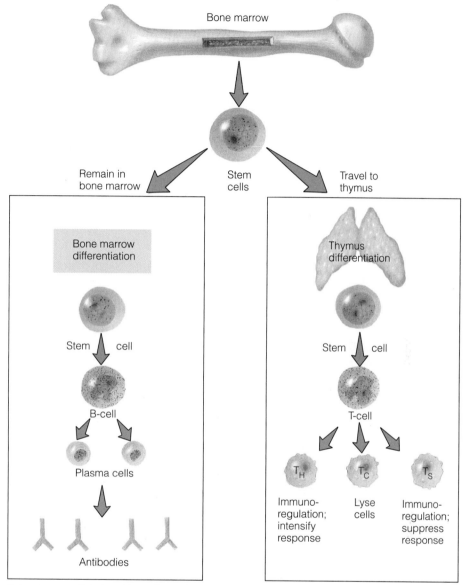

FIGURE 6.3   Origins of B-cells and T-cells.

Source: Introduction to Microbiology (p. 406), by J. L. Ingraham & C. A. Ingraham, 1995, Belmont, CA: Wadsworth. Copyright 1995 by Wadsworth Publishing Company. Reprinted by permission.

many different viruses. Therefore, immunity for colds would require many vaccinations, and such a process has not yet proven practical.

Immune System Disorders

Immune deficiency, an inadequate immune response, may occur for several reasons. For example, it is a side effect of most chemotherapy drugs used to treat cancer. Immune deficiency also occurs naturally. Although the immune system is not fully functional at birth, infants are protected by antibodies they have received from their mothers through the placenta, and infants who breast-feed receive antibodies from their mothers' milk. These antibodies

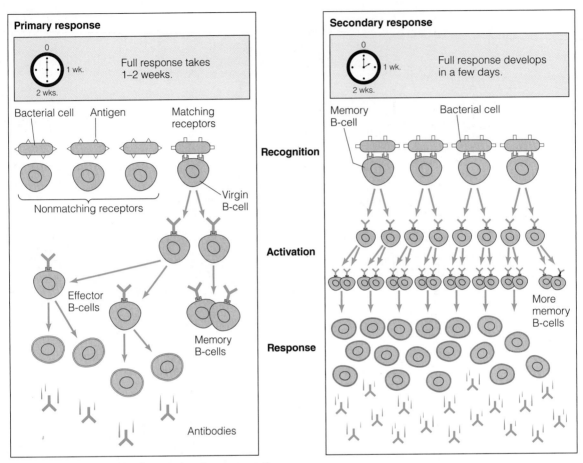

FIGURE 6.4   Primary and secondary immune pathways.

Source: Introduction to Microbiology (p. 414), by J. L. Ingraham & C. A. Ingraham, 1995, Belmont, CA: Wadsworth. Copyright 1995 by Wadsworth Publishing Company. Reprinted by permission.

offer protection until the infant's own immune system develops during the first months of life.

In rare cases, the immune system fails to develop, leaving the child without immune protection. Physicians can try to boost immune function, but the well-publicized "children in plastic bubbles" still show the results of immune deficiency. Exposure to any virus or bacterium can be fatal to these children. They are sealed into sterile quarters to isolate them from the microorganisms that are part of the normal world.

A much more common type of immune deficiency is **acquired immune deficiency syndrome (AIDS)**. This disease is caused by a virus, the human immunodeficiency virus (HIV), which acts to destroy the T-cells and macrophages in the immune system. Those who are infected with HIV may progress to AIDS. The destruction of their immune systems makes them vulnerable to a wide range of bacterial, viral, and malignant diseases. HIV is known to be contagious but not easily transmitted from person to person. The highest concentrations of the virus are found in blood and in semen. Blood transfusions from an infected person, injection with a contaminated needle, sexual intercourse, and transmission during the birth process seem to be the most common routes of infection. Treatment consists of controlling the proliferation of the virus through antiviral drugs and management of the diseases that develop as a result of immune deficiency. As of 2008, a combination of antiviral drugs was capable of slowing the progress of HIV infection, but no treatment was capable of eliminating HIV from an infected person.

Allergies constitute another immune system disorder. An allergic response is an abnormal reaction to a foreign substance that normally elicits little or no immune reaction. People with allergies are hypersensitive to certain substances. A wide range of substances can cause allergic reactions, and the severity of the reactions also varies widely. Some allergic reactions may be life threatening, whereas others merely cause runny noses. Some cases of allergy are treated by introducing regular, small doses of the allergen to desensitize the person to the allergen and diminish or alleviate the allergic response. Other cases of allergy are treated by teaching allergic individuals to recognize and avoid their allergens.

Autoimmune diseases occur when the immune system attacks the body, for reasons not well understood. Part of the function of the immune system is to recognize foreign invaders and mark them for destruction. In some people, the person's own body cells are marked for destruction. In these cases, the immune system appears to have lost the ability to distinguish the body from an invader, and it mounts the same vicious attack against itself that it would against an intruder. Lupus erythematosus, rheumatoid arthritis, and multiple sclerosis are autoimmune diseases.

Transplant rejection is not really an immune disorder, but it is a problem caused by the immune system's activity. When working efficiently, the immune system has the ability to detect foreign substances. With the exception of identical twins, no two humans have the same biochemistry. Therefore, the immune system normally recognizes any foreign tissue as an invader. A transplanted heart, liver, or kidney will be recognized as foreign tissue because the biochemical markers from its donor differ from those of its host. Thus, the host's immune system will try to destroy the transplant. In an effort to prevent this reaction, drugs are administered that suppress immune system function. This strategy often works, but unfortunately the suppression is not specific to the transplanted organ. The entire immune response is affected, leaving the person vulnerable to infection. Currently, people who have received successful organ transplants must adapt their lifestyles to minimize the risk of infection because of their weakened immune system. Modification of lifestyle and compliance with medical regimens are topics of interest to health psychologists and other health professionals who use them in the treatment of organ transplant patients.

According to the **immune surveillance theory**, cancer is also the result of an immune system failure. This view holds that the cellular mutations that initiate cancer occur quite frequently, but that these mutations are normally identified and killed by the T-cells in the immune system. Cancer develops when the immune system fails to identify and destroy mutant cells. This theory is controversial (Forlenza & Baum, 2004), but the immune system does respond to cancer.

IN SUMMARY

If stress can cause disease, it can do so only by affecting biological processes (see Figure 1.4). The most likely candidate for this interaction is the immune system, which is made up of tissues, organs, and processes that protect the body from invasion by foreign material such as bacteria, viruses, and fungi. The immune system also protects the body by eliminating damaged cells. Immune system responses can be either specific or nonspecific. Specific responses attack one particular invader, whereas nonspecific immunity is capable of attacking any invader. Immune system problems can stem from several sources, including organ transplants, allergies, drugs used for cancer chemotherapy, and immune deficiency. The human immunodeficiency virus (HIV) damages the immune system, creating a deficiency that leaves the person vulnerable to a variety of viral and malignant diseases.

PSYCHONEUROIMMUNOLOGY

The previous section examined the function of the immune system as well as its tissues, structure, and disorders. Physiologists have traditionally taken a similar approach, studying the immune system as separate from and independent of other body systems. About 30 years ago, however, evidence began to accumulate suggesting that the immune system interacts with the central nervous system (CNS) and the endocrine system; this evidence showed that psychological and social factors can affect the CNS, endocrine system, and immune system. In addition, immune function can affect neural function, providing the potential for the immune system to alter behavior and thought (Maier, 2003). This recognition led to the founding and rapid growth of the field of **psychoneuroimmunology (PNI),** a multidisciplinary field that focuses on the interactions among behavior, the nervous system, the endocrine system, and the immune system.

History of Psychoneuroimmunology

George Solomon and Rudolph Moos first used the term *psychoneuroimmunology* in a publication in 1964. In that article and in his research in the 1960s, Solomon laid the groundwork for the field of PNI.

An event that dramatically shaped the field of PNI was the 1975 publication of an article by Robert Ader and Nicholas Cohen on classical conditioning of the immune system. This research demonstrated how the nervous system, the immune system, and behavior could interact. Ader and Cohen conditioned rats to associate a novel, conditioning stimulus (CS)—a saccharin and water solution—with an unconditioned stimulus (UCS) that naturally produces an unconditioned response (UCR). In Ader and Cohen's procedure, a drug that suppresses the immune system was the UCS. The rats were allowed to drink the saccharin solution and then were injected with the drug. The response was the expected suppression of the immune system. However, the rats later showed immune suppression when they were given the saccharin solution alone. That is, their immune systems had been conditioned to respond to the saccharin solution in much the same manner that it reacted to the drug. This type of conditioning is not so surprising when one recalls Pavlov's classical experiment in which dogs learned to associate ringing bells with meat powder. But Ader and Cohen demonstrated that the immune system

was subject to the same type of associative learning as other body systems.

Until Ader and Cohen's 1975 report, most physiologists believed that the immune system and the nervous system did not interact, and their results were not immediately accepted (Fleshner & Laudenslager, 2004). After many replications of their findings, physiologists now accept that the immune system and other body systems exchange information in a variety of ways. One mechanism is through **cytokines,** chemical messengers secreted by cells in the immune system (Blalock & Smith, 2007; Maier & Watkins, 2003). One type of cytokine is known as *proinflammatory cytokines* because they promote inflammation. These cytokines, which include several types of *interleukins*, may underlie a number of states, including feelings associated with sickness and depression (Irwin, 2008; Kelley et al., 2003).

The developing knowledge of the connections between the immune and nervous systems spurred researchers to explore the physical mechanisms by which interactions occur. Psychologists began to use measures of immune function to test the effects of behavior on the immune system. During the 1980s, the AIDS epidemic focused public attention (and federal funding) on how behavior influences the immune system and therefore health. The vitality of the new field of psychoneuroimmunology was demonstrated by the appearance in 1987 of a journal, *Brain, Behavior, and Immunity*, devoted to reporting PNI research.

Research in Psychoneuroimmunology

Research in psychoneuroimmunology strives to develop an understanding of the role of behavior in changes in the immune system and the development of disease. To reach this goal, researchers must establish a connection between psychological factors and changes in immune function and also demonstrate a relationship between this impaired immune function and changes in health status. Ideally, research should include all three components—psychological distress, immune system malfunction, and development of disease—to establish the connection between stress and disease (Forlenza & Baum, 2004). This task is difficult for several reasons.

One reason for the difficulty is the less-than-perfect relationship between immune system malfunction and disease. Not all people with impaired immune systems become ill (Segerstrom & Miller, 2004). Disease is a function of both the immune system's competence and the person's exposure to pathogens, the agents that produce illness. The best approach in PNI comes from longitudinal studies that follow people for a period of time after they (1) experience stress that (2) prompts a decline in immunocompetence and then (3) assess changes in their health status. Few studies have included all three components, and most such studies have been restricted to nonhuman animals.

The majority of research in PNI has focused on the relationship between various stressors and altered immune system function. Most studies measure the immune system's function by testing blood samples rather than by testing immune function in people's bodies (Coe & Laudenslager, 2007; Segerstrom & Miller, 2004). Some research has concentrated on the relationship between altered immune system function and the development of disease or spread of cancer (Cohen, 2005; Reiche, Nunes, & Morimoto, 2004), but such studies are in the minority. Furthermore, the types of stressors, the species of animals, and the facet of immune system function studied have varied, resulting in a variety of findings (Forlenza & Baum, 2004).

Some researchers have manipulated short-term stressors such as electric shock, loud noises, or complex cognitive tasks in a laboratory situation; others have used naturally occurring stress in people's lives to test the effect of stress on immune system function. Laboratory studies allow researchers to investigate the physical changes that accompany stress, and such studies have shown correlations between sympathetic nervous system activation and immune responses (Glaser, 2005; Irwin, 2008). This research suggests that sympathetic activation may be a pathway through which stress can affect the immune system. The effect is initially positive, mobilizing resources, but continued stress activates physiological processes that can be damaging.

The naturally occurring stress of school exams provided an opportunity to study immune function in medical students (Kiecolt-Glaser, Malarkey, Cacioppo, & Glaser, 1994). A series of studies showed differences in immunocompetence, measured by numbers of natural killer cells, percentages of T-cells, and percentages of total lymphocytes. A longitudinal assessment of these medical students revealed a trend toward more symptoms of infectious disease immediately before and after exams. More recent research (Chandrashekara et al., 2007) has confirmed that anxious students taking exams experienced a lowering of immune function, which demonstrated that the effect on immune function was specific to the situation and to the students' psychological state.

Exam stress is typically a short-term stress, but chronic stress has even more severe effects on immune competence. Relationship conflict has been shown to relate to immune system suppression for couples that experience marital conflict (Kiecolt-Glaser & Newton, 2001). Indeed, marriage is important in immune function and to a wide range of health outcomes (Graham, Christian, & Kiecolt-Glaser, 2006). For example, effects of marital conflict may include poorer response to immunization and slower wound healing (Ebrecht et al., 2004), and lack of partner support may play a role in increased stress during pregnancy, which raises health risk (Coussons-Read, Okun, & Nettles, 2007).

Other chronic stressors also suppress immune function. For example, people who are caregivers for someone with Alzheimer's disease experience chronic stress (see Chapter 11 for more about the disease and the stress of caregiving). Alzheimer's caregivers experience poorer psychological and physical health, longer healing times for wounds, and lowered immune function (Damjanovic et al., 2007; Kiecolt-Glaser, 1999; Kiecolt-Glaser, Marucha, Malarkey, Mercado, & Glaser, 1995). Furthermore, the death of the Alzheimer's patient fails to improve the stressed caregivers' psychological health or immune system functioning (Robinson-Whelen, Tada, MacCallum, McGuire, & Kiecolt-Glaser, 2001). Both caregivers and former caregivers were more depressed and showed lowered immune system functioning, suggesting that this stress continues after the caregiving is over.

The results of meta-analyses of 30 years of studies on stress and immunity (Segerstrom & Miller, 2004) indicated that substantial evidence exists for a relationship between stress and decreased immune function, especially for chronic sources of stress. The stressors that exert the most chronic effects have the most global influence on the immune system. Refugees, the unemployed, and those who live in high-crime neighborhoods experience the type of chronic, uncontrollable stress that has the most widespread negative effect on the immune system. Short-term stress may produce changes that are adaptive, such as mobilizing hormone production, but chronic stress exerts effects on many types of immune system response that weaken immune system effectiveness.

Some of the PNI research that has most clearly demonstrated the three-way link among stress, immune function, and disease has used stressed rats as subjects, injecting material that provokes an immune system response and observing the resulting changes in immune function and disease (Bowers, Bilbo, Dhabhar, & Nelson, 2008). Some research with human participants has also demonstrated the link among stress, immune function, and disease (Cohen, 2005; Kiecolt-Glaser, McGuire, Robles, & Glaser, 2002). For example, healing time after receiving a standardized wound varies, depending on whether the wound occurs during vacation or during exams. Students under exam stress showed a decline in a specific immune function related to wound healing; the same students took 40% longer to heal during exams than they did during vacation. Thus, some research on human as well as nonhuman subjects has demonstrated that stress can affect immune function and disease processes.

If behavioral and social factors can decrease immune system function, is it possible to *boost* immunocompetence through changes in behavior? Would such an increase enhance health? A number of researchers have conducted interventions designed to increase the effectiveness of the immune system, but a meta-analysis of these studies (Miller & Cohen, 2001) indicated only modest effects. Similarly, a meta-analysis of cognitive behavioral interventions for HIV-positive men (Crepaz et al., 2008) showed significant effects for improvements in anxiety, stress, and depression but limited changes in immune system function. However, even small improvements may be an advantage for these individuals.

Physical Mechanisms of Influence

"Psychosocial factors do not influence disease in some mystic fashion. Rather, the physiological status of the host is altered in some way" (Plaut & Friedman, 1981, p. 5). The previous section presented studies showing that such influence occurs but did not explore the physiology underlying that influence.

The effects of stress can occur through the relationship of the nervous system to the immune system through two routes—the peripheral nervous system and the secretion of hormones. Evidence exists for connection through both routes. In addition, people who are attempting to cope with stress may behave in ways that affect their immune system negatively, such as missing sleep, drinking alcohol, or smoking (Segerstrom & Miller, 2004).

The peripheral nervous system provides connections to immune system organs such as the thymus, spleen, and lymph nodes. The brain can also communicate with the immune system through the production of *releasing factors*, hormones that stimulate endocrine glands to secrete hormones. These hormones travel through the bloodstream and affect target organs, such as the adrenal glands. (Chapter 5 included a description of these systems and the endocrine component of the stress response.) T-cells and B-cells have receptors for the glucocorticoid stress hormones.

When the sympathetic nervous system is activated, the adrenal glands release several hormones. The adrenal medulla releases epinephrine and norepinephrine, and the adrenal cortex releases cortisol. The modulation of immunity by epinephrine and norepinephrine seems to come about through the autonomic nervous system (Dougall & Baum, 2001).

The release of cortisol from the adrenal cortex results from the release of adrenocorticotropic hormone (ACTH) by the pituitary in the brain. Another brain structure, the hypothalamus, stimulates the pituitary to release ACTH.

Elevated cortisol is associated with a number of physical and emotional distress conditions (Dickerson & Kemeny, 2004), and it exerts an anti-inflammatory effect. Cortisol and the glucocorticoids tend to depress immune responses, phagocytosis, and macrophage activation. The nervous system can influence the immune system either through the sympathetic nervous system or through neuroendocrine response to stress.

Communication also occurs in the other direction: the immune system can signal the nervous system by way of cytokines, chemicals secreted by immune system cells (Irwin, 2008; Maier, 2003). Cytokines communicate with the brain, probably by way of the peripheral nervous system. This interconnection makes possible bidirectional interactions of immune and nervous systems and may even enable effects on behavior such as fatigue and depression, which are common symptoms of sickness. Michael Irwin (2008) emphasized the many possibilities for communication between the nervous and immune systems and how behavioral responses are the key to activating processes that influence the immune system. The interrelationship between nervous system and immune system makes it possible for each to influence the other to produce the symptoms associated with stress and disease.

Stress may also "get under the skin" by altering health-related behaviors (Segerstrom & Miller, 2004). For example, people under stress may smoke more cigarettes, drink more alcohol, use illicit drugs, and get less sleep. Each of these behaviors increases risk for a variety of diseases and may influence the immune system in negative ways.

IN SUMMARY

Researchers in the field of psychoneuroimmunology have demonstrated that various functions of the immune system respond to both short-term and long-term psychological stress. The field of psychoneuroimmunology has made progress toward linking psychological factors, immune system function, and disease, but few studies have included all three elements.

Some research has been successful in linking immune system changes to changes in health status; this link is necessary to complete the chain between psychological factors and disease. In addition to establishing links between psychological factors and immune system changes, theorists and researchers in the field of psychoneuroimmunology have attempted to specify the physical mechanisms through which these changes occur. Possible mechanisms include direct connections between nervous and immune systems and an indirect connection through the neuroendocrine system. Chemical messengers called cytokines also allow for communication between immune and nervous system and possible effects on behavior. In addition, stress may prompt people to change their behaviors, adopting less healthy habits that are risk factors for disease.

DOES STRESS CAUSE DISEASE?

Disease is caused by many factors, and stress may be one of those factors. In any consideration of the association between disease and major life events or daily hassles, remember that most people at risk from stressful experiences do *not* develop a disease. Furthermore, in contrast to other risk factors—such as having high cholesterol levels, smoking cigarettes, or drinking alcohol—the risks conferred by life events are usually temporary. Even temporary stress affects some people more than others.

Why does stress affect some people, apparently causing them to get sick, and leave others unaffected? Some high-stress individuals become sick, and others remain healthy. Then, too, some low-stress people develop a disease, and others do not. Why do some people fall ill from stress and other people stay well? The diathesis–stress model offers a possible answer to this question.

The Diathesis–Stress Model

The **diathesis–stress model** suggests that some individuals are vulnerable to stress-related diseases because either genetic weakness or biochemical imbalance inherently predisposes them to those diseases. The diathesis–stress model has a long history in psychology, particularly in explaining the development of psychological disorders. During the 1960s and 1970s, the concept was used as an explanation for the development of psychophysiological disorders (Levi, 1974) as well as schizophrenic episodes, depression, and anxiety disorders (Zubin & Spring, 1977).

Applied to either psychological or physiological disorders, the diathesis–stress model holds that some people are predisposed to react abnormally to environmental stressors. This predisposition (diathesis) is usually thought to be inherited through biochemical or organ system weakness, but some theorists (Zubin & Spring, 1977) have also included acquired propensities as components of vulnerability. Whether inherited or acquired, the vulnerability is relatively permanent. What varies over time is the presence of environmental stressors, which may account for the waxing and waning of illnesses.

Thus, the diathesis–stress model assumes that two factors are necessary to produce disease. First, the person must have a relatively permanent predisposition to the disease, and second, that person must experience some sort of stress. Diathetic individuals respond pathologically to the same stressful conditions with which most people are able to cope. For people with a strong predisposition to a disease, even a mild environmental stressor may be sufficient to produce an illness episode. For example, a study of symptom stress and depression (Schroeder, 2004) revealed that surgical patients with low coping competence were vulnerable to developing depression in the months following their surgery, whereas patients with better coping skills were less vulnerable to depression. Abuse or maltreatment during childhood may create another source of vulnerability to physical and psychological disorders. As adults, these individuals show increased vulnerability to schizophrenia (Rosenberg, Lu, Mueser, Jankowski, & Cournos, 2007), anxiety and depression (Stein, Schork, & Gelernter, 2008), posttraumatic stress disorder (Storr, Lalongo, Anthony, & Breslau, 2007), and infectious disease (Cohen, 2005). Therefore, personal and psychosocial factors have the power to create vulnerabilities to disorders.

The diathesis–stress model may explain why life event scales (see Chapter 5) are so inconsistent in predicting illness. The number of points accumulated on the Holmes and Rahe Social Readjustment Rating Scale or the number of items checked on the Undergraduate Stress Questionnaire is only a weak predictor of illness. The diathesis–stress model holds that a person's diathesis (vulnerability) must be considered along with stressful life events in predicting who will get sick and who will stay well; it allows for a great deal of individual variability in who gets sick and who stays well under conditions of stress (Marsland, Bachen, Cohen, & Manuck, 2001).

In this section, we review the evidence concerning the link between stress and several diseases, including headache, infectious disease, cardiovascular disease, diabetes mellitus, premature birth, asthma, and rheumatoid arthritis. In addition, stress shows some relationship to psychological disorders such as depression and anxiety disorders.

Stress and Disease

What is the evidence linking stress to disease? Which diseases have been implicated? What physiological mechanism might mediate the connection between stress and disease?

Hans Selye's concept of stress (see Chapter 5) included suppression of the immune response, and a growing body of evidence now supports this hypothesis through interactions among the nervous, endocrine, and immune systems (Kemeny & Schedlowski, 2007). These interactions are similar to the responses hypothesized by Selye and provide strong evidence that stress could be involved in a variety of physical ailments. Figure 6.5 shows some possible effects.

Several possibilities exist for pathways through which stress could produce disease (Segerstrom & Miller, 2004). Direct influence could occur through the effects of stress on the nervous, endocrine, and immune systems. Because any or all of these systems can create disease, sufficient physiological foundations exist to provide a link between stress and disease. In addition, indirect effects could occur through changes in health practices that increase risks; that is, stress tends to be related to increases in drinking, smoking, drug use, and sleep problems, all of which can

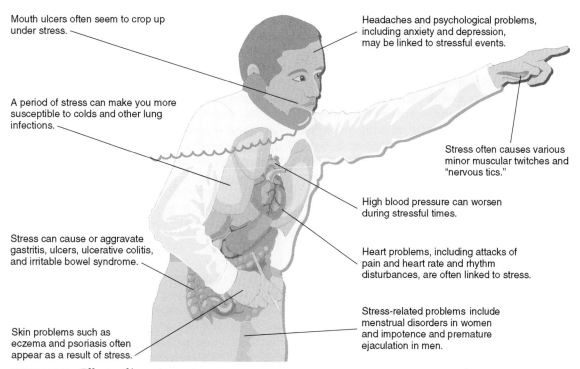

Mouth ulcers often seem to crop up under stress.

Headaches and psychological problems, including anxiety and depression, may be linked to stressful events.

A period of stress can make you more susceptible to colds and other lung infections.

Stress often causes various minor muscular twitches and "nervous tics."

High blood pressure can worsen during stressful times.

Stress can cause or aggravate gastritis, ulcers, ulcerative colitis, and irritable bowel syndrome.

Heart problems, including attacks of pain and heart rate and rhythm disturbances, are often linked to stress.

Skin problems such as eczema and psoriasis often appear as a result of stress.

Stress-related problems include menstrual disorders in women and impotence and premature ejaculation in men.

FIGURE 6.5 Effects of long-term stress.

Source: An Invitation to Health (7th ed., p. 58), by D. Hales, 1997, Pacific Grove, CA: Brooks/Cole. Copyright 1997 by Brooks/Cole Publishing Company. Reprinted by permission.

increase the risk for disease. Thus, possibilities exist for both direct and indirect effects of stress on disease. Does the evidence support these hypothesized relationships?

Headaches Headaches are a common problem; more than 99% of people have experienced headaches at some time in their lives (Smetana, 2000). For most people, headaches are an uncomfortable occurrence, but others experience serious, chronic pain. Headache can signal serious medical conditions, but most often the pain associated with the headache is the problem. This source of pain is one of the leading causes of disability in the world (Andrasik, 2006). The majority of people who seek medical assistance for headaches are plagued by the same sorts of headaches as those who do not; the difference stems from the frequency and severity of the headaches or from personal factors involved in seeking assistance.

Although more than 100 types of headaches have been identified, distinguishing among them

has become controversial, and the underlying causes for the most common types remain unclear (Andrasik, 2001). Nevertheless, diagnostic criteria have been devised for several types of headaches. The most frequent type is *tension headache*, usually associated with increased muscle tension in the head and neck region. Tension is also a factor in migraine headaches, which were believed to originate in the blood vessels in the head, but are now believed to originate in neurons in the brain stem (Silberstein, 2004). These headaches are associated with throbbing pain localized in one side of the head.

Stress is recognized as a factor in headaches; people with either tension or vascular headache named stress as one of the leading precipitating factors (Deniz, Aygül, Koçak, Orhan, & Kaya, 2004; Spierings, Ranke, & Honkoop, 2001). However, a comparison of people with daily headaches and those with infrequent headaches found no difference in stress as measured either by life events or by hassles (Barton-Donovan &

Blanchard, 2005), and a study comparing traumatic life events for headache patients found no difference from a comparison group (de Leeuw, Schmidt, & Carlson, 2005). The type of stress that people associate with headaches tends not to be traumatic life events but rather daily hassles. Students with chronic or frequent headaches reported more hassles than did students with infrequent headaches (Bottos & Dewey, 2004). In addition, stressful events precede periods of headache more often than they precede times with no headache (Marlowe, 1998); stress during a headache intensified the attack.

Nash and Thebarge (2006) discussed the ways through which stress might influence headaches. First, stress may be a predisposing factor that influences the development of headaches. Second, stress may act to transform a person who experiences occasional headaches into one who has chronic

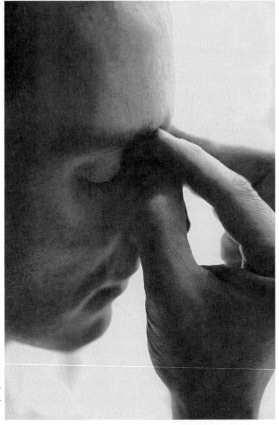

© Royalty-Free/Corbis

Stress is a factor in chronic headaches.

headaches. Third, stress may worsen headache episodes, magnifying the pain. These routes allow for several possibilities through which stress can contribute to the development of a headache and to chronic headaches. Furthermore, stress may decrease the quality of life for those with headaches.

Infectious Disease Are people who are under stress more likely than nonstressed individuals to develop infectious diseases such as the common cold? Research suggests that the answer is yes. An early study (Stone, Reed, & Neale, 1987) followed married couples who kept diaries on their own and their spouse's desirable and undesirable daily life experiences. Results indicated that participants who experienced a decline in desirable events or an increase in undesirable events developed somewhat more infectious diseases (colds or flu) three and four days later. The association was not strong, but this study was the first prospective design to show a relationship between daily life experiences and subsequent disease.

Later studies used a more direct approach, intentionally inoculating healthy volunteers with cold viruses to see who would develop a cold and who would not. Sheldon Cohen and his colleagues (Cohen, 2005; Cohen et al., 1998; Cohen, Tyrrell, & Smith, 1991, 1993) intentionally exposed healthy volunteers to various common cold viruses to determine the role of stress in the development of colds. The results indicated that the higher the person's stress, the more likely it was that the person would become ill.

Cohen and his colleagues (1998) also used the same inoculation procedure to see what types of stressors induce cold symptoms in people exposed to a cold virus. They found that duration of a stressful life event was more important than severity. Acute severe stress of less than one month did not lead to the development of colds, but severe chronic stress (more than one month) led to a substantial increase in colds. This association between stress and cold symptoms could not be explained by increases in epinephrine, norepinephrine, or cortisol or by such factors as social support, personality, or health practices. However, later research showed that susceptibility varied from individual to individual (Marsland,

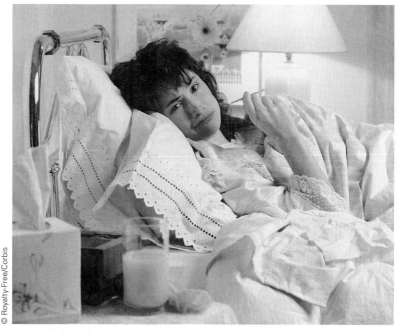

Research has shown that stress can influence development of infectious disease.

Bachen, Cohen, Rabin, & Manuck, 2002); people who were sociable and agreeable developed fewer colds than others after exposure to a cold virus (Cohen, Doyle, Turner, Alper, & Skoner, 2003). A naturalistic study of stress and colds (Takkouche, Regueira, & Gestal-Otero, 2001) showed that high levels of stress were related to increases in infection. People in the upper 25% of perceived stress were about twice as likely as those in the lowest 25% to get a cold, which suggests that stress may be a significant predictor of developing infectious disease.

Stress may also affect the progression of infectious disease. Reviews of psychosocial factors in HIV infection (Cole et al., 2001; Kopnisky, Stoff, & Rausch, 2004) explored the effect of stress on HIV infection; they concluded that stress affects both the progression of HIV infection and the infected person's immune response to antiviral drug treatment. HIV is not the only infectious disease that stress influences. Research has also demonstrated the role of stress in bacterial, viral, and fungal infections, including pneumonia, herpes, hepatitis, and recurrent urinary tract infections

(Levenson & Schneider, 2007). Thus, stress is a significant factor in susceptibility, severity, and progression of infection.

Cardiovascular Disease Cardiovascular disease (CVD) has a number of behavioral risk factors, some of which are related to stress. Chapter 9 examines these behavioral risk factors in more detail; in this section we look only at stress as a contributor to CVD. People who have had heart attacks named stress as the cause of their disorder (Cameron, Petrie, Ellis, Buick, & Weinman, 2005), but the relationship is less direct than they imagine. Two lines of research relate stress to CVD: studies that evaluate stress as a precipitating factor in heart attack or stroke, and studies that investigate stress as a cause in the development of CVD.

Evidence for the role of stress as a precipitating factor for heart attack or stroke in people with CVD is clear; stress increases the risks. Stress can serve as a trigger for heart attacks for people with coronary heart disease (Kop, 2003; Sheps, 2007). Feelings of depression, anger, or tension increase the risk for heart attack. However, even positive stress may create a risk (see Would You Believe . . . ? box). Stress increases the chances of chest pain as well as heart attacks in people with existing CVD (Krantz, Sheps, Carney, & Natelson, 2000). For women with CVD, the stress of marital conflict more than tripled their chances of unstable chest pain or heart attack (Orth-Gomér et al., 2000).

A large cross-cultural study called the INTER-HEART Study compared more than 15,000 people who had experienced a heart attack with almost as many who had not, attempting to identify significant risk factors that held across cultures and continents (Yusuf et al., 2004). This study identified a set of psychological stressors that showed a significant relationship to heart attack, including workplace and home stress, financial problems, major life events in the past year, depression, and external locus of control (Rosengren et al., 2004). These stress factors were significantly related to heart attack and made a substantial contribution to the risk within each population. The individuals who experienced heart attacks may have had long-standing CVD, but stress may also contribute to the development of this disease.

The role of stress in the development of heart disease is indirect but may occur through several routes, including hormone release as a response to stress or as a result of the immune system response (Matthews, 2005). For example, job-related stress (Smith, Roman, Dollard, Winefield, & Siegrist, 2005) and other situations with high demands and low control (Kamarck, Muldoon, Shiffman, & Sutton-Tyrrell, 2007) have been implicated in heart disease. One possible route for this effect is through the action of the immune system, which reacts by releasing cytokines, which promote inflammation. This inflammation is a factor in the development of coronary artery disease (Steptoe, Hamer, & Chida, 2007). The action of stress hormones such as the corticoids also affects the development of diseased arteries, exacerbating artery damage and making the development of arterial plaque more likely. These stress-related responses apply to any source of stress, forming an indirect route to heart disease.

A study that examined blood pressure provides an example of the selective effects of workplace stress (Fauvel, 2001). This study measured blood pressure during a 24-hour period and found that individuals with the combination of high work demands and low job decision latitude showed higher blood pressure during working hours, even though their blood pressure at home was not higher than that of other workers. This finding demonstrates that stressful situations can affect blood pressure and thus the cardiovascular system.

Hypertension "Contrary to the implication of its name, hypertension is not a high level of nervous tension, in terms either of its causes or its manifestations" (Jenkins, 1998, p. 604). Although high blood pressure would seem to be the result of stress, no simple relationship exists between stress and blood pressure. Situational factors such as noise can elevate blood pressure, but most studies have shown that blood pressure returns to normal when the situational stimulus is removed. However, a longitudinal study of blood pressure (Stewart, Janicki, & Kamarck, 2006) showed that the time to return to normal blood pressure after a psychological stressor predicted hypertension over three years. This response is similar to reactivity.

Reactivity The idea that some people react more strongly to stress than others is another possibility for the link between stress and cardiovascular disease. This response, called *reactivity*, may play a role in the development of cardiovascular disease if the response is relatively stable within an individual and prompted by events that occur frequently in the individual's life. Researchers have investigated the stability of reactivity and have also tried to discover those events that prompt it. An array of situations has been considered as stressors and a variety of cardiac responses as reactions.

One study showed that reactivity is related to incidence of stroke (Everson et al., 2001). Men with higher systolic blood pressure reactivity were at greater risk for stroke than men with less blood pressure reactivity. In this study, educational level was also a factor that raised the risk of stroke; other studies have focused on education, ethnicity, and socioeconomic status as factors in reactivity.

The higher rates of cardiovascular disease for African Americans than for European Americans have led researchers to examine differences in reactivity between these two ethnic groups, as well as the stressors that prompt such reaction. Many African Americans experience a continuous struggle to cope with a variety of stressors that relate to their ethnicity, and this struggle may constitute the type of long-term stressor that poses health threats (Bennett et al., 2004). Beginning during childhood and continuing into adolescence, African Americans showed greater reactivity than European Americans (Murphy, Stoney, Alpert, & Walker, 1995); these differences appeared among children as young as 6 (Treiber et al., 1993). In addition, African American children with a family history of cardiovascular disease showed significantly greater reactivity than any other group of children in the study.

Research on the experience of discrimination shows that racist provocations produce reactivity. A study comparing the reactions of African American and European American women (Lepore et al., 2006) showed that African American women who evaluated the stressful situation as racist showed stronger cardiac reactions than women who did not identify the stress as racist. Both European American and African American men who viewed a racist film clip experienced a greater increase in blood pressure than they did while viewing emotionally neutral films (Fang & Myers, 2001). Differences exist in reactivity for African Americans and Caribbean Americans, with both showing higher reactivity than European Americans (Arthur, Katkin, & Mezzacappa, 2004). However, Asian Americans showed lower reactivity than European Americans to a laboratory stressor (Shen, Stroud, & Niaura, 2004). This result is consistent with a lower rate of CVD among Asian Americans.

Another type of stressor that may relate to reactivity is *stereotype threat*. Claude Steele (1997) originated this term to describe situations in which individuals identified with some group are threatened by the negative stereotype associated with that group. Steele and his colleagues (Blascovich, Spencer, Quinn, & Steele, 2001) have demonstrated that members of stereotyped groups such

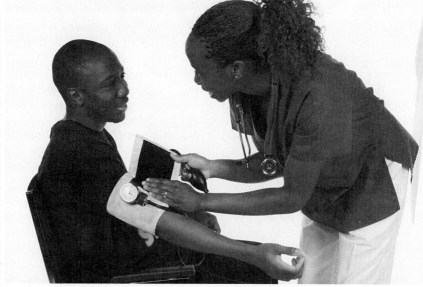

Bobby Deal/RealDealPhoto, 2008/Used under license from Shutterstock.com

Beginning during childhood, African Americans show higher cardiac reactivity than other ethnic groups, which may relate to their higher levels of cardiovascular disease.

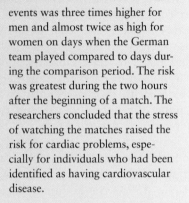

Being a Sports Fan May Be a Danger to Your Health

Would you believe that being a sports fan may endanger your health? A week or so before the 2008 Superbowl, stories appeared in the media suggesting that watching this sports event might present a risk for heart attack. This risk did not stem from the pizza, chips, and beer from Superbowl parties but from the emotional stress and excitement of the game.

The warnings were not based on research on the dangers of American football but rather on the increase in cardiovascular events during the World Cup Soccer championship held in Germany in 2006 (Wilbert-Lampen et al., 2008). Reserchers compared the frequency of cardiac events such as heart attack and cardiac arrythmia during the month of the World Cup championship to the month before and after the playoffs and found an elevated rate during the play-offs. The incidence of such cardiac events was three times higher for men and almost twice as high for women on days when the German team played compared to days during the comparison period. The risk was greatest during the two hours after the beginning of a match. The researchers concluded that the stress of watching the matches raised the risk for cardiac problems, especially for individuals who had been identified as having cardiovascular disease.

as African Americans, Hispanic Americans, and women perform more poorly when they believe that their performance is a reflection of their ethnicity or gender. In addition, African Americans showed higher blood pressure reactivity than European Americans under conditions of stereotype threat, and these elevations persisted even during rest periods. People's tendencies to experience cardiac changes and the circumstances that prompt these changes may be factors that underlie the development of cardiovascular disease. Discrimination and stereotype threat may enhance these factors for African Americans.

Ulcers At one time, stress was widely accepted as the cause of ulcers, but during the 1980s, two Australian researchers, Barry Marshall and J. Robin Warren, proposed that ulcers were the result of a bacterial infection rather than stress (Okuda & Nakazawa, 2004). At the time, their hypothesis seemed somewhat unlikely because most physiologists and physicians believed that bacteria could not live in the stomach environment with its extreme acidity. Marshall (1995) reported that he had trouble obtaining funding to research the possibility of a bacterial basis for ulcers. With no funding for his research and the belief that he was correct, Marshall infected himself with the bacterium to demonstrate its gastric

effects. He developed severe gastritis and took antibiotics to cure himself, providing further evidence that this bacterium has gastric effects. Results of a clinical trial comparing the traditional treatment of acid suppressants and antibiotics (Alper, 1993) revealed that stomach ulcers returned in 50% to 95% of patients who received the acid suppressant, but only 29% of the patients treated with antibiotics experienced a recurrence of ulcers. Positive results for antibiotic treatment changed not only the treatment strategy but also the thinking about ulcers.

However, the psychological component has not disappeared from explanations for the development and reoccurrence of ulcers because *H. pylori* infection does not seem to account for all ulcers (Levenstein, 2000; Watanabe et al., 2002). This infection is very common and related to a variety of gastric problems, yet most infected people do not develop ulcers (Weiner & Shapiro, 2001). Thus, *H. pylori* infection may create a vulnerability to ulcers, which stress or other psychosocial conditions then precipitate. For example, smoking, heavy drinking, caffeine consumption, and use of nonsteroidal anti-inflammatory drugs all relate to ulcer formation. Stress may be a factor in any of these behaviors, providing an indirect link between stress and ulcer formation in infected individuals. In addition, the hormones and altered immune function associated with the experience of chronic stress may be a more direct link. Therefore, behavioral factors play a role in the development of ulcers, but so does *H. pylori* infection, creating a complex interaction of factors in the formation of ulcers.

Other Physical Disorders Besides headache, infectious disease, cardiovascular disease, and ulcers, stress has been linked to several other physical disorders, including diabetes, premature delivery for pregnant women, asthma, and rheumatoid arthritis.

Diabetes mellitus is a chronic disease that shows some relationship to stress. Two kinds of diabetes mellitus are Type 1, or insulin-dependent, and Type 2, or non-insulin-dependent. Type 1 diabetes usually begins in childhood and requires insulin injections for its control. Type 2 diabetes usually appears during adulthood and can most often be controlled by dietary changes. (The lifestyle adjustments and behavioral management required by diabetes mellitus are discussed in Chapter 11.)

Stress may contribute to the *development* of both types of diabetes. First, stress may contribute directly to the development of insulin-dependent diabetes through the disruption of the immune system, possibly during infancy (Sepa, Wahlberg, Vaarala, Frodi, & Ludvigsson, 2005). Immune system measures at age 1 year indicated that those infants who had experienced higher family stress showed more indications of antibodies consistent with diabetes. Second, stress may contribute to the development of Type 2 through its effect on cytokines that initiate an inflammatory process that affects insulin metabolism and produces insulin resistance (Black, 2003; Tsiotra & Tsigos, 2006). Third, stress may contribute to Type 2 through its possible effects on obesity. Research on stress and Type 2 diabetics has shown that stress can be a triggering factor and thus play a role in the age at which people develop Type 2 diabetes.

In addition, stress may affect the *management* of diabetes mellitus through its direct effects on blood glucose (Riazi, Pickup, & Bradley, 2004) and through the indirect route of hindering people's compliance with controlling glucose levels (Farrell, Hains, Davies, Smith, & Parton, 2004). Indeed, compliance, discussed in Chapter 4, is a major problem for this disorder.

Stress during pregnancy has been the topic of research for both human and nonhuman subjects (Kofman, 2002). Research with nonhuman subjects has conclusively demonstrated that stressful environments relate to lower birth weight and developmental delays, and that infants of stressed mothers show higher reactivity to stress. Research with human participants cannot experimentally manipulate such stressors, so the results are not as conclusive, but studies on stress during pregnancy (Roesch, Dunkel-Schetter, Woo, & Hobel, 2004) revealed a tendency for stress to make preterm deliveries more likely and to result in babies with lower birth weights. Both factors are related to a number of problems for the infants. The importance of type and timing of stress remains unclear, but there is some indication that chronic stress may be more damaging than acute stress, and that stress late in pregnancy is riskier than earlier stress.

Asthma is a respiratory disorder characterized by difficulty in breathing due to reversible airway obstruction, airway inflammation, and increase in airway responsiveness to a variety of stimuli (Cohn, Elias, & Chupp, 2004). The prevalence and mortality rate of asthma have increased in recent years for both European American and African American women, men, and children, but poor African Americans living in urban environments are disproportionately affected (Gold & Wright, 2005).

Because inflammation is an essential part of asthma, the proinflammatory cytokines have been hypothesized to play a fundamental (possibly a causal) role in the development of this disease (Wills-Karp, 2004). The link between stress and the immune system presents the possibility that stress plays a role in the development of this disorder, but stress is also involved in asthma attacks (Chen & Miller, 2007).

Physical stimuli such as smoke can trigger an attack, but stressors, such as emotional events and pain, can also stimulate an asthma attack (Gustafson, Meadows-Oliver, & Banasiak, 2008).

Both acute and chronic stress increase the risk of asthma attacks in children with asthma; a population-based study in South Korea (Oh, Kim, Yoo, Kim, & Kim, 2004) found that people who reported more stress were more likely to experience more severe problems with their asthma. Children living in inner-city neighborhoods with parents who have mental problems are at sharply heightened risk (Weil et al., 1999). In addition, even after controlling for inner-city living conditions, exposure to violence appeared as a strong risk for asthma attack (Wright et al., 2004). Thus, stress is a significant factor in triggering asthma attacks.

Rheumatoid arthritis, a chronic inflammatory disease of the joints, may also be related to stress. Rheumatoid arthritis is believed to be an autoimmune disorder in which a person's own immune system attacks itself (Ligier & Sternberg, 2001). The attack produces inflammation and damage to the tissue lining of the joints, resulting in pain and loss of flexibility and mobility. Stress has been hypothesized to be a factor in the development of autoimmune diseases through the production of stress hormones and cytokines (Stojanovich & Marisavljevich, 2008).

A growing body of evidence indicates that stress can make arthritis worse by increasing sensitivity to pain, reducing coping efforts, and possibly affecting the process of inflammation itself. Direct effects of stress on inflammation could occur through neuroendocrine responses to stress (Davis et al., 2008). People with rheumatoid arthritis show lower responding of stress hormones and lower levels of cortisol than healthy people, suggesting a role for stress in this disease. For example, people with rheumatoid arthritis reported more pain on workdays that were stressful (Fifield et al., 2004). Other factors are important for the development of rheumatoid arthritis, but the stress that results from rheumatoid arthritis brings about negative changes in people's lives and requires extensive coping efforts.

Stress and Psychological Disorders

The relationship between stress and mood seems obvious—stress can put people in a bad mood. However, all people experience bad moods, yet most people do not show reactions so severe that they qualify as psychological disorders. Not all people who experience catastrophic life events respond in pathological ways. Therefore, the study of stress as a factor in psychological disorders parallels other research about stress and disease by adopting the diathesis–stress model. This research has concentrated not only on the sources of stress that relate to psychological disorders but also on the factors that create vulnerability.

Another parallel comes from a developing body of research that indicates a relationship between mood and changes in immune function. Such changes may underlie several psychological disorders (Dantzer, O'Connor, Freund, Johnson, & Kelly, 2008; Harrison, Olver, Norman, & Nathan, 2002). Thus, the relationship between stress and psychological disorders may be mediated through processes similar to those involved in other diseases—through the immune system.

Depression Research suggests some relationship between stress and depressive symptoms. This research has focused on the factors that make people vulnerable to depression and the physical mechanisms that translate stress into depression. The research on vulnerability has ranged from a consideration of the effectiveness of coping strategies to genetic vulnerability.

People who can cope effectively are able to avoid depression, even with many stressful events in their lives. Richard Lazarus and his colleagues (Kanner et al., 1981; Lazarus & DeLongis, 1983; Lazarus & Folkman, 1984) regarded stress as the combination of an environmental stimulus with the person's appraisal, vulnerability, and perceived coping strength. According to this theory, people become ill not merely because they have had too many stressful experiences but because they evaluate these experiences as threatening or damaging, because they are physically or socially vulnerable at the time, or because they lack the ability to cope with the stressful event.

Another proposal for vulnerability to depression is the "kindling" hypothesis (Monroe & Harkness, 2005). This view holds that major life stress provides a "kindling" experience that may prompt the development of depression.

This experience then sensitizes people to depression, and future experiences of stress need not be major to prompt recurrences of depression. A meta-analysis of studies on this topic (Stroud, Davila, & Moyer, 2008) showed some support, especially for the hypothesis of stress predicting first episodes of depression.

A negative outlook or the tendency to dwell on problems may exacerbate stress, making people more likely to think in ways that increase depression (Ciesla & Roberts, 2007; Gonzalez, Nolen-Hoeksema, & Treynor, 2003). One particular style of negative thinking—termed rumination—has been implicated. Rumination describes the tendency to dwell on negative thoughts. In support of this view, a longitudinal study of Japanese university students (Ito, Takenaka, Tomita, & Agari, 2006) demonstrated that this type of rumination predicted depression. Thus negative rumination provides a type of vulnerability for depression. Consistent with the diathesis–stress view, more positive ways of thinking or less stress would result in lower risk for depression.

Genetic vulnerability is another type of risk factor for depression. In a longitudinal study of twins (Kendler, Gatz, Gardner, & Pedersen, 2007), stress appeared as a significant factor in depression only under some circumstances. Stress had a higher relationship to depression for early episodes than for later ones, and for people with low rather than high genetic risk. Another longitudinal study (Caspi et al., 2003) demonstrated the interaction between genes and environment in the development of depression. Individuals who inherited a particular version of a gene pair that is involved with the neurotransmitter serotonin developed depression and suicidal thoughts significantly more frequently than did individuals with a different version of this gene pair, but only when the vulnerable individuals experienced stressful life events. These studies suggest that genes furnish the basis for a vulnerability that interacts with stressful life events to precipitate depression.

Some types of stressful situations seem to be greater risks for depression than other events. For example, chronic workplace stress is related to the development of depression, especially for people with low decision-making authority (Blackmore et al., 2007), as is living in a neighborhood where crime and drug use are common (Cutrona et al., 2005). Illness is another type of stress that shows a relationship to depression. Experiencing health problems produces stress both for the sick person and for caregivers. Heart disease (Guck, Kavan, Elsasser, & Barone, 2001), cancer (Spiegel & Giese-Davis, 2003), AIDS (Cruess et al., 2003), and Alzheimer's disease (Dorenlot, Harboun, Bige, Henrard, & Ankri, 2005) have all been related to increased incidence of depression. The relationship between stress and this variety of diseases occurs through the immune system.

Depression that meets the diagnostic criteria for clinical depression (American Psychiatric Association, 2000) is associated with several measures of immune function, with larger effects for older and for hospitalized patients. In addition, the more severe the depression, the greater will be the alteration of immune function. A meta-analysis of depression and immune function (Zorrilla et al., 2001) indicated that depression was significantly related to many facets of immune system function, including reduced T-cells and decreased activity of natural killer cells. This process may develop when prolonged stress disrupts regulation of the immune system through the action of proinflammatory cytokines (Robles, Glaser, & Kiecolt-Glaser, 2005).

The release of proinflammatory cytokines by the immune system (Anisman, Merali, Poulter, & Hayley, 2005; Dantzer et al., 2008) signals the nervous system. Some of their effects are similar to depression, such as fatigue, feelings of listlessness, and a loss of feelings of pleasure. Cytokine production increases when people are depressed, and people undergoing treatments that increase the production of certain cytokines also experience symptoms of depression. Thus, several lines of evidence support the role of cytokines in depression. Indeed, the brain may interpret cytokines as stressors (Anisman et al., 2005), which interact with environmental stressors to create depression.

Anxiety Disorders Anxiety disorders include a variety of fears and phobias, often leading to avoidance behaviors. Included in this category are such conditions as panic attack, **agoraphobia**, generalized anxiety, obsessive-compulsive disorders, and posttraumatic stress disorder (American Psychiatric Association, 2000). This section looks at stress as a possible contributor to anxiety states.

One anxiety disorder that, by definition, is related to stress is **posttraumatic stress disorder (PTSD)**. The *Diagnostic and Statistical Manual of Mental Disorders* (4th ed., text revision; American Psychiatric Association, 2000) defines PTSD as "the development of characteristic symptoms following exposure to an extreme traumatic stressor involving direct personal experience of an event that involves actual or threatened death or serious injury" (p. 463). PTSD can also stem from experiencing threats to one's physical integrity; witnessing another person's serious injury, death, or threatened physical integrity; and learning about death or injury to family members or friends. The traumatic events often include military combat, but sexual assault, physical attack, robbery, mugging, and other personal violent assaults can also trigger posttraumatic stress disorder.

Symptoms of PTSD include recurrent and intrusive memories of the traumatic event, recurrent distressing dreams that replay the event, and extreme psychological and physiological distress. Events that resemble or symbolize the original traumatic event, as well as anniversaries of that event, may also trigger symptoms. People with posttraumatic stress disorder attempt to avoid thoughts, feelings, or conversations about the event and to avoid any person or place that might trigger acute distress. Lifetime prevalence of PTSD in the general population of the United States is around 8% (American Psychiatric Association, 2000).

However, most people who experience traumatic events do not develop PTSD (McNally, 2003), and researchers have sought to understand the risk factors for PTSD. The original conceptualization of PTSD as the result of combat stress was too limited; research has confirmed that many types of experiences are related to the development of this disorder. People who are the victims of crime (Scarpa, Haden, & Hurley, 2006), terrorist attacks (Gabriel et al., 2007), domestic violence or sexual abuse (Pimlott-Kubiak & Cortina, 2003), and natural disasters (Dewaraja & Kawamura, 2006; Norris et al., 2001) are

BECOMING HEALTHIER

Stress may erode people's good intentions to maintain a healthy lifestyle. Stress may underlie people's decisions to eat an unhealthy diet, smoke, drink, use drugs, miss sleep, or avoid exercise. According to Dianne Tice and her colleagues (Tice, Bratslavsky, & Baumeister, 2001), distressed people tend to behave more impulsively. These researchers demonstrated that when distressed, people do things oriented toward making them feel better, and some of those things are health threatening, such as eating high-fat and high-sugar snacks.

Stress is also the rationalization that some people—including Lindsay Lohan—use to smoke (or not quit), have a few drinks, or use drugs.

Some of these indulgences may make people feel better temporarily, but others are poor choices. Maintaining a healthy lifestyle is a better choice. People feel better when they eat a healthy diet, engage in physical exercise, have positive interactions with friends or family, and get enough sleep. Indeed, these steps may be good for your immune system. Social

isolation decreases immune function (Hawkley & Cacioppo, 2003), but social support improves its function (Miyazaki et al., 2003), as does getting enough sleep (Hong, Mills, Loredo, Adler, & Dimsdale, 2005). So, when you are feeling a lot of stress, try to withstand the temptation to indulge in unhealthy behaviors. Instead, prepare to treat yourself with healthy indulgences, such as time with friends or family, more (rather than less) sleep, or participation in sports or other physical activity.

vulnerable. Personal factors and life circumstances also show a relationship to the development of PTSD (McNally, 2003), such as prior emotional problems, but poor social support and reactions to the traumatic event are more important in predicting who will develop PTSD (Ozer, Best, Lipsey, & Weiss, 2003).

The list of experiences that make people vulnerable to PTSD includes more events experienced by women than by men, and women are more likely to show symptoms of the disorder (Pimlott-Kubiak & Cortina, 2003). Hispanic Americans also seem more vulnerable to the disorder than other ethnic groups (Pole, Best, Metzler, & Marmar, 2005). The disorder is not limited to adults; children and adolescents who are the victims of violence or who observe violence are at increased risk (Griffing et al., 2006). PTSD increases the risk for medical disorders; its effects on the immune system may be the underlying reason. PTSD produces long-lasting suppression of the immune system (Kawamura, Kim, & Asukai, 2001) and an increase in proinflammatory cytokines (von Känel et al., 2007).

The relationship between stress and other anxiety disorders is less clear, perhaps because of the overlap between anxiety and depression (Suls & Bunde, 2005). Disentangling symptoms of negative affect presents problems for researchers. However, a study conducted in China (Z. Shen et al., 2003) found that people with generalized anxiety disorder reported more stressful life events than did people with no psychological disorder. Furthermore, those with anxiety disorder showed lower levels of some immune system functioning. Thus, stress may play a role in anxiety disorders, and again the route may be through an effect on the immune system.

IN SUMMARY

Much evidence points to a relationship between stress and disease, but the relationship between stressful life events or daily hassles and disease is indirect and complex. The diathesis–stress model hypothesizes that without some vulnerability, stress does not produce disease; much of the research on stress and various diseases is consistent with this model. Stress plays a role in the development of several physical disorders, including headache and infectious disease. The evidence for a relationship between stress and heart disease is complex. Stress is not directly responsible for hypertension, but some individuals show higher cardiac reactivity to stress, which may contribute to the development of cardiovascular disease. Experiences as a target of discrimination have been implicated as a factor in reactivity. Stress also plays an indirect and minor role in the development of ulcers. Other diseases have a more direct relationship with stress, including diabetes, asthma, and rheumatoid arthritis, as well as some premature deliveries; the influence of stress on the immune system and the involvement of cytokines may underlie all these relationships.

Depression is related to the experience of stressful life events in people who are vulnerable, but not in others. The source of this vulnerability may be genetic, but experiences and attitudes may also contribute to increased vulnerability, especially the experience of abuse or maltreatment during childhood. Posttraumatic stress disorder, by definition, is related to stress, but most people who experience trauma do not develop this disorder. Thus, vulnerability is also a factor for the effect of stress on the development of anxiety disorders.

ANSWERS

This chapter has addressed three basic questions:

1. How does the immune system function?

The immune system consists of tissues, organs, and processes that protect the body from invasion by foreign material such as bacteria, viruses, and fungi. The immune system marshals both a nonspecific response capable of attacking any invader and a specific response tailored to specific invaders. The immune system can also be a source of problems when it is deficient (as in HIV infection) or when it is too active (as in allergies and autoimmune diseases).

2. How does the field of psychoneuroimmunology relate behavior to disease?

The field of psychoneuroimmunology relates behavior to illness by finding relationships among behavior, the central nervous system, the immune system, and the endocrine system. Psychological factors can depress immune function, and some research has linked these factors with immune system depression and severity of physiological symptoms.

3. Does stress cause disease?

Research indicates that stress and illness are related, but as the diathesis–stress model holds, individuals must have some vulnerability for stress to cause disease. Stress is a moderate risk factor for headache and infectious disease. The role of stress in heart disease is complex; reactivity to stress may be involved in hypertension and the development of cardiovascular disease. Most ulcers can be traced to a bacterial infection rather than stress. The experience of stress is one of the many factors that contribute to psychological and mood disorders, but the route through which stress influences the development of these disorders may also be through the immune system.

SUGGESTED READINGS

Cohen, S. (2005). Keynote presentation at the eighth International Congress of Behavioral Medicine. *International Journal of Behavioral Medicine, 12*(3), 123–131. Shelton Cohen summarizes his fascinating research on stress and vulnerability to infectious disease.

Glaser, R. (2005). Stress-associated immune dysregulation and its importance for human health: A personal history of psychoneuroimmunology. *Brain, Behavior, and Immunity, 19*, 3–11. Ronald Glaser and Janice Kiecolt-Glaser have been two of the most prominent researchers in the field of psychoneuroimmunology. Ronald Glaser tells the story of their involvement, summarizing their important research and fitting it into a picture of this developing area.

Irwin, M. R. (2008). Human psychoneuroimmunology: 20 years of discovery. *Brain, Behavior and Immunity, 22*, 129–139. This recent review of the area of psychoneuroimmunology presents an overview of the immune system and the research on the links among psychosocial factors, immune system response, and the development of disease in humans.

Robles, T. F., Glaser, R., & Kiecolt-Glaser, J. K. (2005). Out of balance: A new look at chronic stress, depression, and immunity. *Current Directions in Psychological Science, 14*, 111–115. This short article looks at chronic stress and hypothesizes its relationship to depression through the immune system.

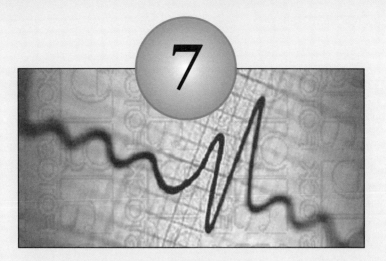

UNDERSTANDING AND MANAGING PAIN

QUESTIONS

This chapter focuses on five basic questions:

1. How does the nervous system register pain?
2. What is the meaning of pain?
3. How can pain be measured?
4. What types of pain present the biggest problems?
5. What techniques are effective for pain management?

Scale Your Pain

Pain is practically a universal experience but not a uniform one. The following questions allow you to understand the role pain plays in your life. To complete the exercise, think of the most significant pain that you have experienced within the past month, or if you have chronic pain, make your ratings with that pain problem in mind.

1. How long did your pain persist? _____ hours and _____ minutes

2. If this pain is chronic, how often does it occur?

   ☐ Less than once a month   ☐ Two or three times a week

   ☐ Once a month   ☐ Daily

   ☐ Two or three times a month   ☐ Throughout most of every day

   ☐ About once a week

3. What did you do to alleviate your pain? (Check all that apply.)

   ☐ Took a prescription drug   ☐ Took an over-the-counter drug

   ☐ Tried to relax   ☐ Tried to ignore the pain

   ☐ Did something to distract you from the pain

4. Place a mark on the line below to indicate how serious your pain was.

   Not at all   Unbearable

0	10	20	30	40	50	60	70	80	90	100

5. Place a mark on the line below to indicate how much this pain interfered with your daily routine.

   Not at all   Completely disrupted

0	10	20	30	40	50	60	70	80	90	100

6. During your pain, what did people around you do? (Check all that apply.)

   ☐ Gave me a lot of sympathy   ☐ Ignored me

   ☐ Did my work for me   ☐ Relieved me of my normal responsibilities

   ☐ Complained when I could not fulfill my normal responsibilities

Completing this assessment will show you something about your own pain experience. Some of the items on this assessment are similar to those on some of the standardized pain scales described in "The Measurement of Pain" later in the chapter.

REAL-WORLD PROFILE OF ASHLYN BLOCKER

As a baby, Ashlyn Blocker never cried, even when one of her eyes was swollen and bloodshot (Morton, 2004). When Ashlyn's mother Tara took her to the pediatrician to have her eye treated, Tara found out that Ashlyn did not cry because she was not able to feel pain. Testing revealed that Ashlyn has *congenital insensitivity to pain*, a rare genetic disorder that prevents her from experiencing pain. She can feel other sensations, such as touch and pressure, but not pain, heat, or cold. Ashlyn is one of only a few hundred people in the world with this disorder.

As a young child, Ashlyn required a lot of supervision. The nurse in her kindergarten examined Ashlyn after each recess, checking for injuries that Ashlyn would never have noticed. Her early childhood photos reveal evidence of injuries she sustained on a regular basis—cuts, scrapes, biting through her lip, knocking out teeth. Ashlyn has learned that if she sees blood, she needs to stop what she is doing, but without pain messages, she has experienced problems learning to protect herself.

Ashlyn's parents worry not only about injuries but also about infection, which could endanger her life. As the case of another person with congenital pain insensitivity shows, this concern is warranted. In the 1950s, a young woman at McGill University was the subject of study because she did not feel pain (Melzack, 1973). This young woman also had a history of injuries and problems as a result of her pain insensitivity. She died of an infection at age 29.

Many people imagine that a life without pain would be wonderful, but examining Ashlyn's experiences reveals a different picture. As Tara Blocker observed, "Pain's there for a reason. It lets your body know something's wrong and it needs to be fixed" (quoted in Morton, 2004). Unlike Ashlyn, most people have a nervous system that relays information about pain as well as other sensations. As Tara Blocker knows, that information helps prevent many injuries. But the experience of pain may also produce problems if the pain persists after the injury heals. This chapter explores some of those problems but first examines how the nervous system registers pain.

PAIN AND THE NERVOUS SYSTEM

All sensory information, including pain, begins with sense receptors on or near the surface of the body. These receptors change physical energy—such as light, sound, heat, and pressure—into neural impulses. We can feel pain through any of our senses, but most of what we think of as pain originates as stimulation to the skin and muscles.

Neural impulses that originate in the skin and muscles are part of the peripheral nervous system (PNS); all neurons outside the brain and spinal cord (the central nervous system, or CNS) are part of the PNS. Neural impulses that originate in the PNS travel toward the spinal cord and brain. Therefore, it is possible to trace the path of neural impulses from the receptors to the brain. Tracing this path is a way to understand the physiology of pain.

The Somatosensory System

The **somatosensory system** conveys sensory information from the body to the brain. All the PNS neurons from the skin's surface and muscles are part of the somatic nervous system. For example, a neural impulse that originates in the right index finger travels through the somatic nervous system to the spinal cord. The interpretation of this information in the brain results in a person's perception of sensations about his or her body and its movements. The somatosensory system consists of several senses, including touch, light and deep pressure, cold, warmth, tickling, movement, and body position.

Afferent Neurons Afferent neurons are one of three types of neurons—afferent, efferent, and interneurons. **Afferent** (sensory) **neurons** relay information from the sense organs toward the brain. **Efferent** (motor) **neurons** result in the movement of muscles or the stimulation of organs or glands; **interneurons** connect sensory to motor neurons. The sense organs contain afferent neurons, called **primary afferents**, with specialized receptors that convert physical energy into neural impulses, which travel to the spinal cord and then to the brain, where that information is processed and interpreted.

Involvement in Pain The skin is the largest of the sense organs, and its numerous receptors provide sensation for the skin. The process of perceiving pain is called *nociception*, and receptors in the skin and organs, called **nociceptors**, are capable of responding to various types of stimulation that may cause tissue damage, such as heat, cold, crushing, cutting, and burning.

Some neurons that convey sensory information (including nociception) are covered with **myelin**, a fatty substance that acts as insulation. Myelinated afferent neurons, called A fibers, conduct neural impulses faster than unmyelinated **C fibers** do. In addition, neurons differ in size, and larger ones conduct impulses faster than smaller ones. Two types of A fibers are important in pain perception: the large **A-beta fibers** and the smaller **A-delta fibers**. The large, myelinated A-beta fibers conduct impulses more than 100 times faster than small, unmyelinated C fibers (Melzack, 1973).

C fibers are much more common, however; more than 60% of all sensory afferents are C fibers (Melzack & Wall, 1982). A-beta fibers are easily stimulated to fire, whereas C fibers require more stimulation. Thus, these different types of fibers respond to different stimulation (Slugg, Meyer, & Campbell, 2000). Stimulation of A-delta fibers produces "fast" pain that is sharp or pricking, whereas stimulation of C fibers often results in a slower developing sensation of burning or dull aching (Chapman, Nakamura, & Flores, 1999).

The Spinal Cord

Protected by the vertebrae, the spinal cord is an avenue for sensory information traveling toward the brain and motor information coming from it. The spinal cord also produces the spinal reflexes. Damage to the spinal cord may interrupt the flow of sensory information, motor messages, or both, creating permanent impairment but leaving spinal reflexes intact. However, the most important role of the spinal cord is to provide a pathway for ascending sensory information and descending motor messages.

The afferent fibers group together after leaving the skin, and this grouping forms a *nerve*. Nerves

may be entirely afferent, entirely efferent, or a mixture of both. Just outside the spinal cord, each nerve bundle divides into two branches (see Figure 7.1). The sensory tracts, which funnel information toward the brain, enter the dorsal (toward the back) side of the spinal cord. The motor tracts, which come from the brain, exit the ventral (toward the stomach) side of the cord. On each side of the spinal cord, the dorsal root swells into a dorsal root ganglion, which contains the cell bodies of the primary afferent neurons. The neuron fibers extend into the **dorsal horns** of the spinal cord.

The dorsal horns contain several layers, or **laminae**. Each lamina receives incoming messages from afferent neurons. In general, the larger fibers penetrate more deeply into the laminae than the smaller fibers do (Melzack & Wall, 1982). The cells in lamina 1 and especially those in lamina 2 receive information from the small A-delta and C fibers; these two laminae form the **substantia gelatinosa**. Ronald Melzack and Peter Wall (1965) hypothesized that the substantia gelatinosa modulates sensory input information, and subsequent research has indicated that they were correct (Chapman et al., 1999). Other laminae also receive

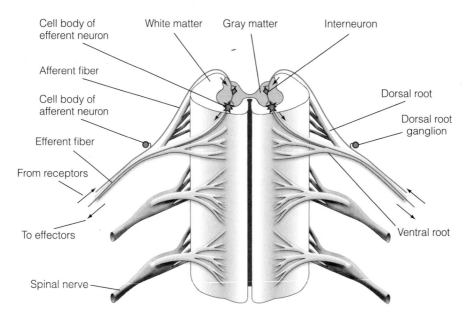

FIGURE 7.1 Cross-section through the spinal cord.

Source: Human Physiology: From Cells to Systems (4th ed.), by L. Sherwood, 2001, p. 164. Pacific Grove, CA: Brooks/Cole. Reprinted by permission.

projections from A and C fibers, as well as fibers descending from the brain and fibers from other laminae. Such connections allow for elaborate interactions between sensory input and the central processing of neural information in the brain.

The Brain

The **thalamus** receives information from afferent neurons in the spinal cord. After making connections in the thalamus, the information is relayed to other parts of the brain, including the **somatosensory cortex** in the cerebral cortex. The primary somatosensory cortex receives information from the thalamus that allows the entire surface of the skin to be mapped onto the somatosensory cortex. However, not all areas of the skin are equally represented. Figure 7.2 shows the area of the primary somatosensory cortex allotted to various regions of the body. Areas that are particularly rich in receptors occupy more of the somatosensory cortex than those areas that are poorer in receptors. For example, even though the back has more skin, the hands have more receptors, and therefore more area of the brain is devoted to interpreting the information these receptors

supply. This abundance of receptors also means that the hands are more sensitive; hands are capable of sensing stimuli that the back cannot.

A person's ability to localize pain on the skin's surface is more precise than it is for internal organs. Internal stimulation can also give rise to sensations, including pain, but the viscera are not mapped in the brain in the same way as the skin, so localizing internal sensation is much less precise. Brain imaging studies (Strigo, Duncan, Boivin, & Bushnell, 2003) have confirmed that visceral pain activates some of the same and some different areas of the brain as pain from the skin's surface. In addition, painful stimulation of the skin produced higher levels of brain activation than stimulation of the viscera did. Intense stimulation of internal organs can result in the spread of neural stimulation to the pathways serving skin senses, creating the perception of visceral pain as originating on the skin's surface. For example, a person who feels pain in the upper arm may not associate this sensation with the heart, but that type of pain is commonly produced by a heart attack. However, people can usually distinguish visceral sensations from skin sensations.

The development of positron emission tomography (PET) and functional magnetic resonance imaging (fMRI) has allowed researchers to study what happens in the brain when people experience pain. These techniques have confirmed neurological activity during the activation of nociceptors, but they paint a complex picture of how pain activates the brain (Apkarian, Bushnell, Treede, & Zubieta, 2005). Studies of brain responses to specific pain stimuli have shown activation in many areas of the brain, including the primary and secondary somatosensory cortices, but also the anterior cingulated cortex, the thalamus, and even the cerebellum in the lower part of the brain (Buffington, Hanlon, & McKeown, 2005; Davis, 2000). Adding to the complexity, an emotional reaction usually accompanies the experience of pain, and the brain imaging studies indicate activation in areas of the brain associated with emotion when people experience pain (Eisenberger, Gable, & Lieberman, 2007; see Would You Believe . . . ? box). Thus, the brain imaging studies using PET and fMRI have not revealed a "pain center" in the

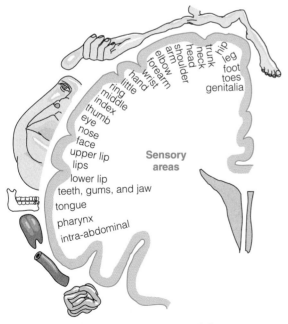

FIGURE 7.2   Somatosensory areas of the cortex.

Emotional and Physical Pain Are Mainly the Same in the Brain

People use the expression "hurt feelings" to describe one type of emotional distress, but this expression may be literally true. Research by Naomi Eisenberger and her colleagues (Eisenberger & Lieberman, 2004; Eisenberger, Lieberman, & Williams, 2003) examined the brains of people whose feelings were "hurt" and found that brains react in similar ways to emotional and physical pain.

Using functional magnetic resonance imaging (fMRI), Eisenberger and her colleagues (2003) examined the patterns of activity in people's brains. This technology allows researchers to measure activity in the brain and to associate various patterns of activity with different stimuli. Through this procedure, researchers can understand which brain structures are activated by various stimuli and situations. The participants in this study

experienced a virtual reality ball-tossing game while their brains were imaged. During the game, the researchers arranged for participants to be excluded from continuing the game by what participants believed to be the decision of two other players. This exclusion represented social rejection, the type of situation in which people get their feelings hurt. Additional research (Eisenberger, Jarcho, Lieberman, & Naliboff, 2006) indicated that individuals who are more sensitive to emotional distress are also more sensitive to pain.

Eisenberger and her colleagues (2003) hypothesized that the anterior cingulate cortex would be activated during the experience of social exclusion, because other brain-imaging studies had indicated that this area of the brain becomes more active when people experience pain. They further

hypothesized that another brain area, the right ventral prefrontal cortex, would be activated during social exclusion, because this area of the brain is involved in modulating the experience of pain. Their findings supported their hypotheses. Participants who were excluded from the game showed higher levels of activation both in the anterior cingulate cortex and in the right ventral prefrontal cortex than participants who believed that they could not play because of technical difficulties with the machinery. The level of activation in the anterior cingulate cortex correlated with the participants' ratings of distress. That is, the experience of social exclusion affected brain activity in a way that was similar to the experience of physical pain, suggesting that the two types of pain are similar in the brain.

brain. Rather, these studies have shown that the experience of pain produces a variety of activation in the brain, ranging from the lower brain to several centers in the forebrain.

Neurotransmitters and Pain

Neurotransmitters are chemicals that are synthesized and stored in neurons. The electrical action potential causes the release of neurotransmitters from neurons, which carries neural impulses across the synaptic cleft, the space between neurons. After flowing across the synaptic cleft, neurotransmitters act on other neurons by occupying specialized receptor sites. Each fits a specialized receptor site in the same way that a key fits into a lock; without the proper fit, the neurotransmitter will not affect the neuron. Sufficient amounts of neurotransmitters will

prompt the formation of an action potential in the stimulated neuron. Many different neurotransmitters exist, and each one is capable of causing an action.

In the 1970s, researchers (Pert & Snyder, 1973; Snyder, 1977) demonstrated that the neurochemistry of the brain plays a role in the perception of pain. This realization came about through an examination of how drugs affect the brain to alter pain perception. Receptors in the brain are sensitive to opiate drugs; that is, some neurons have receptor sites that opiate drugs are capable of occupying and activating. This discovery explained how opiates reduce pain—these drugs fit into brain receptors, modulate neuron activity, and alter pain perception.

The discovery of opiate receptors in the brain raised another question: Why does the brain respond to the resin of the opium poppy? In general, the brain is selective about the types of molecules that it allows to enter; only substances similar to naturally occurring neurochemicals can enter the brain. This reasoning led to the search for and identification of naturally occurring chemicals in the brain that affect pain perception. These neurochemicals have properties similar to those of the opiate drugs (Goldstein, 1976; Hughes, 1975). This discovery prompted a flurry of research that identified more opiate-like neurochemicals, including the **endorphins,** the *enkephalins,* and *dynorphin.*

These neurochemicals seem to be one of the brain's mechanisms for modulating pain. They can be activated by electrical stimulation of the brain as well as by experiences of stress and by suggestion (Turk, 2001). The pain-relieving properties of drugs such as morphine may be coincidental. Perhaps they are effective only because the brain contains its own system for pain relief, which the opiates stimulate.

Neurochemicals also seem to be involved in producing pain. The neurotransmitters *glutamate* and *substance P*, as well as the chemicals *bradykinin* and *prostaglandins,* sensitize or excite the neurons that relay pain messages (Sherwood, 2001). Glutamate and substance P act in the spinal cord to increase neural firings related to pain. Bradykinin and prostaglandins are substances released by tissue damage; they prolong the experience of pain by continuing to stimulate the nociceptors.

In addition, proteins produced by the immune system, *proinflammatory cytokines,* are involved in pain (Watkins et al., 2007; Watkins & Maier, 2003, 2005). Infection and inflammation prompt the immune system to release these cytokines, which signal the nervous system and produce a range of responses associated with sickness, including decreased activity, increased fatigue, and increased pain sensitivity. These responses cause glia in the spinal cord to release these cytokines. Indeed, these cytokines may be involved in the development of chronic pain by sensitizing the structures in the dorsal horn of the spinal cord that modulate the sensory message from the primary afferents (Watkins et al., 2007). Thus, the action of neurotransmitters and other chemicals produced by the body is complex, with the potential to both increase and decrease the experience of pain.

The Modulation of Pain

Research directed toward finding the brain structures involved in pain led to the discovery that one area of the brain, the **periaqueductal gray,** is involved in modulating pain. This brain structure is in the midbrain, close to the center. When it is stimulated, neural activity spreads downward to the spinal cord, and pain relief occurs (Goffaux, Redmond, Rainville, & Marchand, 2007; Sherwood, 2001). Neurons in the periaqueductal gray run down into the reticular formation and the **medulla,** a structure in the lower part of the brain that is also involved in pain perception (Fairhurst, Weich, Dunckley, & Tracey, 2007). These neurons descend into the spinal cord and make connections with neurons in the substantia gelatinosa. The result is that the dorsal horn neurons are kept from carrying pain information to the thalamus.

The inhibition of transmission also involves some familiar neurotransmitters. Endorphins in the periaqueductal gray initiate activity in this descending inhibitory system. Figure 7.3 illustrates this type of modulation. The substantia gelatinosa contains synapses that use enkephalin as a transmitter. Indeed, neurons that contain enkephalin seem to be concentrated in the same parts of the brain that contain substance P, the transmitter that activates pain messages (McLean, Skirboll, & Pert, 1985).

These elaborate physical and chemical systems are the body's way of modulating the neural impulses of pain. The value of pain is obvious, as illustrated by the case of Ashlyn Blocker, the girl whose story began this chapter. Ashlyn experiences daily problems because she cannot feel pain, which should signal tissue damage and provide a built-in motivation to discontinue activity that produces it. Pain after injury is also adaptive, furnishing a reminder of injury and discouraging activity that adds to the damage. In some situations, however, pain modulation is also adaptive. When people or other animals are fighting or fleeing, being able to ignore pain can be an advantage. Thus, the nervous system has complex systems that allow not only for the perception but also for the modulation of pain.

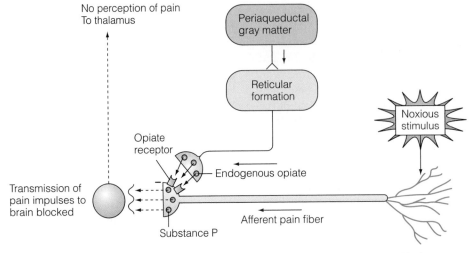

FIGURE 7.3 Descending pathways from the periaqueductal gray prompt the release of endogenous opiates (endorphins) that block the transmission of pain impulses to the brain.

Source: Human Physiology: From Cells to Systems (4th ed.), by L. Sherwood, 2001, p. 181. Pacific Grove, CA: Brooks/Cole. Reprinted by permission.

IN SUMMARY

The activation of receptors in the skin results in neural impulses that move along afferent pathways to the spinal cord by way of the dorsal root. In the spinal cord, the afferent impulses are relayed to the thalamus in the brain. The primary somatosensory cortex includes a map of the skin, with more cortex devoted to areas of the body richer in skin receptors. The A-delta and C fibers are involved in pain, with A-delta fibers relaying pain messages quickly and C fibers sending pain messages more slowly.

The brain and spinal cord also contain mechanisms for modulating sensory input and thereby affecting the perception of pain. One mechanism is through the naturally occurring neurochemicals that relieve pain and mimic the action of opiate drugs, which exist in many places in the central and peripheral nervous systems. The second mechanism is a system of descending control through the periaqueductal gray and the medulla. This system affects the activity of the spinal cord and provides a descending modulation of activity in the spinal cord.

THE MEANING OF PAIN

Until about 100 years ago, pain was most frequently considered a direct consequence of physical injury, specifically related to the degree of tissue damage. Near the end of the 19th century, C. A. Strong and others began to reconceptualize pain. Strong (1895) hypothesized that pain was due to two factors: the sensation and the person's reaction to that sensation. In this view, psychological factors and organic causes were of equal importance. This attention to psychological factors in pain signaled the beginning of a new definition, an altered view of the experience, and new theories of pain.

Definition of Pain

Pain is an almost universal experience. Only those rare people who are insensitive to pain, such as Ashlyn Blocker, escape the experience of pain. Nevertheless, it is remarkably difficult to define. Some experts (Covington, 2000) concentrate on the physiology that underlies the perception of pain, whereas others (Wall, 2000) emphasize the subjective nature of pain. These different views

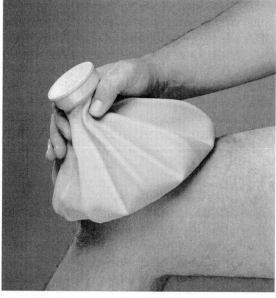

Acute pain is typically the result of injury and does not progress to the stage of chronic pain.

© Royalty-Free/Corbis

reflect the multidimensional nature of pain, which the International Association for the Study of Pain (IASP) has incorporated into its definition. The IASP Subcommittee on Taxonomy (1979, p. 250) has defined pain as "an unpleasant sensory and emotional experience associated with actual or potential tissue damage, or described in terms of such damage." The essence of this definition continues to be acceptable to most pain researchers and clinicians.

Another way to understand the meaning of pain is to see it in terms of three stages: acute, chronic, and prechronic (Keefe, 1982). **Acute pain** is the type of pain that most people experience when injured; it includes pains from cuts, burns, childbirth, surgery, dental work, and other injuries. Its duration is normally brief. This type of pain is ordinarily adaptive; it signals the person to avoid further injury. In contrast, **chronic pain** endures over months or even years. This type of pain may be due to a chronic condition such as rheumatoid arthritis, or it may be the result of an injury that persists beyond the time of healing (Turk & Melzack, 2001). Chronic pain is frequently experienced in the absence of any detectable tissue damage. It is not adaptive, but

rather can be both debilitating and demoralizing and often leads to feelings of helplessness and hopelessness. Chronic pain never has a biological benefit.

Perhaps the most crucial stage of pain is the **prechronic pain** stage, which comes between the acute and the chronic stages. This period is critical because the person either overcomes the pain at this time or develops the feelings of fear and helplessness that lead to chronic pain. These three stages do not exhaust all possibilities of pain. Several other types of pain have been identified, the most common of which is **chronic recurrent pain,** or pain marked by alternating episodes of intense pain and no pain. A common example of chronic recurrent pain is headache pain.

The Experience of Pain

The experience of pain is individual and subjective, but situational and cultural factors have a critical impact on that experience. Acknowledgment of the situational influences on the experience of pain began with reports by Henry Beecher (1946), an anesthesiologist, who observed soldiers wounded at the Anzio beachhead during World War II. Beecher noted that, despite their serious battle injuries, many of these men reported very little pain. What made the experience of pain different in this situation? These men had been removed from the battlefront and thus from the threat of death or further injury. Under these conditions, the wounded soldiers were in a cheerful, optimistic state of mind, whereas surgical patients with comparable injury experienced much more pain and requested more pain-killing drugs (Beecher, 1956). These findings prompted Beecher (1956) to conclude that "the intensity of suffering is largely determined by what the pain means to the patient" (p. 1609) and that "the extent of wound bears only a slight relationship, if any (often none at all), to the pain experienced" (p. 1612). Finally, Beecher (1957) described pain as a two-dimensional experience consisting of both a sensory stimulus and an emotional component. Despite the methodological shortcomings of Beecher's studies, his view of pain as a psychological and physical phenomenon came to be accepted by others working in this field.

Battle wounds are an extreme example of sudden injury, but variable amounts of pain are typical for people with other injuries. For example, most—but not all—people admitted to an emergency room for treatment of injury reported pain (Wall, 2000). Pain was more common among people with injuries such as broken bones, sprains, and stabs than among people with injuries to the skin. Indeed, 53% of those with cuts, burns, or scrapes reported that they felt no pain for at least some time after their injury, whereas only 28% of those with deep tissue injury failed to feel immediate pain. These individual variations of pain contrast with people who have been tortured, all of whom feel pain, even though their injuries may not be as serious as those of people reporting to an emergency room. People who believe that a stimulus will be harmful experience more pain than those who have different beliefs about the situation (Arntz & Claassens, 2004). The threat, intent to inflict pain, and lack of control give torture a very different meaning from unintentional injury and thus produce a different pain experience. These variations in pain perception suggest either individual differences, a cultural component for variations in pain-related behaviors, or some combination of these factors.

Individual Differences in the Experience of Pain Individual factors and personal experience make a difference in the experience of pain. People learn to associate stimuli related to a painful experience with the pain and thus develop classically conditioned responses to the associated stimuli (Sanders, 2006). For example, many people dislike the smell of hospitals or become anxious when they hear the dentist's drill because they have had experiences associating these stimuli with pain. Operant conditioning may also play an important role in pain by providing a means for acute pain to develop into chronic pain. Pioneering pain researcher John J. Bonica (1990) contended that psychological or environmental factors play a central role in chronic pain. He believed that the experience of being rewarded for pain behaviors is important for building acute pain into chronic pain. According to Bonica, people who receive attention, sympathy, relief from normal responsibilities, and disability compensation for their injuries and pain behaviors are more likely to develop chronic pain than are people who have similar injury but receive fewer rewards.

People's beliefs about individual variability tend to be exaggerated; there is no "pain-resistant" personality. Some people endure pain

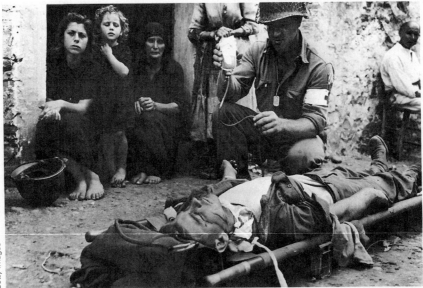

The experience of pain varies with the situation. Wounded soldiers removed from the front lines may feel little pain despite extreme injuries.

with little or no complaint, but nevertheless, these individuals perceive discomfort. They display no sign of their pain because of situational factors, cultural sanctions against the display of emotion, or some combination of these two factors. For example, some Native American, African, and South Pacific island cultures have initiation rituals that involve the silent endurance of pain. These rituals often involve the passage from child to adult status and may include body piercing, cutting, tattooing, burning, or beating. To show signs of pain would result in failure, so individuals are strongly motivated to hide their pain. Individuals may withstand these injuries with no visible sign of distress yet react with an obvious display of pain behavior to an unintentional injury in a situation outside the ritual (Wall, 2000). Other than individuals such as Ashlyn Blocker, who has congenital pain insensitivity, all people perceive pain. However, some people's behaviors reflect pain, whereas other people's behaviors hide their discomfort. These variations in expressions of pain suggest cultural variations in pain behaviors rather than the existence of a pain-resistant personality.

If a pain-resistant personality does not exist, then could there be evidence for a *pain-prone* personality? The concept of a pain-prone personality is also poorly supported by research (Turk, 2001), but individuals who are anxious, worried, and have a negative outlook tend to experience heightened sensitivity to pain (Janssen, 2002). Fear may be part of this negative outlook; individuals who experience a heightened fear of pain and tend to dwell on the most negative consequences of a pain situation also experience more pain (Leeuw et al., 2007). In addition, people with severe chronic pain are much more likely than others to suffer from some type of psychopathology, such as anxiety disorders or depression (McWilliams, Goodwin, & Cox, 2004; Williams, Jacka, Pasco, Dodd, & Berk, 2006). However, the direction of the cause and effect is not always clear (Gatchel & Epker, 1999). Patients suffering from chronic pain are more likely to be depressed, to abuse alcohol and other drugs, and to suffer from personality disorders. Some chronic pain patients develop these disorders as a result of their chronic pain, but others have some

form of psychopathology prior to the beginning of their pain. Thus, individual differences exist in the experience of pain, but cultural and situational factors are more important.

Cultural Variations in Pain Perception Pain sensitivity and the expression of pain behaviors show large cultural differences. In addition, cultural background and social context affect the experience (Cleland, Palmer, & Venzke, 2005) and treatment (Cintron & Morrison, 2006) of pain. These differences come from varying meanings that different cultures attach to pain and from stereotypes associated with various cultural groups.

Cultural expectations for pain are apparent in the pain that women experience during childbirth (Callister, 2003; Streltzer, 1997). Some cultures hold birth as a dangerous and painful process, and women in these cultures reflect these expectations by experiencing great pain. Other cultures expect quiet acceptance during the experience of giving birth, and women in those cultures tend not to show much evidence of pain. Their failure to display signs of pain, however, does not mean that they do not feel pain (Wall, 2000). When questioned about their apparent lack of pain, these women reported that they felt pain but their culture did not expect women to show pain under these circumstances, so they did not.

Since the 1950s, studies have compared pain expression for people from various ethnic backgrounds (Ondeck, 2003; Streltzer, 1997). Some studies have shown differences and others have not, but the studies tend to suffer from the criticism of stereotyping. For example, Italians are stereotyped as people who show a lot of emotion. Consistent with this stereotype, studies have found that Italian Americans express more distress and demand more pain medication than "Yankees" (Americans of Anglo-Saxon descent who have lived in the United States for generations), who have a reputation for stoically ignoring pain. These variations in pain behaviors among different cultures may reflect behavioral differences in learning and modeling, differences in sensitivity to pain, or some combination of these factors.

Laboratory studies of pain perception confirm differences between African Americans and European Americans in sensitivity to painful stimuli; African Americans and Hispanic Americans showed higher sensitivity to pain than European Americans (Rahim-Williams et al., 2007). These sensitivities carry over to clinical pain (Edwards, Fillingim, & Keefe, 2001) and chronic pain (Riley et al., 2002); African Americans reported higher levels of both. Greater sensitivity to pain is doubly unfortunate for African Americans, because physicians are more likely to underestimate their pain (Staton et al., 2007) and to prescribe less analgesia than they do for European Americans as outpatients, in hospitals, and in nursing homes, despite similar complaints about pain (Cintron & Morrison, 2006). Hispanics receive similar treatment—less analgesia in many types of medical settings. This discrimination in treatment is a source of needless pain for patients from these ethnic groups.

Gender Differences in Pain Perception Another common stereotype about pain perception is that women are more sensitive to pain than men (Robinson et al., 2003), and this belief has some research support. Women report pain more readily than men do, but this difference may reflect behavior that is consistent with gender roles rather than differences in perception of pain. However, women experience disabilities and pain-related conditions more often than men do, suggesting that women experience pain more readily than men do (Henderson, Gandevia, & Macefield, 2008).

Other evidence paints a more complex picture of the relationship between gender and pain, beginning during childhood. A nationwide sample of Swedish 9-, 12-, and 15-year-olds (Sundblad, Saartok, & Engström, 2007) revealed more frequent reports of pain from girls than boys and a decrease in pain reports for older boys but an increase among older girls. These changes are consistent with adoption of the male and female gender role; boys may be learning to deny pain, whereas girls are learning that reporting pain is consistent with their gender role. Consistent with this view, men who identified more highly with the male gender role were less likely than other men and less likely than women to report pain in a laboratory experiment (Pool, Schwegler, Theodore, & Fuchs, 2007).

Other research has failed to find dramatic differences between men and women. A study on women and men who had dental surgery (Averbuch & Katzper, 2000) reported that more women than men described their pain as severe but found very small differences between pain reports for men and women and no difference in their responses to analgesic drugs. A similar study with adolescents (Logan & Rose, 2004) showed similar results: Girls reported more pain but used no more analgesics than boys. Another study (Kim et al., 2004) found that women reported pain more readily than men in a laboratory situation but showed similar responses to pain associated with oral surgery. One commonality among these studies was that women reported higher anxiety and threat related to their experiences of pain, which may be an important factor in gender differences in pain perception (Leeuw et al., 2007).

Theories of Pain

How people experience pain is the subject of a number of theories. Of the several models of pain, two capture the divergent ways of conceptualizing pain: the specificity theory and the gate control theory.

Specificity Theory Specificity theory explains pain by hypothesizing that specific pain fibers and pain pathways exist, making the experience of pain virtually equal to the amount of tissue damage or injury (Craig, 2003). The view that pain is the result of transmission of pain signals from the body to a "pain center" in the brain can be traced back to Descartes, who in the 1600s proposed that the body works mechanically (DeLeo, 2006). This mechanistic action of the body is consistent with the notion that transmission of pain signals is relaying information about body damage. Descartes hypothesized that the mind works by a different set of principles, and body and mind interact in a limited way. According to Ronald Melzack (1993), Descartes's view influenced not only the development of a science of physiology and medicine but also the view that pain is a physical experience largely uninfluenced by psychological factors.

Working under the assumption that pain was the transmission of one type of sensory information, researchers tried to determine which type of receptor conveyed what type of sensory information (Melzack, 1973). For example, they tried to determine which type of receptor relayed information about heat, cold, and other types of pain. The attempt to tie specific somatic sensations to specific types of receptors did not succeed. Researchers found that some parts of the body (such as the cornea of the eye) contain only one type of receptor, yet those areas feel a full range of sensations. Some receptors seem specialized to react to specific types of stimulation, but these specialized receptors can also respond to other types of stimuli. Specificity does exist in the different types of receptors and nerve fibers, such as light touch, pressure, itching, pricking, warmth, and cold (Craig, 2003). Pain can come through any of these stimuli, however, so any simple version of specificity theory is not valid. Contemporary theorists who believe in the specificity of pain acknowledge that specificity is limited and that pain is a complex, multidimensional phenomenon.

The Gate Control Theory In 1965, Ronald Melzack and Peter Wall formulated a new theory of pain, which suggests that pain is *not* the result of a linear process that begins with sensory stimulation of pain pathways and ends with the experience of pain. Rather, pain perception is subject to a number of modulations that can influence the experience of pain. These modulations begin in the spinal cord.

Melzack and Wall hypothesized that structures in the spinal cord act as a gate for the sensory input that the brain interprets as pain. Melzack and Wall's theory is thus known as the **gate control theory** (see Figure 7.4). It is based on physiology but explains both sensory and psychological aspects of pain perception.

Melzack and Wall (1965, 1982, 1988) pointed out that the nervous system is never at rest; the patterns of neural activation constantly change. When sensory information from the body reaches the dorsal horns of the spinal cord, that neural impulse enters a system that is already active.

The existing activity in the spinal cord and brain influences the fate of incoming sensory information, sometimes amplifying and sometimes decreasing the incoming neural signals. The gate control theory hypothesizes that these complex modulations in the spinal cord and in the brain are critical factors in the perception of pain.

According to the gate control theory, neural mechanisms in the spinal cord act like a gate that can either increase (open the gate) or decrease (close the gate) the flow of neural impulses. Figure 7.4 shows the results of opening and closing the gate. With the gate open, impulses flow through the spinal cord toward the brain, neural messages reach the brain, and the person feels pain. With the gate closed, impulses are inhibited from ascending through the spinal cord, messages do not reach the brain, and the person does not feel pain. Moreover, sensory input is subject to modulation, depending on the activity of the large A-beta fibers, the small A-delta fibers, and the small C fibers that enter the spinal cord and synapse in the dorsal horns.

The dorsal horns of the spinal cord are composed of several layers (laminae). Two of these laminae make up the substantia gelatinosa, which is the hypothesized location of the gate (Melzack & Wall, 1965). Both the small A-delta and C fibers and the large A-beta fibers travel through the substantia gelatinosa, which also receives projections from other laminae (Melzack & Wall, 1982, 1988). This arrangement of neurons provides the physiological basis for the modulation of incoming sensory impulses. Melzack and Wall hypothesized these mechanisms when they formulated the gate control theory, but later research has confirmed the modulation of afferent messages in the dorsal horns of the spinal cord.

Melzack and Wall (1982) proposed that activity in the small A-delta and C fibers causes prolonged activity in the spinal cord. This type of activity would promote sensitivity, which increases sensitivity to pain. Activity of these small fibers would thus open the gate. On the other hand, activity of the large A-beta fibers produces an initial burst of activity in the spinal cord, followed by inhibition. Activity of these fibers closes the gate. Subsequent research has not confirmed

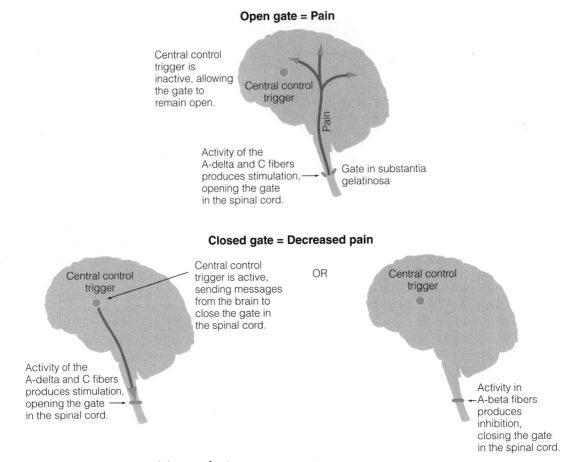

FIGURE 7.4   Gate control theory of pain.

this feature of the gate control theory in a clear way (Turk, 2001). Activity of A-delta and C fibers seems to be related to the experience of pain, but under conditions of inflammation, increased activity of A-beta fibers can increase rather than decrease pain.

The gate may be closed by activity in the spinal cord and also by messages that descend from the brain. Melzack and Wall (1965, 1982, 1988) proposed the concept of a **central control trigger** consisting of nerve impulses that descend from the brain and influence the gating mechanism. They hypothesized that this system consists of large neurons that conduct impulses rapidly. These impulses from the brain affect the opening and closing of the gate in the spinal cord and are affected by cognitive processes. That is, Melzack

and Wall proposed that the experience of pain is influenced by beliefs and prior experience, and they also hypothesized a physiological mechanism that would account for such factors in pain perception. As we discussed, the periaqueductal gray matter furnishes descending controls (Mason, 2005), which is consistent with this aspect of the gate control theory.

According to the gate control theory, then, pain has not only sensory components but also motivational and emotional components. That aspect of the theory revolutionized conceptualizations of pain (Turk, 2001). The gate control theory explains the influence of cognitive aspects of pain and allows for learning and experience to affect the experience of pain. Anxiety, worry, depression, and focusing on an injury can increase pain by affecting the central control trigger, thus opening the gate. Distraction, relaxation, and positive emotions can cause the gate to close, thereby decreasing pain. The gate control theory is not specific about how these experiences affect pain, and other theorists have elaborated on how such psychological factors influence pain perception (Leeuw et al., 2007; Kenntner-Mabiala, Weyers, & Pauli, 2007; Turk, 2001).

Many personal experiences with pain are consistent with the gate control theory. When you accidentally hit your finger with a hammer, many of the small fibers are activated, opening the gate. An emotional reaction accompanies your perception of acute pain. You may then grasp your injured finger and rub it. According to the gate control theory, rubbing stimulates the large fibers that close the gate, thus blocking stimulation from the small fibers and decreasing pain.

The gate control theory also explains how injuries can go virtually unnoticed. If sensory input is sent into a heavily activated nervous system, then the stimulation may not be perceived as pain. A tennis player may turn an ankle during a game but not notice the acute pain because of excitement and concentration on the game. After the game is finished, however, the player may notice the pain because the nervous system is functioning at a different level of activation and the gate is more easily opened.

Although it is not universally accepted, the gate control theory is the most influential theory of pain (Sufka & Price, 2002). This theory allows for the complexities of pain experiences. Melzack and Wall proposed the gate control theory before the discovery of the body's own opiates or of the descending control mechanisms through the periaqueductal gray and the medulla, both of which offer supporting evidence. The gate control theory has been and continues to be successful in spurring research and generating interest in the psychological and perceptual factors involved in pain.

Melzack (1993, 2005) proposed an extension to the gate control theory called the *neuromatrix theory*, which places a stronger emphasis on the brain's role in pain perception. He hypothesized a network of brain neurons that he called the

neuromatrix, "a large, widespread network of neurons that consists of loops between the thalamus and cortex as well as between the cortex and limbic system. I have labeled the entire network, whose spatial distribution and synaptic links are initially determined genetically and are later sculpted by sensory inputs, as a neuromatrix" (Melzack, 2005, p. 86). Normally, the neuromatrix acts to process incoming sensory information, including pain, but the neuromatrix acts even in the absence of sensory input, producing phantom limb sensations. Melzack's neuromatrix theory extends gate control theory but maintains that pain perception is part of a complex process affected not only by sensory input but also by activity of the nervous system and by experience and expectation. The nervous system's capacity for change can also contribute to the development of chronic pain by altering the activity of the neuromatrix (Khalsa, 2004; Melzack, 2005).

IN SUMMARY

Although the extent of damage is important in the pain experience, personal perception is also important. Pain can be classified as acute, prechronic, or chronic, depending on the length of time that the pain has persisted. Acute pain is usually adaptive and lasts for less than six months. Chronic pain continues beyond the time of healing, often in the absence of detectable tissue damage. Prechronic pain occurs between acute and chronic pain. All of these stages of pain appear in pain syndromes, such as headache pain, low back pain, arthritic pain, cancer pain, and phantom limb pain.

Several models have been proposed to explain pain, but specificity theory does not capture the complexity of the pain experience. The gate control theory has been the most influential model of pain. This theory holds that pain can be increased or diminished by mechanisms in the spinal cord and the brain. Since its formulation, increased knowledge of the physiology of the brain and spinal cord has supported this theory. Neuromatrix theory extends the gate control theory by hypothesizing the existence of a set of neurons in the brain that maintain a pattern of activity that defines the self and yet also responds to expectations and to incoming signals such as pain.

THE MEASUREMENT OF PAIN

We have seen that pain has physical and psychological elements, both of which can be quantified and measured. The measurement of pain is important to researchers, who strive to understand the experience of pain and evaluate therapeutic interventions, and to clinicians, who must quantify their patients' pain as part of formulating effective treatment plans.

Asking physicians (Marquié et al., 2003; Staton et al., 2007) or nurses (Wilson & McSherry, 2006) to rate their patients' pain is not a valid approach, because these professionals tend to underestimate patients' pain. Asking people to rate their own pain on a scale would seem be reliable and valid. Who knows better than patients themselves how much pain they are feeling? However, some pain experts (Turk & Melzack, 2001) have questioned both the reliability and the validity of this procedure, stating that people do not reliably remember how they rated an earlier pain. For this reason, pain researchers have developed a number of techniques for measuring pain, including (1) self-reports ratings, (2) behavioral assessments, and (3) physiological measures.

Self-Reports

Self-reports of pain ask people to evaluate and make ratings of their pain on simple rating scales, standardized pain inventories, or standardized personality tests.

Rating Scales Simple rating scales are an important part of the pain measurement arsenal. For example, patients may rate the intensity of their pain on a scale from 0 to 10 (or 0 to 100), with 10 being the most excruciating pain possible and 0 being the complete absence of pain. Such numeric ratings showed advantages over other types of self-reports in a comparison of several approaches to pain assessment (Gagliese, Weizblit, Ellis, & Chan, 2005).

A similar technique is the Visual Analog Scale (VAS), which is simply a line anchored on the left by a phrase such as "no pain" and on the right by a phrase such as "worst pain imaginable." Both the VAS and numerical rating scales are easy to use. For some pain patients, the VAS is superior to word descriptors of pain (Rosier, Iadarola, & Coghill, 2002) and numerical ratings (Bigatti & Cronan, 2002). Visual analog scales have been criticized as sometimes being confusing to patients not accustomed to quantifying their experience (Burckhardt & Jones, 2003b) and difficult for those who cannot comprehend the instructions, such as older people with dementia or young children (Feldt, 2007). Another rating scale is the face scales, consisting of 8 to 10 drawing of faces expressing emotions from intense joy to intense pain. Again, patients merely indicate which illustration best fits their level of pain (Jensen & Karoly, 2001). This type of rating was developed for use with children but is also effective with older adults (Benaim et al., 2007). A limitation of each of these rating scales is that they measure only the intensity of pain; they do not tap into patients' verbal description of their pain, but this approach to pain assessment may be the simplest and most effective for many patients.

Pain Questionnaires Ronald Melzack (1975, p. 278) contended that describing pain on a single dimension was "like specifying the visual world only in terms of light flux without regard to pattern, color, texture, and the many other dimensions of visual experience." Rating scales make no distinction, for example, among pains that are pounding, shooting, stabbing, or hot.

To rectify some of these weaknesses, Melzack (1975) developed the McGill Pain Questionnaire (MPQ), an inventory that provides a subjective report of pain and categorizes it in three dimensions: sensory, affective, and evaluative. *Sensory* qualities of pain are its temporal, spatial, pressure, and thermal properties; *affective* qualities are the fear, tension, and autonomic properties that are part of the pain experience; and *evaluative* qualities are the words that describe the subjective overall intensity of the pain experience.

In addition to these three dimensions of pain, the MPQ has four parts. Part 1 consists of front and back drawings of the human body. Patients mark on these drawings indicating the areas where they feel pain. Part 2 consists of 20 sets of words describing pain, and patients draw a circle around the one word in each set that most accurately describes their pain. These adjectives are ordered from least to most painful—for example, *nagging, nauseating, agonizing, dreadful*, and *torturing*. Part 3 asks how the patient's pain has changed with time. Part 4 measures the intensity of pain on a 5-point scale from *mild* to *excruciating*. This fourth part yields a Present Pain Intensity (PPI) score.

The MPQ has been the most frequently used pain questionnaire (Piotrowski, 1998, 2007), and a short form of the McGill Pain Questionnaire (Melzack, 1987) preserves the multidimensional assessment and correlates highly with scores on the standard MPQ (Burckhardt & Jones, 2003a). The MPQ has been used to assess pain relief in a variety of treatment programs and has demonstrated some validity in assessing multiple pain syndromes (Melzack & Katz, 2001). The short form has grown in use and demonstrates a high degree of reliability (Grafton, Foster, & Wright, 2005). In addition, a computerized, touch-screen administration of this test showed a high degree of consistency with the paper-and-pencil version (Cook et al., 2004).

The Multidimensional Pain Inventory (MPI), also known as the West Haven–Yale Multidimensional Pain Inventory (WHYMPI) is another assessment tool specifically designed for pain patients (Kerns, Turk, & Rudy, 1985). The 52-item MPI is divided into three sections. The first rates characteristics of the pain, interference with patients' lives and functioning, and patients' moods. The second section rates patients' perceptions of the responses of significant others, and the third measures how often patients engage in each of 30 different daily activities. Using this scale allowed researchers (Kerns et al., 1985) to develop 13 different scales that captured different dimensions of the lives of pain patients.

Turk and Rudy (1988) used the statistical technique of cluster analysis to group pain patients into three clusters: (1) dysfunctional, (2) interpersonally distressed, and (3) adaptive copers. Patients in the dysfunctional cluster tend to report higher levels of pain, greater psychological distress, greater interference with their lives, lower levels of activity, and lower levels of perceived control over their lives. The second cluster of patients was called *interpersonally distressed* because they perceived that those around them were failing to provide necessary support. The third cluster—*adaptive copers*—were less troubled by their pain, reporting lower levels of pain severity, lower interference with their lives, lower personal distress, and higher levels of activity and control.

Despite widespread use of this instrument, additional research on the MPI has revealed problems in its interpretation. One team of researchers (Burns, Kubilus, Bruehl, & Harden (2001) found evidence for a fourth cluster—a repressor group. Repressors report high pain and low activity but low distress. They are defensive and tend to repress emotional distress. Other research (Sheffer, Deisinger, Cassisi, & Lofland, 2007) found evidence that the other categories better captured clusters of pain patients taking the MPI. In addition, the classification of pain patients into categories may not be stable (Broderick, Junghaenel, & Turk, 2004); 85% of patients changed categories over a 10-month period. These results suggest that the MPI does not lead to accurate predictions of a patient's category of coping with chronic pain.

Standardized Psychological Tests In addition to the specialized pain inventories, clinicians and researchers also use a variety of standardized psychological tests in assessing pain patients. The most frequently used of these tests is the MMPI-2 (Arbisi & Seime, 2006). The MMPI was not originally designed to assess pain but rather to measure such clinical diagnoses as depression, paranoia, schizophrenia, and other psychopathologies. Research from the early 1950s (Hanvik, 1951) found that different types of pain patients could be differentiated on several MMPI scales, and more recent research (Arbisi & Seime, 2006) has confirmed the use of the MMPI for such assessment. One of the major advantages of using the MMPI-2 for pain assessment is its ability to detect patients who are being dishonest about their experience of pain (Arbisi & Butcher, 2004).

In addition to the MMPI, the Beck Depression Inventory (Beck, Ward, Mendelson, Mock, & Erbaugh, 1961) and the Symptom Checklist–90 (Derogatis, 1977) have been used to measure pain. The Beck Depression Inventory is a short self-report questionnaire that assesses depression; the Symptom Checklist–90 measures symptoms related to various types of behavioral problems. People with chronic pain often experience negative moods, so the relationship between scores on psychological tests and pain is not surprising. However, factor analyses of the Beck Depression Inventory with pain patients (Morley, de C. Williams, & Black, 2002; Poole, Branwell, & Murphy, 2006) indicated that these patients present a different profile of depression than depressed people with no chronic pain. The Symptom Checklist–90 (McGuire & Shores, 2001) demonstrated the ability to differentiate pain patients from those instructed to respond as they thought a pain patient might respond. Thus, these psychological tests may have something to offer in the assessment of pain.

Behavioral Assessments

A second major approach to pain measurement is observation of patients' behavior. Influential researcher Wilbert Fordyce (1974) noted that people in pain often groan, grimace, rub, sigh, limp, miss work, remain in bed, or engage in other behaviors that signify to observers that they may be suffering from pain, including lowered levels of activity, use of pain medication, body posture, and facial expressions. Behavioral observation began as an informal way to assess pain; Fordyce (1976) trained spouses to record pain behaviors, working to obtain a list of between 5 and 10 behaviors that indicate pain for each individual.

Health care professionals tend to underestimate patients' pain (Staton et al., 2007; Wilson & McSherry, 2006) and require extensive training to overcome their bias (Keefe & Smith, 2002; Rapoff, 2003). Another way for health care professionals to attain more accurate assessments is through the development of behavioral observation into a standardized assessment strategy

(Keefe & Smith, 2002). During an observational protocol, pain patients are asked to perform a series of tasks while a trained observer records their body movements and facial expressions, noting signs of pain. For example, patients with low back pain may be asked to sit, stand, walk, and recline during a 1- to 2-minute observation. The session may be videotaped to allow other observers to rate pain-related behaviors such as limping and grimacing. This strategy for collecting information yields data about pain behaviors, and analyses have confirmed that these data are reliable and valid indicators of pain (Keefe & Smith, 2002).

Behavioral observation is especially useful in assessing the pain of those who have difficulty furnishing self-reports—children and some elderly patients. This approach includes assessments of children's pain (von Baeyer & Spagrud, 2007) and a coding system that allows observers to assess the pain of infants by observing five facial movements and two hand actions (Holsti & Grunau, 2007). Many older patients can report on their pain, but some cannot, and behavioral observation of facial expressions allows an assessment of this difficult group (Clark, Jones, & Pennington, 2004; Lints-Martindale, Hadjistavropoulos, Barber, & Gibson, 2007).

Physiological Measures

A third approach to pain assessment is the use of physiological measures (Gatchel, 2005). One approach is through the use of electromyography (EMG), which measures the level of muscle tension. The notion behind this approach is that pain increases muscle tension. Electromyography has been most often used to measure low back pain, headache pain, and neck and jaw pain.

Attaching the measuring electrodes to the surface of the skin provides an easy way to measure muscle tension, but questions have arisen over the validity of this measurement as a pain indicator. For example, Herta Flor (2001) reported little consistency between self-reports of pain and EMG levels. A meta-analysis of EMG assessment of low back pain (Geisser et al., 2005) indicated that EMG was useful in discriminating those with versus those without low back pain, but EMG alone was not an adequate assessment.

Researchers have also attempted to assess pain through several autonomic indices, including such involuntary processes as hyperventilation, blood flow in the temporal artery, heart rate, hand surface temperature, finger pulse volume, and skin resistance level. A systematic evaluation of the relationship between pain and heart rate (Tousignant-Laflamme, Rainville, & Marchand, 2005) revealed a moderately high correlation, but only for men. These assessments have been used for patients who cannot furnish self-reports, but behavioral observation of pain-related behaviors is most often a better choice than physiological measurements for these groups.

IN SUMMARY

Pain measurement techniques can be grouped into three general categories: (1) self-reports, (2) behavioral observation, and (3) physiological measures. Self-reports include rating scales; pain questionnaires such as the McGill Pain Questionnaire and the Multidimensional Pain Inventory; and standardized objective tests such as the Minnesota Multiphasic Personality Inventory and the Beck Depression Inventory. Clinicians who treat pain patients often use a combination of assessments, relying most often on self-report inventories. Behavioral assessments of pain began as informal observation but have evolved into standardized ratings by trained clinicians that are especially useful for individuals, such as young children and people with dementia, who cannot complete self-reports. Physiological measures include muscle tension and autonomic indices such as heart rate, but these approaches are not as reliable or valid as self-reports or behavioral observation.

PAIN SYNDROMES

Acute pain is both an advantage and a disadvantage. The advantages come from the signals it sends about injury and the reminders it conveys to avoid further injury and allow healing. The disadvantage is that it hurts. The advantages outweigh the disadvantages, as the case of Ashlyn Blocker demonstrates. She cannot feel acute pain and has experienced many injuries as a result of this disability.

Chronic pain has no advantages—it signals no injury and causes people to live in misery. More than 10% of the population of the United States (Chen, 2005) and almost 20% of those in Europe (Corasaniti, Amantea, Russo, & Bagetta, 2006) experience chronic or intermittent persistent pain. Pain extracts an enormous personal and economic burden.

Chronic pain is categorized according to **syndrome**, symptoms that occur together and characterize a condition. Headache and low back

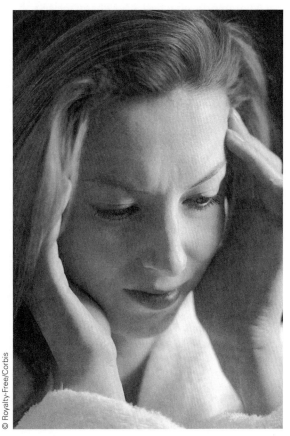

Headache is the most common of all types of pain—more than 99% of people have experienced a headache.

pain are the two most frequently treated pain syndromes, but people also seek treatment for several other common pain syndromes.

Headache Pain

Headache pain is the most common of all types of pain, with more than 99% of people experiencing headache at some time during their lives (Smetana, 2000). Until the 1980s, no reliable classification of headache pain was available to researchers and therapists. Then in 1988, the Headache Classification Committee of the International Headache Society (IHS) published a classification system that standardized definitions of various headache pains (Olesen, 1988). Although the IHS identifies many different kinds of headache, the three primary pain syndromes are migraine, tension, and cluster headaches.

Migraine headaches are characterized by recurrent attacks of pain that vary widely in intensity, frequency, and duration. Originally conceptualized as originating in the blood vessels in the head, migraine headaches are now believed to involve blood vessels but also a complex cascade of reactions that include neurons in the brain stem (Corasaniti et al., 2006) and to have a genetic component (Bigal & Lipton, 2008). The underlying cause and the exact mechanism for producing pain remain controversial. The attacks are associated with loss of appetite, nausea, vomiting, and exaggerated sensitivity to light and sound. Migraine headaches often involve sensory, motor, or mood disturbances. Migraines can be divided into those with aura and those without aura. Those with aura are characterized by identifiable sensory disturbances that precede the headache pain; migraines without aura have a sudden onset and an intense throbbing, usually (but not always) restricted to one side of the head. Brain imaging studies indicate that these two varieties of migraine affect the brain in somewhat different ways (Sánchez del Rio & Alvarez Linera, 2004).

The epidemiology of migraine headaches includes gender differences and variations in prevalence around the world. Women are two to three times more likely than men to have migraine headaches in the United States, Canada, and Europe (Manzoni & Torelli, 2002) as well as in Latin America (Morillo et al., 2005), with rates of 4% to 9% for men and 11% to 25% for women. Rates for non-Western countries are lower. For example, between 3% and 7% of people in Africa report migraines (Haimanot, 2002). However, the experience of migraine is similar; men and women who have chronic migraines have similar experiences of symptoms, frequency, and severity (Marcus, 2001). Most migraine patients experience their first headache before age 30 and some before the age of 10. However, the period for the greatest frequency of migraines is between ages 30 and 50 (Morillo et al., 2005). Few patients have a first migraine after age 40, but people who have migraines continue to do so, often throughout their lives.

Tension headaches have been described as muscular in origin, accompanied by sustained contractions of the muscles of the neck, shoulders, scalp, and face, but current explanations (Fumal & Schoenen, 2008) include mechanisms within the central nervous system. These headaches are characterized by gradual onset; sensations of tightness; constriction or pressure; highly variable intensity, frequency, and duration; and a dull, steady ache on both sides of the head. Nearly 40% of the U.S. population experiences tension headaches (Schwartz, Stewart, Simon, & Lipton, 1998), and people with this pain syndrome reported lost workdays and decreased effectiveness at work, home, and school because of their pain.

A third type of headache is the **cluster headache**, a severe headache that occurs in daily or nearly daily clusters (Favier, Haan, & Ferrari, 2005). Some symptoms are similar to those of migraine, including severe pain and vomiting, but cluster headaches are much briefer, rarely lasting longer than 2 hours (Smetana, 2000). The headache is localized on one side of the head, and often the eye on the other side becomes bloodshot and waters. In addition, cluster headaches are much more common in men than in women, by a ratio of 10:1. Most people who have cluster headaches experience episodes of headache, with weeks, months, or years of no headache (Favier et al., 2005). Cluster headaches are even less understood than other types of headaches, with no clear understanding of risk factors.

Low Back Pain

Low back pain is also very common. As many as 80% of people in the United States experience this type of pain at some time, making the problem extensive but not necessarily serious. Most injuries are not permanent, and most people recover (Leeuw et al., 2007). Those who do not recover quickly have a poor prognosis and are likely to develop chronic pain problems. Health care expenditures for these people total more than $90 billion a year in the United States (Luo, 2004). The incidence of low back pain shows some variation for countries around the world (European Vertebral Osteoporosis Study Group, 2004), but this condition produces direct expenses, such as medical care, and indirect costs, such as lost workdays and disability, affecting people in countries around the world (Dagenais, Caro, & Haldeman, 2008).

Low back pain has many potential causes, including infections, degenerative diseases, and malignancies, but the most frequent cause is probably injury or stress resulting in musculo-skeletal, ligament, and neurological problems in the lower back (Chou et al., 2007). Pregnancy is also a contributor to low back pain, with nearly 90% of pregnant women suffering from low back pain (Hayes et al., 2000). Aging is yet another factor in back pain, because the fluid content and elasticity of the intervertebral disks decrease as one grows older, and arthritis and osteoporosis become more likely. However, fewer than 20% of back pain patients have a definite identification of the physical cause of their pain (Chou et al., 2007), which suggests that psychosocial factors are important in low back pain.

Stress and psychological factors most likely play a role not only in back pain but also in all types of chronic pain. Making the transition from the prechronic stage to chronic pain is a complex process, and physiological and psychological processes accompany this progression. Some researchers (Baliki, Geha, Apkarian, & Chialvo, 2008; Corasaniti et al., 2006) have focused on physical changes in the nervous system that occur when pain becomes chronic. Other researchers (Leeuw et al., 2007; Sanders, 2006) have emphasized psychological factors such as fear, anxiety, depression, a history of trauma and abuse, and reinforcement experiences, all of which are more common among chronic pain patients. However, researchers taking both approaches acknowledge the complexity of the situation and the importance of psychosocial contributions to changes in the nervous system that result in chronic pain.

Arthritis Pain

Rheumatoid arthritis is an autoimmune disorder characterized by swelling and inflammation of the joints as well as destruction of cartilage, bone, and tendons. These changes alter the joint, producing direct pain, and the changes in joint structure lead to changes in movement, which may result in additional pain through this indirect route (Dillard, 2002). Rheumatoid arthritis can occur at any age, even during adolescence and young adulthood, but it is most prevalent among people 40 to 70 years old. Women are more than twice as likely as men to develop this disease (Theis, Helmick, & Hootman, 2007). The symptoms of rheumatoid arthritis are extremely variable. Some people experience a steady worsening of symptoms, but most people face alternating remission and intensification of symptoms. Rheumatoid arthritis interferes with work, family life, recreational activities, and sexuality (Pouchot, Le Parc, Queffelec, Sichère, & Flinois, 2007).

Osteoarthritis is a progressive inflammation of the joints that produces degeneration of cartilage and bone (Goldring & Goldring 2007); it affects mostly older people. This form of arthritis is experienced as a dull ache in the joint area, which is exacerbated by movement; the resulting lack of movement increases joint problems and pain. Osteoarthritis is the most common form of arthritis, which is one of the primary causes of disability in older people, affecting about 50% of those over 70 (Keefe et al., 2002). Older women make up a disproportionate number of those affected. As joints stiffen and pain increases, people with arthritis begin to have difficulties engaging in enjoyable activities and even basic self-care. They often experience feelings of helplessness, depression, and anxiety, which exacerbate their pain.

Fibromyalgia is a chronic pain condition characterized by tender points throughout the

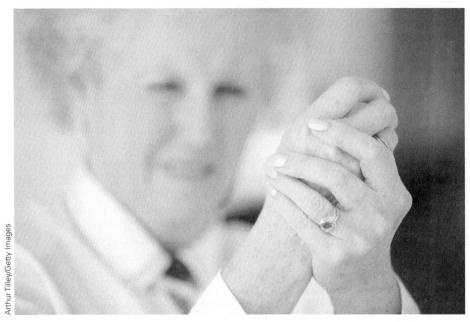

Arthur Tilley/Getty Images

Arthritis is a source of pain and disability for more than 20 million Americans.

body. This disorder also has symptoms of fatigue, headache, cognitive difficulties, anxiety, and sleep disturbances (Chakrabarty & Zoorob, 2007). Although fibromyalgia is not arthritis (Endresen, 2007), some symptoms are common to both, as is a diminished quality of life (Birtane, Uzunca, Tastekin, & Tuna, 2007).

Cancer Pain

More than a million people were diagnosed with cancer in the United States in the year 2005 (USCB, 2007). Cancer can produce pain in two ways: through its growth and progression and through the various treatments to control its growth. Studies have shown that pain is present in 55% of all cancer cases and in 75% or more of terminal cases (van den Beuken-van Everdingen et al., 2007). Some cancers are much more likely than others to produce pain. Head, neck, and cervical cancer patients experience more pain than leukemia patients (Anderson, Syrjala, & Cleeland, 2001). In addition, treatments for cancer may also produce pain; surgery, chemotherapy, and radiation therapy all produce painful effects. Thus, either the disease or its treatment creates pain for most cancer patients. Many also suffer from emotional distress, fear, anxiety, irritability, feelings of hopelessness and helplessness, changes in their relationships with spouses and other family members, or some combination of these conditions (Syrjala & Abrams, 1999).

Phantom Limb Pain

Just as injury can occur without producing pain, pain can occur in the absence of injury. One such type of pain is **phantom limb pain,** the experience of chronic pain in an absent body part. Amputation removes the nerves that produce the impulses leading to the experience of pain, but not the sensations. Most amputees experience some sensations from the amputated limb, and many of these sensations are painful (Czerniecki & Ehde, 2003).

Estimates of the proportion of amputees who experience phantom limb pain have varied. Until the 1970s, phantom pain was believed to be rare, with fewer than 1% of amputees experiencing a painful phantom limb, but more recent research has indicated that the percentage may be as high as 67% (Wall, 2000). The sensations often start soon after surgery as a tingling and then develop into other sensations that resemble actual feelings in the missing limb, including pain. Nor are the sensations of phantom pain limited to limbs. Women who have undergone breast removal also perceive sensations from the amputated breast, and people who have had teeth pulled sometimes continue to experience feelings from those teeth.

Amputees who experience unpleasant sensations from their amputated limbs may feel that the phantom limb is of abnormal size or in an uncomfortable position (Melzack & Wall, 1982). Phantom limbs can also produce painful feelings of cramping, shooting, burning, or crushing. These pains vary from mild and infrequent to severe and continuous. The severity and frequency of the pain tend to decrease over time, but 72% of amputees have pain in their phantom limb eight days after their surgery, 65% have pain six months afterward, and 60% have pain two years later (Melzack & Wall, 1988). Pain is more likely to occur in the missing limb when the person has experienced a great deal of pain before the amputation (Hanley et al., 2007).

The underlying cause of phantom limb pain has been the subject of heated controversy (Melzack, 1992; Woodhouse, 2005). Because surgery rarely relieves the pain, some authorities have hypothesized that phantom limb pain has an emotional basis. Melzack (1992) argued that phantom limb sensation arises within the brain as a result of the generation of a characteristic pattern of neural activity, which he called a *neuromatrix*. Melzack contended that this brain activity constituted "a characteristic pattern of impulses indicating that the body is intact and unequivocally one's own" (p. 123). This neuromatrix pattern continues to operate, even if the neurons in the peripheral nervous system do not furnish input to the brain.

Melzack believed that this pattern of brain activity is the basis for phantom limb sensations, which may include pain, and recent research is consistent with his theory (Woodhouse, 2005). Brain imaging technology has allowed researchers to investigate patterns of brain activation, and such studies have shown that the brain is capable of reorganization after injury, producing changes in the nervous system. Such changes have been observed in the somatosensory and motor cortex of amputees (Flor, Nikolajsen, &

Staehelin Jensen, 2007; Karl, Mühlnickel, Kurth, & Flor, 2004), which is consistent with Melzack's concept of the neuromatrix and its role in phantom limb pain. Therefore, phantom limb pain may be caused by changes that occur in both peripheral and central nervous systems after removal of the limb. Rather than compensating for the loss, the nervous system makes changes that are maladaptive, creating pain.

IN SUMMARY

Acute pain may result from hundreds of different types of injuries and diseases, but chronic pain can be classified according to a limited number of syndromes. A few of these syndromes account for the majority of people who suffer from chronic pain. Headache is the most common type of pain, but only some people experience chronic problems with migraine, tension, or cluster headaches. Most people's experience of low back pain is acute, but for some people the pain becomes chronic and debilitating. Arthritis is a degenerative disease that affects the joints, producing chronic pain. Rheumatoid arthritis is an autoimmune disease that may affect people of any age; osteoarthritis is the result of progressive inflammation of the joints that affects mostly older people. Fibromyalgia is a chronic pain condition characterized by pain throughout the body, sleep disturbances, fatigue, and anxiety. Pain is not an inevitable consequence of cancer, but most people with cancer experience pain either as a result of the progression of the disease or from the various treatments for cancer. One of the most puzzling pain syndromes is phantom limb pain, which constitutes pain without any physical basis. A majority of people with amputations experience this pain syndrome.

MANAGING PAIN

In 2001, an official recognition of inadequate pain control occurred: A jury found a physician guilty of allowing a patient to be in pain when he could have treated that pain (Wilson, 2001). The U.S. Congress passed legislation making the years 2001–2011 the Decade of Pain Control and Research. Patients' pain must now be monitored like other vital signs such as blood pressure and fever. Funding for pain research increased, and the magnitude of the problem and urgency of control were recognized (Nelson, 2003).

Pain presents complex problems for management. Treatment for acute pain is usually straightforward because the source of the pain is clear. However, helping people with chronic pain is a challenge because this type of pain exists without obvious tissue damage. Some people achieve relief through medical treatments, and others experience improvement through behavioral management of their pain.

Medical Approaches to Managing Pain

Drugs are the main medical strategy for treating acute pain. Although drugs are also a choice for some chronic pain syndromes, this strategy carries greater risks. Chronic pain that has not responded to drugs may be treated by surgery, which also presents risks.

Drugs **Analgesic drugs** relieve pain without causing loss of consciousness. Hundreds of different analgesic drugs are available, but almost all fall into two major groups: the opiates and the nonnarcotic analgesics (Julien, 2008). Both types exist naturally as derivatives of plants, and both have many synthetic variations. Of the two, the opium type is more powerful and has a longer history of use, dating back at least 5,000 years (Melzack & Wall, 1982).

Limitations on using opiate drugs for pain control include the development of both tolerance and dependence. **Tolerance** is the body's decreased responsiveness to a drug. When tolerance occurs, larger and larger doses of a drug are required to bring about the same effect. **Dependence** occurs when the drug's removal produces withdrawal symptoms. Because opiates produce both tolerance and dependence, they are potentially dangerous and subject to abuse. As a result, health care professionals are reluctant to prescribe these drugs, and many pain patients are afraid to use them, even when they could relieve severe pain.

How realistic are the fears of drug abuse as a consequence of prescribed opiate drugs? Do patients become addicted while recovering from surgery? What about the dangers to patients with terminal illnesses? According to one study (Porter & Jick, 1980), the risk of addiction is less than 1%. During the late 1990s, prescriptions for opiate analgesics increased dramatically, and publicity about an epidemic of analgesic abuse fueled the fear that increased prescriptions for these drugs were leading to widespread addiction. Despite increases in opiate use and abuse, the number of people who abuse these drugs represents less than 4% of the cases of drug abuse (Joranson, Ryan, Gilson, & Dahl, 2000).

The advantages of opiate drugs outweigh their dangers for some people in some situations; no other type of drug produces more complete pain relief. However, their potential for abuse and their side effects make them more suitable for treating acute pain than for managing chronic pain. The opiate drugs remain an essential part of pain management for the most severe, acute injuries, for recovery from surgery, and for terminal illnesses.

Between 1996 and 2000, the market for prescription analgesic drugs tripled (Raymond et al., 2001), and prescriptions continued to increase through 2005 (USCB, 2007). Much of this increase was for the drugs oxycodone and hydrocodone. Both are opiates with a potential for abuse, which increased during the time when prescriptions increased. Wariness about abuse of these drugs affects both physicians, who are reluctant to prescribe them, and many patients, who are reluctant to take sufficient doses to obtain relief. This reluctance applies to all opiate drugs, even for cancer pain (Reid, Gooberman-Hill, & Hanks, 2008). Thus, people with either acute or chronic pain frequently fail to receive sufficient relief.

One procedure that has overcome the undermedication problem is a system of self-paced administration. Patients can activate a pump attached to their intravenous lines and deliver a dose of medication whenever they wish, within limits that are programmed into the delivery device. Such systems began to appear in the late 1970s and have since gained wide acceptance because patients tend to use less medication, obtain better pain relief (Sri Vengadesh, Sistla, & Smile, 2005), and experience higher satisfaction (Gan, Gordon, Bolge, & Allen, 2007). Because an intravenous line is necessary for this system of drug delivery, it is most commonly used to control postoperative pain. However, a patient-controlled transdermal delivery system is also available (D'Arcy, 2005). This system allows people to self-administer analgesia through a device about the size of a credit card that adheres to their upper arm. These types of self-administered analgesics help prevent undermedication.

Whereas undermedication may be a problem for cancer pain patients, overmedication is often a problem for patients suffering from low back pain. One team of investigators (Von Korff, Barlow, Cherkin, & Deyo, 1994) grouped primary care physicians according to their low, moderate, or high frequency of prescribing pain medication and bed rest for back pain patients. A one- and two-year follow-up found that back pain patients who took less medication and remained active did just as well as those who were told to take more medication and to rest. A more recent study (Rhee, Taitel, Walker, & Lau, 2007) found that back pain patients who took opiate drugs experienced more frequent health problems such as hypertension, anxiety, depression, and arthritis; in addition, they were more likely to make a visit to a hospital emergency room. Both studies indicated that treatment for these patients was more costly than for patients who took other approaches to managing back pain. Thus, low back pain patients who use pain medication have poorer outcomes, more health problems, and higher costs than those who do not.

The nonnarcotic analgesics include a variety of nonsteroidal anti-inflammatory drugs (NSAIDs) as well as acetaminophen. Aspirin, ibuprofen, and naproxen sodium appear to block the synthesis of prostaglandins (Julien, 2008), a class of chemicals released by damaged tissue and involved in inflammation. The presence of these chemicals sensitizes neurons and increases pain. These drugs act at the site of injury instead of crossing into the brain, but they

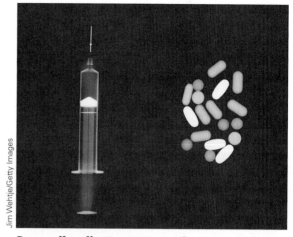

Jim Wehtje/Getty Images

Drugs offer effective treatment for acute pain but are not a good choice to treat chronic pain.

change neurochemical activity in the nervous system and affect pain perception. As a result of their mechanism of action, NSAIDs do not alter pain perception when no injury is present—for example, in laboratory situations with people who receive experimental pain stimuli.

Aspirin and other NSAIDs have many uses in pain relief, including for minor cuts and scratches as well as more severe injuries such as broken bones. But pain that occurs without inflammation is not so readily relieved by NSAIDs. In addition, NSAIDs can irritate and damage the stomach lining, even producing ulcers (Huang, Sridhar, & Hunt, 2002). Aspirin's side effects include the alteration of blood clotting time, and aspirin and other NSAIDs are toxic in large doses, causing damage to the liver and kidneys.

A new type of NSAID, the Cox-2 inhibitor, affects prostaglandins but has lower gastric toxicity. After the approval and heavy marketing of these drugs, their sales skyrocketed, especially among people with arthritis. However, the discovery of increased heart attack risk led to the withdrawal of two Cox-2 inhibitors from the market in the United States and increased caution in the use of this type of NSAID (Shi & Klotz, 2008).

Acetaminophen, another nonnarcotic analgesic, is not one of the NSAIDs. Under brand names such as Tylenol, acetaminophen has become a widely used drug. It has few anti-inflammatory properties but has a pain-relieving capability similar to that of aspirin though somewhat weaker. Acetaminophen does not have the gastric side effects of aspirin, so people who cannot tolerate aspirin find it a good substitute. However, acetaminophen is not harmless. Large quantities of acetaminophen can be fatal, and even nonlethal doses can do serious damage to the liver, especially when combined with alcohol (Julien, 2008).

Analgesic drugs are not the only drugs that affect pain. Antidepressant drugs and drugs used to treat seizures also influence pain perception, and these drugs can be used to treat some types of pain (Maizels & McCarberg, 2005). Antidepressants can be useful in treating low back pain, and some types of anticonvulsant medication can help people with migraine headaches. In addition, drugs have been developed that have some ability to prevent migraine headaches (Peres, Mercante, Tanuri, & Nunes, 2006) and to reduce the inflammation that is a damaging part of rheumatoid arthritis (Iagnocco et al., 2008). Similar developments for other chronic pain syndromes would change the lives of millions of people. Unfortunately, even the variety of drugs and strategies for their use are not adequate for many people with chronic pain. Those individuals may consider surgery or other treatments to attain relief.

Surgery Another traditional medical treatment for pain is surgery, which may be directed toward repairing the source of the pain or altering the nervous system to alleviate the pain. Low back surgery is the most common surgical approach to pain, but surgery is not an option that physicians recommend until other, less invasive possibilities have failed (van Zundert & van Kleef, 2005).

Surgery can also be performed to alter nerves that transmit pain (van Zundert & van Kleef, 2005). This procedure may use heat, cold, or radiofrequency stimulation to change neural transmission and control pain. Complete destruction of nerves is not recommended because this procedure leads to loss of all sensation, which may be more distressing than pain. Another tactic

for altering pain through changing nerve transmission involves stimulation of nerves through implanted wires that stimulate rather than damage nerves. Surgery is required for this approach, which involves implanting devices that can deliver electrical stimulation to either the spinal cord or the brain. Activation of the system produces pain relief by activating neurons and by releasing neurotransmitters that block pain. This process does not destroy neural tissue.

Spinal stimulation is a promising technique for controlling back pain (De Andrés & Van Buyten, 2006), but a related type of stimulation, **transcutaneous electrical nerve stimulation (TENS)**, has proven to be less effective. The TENS system typically consists of electrodes that attach to the skin and are connected to a unit that supplies electrical stimulation. Despite some promising early indications of success, TENS has demonstrated only limited effectiveness in controlling pain (Reeves, Graff-Radford, & Shipman, 2004).

Surgery has at least two limitations as a treatment for pain. First, it does not always repair damaged tissue, and second, it does not provide all patients with sufficient pain relief. Even those for whom surgery is initially successful may experience a return of pain. That is, surgery is not a successful treatment for many people with chronic back pain (Ehrlich, 2003). Thus, this approach is an expensive but unreliable approach to controlling this pain syndrome (Turk & McCarberg, 2005). Also, surgery has its own potential dangers and possibilities for complications, which leads many pain patients to behavioral approaches for managing their pain.

Behavioral Techniques for Managing Pain

Psychologists have been prominent in devising therapies that teach people how to manage pain, and several behavioral techniques have proven effective with a variety of pain syndromes. These techniques include relaxation training, behavioral therapy, cognitive therapy, and cognitive behavioral therapy. Some authorities consider these techniques to be part of mind–body medicine and thus part of alternative medicine (covered in

Chapter 8). Psychologists see these techniques as part of psychology.

Relaxation Training Relaxation has been used as an approach to managing pain and may be the key ingredient in other types of pain management. *Progressive muscle relaxation* consists of sitting in a comfortable chair with no distractions and then systematic tensing and relaxing of muscle groups throughout the body (Jacobson, 1938). After learning the procedure, people can practice this relaxation technique independently.

Relaxation techniques have been used successfully to treat pain problems such as tension and migraine headache (Fumal & Schoenen, 2008; Penzien, Rains, & Andrasik, 2002), rheumatoid arthritis (McCallie et al., 2006), and low back pain (Ostelo et al., 2007). A National Institutes of Health Technology (NIHT) panel evaluated the evidence for progressive muscle relaxation and gave this technique its highest rating in controlling pain (Lebovits, 2007). However, relaxation training typically functions as part of a multicomponent program (Astin, 2004).

Table 7.1 summarizes the effectiveness of relaxation techniques.

Behavioral Therapy The most prominent behavioral therapy is *behavior modification*, which arose from the laboratory research on operant conditioning. **Behavior modification** is the process of shaping behavior through the application of operant conditioning principles. The goal of behavior modification is to shape *behavior*, not to alleviate *feelings* or *sensations* of pain. People in pain usually communicate their discomfort to others through their behavior—they complain, moan, sigh, limp, rub, grimace, and miss work.

Behavior modification strategies for coping with stress and pain are based on the notion that behaviors that are rewarded continue, whereas behaviors that are not rewarded tend to decrease in frequency (Skinner, 1953, 1987). This approach suggests that when complaining, moaning, sighing, limping, and missing work are rewarded, the pain is magnified and is more likely to become chronic. A laboratory study (Jolliffe & Nicholas, 2004) confirmed that verbal reinforcement increased reports of pain, offering confirmation for the underlying premise of a learning theory approach to pain and behavior modification treatment.

Wilbert E. Fordyce (1974) was among the first to emphasize the role of operant conditioning in the perpetuation of pain behaviors. He recognized the *reward* value of increased attention and sympathy, financial compensation, and other **positive reinforcers** that frequently follow pain behaviors. These conditions create what pain expert Frank Andrasik (2003) called pain traps, situations that push people who experience pain toward being trapped in chronic pain. The situations that create chronic pain include attention from family, relief from normal responsibilities,

TABLE 7.1
Effectiveness of Relaxation Techniques

Problem	Findings	Studies
1. Tension and migraine headaches	Relaxation helps in managing headache.	Fumal & Schoenen, 2008; Penzien et al., 2002
2. Rheumatoid arthritis	Progressive muscle relaxation is an effective component in programs to manage these disorders.	McCallie et al., 2006
3. Low back pain	Relaxation is effective in programs to treat low back pain.	Ostelo et al., 2007
4. Variety of chronic pain conditions	Progressive muscle relaxation is effective according to a NIHT review.	Lebovits, 2007

compensation from employers, and medications that people receive from physicians. These reinforcers make it difficult to get better.

Behavior modification works against these pain traps, identifying the reinforcers and training people in the patient's environment to use praise and attention to reinforce more desirable behaviors and to withhold reinforcement when the patient exhibits less desired pain behaviors. In other words, the groans and complaints are now ignored, whereas efforts toward greater physical activity and other positive behaviors are reinforced. Progress is noted by such criteria as amount of medication taken, absences from work, time in bed or off one's feet, number of pain complaints, physical activity, range of motion, and length of sitting tolerance. The strength of the operant conditioning technique is its ability to increase levels of physical activity and decrease the use of medication—two important targets in any pain treatment regimen (Roelofs, Boissevain, Peters, de Jong, & Vlaeyen, 2002). In addition, this approach can also decrease pain intensity (Sanders, 2006). The behavior modification approach does not address the cognitions that underlie and contribute to behaviors, but cognitive therapy focuses on these cognitions.

Cognitive therapy is based on the principle that people's beliefs, personal standards, and feelings of self-efficacy strongly affect their behavior (Bandura, 1986, 2001; Beck, 1976; Ellis, 1962). Cognitive therapies concentrate on techniques designed to change cognitions, assuming that behavior will change when cognitions are altered. Albert Ellis (1962) argued that thoughts, especially irrational thoughts, are the root of behavior problems. He focused on the tendency to "catastrophize," which escalates an unpleasant situation into something worse.

The experience of pain is one that can easily be turned into a catastrophe, and any exaggeration of feelings of pain can lead to maladaptive behaviors and further exacerbation of irrational beliefs. The tendency to catastrophize is associated with the magnification of pain, both acute (Pavlin, Sullivan, Freund, & Roesen, 2005) and chronic (Karoly & Ruehlman, 2007). These findings support Ellis's contention that magnifying an event into a catastrophe will lead to increased emotional distress.

Once irrational cognitions have been identified, the therapist actively attacks these beliefs, with the goal of eliminating or changing them into more rational beliefs. For example, cognitive therapy for pain addresses the tendency to catastrophize, leading people to abandon the belief that their pain is unbearable and will never stop (Thorn & Kuhajda, 2006). Cognitive therapists address these cognitions and work with patients to change them. Rather than concentrating exclusively on thoughts, however, most cognitive therapists working with pain patients address changes in both cognitions and behavior. That is, they practice cognitive behavioral therapy.

Cognitive behavioral therapy (CBT) is a type of therapy that aims to develop beliefs, attitudes, thoughts, and skills to make positive changes in behavior. Like cognitive therapy, CBT assumes that thoughts and feelings are the basis of behavior, so CBT begins with changing attitudes. Like behavior modification, CBT focuses on modifying environmental contingencies and building skills to change observable behavior.

One approach to CBT for pain management is the pain inoculation program designed by Dennis Turk and Donald Meichenbaum (Meichenbaum & Turk, 1976; Turk, 1978, 2001), which is similar to stress inoculation explained in Chapter 5. Pain inoculation includes a cognitive stage, the *reconceptualization* stage, during which patients are led to accept the importance of psychological factors for at least some of their pain and often receive an explanation of the gate control theory of pain. The second stage—*acquisition and rehearsal of skills*—includes learning relaxation and controlled breathing skills. The final, or *follow-through*, phase of treatment includes instructions to spouses and other family members to ignore patients' pain behaviors and to reinforce such healthy behaviors as greater levels of physical activity, decreased use of medication, fewer visits to the pain clinic, or an increased number of days at work. With the help of their therapists, patients construct a posttreatment plan for coping with future pain, and finally, they apply their coping skills to everyday situations outside the pain clinic. A study of laboratory-induced pain (Milling, Levine, & Meunier, 2003) indicated that inoculation training was as effective as hypnosis in helping participants control pain. A study of athletes recovering from knee injury (Ross & Berger, 1996) also found that pain inoculation procedures were effective.

Other CBT programs have demonstrated their effectiveness for a wide variety of pain syndromes. CBT includes strategies for addressing the harmful cognitions that are common among chronic pain patients, such as fear and catastrophizing (Leeuw et al., 2007; Thorn et al., 2007) and a behavioral component to help pain patients behave in ways that are compatible with health rather than illness. Evaluations of cognitive behavioral therapy for low back pain (Hoffman, Papas, Chatkoff, & Kerns, 2007; Ostelo et al., 2007) indicate its effectiveness for this pain syndrome, and studies of CBT with headache patients (Martin, Forsyth, &

Reece, 2007; Nash, Park, Walker, Gordon, & Nicholson, 2004; Thorn et al., 2007) have also demonstrated its benefits. Fibromyalgia patients benefited more from CBT than from a drug treatment (García, Simón, Durán, Canceller, & Aneiros, 2006), and CBT proved beneficial for people with rheumatoid arthritis (Astin, 2004; Sharpe et al., 2001) as well as cancer and AIDS pain (Breibart & Payne, 2001). CBT may even affect the immune system in positive ways (Gaab et al., 2003), an accomplishment that few techniques have achieved (see Chapter 6).

In summary, these studies show that behavior modification and cognitive behavioral therapy can be an effective intervention for pain management for people with a variety of pain syndromes. These techniques are among the most effective types of pain management strategies. Table 7.2 summarizes the effectiveness of these therapies and the problems they can be used to treat.

TABLE 7.2

Effectiveness of Behavioral, Cognitive, and Cognitive Behavioral Therapy

Problem	Findings	Studies
1. Increase in pain behaviors	Verbal reinforcement increases pain behaviors.	Jolliffe & Nicholas, 2004
2. Chronic low back pain	Operant conditioning increases physical activity and lowers medication usage; CBT can also be effective.	Roelofs et al., 2002
3. Pain intensity	Behavior modification decreases pain intensity	Sanders, 2006
4. Catastrophizing the experience of pain	Catastrophizing intensifies acute and chronic pain.	Karoly & Ruehlman, 2007; Pavlin et al., 2005; Thorn & Kuhajda, 2006
5. Laboratory-induced pain	Inoculation training was as effective as hypnosis for pain.	Milling et al., 2003
6. Athletes with knee pain	Pain inoculation reduces pain.	Ross & Berger, 1996
7. Low back pain	CBT was evaluated as effective in a meta-analysis and in a systematic review.	Hoffman et al., 2007; Ostelo et al., 2007
8. Headache pain and prevention	CBT is effective in both management and prevention.	Martin et al., 2007; Nash et al., 2004; Thorn et al., 2007
9. Fibromyalgia	CBT is more effective than drug treatment.	García et al., 2006
10. Rheumatoid arthritis	CBT can relieve some pain.	Astin, 2004; Sharpe et al., 2001
11. Cancer and AIDS pain	CBT helps people cope.	Breibart & Payne, 2000

IN SUMMARY

A variety of medical treatments for pain have demonstrated uses but also limitations. Analgesic drugs offer pain relief for acute pain and can be of use for chronic pain. These drugs include opiates and nonnarcotic drugs. Opiates are effective in managing severe pain, but their tolerance and dependence properties pose problems for use by chronic pain patients, making health care professionals and patients reluctant to use effective doses. Nonnarcotic drugs such as aspirin, nonsteroidal anti-inflammatory drugs (NSAIDs), and acetaminophen are effective in managing mild to moderate acute pain and have some uses in managing chronic pain.

Surgery can alter either peripheral nerves or the central nervous system. Surgical procedures are often done as a last resort in controlling chronic pain, and procedures that involve destruction of nerve pathways are often unsuccessful. Procedures that allow for stimulation of the spinal cord show more promise in pain management, but transcutaneous electrical nerve stimulation (TENS) has not demonstrated effectiveness.

Health psychologists help people cope with stress and chronic pain by using relaxation training, behavioral therapy, cognitive therapy, and cognitive behavioral therapy. Relaxation techniques such as progressive muscle relaxation have demonstrated some success in helping patients manage headache pain, postoperative pain, and low back pain. Behavior modification can be effective in helping pain patients become more active and decrease their dependence on medication, but this approach does not address the negative emotions and suffering that accompany pain. Cognitive therapy addresses feelings and thus helps in reducing the catastrophizing that exacerbates pain. Combined with the behavioral components of operant conditioning, cognitive behavioral therapy has demonstrated greater effectiveness than other therapies.

Cognitive behavioral therapy includes pain inoculation therapy, but other combinations of changes in cognitions concerning pain and behavioral strategies for changing pain-related behavior also fit within this category. These approaches have been successful in treating low back pain, headache pain, rheumatoid arthritis pain, fibromyalgia, and the pain that accompanies cancer and AIDS.

ANSWERS

This chapter has addressed five basic questions:

1. How does the nervous system register pain?

Receptors near the skin's surface react to stimulation, and the nerve impulses from this stimulation relay the message to the spinal cord. The spinal cord includes laminae (layers) that modulate the sensory message and relay it toward the brain. The somatosensory cortex in the brain receives and interprets sensory input. Neurochemicals and the periaqueductal gray can also modulate the information and change the perception of pain.

2. What is the meaning of pain?

Pain is difficult to define, but it can be classified as acute (resulting from specific injury and lasting less than six months), chronic (continuing beyond the time of healing), or prechronic (the critical stage between acute and chronic). The personal experience of pain is affected by situational and cultural factors as well as individual variation and learning history. The meaning of pain can also be understood through theories. The leading model is the gate control theory of pain, which takes both physical and psychological factors into account in the experience of pain.

3. How can pain be measured?

Pain can be measured physiologically by assessing muscle tension or autonomic arousal, but these measurements do not have high validity. Observations of pain-related behaviors (such as limping, grimacing, or complaining) have some reliability and validity. Self-reports are the most common approach to pain measurement; they include rating scales, pain questionnaires, and standardized psychological tests.

4. What types of pain present the biggest problems?

The individual experience of pain can also be defined in terms of syndromes that classify chronic pain according to their symptoms. These syndromes include headache pain, low back pain, arthritic pain, cancer pain, and phantom limb pain; the first two are the most common sources of chronic pain and lead to the most time lost from work or school.

5. What techniques are effective for pain management?

The techniques that health psychologists use in helping people cope with pain include relaxation training and behavioral techniques. Relaxation training can help people cope with pain problems such as headache and low back pain. Behavioral approaches include behavior modification, which guides people to behave in ways compatible with health rather than pain. Cognitive therapy concentrates on thoughts, guiding pain patients to minimize catastrophizing and fear. Cognitive behavioral therapy combines strategies to change cognitions with behavioral application, which is an especially effective approach for pain control.

SUGGESTED READINGS

Baar, K. (2008, March/April). Pain, pain, go away. *Psychology Today, 41*(2), 56–57. This very brief article provides a summary of psychological factors in pain and the treatments psychologists have used successfully to help people manage pain.

Gatchel, R. J. (2005). The biopsychosocial approach to pain assessment and management. In R. J. Gatchel (Ed.), *Clinical essentials of pain management* (pp. 23–46). Washington, DC: American Psychological Association. Gatchel's lengthy article focuses on the biopsychosocial model applied to pain. He devotes much of the article to issues relevant to pain assessment.

Wall, P. (2000). *Pain: The science of suffering.* New York: Columbia University Press. Peter Wall, one of the originators of the gate control theory of pain, tells about his extensive experience in trying to understand this phenomenon. He provides a nontechnical examination of the experience of pain, considering the cultural and individual factors that contribute.

Watkins, L. R., & Maier, S. F. (2003). When good pain turns bad. *Current Directions in Psychological Science, 12,* 232–236. In this brief article, Watkins and Maier summarize their research on the development of chronic pain, which emphasizes the role of neurochemicals and glia as modulators in the nervous and immune systems' response to injury.

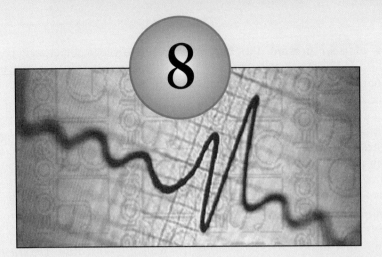

CONSIDERING ALTERNATIVE APPROACHES

QUESTIONS

This chapter focuses on five basic questions:

1. What medical systems represent alternatives to conventional medicine?

2. What alternative practices and products are used in alternative medicine?

3. What is mind–body medicine?

4. Who uses complementary and alternative medicine?

5. What are the effective uses and limitations of alternative treatments?

CHECK YOUR HEALTH CARE PREFERENCES

Check the items that are consistent with your beliefs.

☐ 1. When I am in pain, I go to the medicine cabinet to find something to alleviate my pain.

☐ 2. I believe that herbal treatments can be as effective as drugs in treating pain.

☐ 3. Drug companies should develop a pill to help people deal with stress.

☐ 4. Stress and pain arise from sources outside the person.

☐ 5. If my pain did not respond to medical treatment, I would be willing to try some alternative approach such as hypnosis or acupuncture.

☐ 6. Too many people take drugs to help them cope with their problems.

☐ 7. I would prefer alternative treatment rather than medical treatments for stress and pain problems.

☐ 8. Stress and pain come from an interaction of the person and the situation.

☐ 9. Chiropractic care offers no real benefits.

☐ 10. Alternative treatments cannot be as effective as conventional medical treatments.

☐ 11. Alternative treatments are safer than conventional medical approaches.

☐ 12. I believe that a combination of alternative and conventional medical treatments offers the best approach for pain management.

If you agreed with items 1, 3, 4, 9, and 10, then you probably have a strong belief in traditional medical approaches to treatment, including treatments for stress and pain problems. If you agreed with items 2, 5, 6, 7, 8, 11, and 12, then you show some beliefs that are compatible with alternative and behavioral treatments.

This chapter examines alternative treatments, describes alternative approaches to managing stress and pain, and reviews evidence about the effectiveness of these approaches.

REAL-WORLD PROFILE OF NORMAN COUSINS

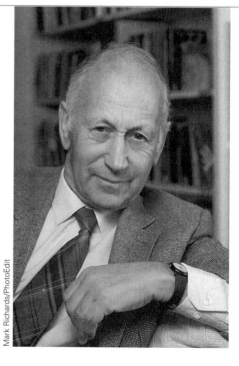

Mark Richards/PhotoEdit

In 1964 Norman Cousins was editor of the influential magazine *Saturday Review* when he was stricken by ankylosing spondylitis, a degenerative, inflammatory disease that affects the connective tissue in the spine. His physician told Cousins that his chances of recovery were 1 in 500 (Cousins, 1979). The treatment involved hospitalization and large doses of anti-inflammatory drugs, which Cousins checked into the hospital and began. However, he decided that he could not remain a passive observer in his health care. Furthermore, he began to question the effectiveness of hospital routine, hospital food, seemingly endless tests, and high doses of drugs. Cousins left the hospital.

Cousins's treatment proceeded, but instead of a hospital room, he chose a nice hotel room. Rather than drugs, Cousins prescribed himself a healthy diet, large doses of vitamin C, an optimistic attitude, and a regimen of laughter from episodes of *Candid Camera* and old Marx brothers movies. His physician was skeptical but agreed to this unusual course of treatment, and to his surprise, Cousins began to improve; eventually, he made a complete recovery. Cousins reported his experience in an article published in 1976 in the *New England Journal of Medicine*, which became the first chapter of his 1979 book, *Anatomy of an Illness as Perceived by the Patient*.

Cousins became a vocal advocate for the power that lies within people to heal themselves. He argued for the necessity of broadening medicine to focus on the patient and including psychological factors in the healing process. By accepting the position of Adjunct Professor of Medical Humanities at the University of California at Los Angeles, Cousins was able to work within conventional medicine to advocate for alternatives to that approach. He spoke and wrote about the possibilities for the healing power of positive emotions until his death in 1990. Cousins helped move medical care from one dominated by the biomedical model based on the concept of pathogens as the underlying cause of disease to a biopsychosocial model that includes social, cultural, and psychological factors.

The biopsychosocial model is an expansion of the biomedical view, but other conceptualizations of illness differ so much from mainstream medicine that they fall into the category of **alternative medicine**, which is a group of diverse medical and health care systems, practices, and products that are not currently considered part of conventional medicine (National Center for Complementary and Alternative Medicine [NCCAM], 2002). Alternatives to conventional medicine come from systems of medicine that arose in different cultures, such as traditional Chinese medicine; from practices that are not yet accepted in mainstream medicine, such as chiropractic treatment and massage therapy; and from products that are not yet recognized as having medicinal value, such as megadoses of vitamins or herbal remedies. These practices and products may be used as alternatives to conventional medicine— for example, when a person seeks chiropractic treatment or massage therapy for pain rather than taking an analgesic drug. However, people usually combine alternative with conventional treatments (Barnes et al., 2004). In such circumstances, the term **complementary medicine** applies—for example, when a person uses both massage and analgesic drugs to control pain. The group of systems, practices, and products is often termed *complementary and alternative medicine (CAM)*.

ALTERNATIVE MEDICAL SYSTEMS

The classification of procedures and products as complementary or alternative depends not only on cultural context but also on time period. In the United States 150 years ago, surgery was an alternative treatment not well accepted by established medicine (Weitz, 2007). As surgical techniques improved and evidence began to accumulate that surgery was the best treatment for some conditions, it became part of conventional medicine. More recently, the value of whole grain diets made the transition from alternative medicine to mainstream medical recommendation when evidence about the health value of high-fiber diets began to accumulate (Hufford, 2003). Some of the techniques that are now considered CAM will, with research and time, become part of conventional medicine.

Making the transition from CAM to conventional medicine requires demonstrating the effectiveness of the procedure or substance through scientific research (Berman & Straus, 2004; Committee on the Use of Complementary and Alternative Medicine, 2005). The U.S. Congress created an agency that became the National Center for Complementary and Alternative Medicine, which has provided funding and sponsored research. Beginning in 1992, this agency has sponsored research on CAM in an attempt to determine which of these approaches is effective for what conditions, as well as who uses CAM and for what conditions. Before considering the findings on CAM approaches for managing stress, pain, and other conditions, we will review some of the major CAM approaches and techniques.

The health care most people receive in North America, Europe, and other places around the world comes from physicians, surgeons, nurses, and pharmacists who represent the biomedical system of medicine. Various alternative systems have arisen at different times and places; some have evolved during the same time frame as what we consider to be conventional medicine (NC-CAM, 2004d). Each of these alternative systems includes a complete theory of disease (and possibly of health as well) and a description of what constitutes appropriate medical practice. In the United States, about 8% of people have used a treatment based on at least one of these systems (Barnes et al., 2004).

Traditional Chinese Medicine

Traditional Chinese medicine (TCM) originated in China at least 2,000 years ago (NCCAM, 2004d) and remains a major treatment approach in China and other Asian countries. The system of TCM holds that a vital force, called *qi* (pronounced "chee" and sometimes written *chi*) animates the body, flowing through channels in the body called *meridians* (Traditional Chinese Medicine World Foundation [TCMWF], 2005–2008). These meridians connect parts of the body to each other and to the universe as a whole. If the qi is blocked or becomes stagnant, health impairment and disease can develop. Keeping the qi in balance is important to maintaining and restoring health.

The body exists in a balance between two opposing energies or forces, *yin* and *yang* (TCMWF, 2005–2008). Yin represents cold, passive, and slow energy, whereas yang is seen as hot, active, and rapid. The two always operate together, and achieving a balance between the two is essential for health; attaining a harmony is ideal. Imbalances may occur through physical, emotional, or environmental events, and thus TCM takes a holistic approach to diagnosis and treatment. Practitioners have a variety of techniques to help individuals revitalize and unblock qi, bring yin and yang into balance, and restore health. These techniques include acupuncture, massage, herbal preparations, diet, and exercise.

Acupuncture became the first component of traditional Chinese medicine to gain widespread publicity in the West in 1971, when *New York Times* journalist James Reston experienced and reported on acupuncture treatment he received in China (Harrington, 2008). Reston had accompanied Secretary of State Henry Kissinger to China as Kissinger worked toward a meeting between Chinese leader Mao Tse-Tung and U.S. President

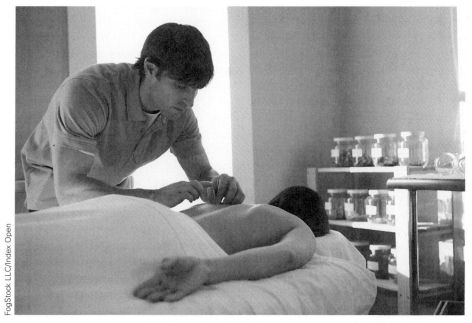

FogStock LLC/Index Open

Acupuncture originated within traditional Chinese medicine and has become a popular alternative treatment.

Richard Nixon, who wanted to establish diplomatic relations with China. Reston's story about the success of acupuncture in controlling his postoperative pain captured the interest of many people and led the way toward acupuncture's becoming well known as a treatment in alternative medicine. Acupuncture holds an important place in the system of traditional Chinese medicine.

Acupuncture consists of inserting needles into specific points on the skin and continuously stimulating the needles (NCCAM, 2007c). The stimulation can be accomplished electrically or by twirling the needles. About 4% of people in the United States have used acupuncture (Barnes et al., 2004). **Acupressure** is a manipulative technique that involves the application of pressure rather than needles to the points used in acupuncture. In the system of traditional Chinese medicine, acupuncture and acupressure help to unblock the flow of qi along the meridians and thus restore health. In addition, massage called *tui na* is used to stimulate or subdue qi (TCMWF, 2005–2008). To determine which of two types of tui na is appropriate, practitioners feel the patient's pulse. The application of massage is believed to regulate the nervous system, boost immune function, and help flush wastes out of the system.

The Chinese *Materia Medica* is a reference guide to the use of herbs and herbal preparations in treatment (NCCAM, 2004d). Herbs such as ginseng and ginger are common, but many other plant, mineral, and even animal preparations are part of herbal remedies. The ingredients are ground into a powder and either made into tea or formed into pills.

Diet and exercise are also part of traditional Chinese medicine. Rather than aiming for a diet with a balance of carbohydrates, protein, and fats, recommendations in TCM strive to remedy imbalances in yin and yang by eating certain foods and avoiding others (TCMWF, 2005–2008). Some foods and methods of preparation are seen as cool and moist (properties of yin), and people with conditions in which cold and moisture predominate should avoid these foods. Rather, these individuals should eat warming foods that stimulate circulation. The exercise that has therapeutic properties is *qi gong*, which consists of a series of movements and breathing techniques that help with the circulation of qi.

Some of these practices from TCM, such as acupuncture and qi gong, as well as products such as herbal preparations, have been used as alternative treatments for specific problems. However, traditional Chinese medicine consists of an integrated theory of health and disease. Ayurveda is another system of medicine that emphasizes balance.

Ayurvedic Medicine

Ayurveda, or Ayurvedic medicine, is an ancient system that arose in India; the first written texts appeared more than 2,000 years ago (NCCAM, 2005). The term originated in two Sanskrit words, the combination of which means "science of life." The goal of Ayurvedic medicine is to integrate and balance the body, mind, and spirit. These three elements are believed to be an extension of the relationship among all things in the universe. Humans are born in a state of balance, but events can disrupt this balance. When these elements are out of balance, health is endangered; bringing them back into balance restores health.

Ayurvedic practitioners diagnose patients through examinations that include observation of physical characteristics as well as questions about lifestyle and behavior (NCCAM, 2005). Formulating a treatment plan may require consultation with family members as well as the patient. The goals of treatment are to eliminate impurities and to increase harmony and balance, which are achieved through changes to diet and exercise. These changes may include special diets or fasting to eliminate impurities in the body and yoga exercises. Massage to vital points on the body is also part of Ayurvedic medicine as a form of pain relief and improvement to circulation. The use of herbs, medicated oils, spices, and minerals is extensive; more than 5,000 products exist in Ayurvedic medicine. Patients may also be directed to change behaviors to reduce worry and increase harmony in their lives, and yoga practice may be part of this element. About 0.4% of people in the United States have sought Ayurvedic treatment, making it much less common than traditional Chinese medicine (Barnes et al., 2004).

Naturopathy

Naturopathy, or naturopathic medicine, is a medical system that arose in Europe during the 19th century (NCCAM, 2007e). Its central belief is that nature contains the power to heal, and the human body has the ability to maintain and to return to a state of health. Table 8.1 lists the key principles of naturopathy.

This system was especially popular in Germany and came to the United States when an enthusiastic patient, Benedict Lust, immigrated (NCCAM, 2007e). Lust had been diagnosed with tuberculosis and treated by a priest and healer who advocated wholesome diet, light exercise, fresh air, and exposure to sunlight. *Hydrotherapy*, using hot and cold baths, was also popular and included in some naturopathic treatments. Lust named the movement *naturopathy* and dedicated himself to promoting it, founding a professional society and a college for training naturopathic practitioners in the United States.

Some naturopathic practitioners are physicians who train in one of the four naturopathic colleges in the United States and receive a doctor of naturopathy (ND) degree (NCCAM, 2007e). These naturopathic physicians may prescribe some drugs, perform minor surgery, and deliver babies. Other practitioners do not have doctoral degrees. Their practices emphasize a healthy lifestyle and reject medicines, X rays, and surgery as treatments. Both types of naturopathic practitioners rely on an extensive diagnostic interview and make recommendations about dietary and lifestyle changes to those who consult them. They may recommend vitamin and herbal supplements, exercise, hydrotherapy, massage, yoga, and meditation. A bit less than 1% of people in the United States have sought naturopathic treatment (Barnes et al., 2004).

Homeopathy

Homeopathy is another medical system that diverges from the background and assumptions of conventional medicine. Samuel Christian Hahnemann developed this system in Germany in the late 1700s (NCCAM, 2004c). Hahnemann envisioned treatment that was less harsh than the bloodletting, purging, and blistering that were common medical practice at the time. He developed the hypothesis that "like cures like"; that is, substances have curative power when they produce symptoms that are similar to those of the disease. Hahnemann added two other principles to his system. One principle was *potentization*, the notion that systematically diluting a substance and shaking it vigorously after each dilution makes the mixture more rather than less potent. Hahnemann's final principle was that a treatment should be selected for the entire patient rather than for the patient's symptoms. Thus, homeopathy originated as a type of holistic health care.

An American doctor, Hans Burch Gram, studied homeopathy in Europe and brought it to the United States in 1825, where it gained popularity (NCCAM, 2004c). A college to train homeopaths was established in 1835, and homeopathic hospitals arose during the 19th century. By 1900, homeopathy was widespread in the United States. The practice declined with the growing dominance of conventional medicine, beginning in the 1930s, but interest increased during the 1960s.

Homeopathic treatment relies on *remedies*, the diluted substances formed from potentization. In the United States, these remedies are over-the-counter drugs regulated by the Food and Drug Administration (NCCAM, 2004c). People may select remedies for themselves or consult a homeopath. A consultation typically includes an in-depth interview that allows the selection of remedies. Additional visits to the practitioner allow for an evaluation of response and progress. About 3.6% of

TABLE 8.1

Key Principles of Naturopathy

1. Promote the healing power of nature.
2. First do no harm.
3. Treat the whole person.
4. Treat the cause rather than the symptoms.
5. Prevention is the best cure.
6. The physician is a teacher, helping patients in taking responsibility for their own health.

Source: National Center for Complementary and Alternative Medicine. (2007). *An Introduction to Naturopathy.* Bethesda, MD: Author, p. 3.

people in the United States have used homeopathic treatments (Barnes et al., 2004).

All of the alternative medical systems propose a unified view of disease and health, complete with treatments to restore health and a rationale for their use. All the systems are holistic, considering psychological and emotional as well as physical factors that affect health. Many also share the concept of a vital energy that has healing power. In addition to alternative systems of health, CAM includes other practices and products that lie outside conventional medicine.

IN SUMMARY

Alternative medicine consists of a group of health care systems, practices, and products that are not currently part of conventional medicine but that people use rather than (alternative medicine) or along with conventional treatments (complementary medicine).

Alternative health care systems include traditional Chinese medicine (TCM), Ayurvedic medicine, naturopathy, and homeopathy. TCM and Ayurvedic medicine are ancient; naturopathy and homeopathy arose in the 19th century. Each of these systems presents a theory of health and disease as well as practices for diagnosis and treatment.

TCM holds that the body contains a vital energy called qi; keeping this energy in balance is essential to health. Technqiues such as acupuncture and acupressure, herbal remedies, massage (called tui na), and the energy-channeling practices of qi gong and tai chi are aimed at achieving this balance. Ayurvedic medicine accepts the notion of vital energy and holds that the integration of body, mind, and spirit is essential to health. Diet and herbal preparations are part of Ayurvedic medicine, and so is exercise, including yoga. Naturopathy holds that the body is capable of healing itself, with the help of diet, exercise, and fresh air. Homeopathy assumes that substances have curative power when they produce symptoms that are similar to those of the disease. Homeopathic remedies are diluted mixtures of these substances.

ALTERNATIVE PRACTICES AND PRODUCTS

Alternative practices lie outside of conventional medicine but do not constitute entire medical systems. Rather, they consist of practices oriented toward symptom relief or treatment of disease conditions. The most common alternative practices are chiropractic treatment, massage, and specific diets. These practices are among the most popular alternative treatments, accounting for more than half of CAM usage (Barnes et al., 2004). The practice of energy healing is much less common (NCCAM, 2007b). Natural products such as echinacea and ginseng are also popular, as is the use of megavitamins and some herbal treatments. More than 30% of people in the United States have used one or more of these alternative practices and products (Barnes et al., 2004).

Chiropractic Treatment

Chiropractic was founded by Daniel David Palmer in 1895 (NCCAM, 2007d). Palmer believed that manipulation of the spine was the key not only to curing illness but also to preventing it. That focus forms the basis for chiropractic care—performing adjustments to the spine and joints to correct misalignments that underlie health problems. Chiropractic adjustments involve applying pressure with the hands or with a machine that forces a joint to move beyond its passive range of motion. Chiropractors may also use heat, ice, and electric stimulation as part of treatment; they may also prescribe exercise for rehabilitation, dietary changes, or dietary supplements. With these problems corrected, the body can heal itself (NCCAM, 2004a).

Palmer founded the first chiropractic school in 1896, and chiropractic began to spread in the United States during the early 20th century (Pettman, 2007). Students are accepted into schools of chiropractic training after completing at least 90 hours in undergraduate college courses, focusing on science (NCCAM, 2004a). Chiropractic training requires an additional four years of study in one of the schools accredited by the Council of Chiropractic Education. The program involves coursework and patient care. All 50 states of the United States license chiropractors after they finish their course of study and undergo board examinations.

Almost from the beginning of chiropractic, physicians attacked the practice, having chiropractors prosecuted for practicing medicine without a license (Pettman, 2007). The American Medical Association waged a bitter battle against chiropractic throughout the mid-20th century, but the chiropractors prevailed. Chiropractic is in the process of becoming integrated into conventional medicine; for example, requests by athletes for chiropractic treatment has encouraged its integration into sport medicine (Theberge, 2008). Chiropractic treatment is also available for clients served through the U.S. Department of Defense and the Department of Veterans Affairs (2004a). Indeed, chiropractic treatment has become so well accepted that many insurance plans pay for these services. About 8% of people in the United States (Barnes et al., 2004) and about 11% of those in Canada (Park, 2005) used chiropractic in 2002 or 2003. Considering lifetime use, almost 20% of people in the United States have sought chiropractic treatment, mostly for back, neck, and headache pain (Barnes et al, 2004).

Massage

Chiropractic manipulation focuses on the spine and joints, but massage manipulates soft tissue to produce health benefits. Considered a luxury a few years ago, massage is now recognized as an alternative therapy used to control stress and pain. This approach dates back thousands of years and arose in many cultures (Moyer, Rounds, & Hannum, 2004). Records of massage date back to 2000 B.C., and early healers such as Hippocrates and Galen wrote about its benefits. Today, about 5% of people in the United States have used massage as CAM (Barnes et al., 2004).

Several different types of therapeutic massage exist. Although Per Henrik Ling is often credited, it was Johan Mezger who developed the massage techniques during the 19th century that became known as Swedish massage (Pettman, 2007). This type of massage uses light strokes in one direction combined with kneading muscles using deeper

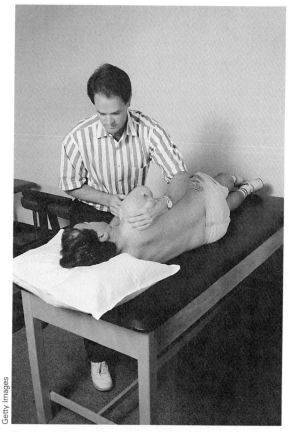

Getty Images

Manipulating the spinal cord or muscles can be effective in helping to relieve pain.

pressure in the opposite direction to achieve relaxation (NCCAM, 2006a). Originally part of physical therapy and rehabilitation, this approach to massage is now also practiced as an independent therapy for stress and pain management.

Other types of massage come from other systems of medicine, including traditional Chinese medicine (TCM), Ayurveda, and naturopathy. Acupressure and tui na are both manipulative techniques originating in TCM (NCCAM, 2004d). Acupressure involves the application of pressure to meridians on the body, with the goal of unblocking the flow of qi. *Shiatsu massage* is the Japanese counterpart of acupressure. Tui na is another approach from TCM for allowing the qi to flow freely throughout the body. It may involve pushing the qi along specific meridians using one finger or thumb, which is also similar to shiatsu massage. The use of massage in naturopathic treatment may be similar to massage in TCM, with the goal of releasing the body's natural healing power. The rationale for Ayurvedic massage is similar, holding that manipulating specific points on the body will channel healing energy within the body. Its practice often involves medicinal oils to decrease friction and to help with the healing. Thus the practice of massage is common among CAM, arising from several systems and used as an independent healing practice.

Energy Healing

The view that energy can heal the body or that the body contains vital, healing energy is common to many alternative systems and practices. One version of energy healing employs some type of physical energy applied to the body for health purposes. This energy may be vibration such as sound or some form of electromagnetic energy such as light, magnetism, or lasers (NCCAM, 2007b). Other versions of energy healing seek to prompt or channel the body's healing energy. An example of this approach is the concept of qi from traditional Chinese medicine; the techniques of qi gong and tui na are intended to remedy problems with the flow of qi. About 1% of people in the United States have used some form of energy healing (Barnes et al., 2004).

Japanese traditional medicine, Ayurveda, homeopathy, and naturopathy all contain techniques for directing energy for healing (NCCAM, 2007b). The Japanese technique of Reiki appears to be a version of massage, but the concept behind this manipulation is a directing of energy from the universe through the hands of a practitioner and to the body of the recipient. The technique of Therapeutic Touch involves manipulating the energy fields that emanate from the body to redirect its vital energy. In the application of Therapeutic Touch, practitioners do not actually touch patients but instead perform movements a few inches from their bodies to get in touch with and redirect their energy. The failure to measure this vital energy reliably has made energy healing one of the most controversial of alternative treatments. However, one of the most widely used alternative practices fits into this controversial

category—prayers for health improvement (see Would You Believe . . . ? box).

Diets

Another strategy for improving health involves following specific diets for health benefits, which may include weight loss. Such diets include vegetarian, macrobiotic, Atkins, Pritikin, Ornish, and Zone diets. About 7% of people in the United States have followed one of these diets (Barnes et al., 2004).

Several varieties of vegetarian diets exist (Mayo Clinic Staff, 2008). All vegetarian diets restrict meat and fish and focus on vegetables, fruits, grains, legumes, seeds, and plant-based oils. Lacto-vegetarian diets allow dairy products, ovo-lacto vegetarian diets allow dairy products and eggs, whereas vegan diets allow neither dairy nor egg products. Diets that restrict meat and meat products tend to be lower in fat and higher in fiber than other diets, which makes them beneficial for people with health problems such as high cholesterol levels. The American Heart Association and the American Cancer Society have recommended limiting meat consumption for health reasons. The American Dietetic Association (Mangels, Messina, & Melina, 2003) has analyzed all three varieties of vegetarian diets and pronounced all capable of furnishing adequate nutrition for people in all stages of development, but vegetarians must plan their meals carefully to assure that they receive adequate protein, calcium, and other nutrients.

Those who follow a *macrobiotic diet* must be even more careful than other vegetarians to obtain adequate nutrients (American Cancer Society, 2007). This diet was developed by Japanese philosopher George Ohsawa in the 1930s as a way to integrate Asian and Western religion and medicine. The macrobiotic diet is largely vegetarian but restricts food choices to grains, cereals, cooked vegetables, and a limited amount of fruit and fish.

The Atkins, Pritikin, Ornish, and Zone diets vary in terms of the amount of carbohydrates and fats allowed and also vary in their overall goals (Gardner et al., 2007). The Atkins diet is a weight loss program that limits carbohydrates but not

WOULD YOU BELIEVE . . . ?

Religious Involvement May Improve Your Health

Beginning with Emile Durkheim (1912/1967) nearly a century ago, social scientists have pondered and debated the health benefits of religious involvement. Recently, researchers have begun to study this relationship, and a major meta-analysis (McCullough, Hoyt, Larson, Koenig, & Thoresen, 2000) found that religious involvement was related to lower rates of hypertension, heart disease, stroke, and cancer. This conclusion is consistent with the practice of a substantial percentage of people in the United States: A survey of adults in the United States (McCaffrey, Eisenberg, Legedza, Davis, & Phillips, 2004) found that 35% had used prayers for health within the past year. A large majority of those people rated the prayers as helpful.

However, finding prayer helpful is not the same as being helped by prayers for health. In a controlled study of prayer (Palmer, Katerndahl, & Morgan-Kidd, 2004) and

two meta-analyses of such studies (Masters & Spielmans, 2007; Masters, Spielmans, & Goodson, 2005), the results indicated that people who were the objects of prayers did not differ significantly from those who were not. That is, having others pray for the improvement of a person's problem did not diminish the problem significantly. However, people's beliefs in being able to solve the problem were related to improvement. When people are the object of prayers for their health but do not know about the intercession, their health remains the same. However, this situation is not typical—most people know when others are praying for their health.

The knowledge that someone is praying for one's health is a type of social support, and social support constitutes one of the important ways in which religion may affect health (Oman & Thoresen, 2002). In addition, many religions offer

guidelines for behavior such as moderation in lifestyle choices, which could also contribute to health. Another route of influence is through spirituality, which can lead people to enhanced positive mental states that may affect the immune system and thus influence health. Indeed, spirituality is one path that people follow to find meaning in their misfortunes, and this strategy allows people to develop feelings of optimism and hope (Ai, Peterson, Tice, Bolling, & Koenig, 2004).

Despite widespread beliefs that prayer can affect health directly, research offers little support for this possibility. However, research has confirmed health and longevity advantages for religious involvement (McCullough et al., 2000). These effects may occur through several routes, including enhanced social support, encouragement of healthy lifestyles, and feelings of optimism and meaning in life.

---

fat or calories. The Zone diet is also a weight loss diet that limits carbohydrate consumption, but it aims to balance carbohydrates, proteins, and fats to specified percentages of caloric intake. The Ornish and Pritikin programs strive to limit fat intake to 10% of calories, which represents a very low level of fat consumption. Because of the severe fat restriction, both diets are almost entirely vegetarian. Neither of these diets is specifically aimed at weight loss; rather, both were designed as beneficial for cardiovascular health. However, both tend to produce weight loss as a result of the very low fat intake, and weight loss may be desirable for some people at high risk.

Another strategy to improve or enhance health involves supplementing the diet with vitamins, minerals, herbs, or other products. This

approach may be used in connection with or as an alternative to adopting a specific diet.

Dietary Supplements

People supplement their diets with a wide variety of vitamins, minerals, herbs, amino acids, extracts, and special foods. In the United States, the Food and Drug Administration regulates dietary supplements as food rather than as drugs; such products are sold without restriction, without evaluations of effectiveness, but with evaluations of safety (NCCAM, 2007a).

The practice of supplementing the diet to improve health is ancient (NCCAM, 2007a). An examination of the mummified remains of the "Ice Man" found in the Alps in 1991 indicated that he carried medicinal herbs with him. The practice of using dietary supplements arose in many cultures and exists in many variations. People use vitamin and mineral supplements primarily to preserve their health and to promote wellness. Almost half the people in the United States take a multivitamin supplement, but only about 4% take very large doses of vitamins (Barnes et al., 2004). Some supplements are used to treat diseases and conditions. For example, echinacea is used as a treatment for colds and flu, Saint-John's-wort for depression, calcium supplements for bone mineral loss, and glucosamine for osteoarthritis (NCCAM, 2007a). In addition, some people supplement their diets with *functional foods*, components of a normal diet that have biologically active components, such as fish oil, soy, chocolate, and cranberries. Within the past 20 years, vitamin supplements have grown in popularity, but enthusiasm for herbal supplements has decreased. Sales of dietary supplements amount to billions of dollars each year in the United States, and supplements are among the most widely used types of alternative medicine (Barnes et al., 2004).

IN SUMMARY

Alternative practices and products include chiropractic treatments, massage, energy healing, diets, and dietary supplements. Chiropractic focuses on spinal alignment and the joints, using adjustment techniques to bring the spine back into alignment. Massage is also a manipulation technqiue, but massage focuses on the soft tissue. Several different types of massage exist, but many share the underlying premise that this type of manipulation helps the body to heal itself. Energy healing shares some characteristics of massage, especially Reiki, the Japanese method of directing healing energy through massage. Another common procedure is following a specialized diet. Many diets are oriented to weight loss or lowering cholesterol levels, such as the Atkins, Ornish, or Zone diets; other diets have the goal of improving health, such as vegetarian and macrobiotic diets. People supplement their diets with a wide variety of vitamins, minerals, herbs, amino acids, extracts, and special foods to improve health or to treat specific conditions.

MIND–BODY MEDICINE

Mind–body medicine is the term applied to a variety of techniques that are based on the notion that the brain, mind, body, and behavior interact in complex ways and that emotional, mental, social, and behavioral factors exert important effects on health (NCCAM, 2004b). Some of these techniques are associated with psychology and some with conventional medicine, but all share the notion that mind and body represent a holistic system of dynamic interactions. Norman Cousins, whose story began this chapter, was an enthusiastic proponent of this view. However, this conception is not recent; it forms the basis for traditional Chinese medicine, Ayurvedic medicine, and many other systems of traditional and folk medicine. This notion was also prominent in Europe until the 17th century, when French philosopher René Descartes proposed that the mind and the body work according to different principles. Descartes' pronouncement promoted the view that the body functions according to mechanistic principles, which was important in the development of Western medicine but discounted the importance of the mind in physical health.

Those who accept mind–body medicine seek to understand the interaction of mind and body and its relationship to health. Some of the techniques of mind–body medicine come from those systems that originated a holistic view, such as traditional Chinese medicine and Ayurvedic medicine. However, the techniques include not only those that arose within those systems of medicine, such as meditation, tai chi, qi gong, and yoga, but also guided imagery, hypnosis, and biofeedback.

Meditation and Yoga

Most approaches to meditation originated in Asian religions, but the mind–body approaches to meditation typically have no religious connotations (NCCAM, 2006b). Many variations of meditation exist, but all involve a quiet location, a specific posture, a focus of attention, and an open attitude. Two prominent types of meditation are transcendental meditation and mindfulness meditation. About 10% of people in the United States have used meditation (Barnes et al., 2004).

Transcendental Meditation Transcendental meditation originated in the Vedic tradition in India (NCCAM, 2006b). Participants who practice this type of meditation usually sit with eyes closed and muscles relaxed. They then focus attention on their breathing and silently repeat a sound, such as "om" or any other personally meaningful word or phrase, with each breath for about 20 minutes. Repetition of the single word is intended to prevent distracting thoughts and to sustain muscle relaxation. Meditation requires a conscious motivation to focus attention on a single thought or image along with effort not to be distracted by other thoughts.

Mindfulness Meditation Mindfulness meditation has roots in ancient Buddhist practice but has been adapted as a modern stress-reduction practice. In mindfulness meditation, people usually sit in a relaxed, upright posture and focus on any thoughts or sensations as they occur, trying to enhance their own awareness of their perceptions and thought processes in a nonjudgmental way (Kabat-Zinn, 1993). If unpleasant thoughts or sensations occur, meditators are encouraged not to ignore them, but to let them pass and to concentrate on the breath. By noting thoughts objectively, without censoring or editing them, people can gain insight into how they see the world and what motivates them.

Mindfulness meditation has been adapted into a program of mindfulness-based stress reduction (Kabat-Zinn, 1993). This procedure involves an eight-week course of training, which typically occurs for at least two hours per day and may also include an intensive retreat to develop meditation skills. This procedure has been used in a wide variety of settings to help people control anxiety and manage chronic disease and pain conditions. Research into the nature of mindfulness training (Jha, Krompinger, & Baime, 2007) suggests that it improves attention processes by altering the subcomponents of attention such as orienting attention and alerting attention.

Guided Imagery Guided imagery has some elements in common with meditation, but it also has important differences. In guided imagery, people conjure up a calm, peaceful image, such as the repetitive rhythmic roar of an ocean or the quiet beauty of a pastoral scene. They then concentrate on that image for the duration of a situation, often one that is painful or anxiety provoking. The assumption underlying guided imagery is that a person cannot concentrate on more than one thing at a time. Therefore, imagining an especially powerful or delightful scene will divert attention from the painful experience (see Becoming Healthier box). About 3% of people in the United States have used guided imagery (Barnes et al., 2004).

Yoga Yoga has its origins in ancient India but is now part of mind–body practice (NCCAM, 2004b). It includes physical postures, breathing, and meditation, and its goal is to balance body, mind, and spirit. Of the various schools of yoga, Hatha yoga is the most common in the United States and Europe. The many postures of yoga furnish ways to move and concentrate energy in the body. This concentration of attention on the body permits people to ignore other situations and problems and to live in their bodies in the moment. Controlled breathing fosters relaxation. About 7.5% of people in the United States have practiced yoga (Barnes et al., 2004).

Qi Gong and Tai Chi

Traditional Chinese medicine includes movement-based approaches to unblock qi and improve health. The basic technique is *qi gong* (also written *qigong*, *chi gung*, and *chi gong*), which consists of a series of exercises or movements that are intended to concentrate and balance the body's vital energy (Sancier & Holman, 2004). Its practice promotes relaxation. Tai chi or tai chi chuan originated as one of the martial arts but evolved into a set of movements used for therapeutic benefits (Gallagher, 2003).

Qi Gong Qi gong involves the practice or cultivation (gong) of the qi (energy) by postures and simple movements that channel vital energy and restore balance in the body. It is one of the basic practices of traditional Chinese medicine (TCMWF, 2005–2008). "At its core qigong is the manipulation of the regulation of the body, breath, and mind into

BECOMING HEALTHIER

One technique that helps people manage and minimize pain is guided imagery. This technique involves creating an image and being guided (or guiding yourself) through it. The process can be helpful in dealing with both chronic pain and acute pain, such as medical or dental procedures. Those who are not experienced at guided imagery will benefit from putting the guided imagery instructions on an audiotape or digital recorder.

To practice guided imagery, choose a quiet place where you will not be disturbed and where you will be comfortable. Prepare for the experience by placing the tape player or recorder where you can turn it on, seating yourself in a comfortable chair, and taking a few deep breaths. Turn on the player, close your eyes, and follow the instructions you have recorded.

The instructions should include a description of a special place, one that you either imagine or have experienced, where you feel safe and at peace. Tailor the place to fit with your life and experiences—one person's magic place may not be so attractive to another person, so think about what will be appealing to you. Many people enjoy a beach scene, but others like woods, fields, or special rooms. The goal is to imagine somewhere that you will feel relaxed and at peace.

Put instructions on your recording concerning this place and its description. Spend time in this place and experience it in detail. Pay attention to the sights and sounds, but do not neglect the smells and skin senses associated with the place. Spend time imagining each of these sensory experiences, and include instructions to

yourself about the feelings. You should feel relaxed and peaceful as you go though this scene. Linger over the details and aim to allow yourself to become completely absorbed in the experience.

Include some instructions for relaxed breathing in your tour of your special place. Your goal is to achieve peace and relaxation that will replace the anxiety and pain that you have felt. As you repeat the guided imagery exercise, you may want to revise the recording to include more details. The recording should include at least 10 minutes of guided instructions, and you may want to redo the recording into a longer version as you become more proficient in the exercise. Eventually, you will not need the recording, and you will be able to use this technique wherever you go.

an integrative whole, with the breath as the key regulator practice to make this happen" (Shinnick, 2006, p. 351). These postures and movements may be practiced individually or integrated into a sequence, called a *form*. Within traditional Chinese medicine, the practice of qi gong increases health and decreases the need for treatments such as acupuncture and herbal remedies.

Although qi gong fits within the philosophy of traditional Chinese medicine, its practice has been adapted to be compatible with Western medicine, under the name *medical qi gong* (He, 2005; Sancier & Holman, 2004). Researchers have investigated the physical existence of qi, with claims that the practice of qi gong creates measurable changes in thermal and electrical energy (Shinnick, 2006). Evidence also exists that qi gong training produces changes in the function of the immune system (Lee, Kim, & Ryu, 2005),

which allows for a specific route through which qi gong might affect health. The practice of medical qi gong seeks to prevent disease, promote long life, and treat specific disease conditions such as hypertension, diabetes, and heart disease as well as stress and pain. The practice of qi gong is not common in the United States; fewer than 1% of people in the United States have practiced qi gong (Barnes et al., 2004).

Tai Chi Tai chi (or tai chi chuan) is one category of qi gong form, which has evolved from a martial art with a long but controversial history. Some advocates trace its history back thousands of years, whereas others point to a history of only several hundred years (Kurland, 2000). The key figures in its development are also the subject of debate, but a commonly cited story involves a Shaolin monk who noticed the struggle between

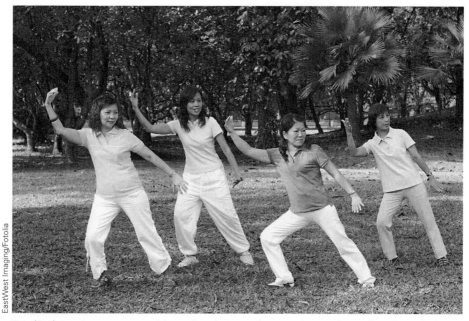

Tai chi chuan is a movement-based technique that produces physical and psychological benefits.

a snake and a crane and adapted their movements to a form of defense. Over time, the practice of tai chi became increasingly popular as a way to promote health, spreading throughout China and around the world. As one of the practices of traditional Chinese medicine, tai chi cultivates balance between the yin and yang energies and thus promotes health.

Tai chi involves slow, gentle movements that shift the weight while the person maintains an upright yet relaxed posture and controlled breathing (NCCAM, 2006d). One movement flows into another, and those who practice tai chi strive to maintain a steady rate of movement while coordinating the breath with the movements, creating a "moving meditation." The history of tai chi includes the development of many different styles, originally perpetuated within families. Currently, the Yang style is the most common in China and among those who practice tai chi as alternative medicine. All of the variations in styles include a set of movements connected together into a sequence, called a form. The Yang long form consists of 108 movements, but shorter forms exist, with some having as few as 12 movements. Tai chi

provides moderate intensity aerobic exercise equivalent to brisk walking and a low-impact form of exercise that is appropriate for a wide variety of individuals (Taylor-Piliae, Haskell, Waters, & Froelicher, 2006). Tai chi is more widely practiced in the United States than is qi gong; 2.5% report its use (Barnes et al., 2004).

Biofeedback

Until the 1960s, most people in the Western world assumed that it was impossible to consciously control physiological processes such as heart rate, the secretion of digestive juices, and the constriction of blood vessels. These biological functions do not require conscious attention for their regulation, and conscious attempts at regulation seem to have little effect. Then, during the late 1960s, a number of researchers began to explore the possibility of controlling biological processes traditionally believed to be beyond conscious control. Their efforts culminated in the development of **biofeedback**, the process of providing feedback information about the status of biological systems. Early experiments indicated that biofeedback made possible the control of some otherwise automatic functions. In 1969, Neal E. Miller reported a series of experiments in which he and his colleagues altered the levels of animals' visceral response through reinforcement. Some subjects received rewards for raising their heart rate and others for lowering it. Within a few hours, significant differences in heart rate appeared. After other investigators demonstrated that biofeedback could be used with humans (Brown, 1970; Kamiya, 1969), interest in this procedure became widespread.

In biofeedback, biological responses are measured by electronic instruments, and the status of those responses is immediately available to the person being tested. By using biofeedback, a person gains information about changes in biological responses as they are taking place. This feedback allows the person to alter physiological responses that cannot be voluntarily controlled without the biofeedback information.

Several types of biofeedback are found in clinical use, including electromyography and thermal biofeedback; 1% of people in the United States reported that they have used biofeedback (Barnes et al., 2004). **Electromyograph (EMG) biofeedback** reflects the activity of the skeletal muscles by measuring the electrical discharge in muscle fibers. The measurement is taken by attaching electrodes to the surface of the skin over the muscles to be monitored. The level of electrical activity reflects the degree of tension or relaxation of the muscles. The machine responds with a signal that varies according to that muscle activity. Biofeedback can be used to increase muscle tension in rehabilitation or to decrease muscle tension in stress management. The most common use of EMG biofeedback is in the control of low back pain and headaches.

Thermal biofeedback, which may also be used to help people cope with stress and pain, is based on the principle that skin temperature varies in relation to levels of stress. Stress tends to constrict blood vessels, whereas relaxation opens them. Therefore, cool surface skin temperature may indicate stress and tension; warm skin temperature suggests calm and relaxation. Thermal biofeedback involves placing a **thermister**— a temperature-sensitive resistor—on the skin's surface. The thermister signals changes in skin temperature, thereby furnishing the information that allows control. The feedback signal, as with EMG biofeedback, may be auditory, visual, or both.

Hypnotic Treatment

Although trancelike conditions are probably older than human history, modern hypnosis is usually traced to the last part of the 18th century, when Austrian physician Franz Anton Mesmer conducted elaborate demonstrations in Paris. Although Mesmer's work was attacked, modifications of his technique, known as *mesmerism*, soon spread to other parts of the world. By the 1830s, mesmerism was being used by some surgeons as an anesthetic during major operations (Hilgard & Hilgard, 1994).

With the discovery of chemical anesthetics, the popularity of hypnosis waned, but during the late 19th century, many European physicians, including Sigmund Freud, employed hypnotic procedures in the treatment of mental illness. Since the beginning of the 20th century, the popularity of hypnosis as a medical and psychological tool has continued to wax and wane. Its present position is still somewhat controversial, but a significant number of practitioners within medicine and psychology are using hypnotherapy to treat health-related problems, especially pain. The technique remains in limited use; fewer than 2% of people in the United States have used hypnosis (Barnes et al., 2004).

Not only is the use of hypnotic processes still controversial, but the precise nature of hypnosis is also debatable. Some authorities, such as Joseph Barber (1996) and Ernest Hilgard (1978), regard hypnosis as an altered *state* of consciousness in which a person's stream of consciousness is divided or dissociated. Barber argued that hypnotic analgesia works through a process of negative hallucination—not perceiving something that one would ordinarily perceive. To Hilgard, the process of **induction**—that is, being placed into a hypnotic state—is central to the hypnotic process. After induction, the responsive person enters a state of divided or dissociated consciousness that is essentially different from the normal state. This altered state of consciousness allows people to respond to suggestion and to control physiological processes that they cannot control in the normal state of consciousness.

The alternative view of hypnosis holds that it is a more generalized *trait*, or a relatively permanent characteristic of some people who respond well to suggestion (T. X. Barber, 1984, 2000). Those who hold this view reject the basic conception that hypnosis is altered consciousness. Rather, they argue that hypnosis is nothing more than relaxation, induction is not necessary, and suggestive procedures can be just as effective without entering a trancelike state.

Research has not resolved this controversy. Brain imaging studies (De Benedittis, 2003; Rainville & Price, 2003) tend to support the view that hypnosis is an altered state of consciousness. However, in a study comparing hypnotic to nonhypnotic suggestion (Milling, Kirsch, Allen, & Reutenauer, 2005), both types were comparably effective. That is, expectancy and suggestion led to a reduction of pain whether participants were hypnotized or not.

IN SUMMARY

Mind–body medicine is a term applied to a variety of techniques that people use to improve their health or treat health problems, including meditation, guided imagery, yoga, qi gong, tai chi, biofeedback, and hypnosis. Transcendental meditation directs people to focus on a single thought or sound to achieve relaxation, whereas mindfulness meditation encourages practitioners to focus on the moment, becoming mindful of the details of their current experience. Guided imagery encourages people to create a pleasant scene to achieve relaxation. Yoga uses physical postures, breathing, and meditation, with the goal of balancing body, mind, and spirit. The movement-based practices of qi gong and tai chi originated in traditional Chinese medicine. Qi gong and tai chi involve postures and movements intended to direct and balance the body's vital energy.

Biofeedback is the process of providing feedback information about the status of biological systems with the goal of controlling them. Many types of biofeedback exist, but learning to control muscle tension through electromyograph biofeedback and skin temperature through thermal biofeedback have the widest clinical applications. Hypnotic treatment is controversial, with some authorities arguing that it represents an altered state of consciousness that boosts relaxation and suggestibility, whereas others contend that it is a trait of some individuals. In either case, the relaxation and suggestibility both have the potential to improve health.

WHO USES COMPLEMENTARY AND ALTERNATIVE MEDICINE?

People use techniques from complementary and alternative medicine to enhance health, prevent disease, and manage health problems. Table 8.2 summarizes the most commonly used types of CAM in the United States. Many of the techniques from CAM are applicable and widely used in managing anxiety, stress, and pain. Indeed, a great deal of the research funded by the U.S. National Center for Complementary and Alternative Medicine is oriented toward assessing the effectiveness of these approaches for these conditions. In addition, a growing number of people find these techniques appealing, and an increasing number of people use CAM.

Assessing the prevalence of CAM use depends on what techniques are included within the definition. For example, when prayers for health were included, the percentage of CAM users in the United States was 62%; excluding prayer yielded a figure of 36% of people who used some form of CAM within the year before the survey (Barnes et al., 2004). These people used a variety of CAM techniques. The most common reason they gave was that they thought the technique would be a good addition to what they were doing to manage their problem. That is, most people (54.9%) indicated that they were using the technique as complementary rather than alternative medicine, which is similar to CAM use in Europe (Rössler et al., 2007) and Canada (Foltz et al., 2005). Only 28% of U.S. residents were using CAM because they believed that conventional medicine would not help their condition (Barnes et al., 2004).

TABLE 8.2

Most Frequently Used CAM Therapies Among U.S. Adults

Technique	Percentage of Adults Who Used This Approach
Prayer for one's health	43.0%
Prayers of others for one's health	24.4
Natural products: echinacea, ginseng, ginkgo biloba, garlic	18.9
Deep-breathing exercises	11.6
Participation in prayer group for one's health	9.6
Meditation	7.6
Chiropractic care	7.5
Yoga	5.1
Massage	5.0
Diet-based therapies: Atkins diet, vegetarian diet	3.5
Any CAM technique	62.1%

Source: Data from "Complementary and Alternative Medicine Use Among Adults: United States, 2002," by P. M. Barnes, E. Powell-Griner, K. McFann, & R. L. Nahin, 2004, *Advance Data from Vital and Health Statistics,* no. 343. Hyattsville, MD: National Center for Health Statistics.

Culture, Ethnicity, and Gender

The use of CAM varies among countries to some extent. In a population study in Australia, 68.9% of people reported using some form of CAM (Xue, Zhang, Lin, Da Costa, & Story, 2007). This study did not include prayers for health as a CAM category; thus, the percentage of people seeking CAM in Australia is substantially higher than in the United States. In addition, the Australian government has integrated CAM into health care delivery to a greater extent than in most other English-speaking countries (Baer, 2008).

In Europe, the percentage of users varies by country. Some countries are similar to the United States, whereas others use CAM as frequently as Australians do (di Sarsina, 2007). The types of treatments and demographics of users are similar among these three geographic areas. Nutritional supplements such as vitamins as well as massage therapy, meditation, chiropractic treatments, yoga, and acupuncture are among the most popular CAM therapies (Xue et al., 2007). Individuals who seek CAM tend to be female, well-educated, and in the upper income brackets. The availability of CAM varies by European country. In some countries, such as Sweden, the availability is limited; the Swedish health service does not consider

offering CAM treatments because of insufficient evidence of their effectiveness (di Sarsina, 2007). In other countries, such as Germany and the United Kingdom, CAM is integrated into medical practice, with physicians receiving training in CAM and referring patients to CAM practitioners. In countries in which CAM is integrated into the health services, users tend to come from a wider variety of socioeconomic backgrounds than in countries such as the United States, where most CAM users must pay out-of-pocket for such treatment.

CAM use varies with ethnicity in the United States, but not in ways that correspond to stereotypes (Keith, Kronenfeld, Rivers, & Liang, 2005). The stereotypical association of CAM with ethnic minorities and recent immigrants is largely incorrect: European Americans are more likely than African Americans or Hispanic Americans to use CAM. Indeed, recent immigrants are *less* likely to use CAM than immigrants who have been in the United States for years (Su, Li, & Pagán, 2008). A similar finding emerged from a study of Asian Americans (Hsiao, Wong, et al., 2006); acculturation did not predict CAM usage. However, Asian Americans used CAM at higher rates than non-Hispanic European Americans. Chinese

Americans' usage of CAM was higher than that of other Asian Americans, and their usage tended to correspond to their culture: Chinese Americans were more likely than other Asian Americans to use herbal products (Hsiao, Wong, et al., 2006) and to seek acupuncture treatment (Burke, Upchurch, Dye, & Chyu, 2006).

In all ethnic groups and in various countries, women are more likely than men to use CAM. In the United States, well-educated European American women are more likely than others to use CAM (Barnes et al., 2004). The willingness of women to use CAM may relate to personal beliefs or health concerns (Furnham, 2007). The importance of personal beliefs and the compatibility of CAM with one's beliefs may explain why some people seek alternative treatments whereas others do not.

Motivations for Seeking Alternative Treatment

Although culture, ethnicity, and gender each shows a relationship to CAM use, other factors are probably more important. One of those important factors is acceptance of the underlying values of CAM. Research findings suggest that people use CAM when the techniques are compatible with their personal worldviews and concerns about health (Astin, 1998). For example, young men who expressed strong beliefs in science were less likely to use CAM than other people (Furnham, 2007). People who have less faith in conventional medicine and stronger beliefs in the role of attitude and emotion in health are more likely to try CAM. Thus, an openness to different worldviews, an acceptance of the value in holistic treatment, and a belief in the contribution of biopsychosocial factors to health are more typical of CAM users than of those who stay with conventional treatments exclusively.

A person's current health status is also an important predictor of CAM usage. People tend to seek alternative treatments when conventional medicine has not offered relief for their conditions. Those who use CAM may not be dissatisfied with conventional medicine (Astin, 1998; Barnes et al., 2004); people tend to add alternative treatments to the conventional ones they are

using rather than replace conventional treatments with alternative ones. However, individuals who experience chronic health problems that have not responded well to conventional treatments may be open to the possibilities of alternative treatment. Therefore, poor health status is a significant predictor of CAM usage (Astin, 1998; Burke et al., 2006; Feinglass et al., 2007; Shmueli & Shuval, 2006). Reasonably enough, people who are unwell and continue to experience distressing symptoms are motivated to find some effective treatment and to consider alternative medicine.

Within both conventional and alternative medicine lie concerns about effectiveness and safety for the various products and practices that fall within CAM. What is the evidence of success for these alternative approaches?

IN SUMMARY

Most people who use CAM use it as a complementary rather than an alternative treatment. People in the United States and other countries use a great variety of CAM products and practices, including prayers for health, vitamin supplements, natural products, meditation, chiropractic, massage, and yoga. People in Australia and some European countries use CAM more often than people in the United States, but the assortment of techniques is similar. Ethnicity is a factor in CAM use in the United States, but ethnic stereotypes of recent immigrants' using traditional remedies is incorrect. CAM usage is associated with being European American, well educated, in a high income bracket, and being female. These demographic characteristics apply to CAM use in Australia and some European countries as well.

People are motivated to use CAM if their worldviews are compatible with the philosophies that underlie CAM. Those who accept a biopsychosocial view of health are more likely to seek CAM than those who endorse the biomedical view. Health status is also a motivation for seeking CAM; people who have health problems that have not responded to conventional treatments are motivated to seek CAM.

How Effective Are Alternative Treatments?

Alternative treatments are classified as *alternative* because insufficient evidence exists for their effectiveness. Evaluating the effectiveness of alternative treatments has proven to be one of the most controversial areas related to alternative medicine, spurring bitter arguments. Advocates of conventional medicine contend that little evidence exists for the effectiveness of alternative treatments and that the dangers remain unevaluated (Berman & Straus, 2004). According to this view, the only acceptable method of establishing effectiveness is the randomized, controlled trial in which participants are assigned randomly to a treatment group or a placebo control group in a design using the double-blind method in which neither practitioner nor participants know to which treatment condition participants belong.

Using the randomized, controlled method of conducting experiments allows researchers to minimize the influence of bias and expectation. Both of these factors are important in evaluating treatment studies (as discussed in Chapter 2). People who have expectations concerning CAM will bring this bias into treatment, which may affect the outcome. For example, a study on acupuncture (Linde et al., 2007) assessed participants' attitudes about the effectiveness of acupuncture at the beginning of the study. The results indicated that those who expressed belief that acupuncture was an effective treatment experienced greater pain relief from an eight-week course of treatment than did those who had lower expectations for success. Although expectations for success boost treatment effectiveness, these expectations are a placebo response rather than a response to the treatment. Thus, randomized controlled trials represent an important part of research evidence for effectiveness. Advocates of conventional medicine consider a study to be of lesser quality and thus less convincing when studies lack random assignment or "blinding." In systematic reviews of research on specific treatments, those treatments that have few randomized controlled trials yield judgments of insufficient evidence to make conclusions of effectiveness, regardless of the number of other types of studies.

CAM advocates have made several arguments that CAM treatments are being judged inappropriately. One line of argument comes from the contention that demonstrating effectiveness through randomized controlled trials is the standard of conventional medicine, not alternative medicine (Clark-Grill, 2007). Performing such studies is consistent with the biomedical model, which CAM seeks to replace with the biopsychosocial model. Another argument comes from the examination of the method of locating studies for systematic reviews (Pilkington, 2007). An examination of the databases that furnish this information revealed omissions in all sources, which could lead to erroneous conclusions in these systematic reviews of CAM. A third type of objection comes from the assumption that treatments within conventional medicine are based on the type of evidence demanded of CAM. Kenneth Pelletier (2002) argued that many of the treatments used in conventional medicine have not submitted this type of evidence. That is, much of the practice of conventional medicine has not come to be accepted through evidence from randomized controlled trials. Many of the standard treatments in medicine and surgery have evolved through clinical practice and observation of what works rather than through experimental evidence of effectiveness. The concept of evidence-based medicine is relatively recent, but this standard is being applied to CAM more stringently than to treatments within conventional medicine.

Despite these challenges, CAM researchers strive to conduct research that demonstrates effectiveness and safety; this route allows for greater acceptability of CAM treatments. Some evidence indicates success. A comparison of the evidence base in 2000 versus 2005 indicated that the quality of evidence has improved for mind–body treatments (Ernst, Pittler, Wider, & Boddy, 2007b) and massage (Ernst, Pittler, Wider, & Boddy, 2007a). What does the evidence say about alternative treatments? Which have demonstrated that they are effective, and for what conditions?

Alternative Treatments for Anxiety, Stress, and Depression

Many CAM modalities have targeted anxiety, stress, and depression, and some have demonstrated their effectiveness for these conditions. Meditation is an obvious choice for these problems, and the research evidence confirms its effectiveness. Brain imaging studies have helped clarify what happens when a person relaxes and meditates, and the developing picture is consistent with other knowledge about brain activity related to emotions (Davidson et al., 2003). During mindfulness meditation, the left frontal lobe of the brain becomes more active and the right less so, indicating an increase in the experience of positive emotions. Such improvements should indicate stress reduction, and a meta-analysis of mindfulness-based stress reduction (Grossman, Niemann, Schmidt, & Walach, 2004) showed that this approach was effective for a wide variety of people and for several stress-related problems. The analysis also indicated that mindfulness meditation can help not only people with stress-related and anxiety disorders but also people who do not have clinical problems but are seeking a way to manage the stresses in their lives. Those who practiced the technique more also received greater benefits, indicating a dose–response relationship (Carmody & Baer, 2008).

Systematic reviews have offered additional confirmation for the effectiveness of meditation in managing anxiety and depression. A systematic review devoted to an evaluation of the effectiveness of mindfulness meditation (Ivanovski & Malhi, 2007) showed that this type of meditation is effective for the treatment of anxiety disorders and depression. However, another systematic review of mindfulness-based treatments (Toneatto & Nguyen, 2007) found only equivocal support for mindfulness-based stress reduction as a treatment for anxiety disorders and depression. Yet another systematic review led to a conclusion that meditation is effective for anxiety and mood disorders (Arias, Steinberg, Banga, & Trestman, 2006). As one critic of systematic reviews pointed out (Pilkington, 2007), such reviews do not always come to the same conclusions.

Studies on transcendental meditation have also been the focus of a systematic review (Krisanaprakornkit, Krisanaprakornkit, Piyavhatkul, & Laopaiboon, 2006), which indicated that this type of meditation is similar to other relaxation

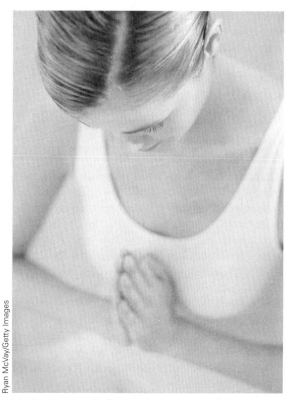

Ryan McVay/Getty Images

Meditation can help people cope with depression and a variety of stress-related problems.

modalities in helping people with anxiety disorders. The problem of sparse studies prevented a systematic review of yoga from determining that it is an effective strategy for dealing with anxiety, but the analysis indicated encouraging results (Kirkwood, Rampes, Tuffrey, Richardson, & Pilkington, 2005). Thus, the majority of evidence indicates that meditation is an effective treatment for anxiety and depression, and the evidence for yoga is encouraging.

As the meta-analysis of mindfulness-based stress reduction (Grossman et al., 2004) indicated, meditation is also helpful in dealing with stress. Studies with students have demonstrated that meditation is effective in helping control exam stress and may extend to overall improvements in academic performance. A study with medical students who used deep-breathing meditation as a stress reduction technique showed positive results (Paul, Elam, & Verhulst, 2007). Chinese college students exhibited reduced levels of stress hormones and increased immune system effectiveness after participating in a meditation program (Tang, Eslick, Nowson, Smith, & Bensoussan, 2007). Thus, the evidence indicates that meditation is effective in stress management.

The movement-based practices of qi gong and tai chi also show stress-reducing effects. A number of physiological measurements indicate that the practice of qi gong reduces stress (Sancier & Holman, 2004). A study of older Chinese immigrants at risk for cardiovascular disease showed improvements in mood and stress after practicing tai chi for 12 weeks (Taylor-Piliae et al., 2006).

Acupuncture holds some promise in treating depression. In a systematic review (Leo & Ligot, 2007), acupuncture was found to be comparable to antidepressant drugs in relieving symptoms of depression. The number and quality of studies was limited, but the results are promising for this alternative treatment. Yoga has also been used successfully as a complementary treatment for depressed people who did not experience a complete response to antidepressant drugs (Shapiro et al., 2007). Another effective alternative treatment for depression is the herbal remedy Saint-John's-wort. A meta-analysis of randomized controlled trials indicated that an extract of this herb alleviates mild to moderate clinical depression, with effectiveness similar to that of antidepressant drugs (Szegedi, Kohnen, Dienel, & Kieser, 2005).

Therefore, a variety of alternative medicine approaches have demonstrated effectiveness in treating anxiety, stress, and depression. Table 8.3 summarizes the evidence for alternative treatments for anxiety, stress, and depression.

Alternative Treatments for Pain

As we discussed in Chapter 7, chronic pain presents problems for those who experience it and for those who attempt to treat it. Conventional medicine often fails to control pain adequately, which motivates many people to seek alternative treatments (Cherkin, Sherman, Deyo, & Shekelle, 2003). A variety of alternative treatments have been applied to the problem of pain, but the CAM techniques that are successful in managing pain vary somewhat from those that are effective in managing anxiety, stress, and depression.

Meditation and the related technique of guided imagery received a strong endorsement from a National Institutes of Health Technology panel review, which concluded that these interventions were effective in managing chronic pain (Lebovits, 2007). Guided imagery has also been described as a best practice for the pain associated with pregnancy and childbirth (Naparstek, 2007). This technique is also effective in managing headaches (Tsao & Zeltzer, 2005) and for reducing postoperative pain in children (Huth, Broome, & Good, 2004) and in older people (Antall & Kresevic, 2004).

Techniques derived from traditional Chinese medicine have been applied to pain control, including tai chi, qi gong, and acupuncture. Tai chi demonstrated its effectiveness in helping adults with tension headache manage their pain (Abbott, Hui, Hays, Li, & Pan, 2007). Qi gong has been applied to pain management more extensively than tai chi. A systematic review of studies of qi gong (Lee, Pittler, & Ernst, 2007) found encouraging evidence regarding its effectiveness in treating chronic pain. A controlled randomized trial (Haak & Scott, 2008) showed that qi gong provided relief from pain and improvement in quality of life for people with fibromyalgia.

Acupuncture is better established as a pain treatment than either tai chi or qi gong. A study of the brain changes in connection with acupuncture (Napadow et al., 2007) revealed that participants who received acupuncture, compared with those who received sham acupuncture, showed changes in brain activity that were consistent with decreases in pain perception. Acupuncture also produces complex reactions in the somatosensory system and in the neurochemistry of the central nervous system, which is likely related to its analgesic effects (Dhond, Kettner, & Napadow, 2007). A large-scale research project (Witt, Brinkhaus, Reinhold, & Willich, 2006) examined the benefits of integrating acupuncture into standard medical care for chronic pain. Low back pain, osteoarthritis of the hip and knee, neck pain, and headache were among the types of pain included in treatment. The study found that acupuncture was effective in addition to the benefit obtained from

TABLE 8.3

Effectiveness of Alternative Treatments for Anxiety, Stress, and Depression

Problem	Findings	Studies
1. Anxiety and stress	Mindfulness meditation is effective, according to a meta-analysis.	Grossman et al., 2004
2. Anxiety disorders and depression	Mindfulness meditation is effective, according to a systematic review.	Ivanovski & Malhi, 2007
3. Stress	Mindfulness-based stress reduction is more effective if practiced more frequently.	Carmody & Baer, 2008
4. Anxiety disorders and depression	Mindfulness-based stress reduction received equivocal support in a systematic review.	Toneatto & Nguyen, 2007
5. Anxiety and mood disorders	Meditation is effective, according to a systematic review.	Arias et al., 2007
6. Anxiety disorders	Transcendental meditation is comparable to relaxation training, according to a systematic review.	Krisanaprakornkit et al., 2006
7. Anxiety	Yoga may be effective, but too few quality studies exist for a systematic review to form conclusions.	Kirkwood et al., 2005
8. Stress	Deep-breathing meditation was effective for medical students.	Paul et al., 2007
9. Stress	Meditation was effective for Chinese college students.	Tang et al., 2007
10. Stress	Qi gong reduces physiological indicators of stress.	Sancier & Holman, 2004
11. Stress and negative mood	Tai chi practice improves stress and mood among older Chinese immigrants.	Taylor-Piliae et al., 2006
12. Depression	Acupuncture showed effectiveness comparable to antidepressant drugs in a systematic review.	Leo & Ligot, 2007
13. Depression	Yoga is a successful complementary treatment for people taking antidepressants.	Shapiro et al., 2007
14. Depression	Saint-John's-wort is as effective as antidepressant drugs, according to a systematic review.	Szegedi et al., 2005

standard medical care. That is, acupuncture was an effective complementary therapy for a variety of pain syndromes. Other studies have examined acupuncture as an alternative treatment.

A meta-analysis of acupuncture for low back pain (Manheimer, White, Berman, Forys, & Ernst, 2005) indicated that this treatment is more effective for short-term relief of chronic back pain than sham acupuncture or no treatment. In a systematic review that considered all types of treatment for back pain (Keller, Hayden, Bombardier, & van Tulder, 2007), acupuncture was among the most effective treatments. Although none of the treatments revealed a high degree of effectiveness,

acupuncture was similar to nonsteroidal anti-inflammatory drugs in relieving back pain. This result may point to an answer to some of the confusion concerning the effectiveness of acupuncture (Johnson, 2006): When compared to other treatments, acupuncture may fail to show advantages. When compared to no treatment, the effects may be small. However, none of the available treatment for this condition is very effective. Therefore, acupuncture may be as effective a treatment as any for low back pain.

A systematic review of acupuncture for pelvic and back pain during pregnancy indicated limited effectiveness (Ee, Manheimer, Pirotta, & White,

2008), but a meta-analysis of acupuncture for osteoarthritis of the knee suggested that this treatment is effective for this condition (Pittler & Ernst, 2008). A critical review of studies on acupuncture as a treatment for migraine headaches in adults (Griggs & Jensen, 2006) found conflicting results, studies of poor quality, and therefore no conclusions regarding effectiveness. Thus, acupuncture seems to have demonstrated effectiveness for several pain syndromes, both as an alternative and as a complementary treatment, but it is not equally effective for all types of pain.

Massage is another treatment that is effective for several types of pain, but less effective for others. A review of massage for all types of chronic pain except cancer pain (Tsao, 2007) indicated varying effectiveness for different pain syndromes. The strongest evidence of effectiveness came from studies on low back pain, whereas the evidence for shoulder and headache pain was more modest. Evidence was too limited to come to conclusions concerning the effectiveness of massage for fibromyalgia, neck pain, and carpal tunnel syndrome. Because of a lack of high-quality studies, a review of massage for musculoskeletal pain (Lewis & Johnson, 2006) failed to reach conclusions concerning effectiveness.

Chiropractic manipulation has also been the subject of systematic review. This type of CAM is most often used for back and neck pain, and a review indicated that it is effective for these conditions (Cherkin et al., 2003). A review of studies on spinal manipulation for musculoskeletal pain (Perram, 2006) indicated that chiropractic treatment was superior to conventional medical treatment for this type of pain. However, chiropractic manipulation did not appear to be effective in treating tension headaches (Lenssinck et al., 2004).

Early research on the effectiveness of biofeedback (Blanchard et al., 1990) looked promising: Thermal biofeedback with relaxation showed its effectiveness as a treatment for migraine and tension headaches. Later research painted a less optimistic picture, as biofeedback demonstrated no greater effects than relaxation training in preventing migraine headaches (Stewart, 2004). A meta-analysis of biofeedback studies in the treatment of migraine (Nestoriuc & Martin, 2007) indicated a medium-sized effect. EMG biofeedback is recognized as an appropriate treatment for tension headache (Astin, 2004), but its effects are no greater than those of relaxation training or hypnosis. For low back pain, EMG biofeedback shows little evidence of benefit (Roelofs, Boissevain, Peters, de Jong, & Vlaeyen, 2002). EMG biofeedback has thus demonstrated some effectiveness for several problems but few advantages over relaxation. The added expense associated with providing biofeedback is a drawback for this CAM. On balance, then, biofeedback shows more limited benefits than do some other CAM treatments.

Hypnotic treatment also has some applications in controlling pain, and the list of pains that are responsive to hypnotic procedures is extensive. A meta-analysis (Montgomery, DuHamel, & Redd, 2000) showed that hypnotic suggestion is equally effective in reducing both experimental pain induced in the laboratory and clinical pain that people experience in the world for about 75% of participants. Recent research exploring brain activity during hypnosis (Röder, Michal, Overbeck, van de Ven, & Linden, 2007) showed that hypnosis altered the brain response to painful stimulation in areas that underlie both the sensory and emotional responses to pain. Indeed, the effectiveness of hypnosis in managing pain may be its power to change the fear that often accompanies pain (De Benedittis, 2003).

Hypnosis is not equally effective with all types of clinical pain; it is more effective in controlling acute pain than in managing chronic pain (Patterson & Jensen, 2003). Hypnosis is most effective in helping people manage pain associated with invasive medical procedures, postoperative recovery, and burns. For example, research shows that hypnosis was effective in reducing the need for preoperative medication in children (Calipel, Lucaspolomeni, Wodey, & Ecoffey, 2005), in stabilizing the pain of invasive surgical procedures, and in reducing surgery patients' need for analgesic drugs (Lang et al., 2000). Burns are notoriously difficult to treat because they involve severe pain and suffering. An early review of the effectiveness of hypnosis in treating the pain associated with burns (Van der Does & Van Dyck, 1989) examined 28 studies that used hypnosis with burn patients and found consistent evidence of its benefits. More recent research (Askay, Patterson, Jensen, & Sharar, 2007; Harandi, Esfandani, & Shakibaei, 2004) has confirmed those benefits.

Although hypnotic treatment is effective with many types of acute pain, chronic pain is a more difficult management issue, and hypnosis is not as successful with chronic pain such as headache and low back pain as it is with acute pain (Patterson & Jensen, 2003). Hypnosis is also more effective with some people than with others. Individual differences in susceptibility to hypnosis are a factor in the analgesic effects of hypnosis—highly suggestible

people may receive substantial analgesic benefits from this technique, whereas others receive limited benefits. Thus, hypnosis can be very effective with some people for some pain problems.

Table 8.4 summarizes the effectiveness of CAM treatments for pain. Although the studies on pain management using CAM could benefit from better design, evaluations of the results indicate that several of these techniques are effective for a variety of pain problems. Conventional medicine has not been very successful for many patients in pain, and the conventional treatments tend to have many side effects, a criticism that is uncommon for CAM and thus a benefit in addition to effectiveness.

TABLE 8.4
Effectiveness of Alternative Therapies for Pain

Problem	Findings	Studies
1. Chronic pain	Meditation is effective, according to a National Institutes of Health Technology panel review.	Lebovits, 2007
2. Pain associated with pregnancy and childbirth	Guided imagery is a best practice for this type of pain.	Naparstek, 2007
3. Headache pain	Guided imagery is effective in managing headache pain.	Tsao & Zeltzer, 2005
4. Postoperative pain in children	Guided imagery reduces postoperative pain.	Huth et al., 2004
5. Postoperative pain in older people	Guided imagery reduces postoperative pain.	Antall & Kresevic, 2004
6. Tension headache pain in adults	Tai chi was effective in a randomized controlled trial.	Abbott et al., 2007
7. Chronic pain	Qi gong was evaluated as promising in a systematic review.	Lee et al., 2007
8. Fibromyalgia	Qi gong provided pain relief and lowered distress in a randomized controlled trial.	Haak & Scott, 2008
9. Low back pain, osteoarthritis, neck pain, and headache	Acupuncture was effective as a complementary treatment.	Witt et al., 2006
10. Low back pain	Acupuncture was effective for short-term relief of chronic pain.	Manheimer et al., 2005
11. Low back pain	Acupuncture was one of the most effective treatments.	Keller et al., 2007
12. Pelvic and back pain during pregnancy	Acupuncture has limited effectiveness, according to a systematic review.	Ee et al., 2008
13. Osteoarthritis of the knee	Acupuncture was judged effective in a systematic review.	Pittler & Ernst, 2008
14. Migraine headache in adults	Acupuncture showed conflicting results in a critical review.	Griggs & Jensen, 2006

(Continued)

TABLE 8.4 Effectiveness of Alternative Therapies for Pain—*Continued*

Problem	Findings	Studies
15. Low back pain, shoulder pain, headache pain	Massage was effective for low back pain and modestly effective for shoulder and headache pain.	Tsao, 2007
16. Fibromyalgia, neck pain, carpal tunnel syndrome	Massage studies are too limited to allow conclusions of effectiveness.	Tsao, 2007
17. Musculoskeletal pain	Massage studies are too limited to allow conclusions of effectiveness.	Lewis & Johnson, 2006
18. Back and neck pain	Chiropractic manipulation is effective, according to a systematic review.	Cherkin et al., 2003
19. Musculoskeletal pain	Chiropractic manipulation was more effective than conventional medical treatment.	Perram, 2006
20. Tension headache	Chiropractic manipulation was not found effective.	Lenssinck et al., 2004
21. Migraine and tension headache	Thermal biofeedback plus relaxation produced a significant reduction in headache activity.	Blanchard et al., 1990; Astin, 2004
22. Migraine headache prevention	Thermal biofeedback is comparable to other preventive treatments.	Stewart, 2004
23. Migraine headache	Biofeedback produced a medium-sized effect, according to a systematic review.	Nestoriuc & Martin, 2007
24. Low back pain	EMG biofeedback was not effective.	Roelofs et al., 2002
25. Experimental and clinical pain	Hypnotic suggestion is effective for clinical and experimental pain.	Montgomery et al., 2000
26. Fear and anxiety associated with pain	Hypnosis is especially effective.	De Benedittis, 2003
27. Clinical pain	Hypnosis is more effective in controlling acute than in managing chronic pain.	Patterson & Jensen, 2003
28. Preoperative distress	Hypnosis reduces preoperative distress better than medication.	Calipel et al., 2005
29. Surgery pain	Self-hypnosis decreases postoperative pain and reduces need for drugs.	Lang et al., 2000
30. Burn pain	Hypnosis is a valuable component in treating severe burn pain.	Askay et al., 2007; Van der Does & Van Dyck, 1989

Alternative Treatments for Other Conditions

Although anxiety, stress, depression, and pain are the most common problems for which people use CAM, some products and procedures have been found effective for other conditions. Both the products and procedures and the conditions for which they are effective vary widely; CAM has been used to achieve more rapid healing, to lower blood pressure, and to improve balance. For example, use of aloe vera speeds burn wound healing significantly (Maenthaisong, Chaiyakunapruk, Niruntraporn, & Kongkaew, 2007). Although biofeedback is not as effective as other CAM for stress and pain, thermal biofeedback is effective in the management of **Raynaud's disease**, a disorder that involves painful constriction of peripheral blood vessels in the hands and feet (Karavidas, Tsai, Yucha, McGrady, & Lehrer, 2006). Hypnosis was found to be effective in controlling nausea and vomiting associated with chemotherapy in children (Richardson et al., 2007). The practice of transcendental meditation has been evaluated as effective in controlling risk factors such as high blood pressure and some of the physiological changes that underlie cardiovascular disease, and thus may offer protection (Walton et al., 2002). Yoga may help not only to control some of the risks for Type 2 diabetes (Innes & Vincent, 2007) but also to prevent cardiovascular complications in these diabetics. A mindfulness-based meditation program was successful with male and female prisoners in improving mood and decreasing hostility (Samuelson, Carmody, Kabat-Zinn, & Bratt, 2007). This assortment of effective treatments represents many different complementary and alternative interventions, but some systems of alternative medicine have yielded successful treatments for a number of problems.

Traditional Chinese medicine includes acupuncture, qi gong, and tai chi, all of which produce a wide range of health benefits and effective treatments. For example, acupuncture (Ezzo, Streitberger, & Schneider, 2006) has been found to be effective in controlling nausea and vomiting associated with postoperative symptoms. Also, a systematic review showed that acupuncture was effective in treating insomnia (H. Y. Chen et al., 2007). Improvements in blood pressure appeared in a systematic review of qi gong practice (Guo, Zhou, Nishimura, Teramukai, & Fukushima, 2008). Although the practice of qi gong was superior to no treatment or placebo, it was not superior to drug treatment. Qi gong was also evaluated as effective in managing the risk factors for diabetes such as oral glucose tolerance and blood glucose (Xin, Miller, & Brown, 2007).

Qi gong and the related practice of tai chi seem to have the ability to improve immune system function, which would give these practices the potential for many health benefits. Compared with healthy control participants who did not practice qi gong or tai chi, the immune system response of those who practiced qi gong was enhanced in ways that would resolve inflammation more rapidly (Li, Li, Garcia, Johnson, & Feng, 2005). Older adults who practiced qi gong or tai chi showed an enhanced immune system response to influenza immunization (Yang et al., 2007). Indeed, the immune response was sufficiently strong to produce positive health consequences before

immunization. In a randomized controlled trial (Irwin, Pike, Cole, & Oxman, 2003), older adults who practiced tai chi exhibited an enhanced immune response to the herpes zoster (shingles) virus, even before they received the immunization for this virus. Thus, the practice of qi gong and tai chi seems to confer some immune system benefits that have been researched most extensively with older people but may apply to all.

The most common applications of tai chi have been among older people to improve balance and flexibility and to decrease falls. A systematic review of older people's fear of falling (Zijlstra et al., 2007) and balance (Komagata & Newton, 2003) revealed positive effects for the practice of tai chi. However, the evidence concerning falling is mixed. One review (Komagata & Newton, 2003) found no improvement among tai chi practitioners, but a large randomized controlled trial (Voukelatos, Cummings, Lord, & Rissel, 2007) found a decrease in falls among healthy, community-dwelling older adults. Tai chi does not seem to be effective for preventing the progress of osteoporosis, an underlying factor in falls (Lee, Pittler, Shin, & Ernst, 2008). However, another CAM treatment is effective in slowing bone mineral loss: calcium and vitamin D supplements help people over age 50 retain bone minerals (Tang et al., 2007).

Reasoning that the benefits of tai chi for balance and flexibility might apply to individuals with multiple sclerosis and rheumatoid arthritis, researchers have tested those benefits. A systematic review of the research on rheumatoid arthritis (Han et al., 2004) indicated no effect on the progression of the disease, but individuals who practiced tai chi experienced improved flexibility and greater enjoyment of this form of physical activity. Rheumatoid arthritis produces pain associated with movement, but individuals with this disorder benefit from activity, so an enjoyable physical activity is a positive factor in management of this condition. The study assessing the benefits of tai chi for people with multiple sclerosis was a small one (Mills, Allen, & Morgan, 2000), and thus its findings must be considered as preliminary. However, individuals who practiced tai chi for two months experienced improvements in balance, which is a major problem for people with this disorder.

The alternative medical systems of homeopathy, naturopathy, and Ayurvedic medicine have been subjected to few rigorous experimental evaluations, and thus few reviews exist of their effectiveness. However, one review of homeopathy (Jonas, Kaptchuk, & Linde, 2003) examined the evidence concerning the effectiveness of homeopathic remedies and found that such remedies showed some benefit for treating influenza, allergies, and childhood diarrhea but not for migraine headache, muscle soreness, or influenza prevention. An extensive review of research on naturopathy (S. B. Myers et al., 2006) found no overall evaluation of this system. Instead, many reviews were available for the effectiveness of specific herbal preparations that fall within this system but are also part of other systems and used individually. The practice of Ayurvedic medicine encompasses yoga and herbal preparations, but Ayurveda also exists as a complete system of health and health care. Many evaluations have been conducted on the effectiveness of yoga and of some herbal preparations, but the lack of systematic evaluations of Ayurveda prohibits any conclusions as to its overall effectiveness (NCCAM, 2005).

Thus, CAM interventions are effective for a variety of problems. The most persuasive evidence comes from traditional Chinese medicine and from mind–body medicine, but an assortment of products and procedures have demonstrated their effectiveness in randomized controlled trials, in meta-analyses, and in systematic reviews. Table 8.5 summarizes these treatments. Despite some impressive evidence for effectiveness, treatments within complementary and alternative medicine also have limitations.

Limitations of Alternative Therapies

All forms of therapy have limitations, including CAM. One of the primary limitations is the reason any technique is considered *alternative*: the lack of information on its effectiveness. As we have seen, this deficit may be due to the sparseness of research rather than a lack of effectiveness. The growing interest in CAM and the funding for research through the U.S. National Center for Complementary and Alternative Medicine is beginning to solve this problem, revealing that some products and procedures are effective, whereas others are not. Both conventional and alternative treatments are limited by their success for some conditions and not others. However, specific CAM techniques have limitations and even dangers.

Herbal remedies and botanicals are part of many CAM systems, including Ayurvedic medicine, traditional Chinese medicine, naturopathy, and homeopathy. Nutritional supplements are among the most commonly used CAM approaches (Barnes et al., 2004). Like drug treatments, herbal, botanical, and nutritional supplements carry risks of adverse reactions and interactions with over-the-counter and prescription drugs (Firenzuoli & Gori, 2007; NCCAM, 2007a). Unlike drugs, herbal and dietary supplements are considered to be food by the U.S. government, so these products are not evaluated for effectiveness but only for safety. People often consider natural herbs and botanicals to be safe and even if not effective, then at least harmless. Such is not always the case. Sometimes, evidence of dangers accumulates only after these products have been available for some time. The case of ephedra, a weight loss supplement, is an example. The U.S. Food and Drug Agency banned ephedra in response to accumulated evidence of its dangers.

Also like drug treatments, massage has benefits that are significant for the duration of treatments but do not last beyond them (Field, 1998; Hasson, Arnetz, Jelveus, & Edelstam, 2004). In addition, massage is not suitable for people with arthritis or other pain problems related to joints, weakened bones, damaged nerves, a tumor, an open wound, or infection, or for people with bleeding disorders or those who are taking blood thinning agents (NCCAM, 2006a). Chiropractic treatment may do harm when applied to individuals with broken bones or infection, and treatment may produce headache or other discomfort (NCCAM, 2007d).

Acupuncture and acupressure do not work for everyone. Some people do not respond, some types of manipulation of the needles are more effective than others, and some needle placements work better than others (Martindale, 2001). Needles

TABLE 8.5

Effectiveness of Alternative Treatments for Other Conditions

Problem	Findings	Studies
1. Burn healing	Aloe vera speeds healing.	Maenthaisong et al., 2007
2. Raynaud's disease	Thermal biofeedback is an effective treatment.	Karavidas et al., 2006
3. Cardiovascular disease risk factors	Transcendental meditation is effective in controlling risk factors.	Walton et al., 2002
4. Nausea and vomiting associated with chemotherapy	Hypnosis is effective in controlling these symptoms.	Richardson et al., 2007
5. Hostility	Mindfulness meditation is effective in moderating hostility among prisoners.	Samuelson et al., 2007
6. Risks for Type 2 diabetes	Yoga is effective in controlling risks and in decreasing CVD complications.	Innes & Vincent, 2007
7. Postoperative nausea and vomiting	Acupuncture is effective.	Ezzo et al., 2006
8. Insomnia	Acupuncture is effective.	H. Y. Chen et al., 2007
9. High blood pressure	Qi gong practice lowered blood pressure, but not as much as drugs.	Guo et al., 2008
10. Risk factors for diabetes	Qi gong was effective in lowering risk.	Xin et al., 2007
11. Immune system function	Qi gong altered immune function in ways that decreased inflammation.	Li et al., 2005
12. Immune system function	Qi gong and tai chi enhanced immune system response to influenza vaccination in older adults.	Yang et al., 2007
13. Immune system function	Tai chi practice enhanced older adults' immune system response to herpes zoster before and after immunization.	Irwin et al., 2003
14. Fear of falling and balance	Tai chi practice decreased fear of falling and increased balance among older adults.	Zijlstra et al., 2007; Komagata & Newton, 2003
15. Falling	Tai chi showed mixed results.	Komagata & Newton, 2003; Voukelatos et al., 2007
16. Osteoporosis	Tai chi practice failed to slow bone loss.	Lee et al., 2008
17. Osteoporosis	Calcium and vitamin D supplements slowed bone mineral loss in people over age 50.	Tang et al., 2007
18. Rheumatoid arthritis	Tai chi did not slow disease progression but increases joint flexibility.	Han et al., 2004
19. Multiple sclerosis	Tai chi practice improved balance.	Mills et al., 2000
20. Influenza and influenza prevention, allergies, childhood diarrhea, and migraine headache	Homeopathic remedies were effective for influenza, allergies, and childhood diarrhea, but not for influenza prevention or migraine headaches.	Jonas et al., 2003

should be sterile and inserted properly; improper insertion and needles that are not sterile can cause damage and infection (NCCAM, 2007c). Tai chi and qi gong are generally safe, but people with severe osteoporosis, sprains, fractures, or joint problems should exercise caution or modify the positions (NCCAM, 2006d). Meditation carries few health risks (NCCAM, 2006b).

People should exercise caution in using any CAM treatment as an alternative to conventional medical care. People who trust alternative approaches and mistrust conventional medicine may fail to seek treatment that could be more effective. For example, yoga may help to control some of the risks for Type 2 diabetes (Innes & Vincent, 2007), but for most people, yoga will not be sufficient to control diabetes. The majority of people who use CAM recognize the limitations of these therapies and use them as additions to conventional medical care. However, many people who use some CAM modality fail to tell their conventional medical practitioner that they are using an alternative as a well as conventional treatment (Barnes et al., 2004). This failure may present risks due to interactions between the two treatments.

Another limitation for CAM is its accessibility. Not everyone who is interested in CAM may be able to find or to afford CAM treatment. Many CAM treatments are limited by the number of qualified practitioners and by their geographic location. For example, an examination of acupuncture use (Burke & Upchurch, 2006) suggested that accessibility was a factor that limited its use. The same study also found that 60% of those people who used acupuncture were not reimbursed for the services they received. The failure to include CAM services in insurance reimbursement is typical in the United States (NCCAM, 2006c). One way to remove this barrier is to increase the presence of alternative treatments in conventional medical settings. Moving complementary and alternative medicine to group practices, hospitals, and clinics would improve accessibility. This strategy is the focus of integrative medicine.

Integrative Medicine

Integrating conventional and alternative medicine is what Norman Cousins, whose story began this chapter, envisioned for health care and treatment. Cousins's experience with a debilitating disease and cure through a very unorthodox treatment prompted him to work toward changes to conventional medicine. As Cousins said,

It becomes necessary therefore to create a balanced perspective, one that recognizes that attitudes such as a strong will to live,

high purpose, a capacity for festivity, and a reasonable degree of confidence are not an alternative to competent medical attention, but a way of enhancing the environment of treatment. The wise physician favors a spirit of responsible participation by the patients in a total strategy of medical care. (UCLA Cousins Center, 2007, ¶ 1)

One way to overcome the limitations of both conventional medicine and CAM is to integrate them, providing a mixture of both types of treatment, called **integrative medicine**. This approach is what most patients attempt when they use alternative treatments; few completely reject conventional medicine. Rather, they choose to combine the techniques from each that they believe will help them manage their problem, but they do so on their own rather than under the direction of their physician (Barnes et al., 2004).

Not only do many people who use CAM do so without the guidance of their physician, but they often do so without informing their physician (Hsiao, Ryan, et al., 2006). These people may feel reluctant to discuss their use of alternative treatment with their physician because the response from conventional medicine has often been opposition to CAM (Kaptchuk & Miller, 2005). Despite growing evidence of the effectiveness of these techniques, physicians in the United States do not often refer their patients to acupuncturists or other CAM practitioners (Barnes et al., 2004). Integrative medicine requires conventional and alternative medicine practitioners to accept the effectiveness of both approaches and to work together. Both the acceptance and the cooperation present challenges.

Conventional medicine holds different assumptions than alternative medicine, leading to basic differences in the way that practitioners view health and treatment (Lake, 2007). For example, the assumptions of traditional Chinese medicine, chiropractic, and homeopathy have been difficult for many physicians trained in Western medicine to accept. Recent research (Klimenko & Julliard, 2007) indicated that conventional medical practitioners remain resistant to integrating alternative treatments. Practitioners whose training has not included alternative treatments are more resistant than those who have training in CAM (Hsiao, Ryan, et al., 2006). Students in a variety of professional schools of health care have a great interest in CAM (Nedrow et al., 2007; Song, John, & Dobs, 2007), and the increasing number of medical schools with CAM departments and curricula (Mosquera, 2008) holds promise for integrating alternative medicine with conventional medicine.

Such integration is more common in some areas of practice than others, such as pain treatment and cancer care. Patients who visit an integrative pain clinic tend to be people with chronic pain problems who have tried many different approaches from conventional medicine and perhaps some from alternative medicine, none of which have been entirely successful. In pain clinics, pain is the problem, and treatment is oriented toward managing it and not the condition that originally caused it. Such a clinic should include health care professionals from several specialties (Dillard, 2002), including (1) a physician trained in neurology, anesthesia, rehabilitation, or psychiatry; (2) a physical rehabilitation expert; (3) a psychiatrist or psychologist; and (4) a chiropractor, massage therapist, or acupuncturist (or all three). This range of health care providers can offer techniques from both conventional and alternative medicine, consult with one another, and tailor the treatment to fit each individual's situation and needs.

Integrative oncology also involves treatment by a team of providers. In addition to conventional treatments for cancer such as chemotherapy, radiation, and surgery, patients may participate in interventions aimed at pain control, stress management, nutrition, and physical activity. Stress management, healthy diet, and exercise represent changes that improve the quality of life for most people, but these lifestyle changes may also affect the progression of cancer (Boyd, 2007). About 26% of cancer patients seek some type of CAM treatment, most often to help with musculoskeletal problems (Lafferty, Tyree, Devlin, Andersen, & Diehr, 2008). Some cancer patients look to CAM to help them become actively involved in their treatment to "fight" their cancer (Evans et al., 2007). A systematic review of studies using mindfulness-based stress reduction for individuals with cancer (Smith, Richardson, Hoffman, & Pilkington, 2005) found evidence for stress reduction and improved mood and sleep quality. Thus, integrative oncology holds potential for providing a wider range of treatments and improving the quality of life for cancer patients.

Such improvements could apply to many chronic diseases. The growing consumer interest in CAM and the increasing acceptance of CAM by health care professionals suggest that integrative medicine will overcome the barriers to combining alternative with conventional medicine.

IN SUMMARY

For alternative treatments to be accepted by conventional medicine, research evidence must confirm their effectiveness. The standard for this evidence is controversial. Should CAM be held to the standard of effectiveness as demonstrated by randomized, controlled trials? Some in conventional medicine say so, but some in alternative medicine argue that most treatments in conventional medicine fail to meet this criterion. Nonetheless, evidence is accruing concerning effectiveness for CAM.

Both transcendental meditation and mindfulness meditation have demonstrated effectiveness for anxiety, and mindfulness-based stress reduction is effective in managing stress. The movement-based practices of qi gong and tai chi are also effective in helping to manage stress. Acupuncture and yoga show some promise of reducing depression, and the herbal remedy Saint-John's-wort has also been found to reduce depression.

Guided imagery seems to be an effective intervention in helping people manage several types of pain. Techniques from traditional Chinese medicine have been successful in pain management, including qi gong, tai chi, and acupuncture. Qi gong and tai chi may be good choices for people with chronic pain problems such as headache and fibromyalgia. Acupuncture can be effective for easing low back pain and the pain that accompanies osteoarthritis. Research also indicates that massage is effective for low back pain; chiropractic manipulation is effective for low back, neck, and musculoskeletal pain. However, biofeedback is no more effective for managing headache or low back pain than relaxation training. Hypnosis is effective for a variety of types of pain but is more effective for acute pain such as postsurgical and burn pain than for chronic pain.

Techniques from CAM are also effective for a variety of other conditions, including speeding burn healing (aloe vera), treating insomnia (acupuncture), controlling nausea and vomiting (hypnosis and acupuncture), managing Raynaud's disease (thermal biofeedback), and lowering risk for cardiovascular disease (meditation) and diabetes (qi gong). Research has indicated that the practice of qi gong and tai chi can alter the immune system in beneficial ways, and tai chi decreases fear of falling and improves balance and flexibility in older adults.

Like all treatments, CAM has limitations and even dangers. Some herbal remedies and botanical products may be toxic or may interact with each other or with over-the-counter or prescription drugs. Individuals with some conditions should avoid some treatments; for example, people with weakened bones should be cautious in seeking massage or chiropractic treatment. Another limitation for CAM is its accessibility, in terms of both availability and cost of treatments.

Integrative medicine is the integration of alternative and conventional medicine, which should provide the best of both approaches. The challenges for achieving such integration include melding the two discrepant traditions and training practitioners who will refer patients to each other when appropriate. Two areas in which integrative medicine is advancing most rapidly are pain management and cancer treatment.

ANSWERS

This chapter has addressed five basic questions:

1. **What medical systems represent alternatives to conventional medicine?**

The alternative medical systems include traditional Chinese medicine (TCM), Ayurvedic medicine, naturopathy, and homeopathy. TCM and Ayurvedic medicine are ancient; naturopathy and homeopathy arose in the 19th century and gained popularity in the early 20th century. Each of these systems presents a theory of health and disease as well as practices for diagnosis and treatment. All of the alternative systems share the concept of vital energy and the notion that bringing the mind and body together is important to health.

2. **What alternative practices and products are used in alternative medicine?**

Alternative medicine includes a wide variety of practices and products for improving or restoring health. Manipulative techniques include chiropractic and massage; chiropractic manipulation focuses on adjusting the spine and joints, whereas massage manipulates soft tissue.

Energy healing is another alternative practice; the several varieties of energy healing all accept that the body produces or is sensitive to healing energy. Diets such as the Atkins, Ornish, Zone, and Pritikin diets may be undertaken for weight loss or to control risk factors for heart disease. Alternative products include dietary supplements such as vitamins, minerals, herbs, extracts, and special foods that people typically take to improve their health but may be used to prevent or cure specific conditions.

3. **What is mind–body medicine?**

Mind–body medicine is the term applied to a variety of techniques that are based on the notion that the brain, mind, body, and behavior interact in complex ways and that emotional, mental, social, and behavioral factors exert important effects on health. These techniques share the view that mind and body form a holistic system of dynamic interaction, with each influencing the other. According to mind–body medicine, overlooking psychological factors will lead to an incomplete form of health treatment and lose the power that can come from enlisting mind and emotions in treatment. The techniques included within mind–body medicine are meditation, guided imagery, yoga, qi gong, tai chi, biofeedback, and hypnosis.

4. **Who uses complementary and alternative medicine?**

People in industrialized nations show an increasing interest and participation in CAM. Countries vary in CAM usage, and within countries, some demographic factors predict CAM use. Australia and some European countries show higher percentages of the population seeking CAM treatments than in the United States. Within the United States, ethnicity shows some relationship to CAM use, with European American, well-educated, and upper-income groups using CAM more often than others. In all countries, women are more likely than men to use CAM. Personal attitudes of acceptance of the underlying philosophy of CAM also predicts use, as does health status—people who have a persistent health problem that conventional medicine has not helped are more likely to seek alternative treatment.

5. **What are the effective uses and limitations of alternative treatments?**

A variety of techniques are available to help people manage anxiety, stress, depression, pain, and other problems, and an increasing body of research indicates that some alternative treatments are effective in managing these problems. Both transcendental and mindfulness meditation are effective in managing anxiety; mindfulness-based stress reduction helps in coping with stress. Different alternative treatments have been found to be effective in managing various types of pain; no one technique is effective for all pain situations. Manipulation techniques such as massage, chiropractic treatment, and acupuncture seem to be as effective as any treatment for the difficult problem of chronic low back pain. The movement-based approaches of qi gong and tai chi show promise of helping to manage headaches and fibromyalgia. In addition, these practices influence the immune system in beneficial ways that may affect health in a variety of ways. However, their primary therapeutic use is to help older people maintain balance and flexibility. Hypnosis also has benefits for pain control, but these benefits apply more to acute pain than to chronic pain.

Lack of rigorous research has limited evidence concerning the effectiveness of CAM, but that situation is changing. Other limitations are similar to those of treatments in conventional medicine—hazards for some individuals using some treatments and drug interactions arising from the use of herbal treatments or dietary supplements. Availability and cost of treatments are other limitations of CAM.

SUGGESTED READINGS

Harrington, A. (2008). *The cure within: A history of mind–body medicine*. New York: Norton. Harrington's book takes a social and historical perspective on the status of alternative medicine, weaving together a wide collection of information concerning the interaction between mind and body.

Lake, J. (2007). Philosophical problems in medicine and psychiatry, part II. *Integrative Medicine: A Clinician's Journal, 6*(3), 44–47. This brief article takes a historical and philosophical perspective in explaining the underlying differences in assumptions and worldviews between advocates of conventional and alternative medicine and how these differences present barriers to integrating the two types of medical care.

National Center for Complementary and Alternative Medicine (NCCAM). (2002). *What is complementary and alternative medicine?* NCCAM Publication No. D156. Retrieved June 3, 2005, from http://nccam.nih.gov/health/whatiscam/. For those who want an introduction to complementary and alternative medicine, the website for the National Center for Complementary and Alternative Medicine offers this summary as well as information on other CAM topics.

Pelletier, K. R. (2002). Mind as healer, mind as slayer: Mind–body medicine comes of age. *Advances in Mind–Body Medicine, 18*, 4–15.

This provocative review not only evaluates the evidence concerning the effectiveness of mind–body interventions but also critiques the criteria for such an evaluation.

Wallis, C. (2005, February 28). The right (and wrong) way to treat pain. *Time, 165,* 46–57. This magazine article presents the range of options for pain control, including conventional medical treatments as well as complementary and alternative techniques. The article gives good advice for those experiencing pain about how to find a treatment tailored to each individual's needs.

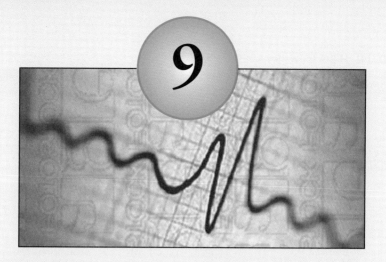

9

BEHAVIORAL FACTORS IN CARDIOVASCULAR DISEASE

QUESTIONS

This chapter focuses on four basic questions:

1. What are the structures, functions, and disorders of the cardiovascular system?

2. What are the risk factors for cardiovascular disease?

3. How does lifestyle relate to cardiovascular health?

4. What behaviors allow people to lower their cardiovascular risks?

CHECK YOUR HEALTH RISKS

Check the items that apply to you.

☐   1. Someone in my immediate family (a parent, sibling, aunt, uncle, or grandparent) died of heart disease before the age of 55.

☐   2. I am diabetic.

☐   3. I am female.

☐   4. I am African American.

☐   5. My blood pressure is less than 130 over 80.

☐   6. My total cholesterol level is between 170 and 200.

☐   7. My HDL is less than 40.

☐   8. The ratio of my total cholesterol to HDL is 6 to 1 or higher.

☐   9. I have never been a smoker.

☐   10. I am less than 30 years old.

☐   11. I eat four or more serving of fruits and vegetables every day.

☐   12. My diet contains lots of red meat.

☐   13. I almost never eat fish.

☐   14. My diet is high in fiber.

☐   15. I am an unmarried man.

☐   16. I frequently get angry, and when I do, I let everyone around me know about it.

☐   17. I frequently get angry, and when I do, I keep my anger to myself.

☐   18. I do not participate in regular physical activity.

☐   19. I eat "fast food" at least three times a week.

Each of these topics is either a known risk factor for some type of cardiovascular disease or has the potential to protect against it. Conditions consistent with items 3, 5, 6, 9, 10, 11, and 14 may offer some protection against cardiovascular disease. If you checked none or only a few of these items and a large number of the remaining items, you may be at risk for heart disease or stroke.

REAL-WORLD PROFILE OF PRESIDENT BILL CLINTON

In early September 2004, former President Bill Clinton went to the hospital because he experienced chest pains and shortness of breath (King & Henry, 2004). Extensive testing revealed that his coronary arteries were blocked, and the former president was scheduled for coronary bypass surgery. Clinton did not have a heart attack, but he believed that he would have if he had not obtained treatment. He understood that many people who have heart attacks experience no symptoms beforehand, so he considered himself fortunate to have a warning of coronary problems. Clinton viewed the experience of diagnosis and treatment as an opportunity to avoid a heart attack and to have additional years of healthy life. His optimistic outlook may have played a role in his recovery.

Clinton also speculated about the underlying cause of his heart problems. He mentioned a history of heart disease in his family, but during his presidency, Clinton was the target of jokes about his fondness for high-fat fast food. He acknowledged, "I may have done

President Bill Clinton discovered that his coronary arteries were blocked, and he underwent successful bypass surgery.

© Mike Segar/Corbis

some damage in those years when I was too careless about what I ate" ("Clinton," 2004). Experts have pointed out that his eating habits were more than a little careless; Clinton's unhealthy diet during his White House years was "legendary" (Templeton, 2008). Clinton also discussed his history of treatment for high blood pressure and high cholesterol. All of these factors are risks for heart disease, but Clinton also behaved in ways that were protective and received years of good health reports. For example, he had been a jogger for years, remaining physically active throughout his presidency and afterwards. He has struggled to maintain a healthy weight, but after leaving the presidency, he dieted to a weight that seemed nearly ideal. Those protective measures may have been too little and too late—the basis for heart disease grows over years and is not easy to detect (Templeton, 2008).

Clinton looked healthy, but despite the appearance of health, his coronary arteries were seriously blocked—one more than 90% (Associated Press, 2004). He was not a candidate for surgery that would unblock his arteries; instead, the former president

underwent quadruple coronary bypass surgery. As his physicians predicted, Clinton recovered from his surgery, but additional surgery was required six months later to remove scar tissue (K. Matthews, 2005). Clinton's experience turned him into an advocate for prevention of heart disease (Clinton, 2005). He joined with the American Heart Association to begin an initiative to combat childhood obesity, including urging fast-food restaurants to provide healthier menu choices for children.

This chapter examines the behavioral risks for cardiovascular disease—the most frequent cause of death in the United States and other industrialized nations—and looks at Bill Clinton's risk from both inherent and behavioral factors. But first it describes the cardiovascular system and methods of measuring cardiovascular function.

THE CARDIOVASCULAR SYSTEM

The **cardiovascular system** consists of the heart, arteries, and veins. By contracting and relaxing, the heart muscle pumps blood that circulates throughout the body, providing a rapid-transit system to carry oxygen to body cells and to remove carbon dioxide and other wastes from cells. During normal functioning, the cardiovascular, respiratory, and digestive systems are integrated: The digestive system produces nutrients and the respiratory system furnishes oxygen, both of which circulate through the blood to various parts of the body. In addition, the endocrine system affects the cardiovascular system by stimulating or depressing the rate of cardiovascular activity. Although the cardiovascular system can be analyzed in isolation, it does not function that way.

The blood's route through the body appears in Figure 9.1. The entire circuit takes about 20 seconds when the body is at rest, but exertion speeds the process. Blood travels from the right ventricle of the heart to the lungs, where hemoglobin (one of the components of blood) becomes saturated with oxygen. From the lungs, oxygenated blood

travels back to the left atrium of the heart, then to the left ventricle, and finally out to the rest of the body. The **arteries** carry the oxygenated blood branch into vessels of smaller and smaller diameter, called **arterioles**, and finally terminate in tiny **capillaries** that connect arteries and **veins**. Oxygen diffuses out to body cells, and carbon dioxide and other chemical wastes pass into the blood so they can be disposed of. Blood that has been stripped of its oxygen returns to the heart by way of the system of veins, beginning with the tiny **venules** and ending with the two large veins that empty into the right atrium, the upper right chamber of the heart.

This section briefly considers the functioning of the cardiovascular system, concentrating on the physiology underlying **cardiovascular disease** (**CVD**), a general term that includes coronary artery disease, coronary heart disease, and stroke.

The Coronary Arteries

The coronary arteries supply blood to the heart muscle, the **myocardium**. The two principal coronary arteries branch off from the aorta (see Figure 9.2), the main artery that carries oxygenated blood from the heart. Left and right coronary arteries divide into smaller branches, providing the blood supply to the myocardium.

With each beat, the heart makes a slight twisting motion, which moves the coronary arteries. The coronary arteries, therefore, receive a great deal of strain as part of their normal function. This movement of the heart has been hypothesized to almost inevitably cause injury to the

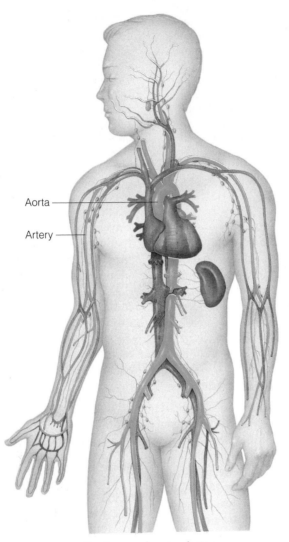

FIGURE 9.1   Cardiovascular circulation.

Source: Introduction to Microbiology (p. 671), by J. L. Ingraham &
C. A. Ingraham, 1995, Belmont, CA: Wadsworth. Copyright 1995 by
Wadsworth Publishing Company. Reprinted by permission.

coronary arteries (Friedman & Rosenman, 1974).
The damage can heal in two different ways. The
preferable route involves the formation of small
amounts of scar tissue and results in no serious
problem. The second route involves the formation of **atheromatous plaques,** deposits composed
of cholesterol and other lipids (fats), connective
tissue, and muscle tissue. The plaques grow and
calcify into a hard, bony substance that thick-
ens the arterial walls (Kharbanda & MacAllister,

2005). This process also involves inflammation
(Abi-Saleh, Iskandar, Elgharib, & Cohen, 2008).
The formation of plaques and the resulting oc-
clusion of the arteries is called **atherosclerosis,**
shown in Figure 9.3.

A related but different problem is **arteriosclerosis,** or the loss of elasticity of the arteries. The beating of the heart pushes blood
through the arteries with great force, and arterial
elasticity allows adaptation to this pressure.

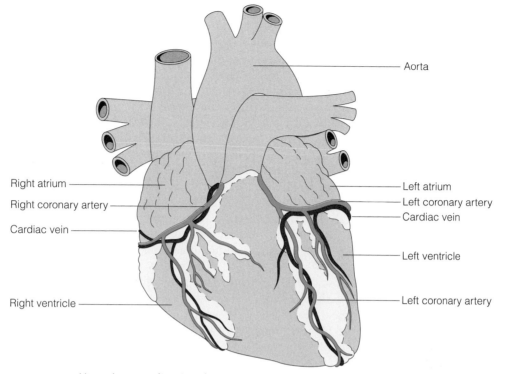

FIGURE 9.2   Heart (myocardium) with coronary arteries and veins.

Loss of elasticity tends to make the cardiovascular system less capable of tolerating increases in cardiac blood volume. Hence, a potential danger exists during strenuous exercise for people with arteriosclerosis.

The formation of arterial plaques (atherosclerosis) and the "hardening" of the arteries (arteriosclerosis) often occur together. Both can affect

any artery in the cardiovascular system, but when the coronary arteries are affected, the heart's oxygen supply may be threatened.

Coronary Artery Disease

Coronary artery disease (CAD) arises as a result of atherosclerosis and arteriosclerosis in the coronary arteries. No clearly visible outward

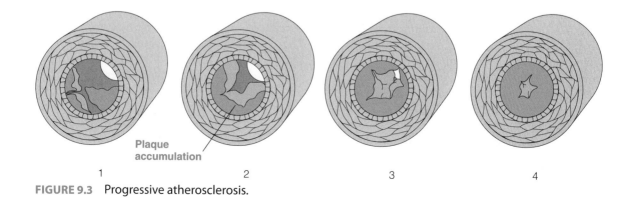

FIGURE 9.3   Progressive atherosclerosis.

symptoms accompany the buildup of plaques in the coronary arteries, as Bill Clinton discovered. CAD can be developing while a person remains totally unaware of its progress, but the plaques narrow the arteries and restrict the supply of blood to the myocardium. Deposits of plaque may also rupture, and such ruptures tend to collect blood platelets, which form blood clots around the plaques. These blood clots can transform the partially obstructed artery into a completely closed one. If the coronary arteries do not allow enough blood to reach the heart muscle, the heart, like any other organ or tissue deprived of oxygen, will not function properly. Restriction of blood flow is called **ischemia**. Bill Clinton's symptoms of chest pain and shortness of breath were likely due to ischemia.

The term **coronary heart disease (CHD)** is sometimes used interchangeably with coronary artery disease. Technically, coronary heart disease refers to any damage to the myocardium as a result of insufficient blood supply, whereas coronary artery disease refers to damage to the coronary arteries, typically through the processes of atherosclerosis and arteriosclerosis. Clinton had coronary artery disease, but the disease had not damaged his heart when he experienced symptoms and sought treatment.

Complete blockage of either coronary artery shuts off the blood flow and thus the oxygen supply to the myocardium. Like other tissue, the myocardium cannot survive without oxygen; therefore, coronary blockage results in the death of myocardial tissue, an infarction. **Myocardial infarction** is the medical term for the condition commonly referred to as a heart attack. During myocardial infarction, the damage may be so extensive as to completely disrupt the heartbeat. In less severe cases, heart contractions may become less effective. The signals for a myocardial infarction include a feeling of weakness or dizziness combined with nausea, cold sweating, difficulty in breathing, and a sensation of crushing or squeezing pain in the chest, arms, shoulders, jaw, or back. Rapid loss of consciousness or death may occur, but the victim sometimes remains quite alert throughout the experience. The severity of symptoms depends on the extent of damage to the heart muscle.

In those people who survive a myocardial infarction (somewhat more than half do), the damaged portion of the myocardium will not regrow or repair itself. Instead, scar tissue forms at the infarcted area. Scar tissue does not have the elasticity and function of healthy tissue, so a heart attack lessens the capacity of the heart to pump blood efficiently. A myocardial infarction can limit the type and vigor of activities that a person can safely do, prompting some lifestyle changes. Frequently, these changes result from cardiac patients' uncertainty about which activities are safe and from their fears about suffering another attack. Such fears have some basis. The coronary artery disease that caused a first attack can cause another, but future infarctions are not a certainty.

The process of **cardiac rehabilitation** often involves psychologists, who help cardiac patients adjust their lifestyle to minimize risk factors and lessen the chances of future attacks. Because heart disease is the most frequent cause of death in the United States, preventing heart attacks and furnishing cardiac rehabilitation are major tasks for the health care system.

A less serious result of restriction of the blood supply to the myocardium is **angina pectoris**, a disorder with symptoms of crushing pain in the chest and difficulty in breathing—the symptoms Bill Clinton experienced. Angina is usually precipitated by exercise or stress because these conditions increase demand on the heart. Clinton had experienced such symptoms during exercise and was not distressed, but when he had difficulty in breathing and tightness across the chest during his normal activities, he sought medical attention (Clinton, 2005). With oxygen restriction, the reserve capacity of the cardiovascular system is reduced, and heart disease becomes evident. The uncomfortable symptoms of angina rarely last more than a few minutes, but angina is a sign of obstruction in the coronary arteries.

Former president Clinton's symptoms led to a diagnosis of CAD, and his treatment was bypass surgery, one of the common treatments for this disorder. This procedure replaces the blocked portion of the coronary artery (or arteries) with grafts of healthy sections of the coronary arteries (see Figure 9.4). Bypass surgery is expensive, carries some risk of death, and may not extend

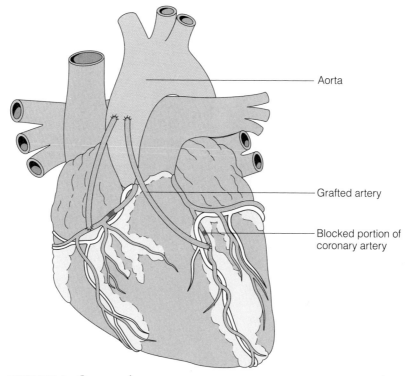

FIGURE 9.4   Coronary bypass.

the patient's life significantly, but it is generally successful in relieving angina and improving quality of life, as it has been for Clinton.

Unfortunately, the disease processes that led to the initial blockage of the coronary arteries often lead to obstruction of the replacement vessels. Therefore, people who have coronary bypass surgery may redevelop CAD (Ketonen et al., 2008); these patients must change their lifestyle if they are to prevent blockage of the replacement arteries. Bill Clinton seems aware of his risks for additional CAD, and almost immediately, he began a commitment to maintaining a healthier lifestyle (K. A. Matthews, 2005). Lifestyle factors are important for both the development and prevention of cardiovascular disease and in cardiac rehabilitation programs.

Stroke

Atherosclerosis and arteriosclerosis can also affect the arteries that serve the head and neck, thereby restricting the blood supply to the brain. That is, the same disease process that causes CAD and

CHD may affect the brain. Any obstruction in the arteries of the brain will restrict or completely stop the flow of blood to the area of the brain served by that portion of the system. A piece of material too small to obstruct an arteriole might completely block a capillary. Oxygen deprivation causes the death of brain tissue within 3 to 5 minutes. This damage to the brain resulting from lack of oxygen is called a **stroke**, the third most frequent cause of death in the United States. But strokes have other causes as well—for example, a bubble of air (air embolism) or an infection that impedes blood flow in the brain. In addition, the weakening of artery walls associated with arteriosclerosis may lead to an *aneurysm*, a sac formed by the ballooning of a weakened artery wall. Aneurysms may burst, causing a *hemorrhagic stroke* or death (see Figure 9.5).

A stroke damages neurons in the brain, and these neurons have no capacity to replace themselves. Therefore, death of any neuron results in the loss of its function. The brain, however, contains billions of neurons. People rarely experience

A common stroke is caused by a clot. Most often, as in this illustration, the clot forms where an artery has been narrowed by fatty deposits.

A hemorrhagic stroke is caused by bleeding in the brain due to a rupture of a weakened artery.

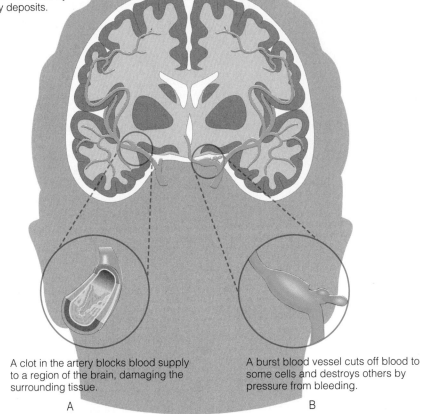

A clot in the artery blocks blood supply to a region of the brain, damaging the surrounding tissue.

A burst blood vessel cuts off blood to some cells and destroys others by pressure from bleeding.

A   B

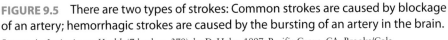

FIGURE 9.5   There are two types of strokes: Common strokes are caused by blockage of an artery; hemorrhagic strokes are caused by the bursting of an artery in the brain.

Source: An Invitation to Health (7th ed., p. 379), by D. Hales, 1997, Pacific Grove, CA: Brooks/Cole.

strokes that kill *all* neurons controlling a particular function. More commonly, some of the neurons devoted to a particular function are lost, impairing brain function. Even though neurons are not replaced, the remaining healthy neural tissue compensates to some extent. For example, specific areas of the brain control speech production. If these areas are completely damaged by a stroke, the victim can no longer speak (but may still comprehend speech). A stroke that damages some of these neurons results in loss of speech fluency and produces some difficulty in speaking. The extent

of the loss is related to the amount of damage to the area; more extensive damage results in greater impairment. This same principle applies to other types of disabilities caused by stroke. Damage may be so extensive—or in such a critical area—as to bring about immediate death, or damage may be so slight as to go unnoticed.

Degenerative diseases of the cardiovascular system, such as atherosclerosis and arteriosclerosis, are not the only cause of stroke. Blood clots can form around internal wounds in the process of healing and break away to float through the

TABLE 9.1

Ranges of Blood Pressure (expressed in mm of Hg)

	Systolic		Diastolic
Normal	<120	and	<80
Prehypertension	120–139	or	80–89
Stage 1 Hypertension	140–159	or	90–99
Stage 2 Hypertension	≥160	or	≥100

Source: Adapted from *The Seventh Report of the Joint National Committee on Prevention, Detection, Evaluation and Treatment of High Blood Pressure* (NIH Publication No. 03–5233), 2003, by U.S. Department of Health and Human Services (USDHHS). Washington, DC: Author. Table 1.

circulatory system. However, the most common cause of stroke is similar to that of heart attack—atherosclerosis, the rupture of plaques, and the formation of blood clots. Such clots form a floating hazard in the cardiovascular system that may result in a debilitating or deadly stroke.

Blood Pressure

When the heart pumps blood, the force must be substantial to power circulation for an entire cycle through the body and back to the heart. In a healthy cardiovascular system, the pressure in the arteries is not a problem because arteries are quite elastic. In a cardiovascular system diseased by atherosclerosis and arteriosclerosis, however, the pressure of the blood in the arteries can produce serious consequences. The narrowing of the arteries that occurs in atherosclerosis and the loss of elasticity that characterizes arteriosclerosis both tend to raise blood pressure. In addition, these disease processes make the cardiovascular system less capable of adapting to the demands of heavy exercise and stress.

Blood pressure measurements are usually expressed by two numbers. The first number represents **systolic pressure**, the pressure generated by the heart's contraction. The second number represents **diastolic pressure**, or the pressure experienced between contractions, reflecting the elasticity of the vessel walls. Both numbers are measured by determining how high in millimeters (mm) a column of mercury (Hg) can be raised in a glass column.

Elevations of blood pressure can occur through several mechanisms. Some elevations in blood pressure are normal and even adaptive.

Activation of the sympathetic nervous system, for example, increases heart rate and also causes constriction of the blood vessels, both of which raise blood pressure. The parasympathetic division blocks sympathetic action and returns blood pressure to its baseline rate, so sympathetic activation should not result in permanent increases in blood pressure. Other elevations in blood pressure, however, are neither normal nor adaptive—they are symptoms of cardiovascular disease.

Millions of people in the United States have **hypertension**—that is, abnormally high blood pressure. This "silent" illness is the single best predictor of both heart attack and stroke, but it can also cause eye damage and kidney failure (see Figure 9.6). Hypertension is of two types—primary or essential hypertension and secondary hypertension. **Essential hypertension** refers to a chronic elevation of blood pressure, which has both genetic and environmental causes (Staessen, Wang, Bianchi, & Birkenhager, 2003). This condition affects 25–35% of people in the United States and other developed countries, for a total of about 50 million in the United States and 1 billion worldwide (USDHHS, 2003). It is strongly related to aging but also to such factors as African American ancestry, weight, sodium intake, tobacco use, and lack of exercise. **Secondary hypertension** is much less common than essential hypertension; it stems from other diseases such as kidney disorders and some disorders of the endocrine system.

Table 9.1 shows the ranges for normal blood pressure, prehypertension, and Stage 1 and Stage 2 hypertension. Despite beliefs to the contrary, people with hypertension cannot diagnose their

Eye damage
Prolonged high blood
pressure can damage
delicate blood vessels on
the retina, the layer of cells
at the back of the eye. If
the damage, known as
retinopathy, remains
untreated, it can lead to
blindness.

Stroke
High blood pressure can damage vessels
that supply blood to the brain, eventually
causing them to rupture or clog. The
interruption in blood flow to the brain
is known as a stroke.

Heart attack
High blood pressure
makes the heart work
harder to pump sufficient
blood through narrowed
arterioles (small blood
vessels). This extra effort
can enlarge and weaken
the heart, leading to
heart failure. High
blood pressure
also damages the
coronary arteries
that supply blood to
the heart, sometimes
leading to blockages that
can cause a heart attack.

Kidney failure
Prolonged high blood
pressure can damage blood
vessels in the kidney, where
wastes are filtered from the
bloodstream. In severe
cases, this damage can
lead to kidney failure
and even death.

Damage to artery walls
Artery walls are normally smooth, allowing blood
to flow easily. Over time, high blood pressure can
wear rough spots in artery walls. Fatty deposits
can collect in the rough spots, clogging arteries
and raising the risk of a heart attack or stroke.

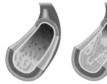

Rough
artery walls

Clogged
artery

FIGURE 9.6   The consequences of high blood pressure.

Source: An Invitation to Health (7th ed., p. 370), by D. Hales, 1997, Pacific Grove, CA: Brooks/Cole.

own blood pressure reliably (Meyer, Leventhal, & Gutman, 1985). Therefore, people can have dangerously elevated blood pressure and remain completely unaware of their vulnerability to heart attack and stroke.

In younger individuals, high diastolic pressure is most strongly related to cardiovascular risk, but in older individuals, elevated systolic pressure is a better predictor (Staessen et al., 2003). Incremental increases in blood pressure are proportionally related to elevated risk. Each 20 mm Hg increase in systolic blood pressure doubles the risk of cardiovascular disease (USDHHS, 2003). Systolic pressure that exceeds 200 mm Hg presents a danger of rupture in the arterial walls (Berne & Levy, 2000). A rupture of the aorta is usually fatal; a rupture of a cerebral artery results in a stroke that may be fatal. Diastolic hypertension tends to result in vascular damage that may injure organs served by the affected vessels, most commonly the kidneys, liver, pancreas, brain, and retina.

Because the underlying cause of essential hypertension is complex and not fully understood, no treatment exists that will remedy its basic cause. Treatment tends to be oriented toward drugs or changes in behavior and lifestyle that can lower blood pressure (USDHHS, 2003). Because part of the treatment of hypertension involves behavioral changes, health psychologists have a role to play in encouraging such behaviors as controlling weight, maintaining a regular exercise program, and restricting sodium intake. Adherence to these behaviors is important for controlling blood pressure.

IN SUMMARY

The cardiovascular system consists of the heart and blood vessels. The heart pumps blood, which circulates throughout the body, supplying oxygen and removing waste products. The coronary arteries supply blood to the heart itself, and when atherosclerosis affects these arteries, coronary artery disease (CAD) occurs. In this disease process, plaques form within the arteries, restricting the blood supply to the heart muscle. The restriction can cause angina pectoris, with symptoms of chest pain and difficulty in breathing. Blocked coronary arteries can also lead to a myocardial infarction (heart attack). When the oxygen supply to the brain is disrupted, stroke occurs. Stroke can affect any part of the brain and can vary in severity from minor to fatal. Hypertension—high blood pressure—is a predictor of both heart attack and stroke. Both behavioral and medical treatments can lower hypertension as well as other risk factors for cardiovascular disease.

THE CHANGING RATES OF CARDIOVASCULAR DISEASE

The current mortality rate from CVD for people in the United States is lower than the rate in 1920. However, between 1920 and 2002, the death rates changed dramatically. Figure 9.7 reveals a sharp rise in CVD deaths from 1920 until the 1950s and 1960s, followed by a decline that continued throughout the century and into this one. By 2003, the mortality rate was lower than it was in 1920. Currently, 33% of all deaths in the United States are from cardiovascular disease (USCB, 2007).

In 1920, the rate of deaths due to heart disease was similar for women and men. Overall, the rates of death from CVD remain similar, but the pattern of deaths began to differ when CVD rates began to rise. During the middle of the 20th century, men died from CVD at younger ages than women, creating a gender gap in heart disease.

Reasons for the Decline in Death Rates

The decline in cardiac mortality in the United States is due largely to two causes: improved emergency coronary care and changes in risk factors for CVD (Ford et al., 2007; Wise, 2000). Beginning in the 1960s, many people in the United States began to change their lifestyle. They began to smoke less, be more aware of their blood pressure, control serum cholesterol, watch their weight, and follow a regular exercise program.

Many of these lifestyle changes were prompted by the publicity given to two monumental studies. The first was the Framingham Heart Study that began to issue reports during the 1960s, implicating cigarette smoking, high cholesterol, hypertension, a sedentary lifestyle, and obesity as risk factors in cardiovascular disease (Levy & Brink, 2005). The second study was the highly publicized 1964 Surgeon General's report (U.S. Public Health Service [USPHS], 1964), which found a strong association between cigarette smoking and heart disease. Many people became aware of these studies and began to alter their way of living.

Although these lifestyle changes closely parallel declining heart disease death rates, they offer no proof of a causal link between behavior changes and the drop in cardiovascular mortality. During this same period, medical care and technology continued to improve, and many cardiac patients who in earlier years would have died were saved by better and faster treatment.

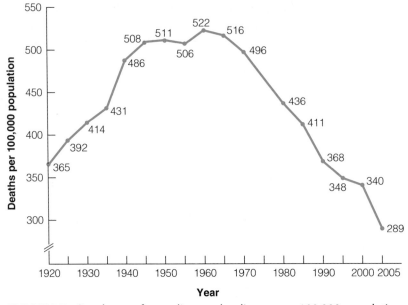

FIGURE 9.7 Death rates for cardiovascular disease per 100,000 population, United States, 1920–2005.

Sources: U.S. Public Health Service, *Vital Statistics of the United States*, annual, Vol. I and Vol. II (1900–1970); U.S. National Center for Health Statistics, *Vital Statistics of the United States*, annual (1971–2001); *National Vital Statistics Report*, monthly (2002–2005). Retrieved August 21, 2008, from http://www.infoplease.com/ipa/A0922292.html

Which factor—lifestyle changes or better medical care—has contributed more to the declining death rate from heart disease? An analysis of both medical care and risk factor reduction (Ford et al., 2007) indicated that each of these improvements contributed to the decline, in approximately equal proportions. About 47% of the decline in CHD was due to improvements in treatment and 44% to changes in risk factors. Thus, the declining rate of death from heart disease is due about as much to changes in behavior and lifestyle as it is to improved medical care.

Heart Disease Throughout the World

Heart disease is the leading cause of death, not only in the United States but worldwide. This situation is not true for every country—in some countries, infectious diseases kill more people than CVD—but the total number of deaths from heart disease and stroke accounts for about 30% of all deaths (Mackay & Mensah, 2004). The

United States is only one of many high-income Western countries that have seen lifestyle changes and dramatic reductions in cardiovascular deaths among its population (World Health Organization [WHO], 2008b).

In Finland, CVD rates fell more than 70% from the 1970s through the 1990s (Puska, 2002; Puska, Vartiainen, Tuomilehto, Salomaa, & Nissinen, 1998). Part of this decrease was the result of a countrywide effort to change risk factors. That effort began with a community intervention that targeted an area of Finland with particularly high rates of CVD and attempted to change diet, hypertension, and smoking. An analysis of the contributions of improved medical care and lowered risk profiles (Laatikainen et al., 2005) indicated that lowering risk factors was responsible for the majority of the reduction.

A very different situation has occurred in countries that were once part of the Soviet Union (Weidner, 2000; Weidner & Cain, 2003); in these countries, heart disease has increased. Since

1990, this epidemic has affected middle-aged men more than other groups, and the gender gap in heart disease is larger in Russia than in any other country. The risk of premature death from heart disease is four times greater for a Russian man than for one in the United States. In some countries in Eastern Europe, coronary heart disease accounts for 80% of deaths; the average life expectancy has decreased and is not expected to increase in the near future. The reasons for this plague of heart disease are not completely understood. Many risk factors are similar to those in other locations, but lack of social support, stress, smoking, and alcohol abuse are higher, and these psychosocial and behavioral differences may underlie the increased rates of CVD (Weidner & Cain, 2003).

People associate CVD with industrialized countries, but heart disease and stroke are also leading causes of death in developing and underdeveloped countries, which have experienced an increase in heart disease and stroke that promises to continue (WHO, 2008b). These countries will not undergo a decline in CVD; instead, as tobacco smoking, obesity, physical activity, and dietary patterns become more like those of developed nations, CVD will increase in developing nations. In these countries, CVD affects people at a younger age than in more developed nations, presenting an even greater burden of disease to the workforces of these countries. Thus, the worldwide burden of CVD is immense.

<hr>

IN SUMMARY

Since the mid-1960s, deaths from coronary artery disease and stroke have steadily declined in the United States and most (but not all) other high-income nations. Although some of that decline is a result of better and faster coronary care, most authorities believe that lifestyle changes account for 50% or more of this decrease. During the past four decades, millions of people in the United States have made changes in their lifestyles that decreased their risk for CVD. In low-income countries around the world, the opposite has occurred: Smoking and obesity have increased, and

physical activity has decreased. These habits have increased risks for CVD, which will grow in these countries in the coming years.

RISK FACTORS IN CARDIOVASCULAR DISEASE

Medical research has no exact answers as to what causes dangerous buildup of atheromatous plaques in the arteries of some people but not in others, or what causes some plaques to rupture whereas others do not. However, research has linked several risk factors to the development of cardiovascular disease. In Chapter 2, we defined a *risk factor* as any characteristic or condition that occurs with greater frequency in people with a disease than in people free from that disease. The risk factor approach does not reveal the underlying physiology in the development of the disorder; that is, it does not allow for the identification of a cause. Nor does it allow a precise prediction of who will be affected and who will remain healthy. The risk factor approach simply yields information concerning which conditions are associated—directly or indirectly—with a particular disease or disorder.

The risk factor approach to predicting heart disease began with the Framingham Heart Study in 1948, an investigation of more than 5,000 people in the town of Framingham, Massachusetts (Levy & Brink, 2005). The study was a prospective design; thus, all participants were free of heart disease at the beginning of the study. The original plan was to follow these people for 20 years to study heart disease and the factors related to its development. The results proved so valuable that the study has continued now for more than 50 years and includes both second- and third-generation offspring of the original participants.

During its early years, the Framingham study uncovered a number of risk factors for cardiovascular disease. At the time of their discovery, medicine had not considered some of these factors to be particularly dangerous. Cigarette smoking, high-fat diet, overweight, high cholesterol, elevated blood pressure, and lack of exercise were part of the typical American lifestyle (Levy & Brink, 2005). Prompted by the growing epidemic of heart disease in the 1950s, the Framingham study revealed that these risk factors are reliably related to the development of heart disease and stroke. Research has identified a host of other risk factors for cardiovascular disease, including diabetes, family history, gender, and ethnic background as well as psychosocial factors such as phobic anxiety, marital status, employment, hostility, and anger.

Cardiovascular risk factors include those that are inherent and cannot be changed but can be monitored, physiological conditions such as hypertension and high serum cholesterol level that are indirectly related to behavior and lifestyle, behavioral factors such as smoking and diet, and a variety of psychosocial factors.

Inherent Risk Factors

Inherent risk factors result from genetic or physical conditions that cannot be readily modified. Although inherent risk factors cannot be changed, people with these risk factors are not necessarily destined to develop cardiovascular disease. Identifying people with inherent risk factors enables these high-risk individuals to minimize their overall risk profile by controlling the things that they can, such as hypertension, smoking, and diet. Inherent risk factors for CVD include advancing age, family history, gender, and ethnic background.

Advancing Age Advancing age is the primary risk factor for cardiovascular disease as well as for cancer and many other diseases. As people become older, their risk for cardiovascular death rises sharply. Figure 9.8 shows that for every 10-year increase in age, both men and women more than double their chances of dying of cardiovascular disease. For example, men 85 and older are about 2.7 times as likely to die of cardiovascular disease as men between the ages of 75 and 84, and women 85 and older are about 3.7 times as likely as women 75 to 84 to die from cardiovascular disease.

Family History Family history is also an inherent risk factor for CVD. People with a history of cardiovascular disease in their family are more likely to die of heart disease than those with no

such history. Bill Clinton mentioned his family history as a factor that put him at risk for cardiovascular disease. This familial risk is likely to occur through the action of many genes and their interactions with environmental factors in people's lives (Doevendans, Van der Smagt, Loh, De Jonge, & Touw, 2003). Like other inherent risk factors, genes cannot be altered through lifestyle changes, but people with a family history of heart disease can lower their risk by changing those behaviors and lifestyles that can be altered.

Gender Gender is another risk factor that may be inherent. Biological sex is an inherent factor, but many behaviors and social conditions are related to gender. Thus, the differing risk for women and men may or may not be inherent.

Heart disease is the leading cause of death in the United States (and other high-income, industrialized nations) for both women and men (Pilote et al., 2007). Men have a higher rate of death from CVD than women, and this discrepancy shows most prominently during the middle-age years. Figure 9.8 shows that the rate of men's death from cardiovascular disease is about double that of women for ages 35 to 74. After that age, the percentage of women's deaths due to CVD increases sharply, and a larger number of older women than older men die of cardiovascular disease; nonetheless, the *rate* of death from CVD remains higher for men.

What factors explain this gender gap? Both physiology and lifestyle contribute (Pilote et al., 2007). Before menopause, women experience a lower rate of CVD than men. At one time, estrogen was believed to furnish protection, but the failure to produce any benefit in a large-scale hormone replacement trial engendered doubt (Writing Group for the Women's Health Initiative Investigators, 2002). A recent focus has been on androgens, including the possibility that these hormones may involve both protections and risks for both men and women (Ng, 2007). However, lifestyle must be responsible for some of the discrepancy, because differences among countries are greater than the difference between women and men. For example, Russia has the widest

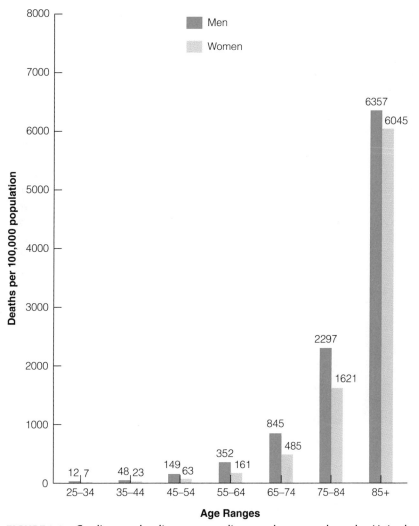

FIGURE 9.8   Cardiovascular disease mortality rates by age and gender, United States, 2004.

Source: Health United States, 2007, by National Center for Health Statistics, 2007, Hyattsville, MD: U.S. Government Printing Office, pp. 201, 204.

gender gap in life expectancy in the world—71 years for women and 58 for men—and most of the discrepancy comes from higher rates of CVD among men (Weidner & Cain, 2003). Russian men's health habits include more smoking and drinking, and they show poorer coping skills for dealing with stress. In other countries, such as Iceland, the gender difference in CVD rate is small (Weidner, 2000). The fact that gender differences in CVD mortality are much greater in some countries than in others suggests that inherent biological differences do not explain the CVD mortality discrepancy between men and women.

In addition, if gender is truly an inherent risk factor for CVD, then the differences between men and women should be similar not only from country to country but throughout history.

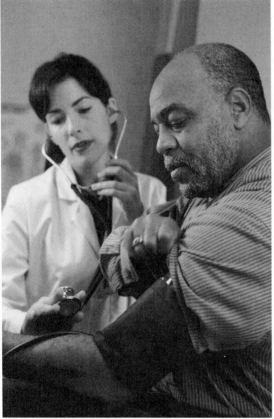

Charles Thatcher/Getty Images

African Americans are more likely to have hypertension than European Americans.

Evidence suggests that the gender gap in heart disease in the United States was small until the 1920s (Nikiforov & Mamaev, 1998). Until that time, CVD deaths for men ages 25 to 74 years were only about 20% higher than for women, and these differences remained modest until the 1960s. At that time, however, the gap between men and women began to expand as middle-aged men's rates increased while women's rates declined. As a consequence, men now have twice the cardiovascular mortality as women during middle age (see Figure 9.8). This historical perspective suggests that factors other than biology are at work in creating the gender gap, but it leaves the discrepancy unexplained. However, African American women are at elevated risk compared to European American women (NCHS, 2007), which suggests that ethnicity is also a factor in CVD.

Ethnic Background A fourth inherent risk for cardiovascular disease is ethnic background. In the United States, African Americans have more than a 30% greater risk for cardiovascular death than European Americans, but Native Americans, Asian Americans, and Hispanic Americans have lower rates (NCHS, 2007). The increased risk for African Americans may be related to social, economic, or behavioral factors rather than to any biological basis, because a worldwide study (Yusuf et al., 2004) indicated that the risk factors for heart disease are the same for people in countries around the world. However, some individuals and even some groups may experience higher levels of these risks.

African Americans follow that pattern: They have the same categories as but higher levels of risk factors for heart disease than European Americans, Hispanics, Asians, and Native Americans. The strongest risk for African Americans is high blood pressure (Jones et al., 2002), but psychosocial risks such as low income and low educational level also have a major impact (Karlamangla et al., 2005; Pilote et al., 2007). The higher rates of cardiovascular death among African Americans may relate to their higher rate of hypertension, which may relate to greater cardiac reactivity, which in turn may relate to racial discrimination. Even threats of discrimination can raise blood pressure in African Americans (Blascovich et al., 2001). The tendency to react to stress and threats of stress with increased cardiac reactivity is probably not inherent; rather, it springs from years of racial discrimination, a discrimination most likely to be experienced by dark-skinned people. For example, Elizabeth Klonoff and Hope Landrine (2000) found that dark-skinned African Americans were 11 times more likely than light-skinned African Americans to experience frequent racial discrimination. This finding suggests that the high blood pressure ratings of African Americans may be influenced by color discrimination. Thus, racial discrimination seems to be a factor in the increased blood pressure levels among African Americans, but these responses are classified as psychosocial risks that relate to ethnicity rather than as a risk that is inherent in ethnic differences.

Physiological Conditions

A second category of risk factors in cardiovascular disease includes the physiological conditions of hypertension, serum cholesterol level, problems in glucose metabolism, and inflammation.

Hypertension Other than advancing age, hypertension is the single most important risk factor for cardiovascular disease, yet millions of people with high blood pressure are not aware of their vulnerability. Unlike most disorders, hypertension produces no overt symptoms, and dangerously elevated blood pressure levels commonly occur with no signals or symptoms. Most people believe that if their blood pressure were high, they would be aware of it (Meyer et al., 1985). They are wrong; hypertension ordinarily has no discernible symptoms.

Although the Framingham Heart Study was not the first to suggest that people with high blood pressure have more cardiovascular problems than those with normal blood pressure, it provided solid evidence of the risks of hypertension (Levy & Brink, 2005). Regardless of people's age or gender, results from the Framingham study indicated that their risk of cardiovascular disease increased with increases in blood pressure. Since that early research, the importance of blood pressure has become unquestionably evident. As a U.S. government report stated, "The risk between BP and risk of CVD events is continuous, consistent, and independent of other risk factors. The higher the BP, the greater the chance of heart attack, heart failure, stroke, and kidney disease" (USDHHS, 2003, p. 2).

Serum Cholesterol Level A second physiological condition related to cardiovascular disease is high serum cholesterol level. *Serum* or *blood cholesterol* is the level of cholesterol circulating through the bloodstream; this level is related (but not perfectly related) to *dietary cholesterol*, or the amount of cholesterol in one's food. Cholesterol is a waxy, fatlike substance that is essential for human life as a component of cell membranes. Dietary cholesterol comes from animal fats and oils but not from vegetables or vegetable products. Although cholesterol is essential for life, too much may contribute to the process of developing cardiovascular disease.

After a person eats cholesterol, the bloodstream transports it as part of the process of digestion. A measurement of the amount of cholesterol carried in the serum (the liquid, cell-free part of the blood) is typically expressed in milligrams (mg) of cholesterol per deciliters (dl) of serum. This measurement is a ratio, but it is generally abbreviated to the cholesterol count. Thus, a cholesterol reading of 210 means 210 mg of cholesterol per deciliter of blood serum. But what does a cholesterol level of 210 mean? Is that number good or bad?

High cholesterol levels are related to total mortality for men in the United States and many (but not all) other countries (Cai et al., 2004). However, the relationship is more complex for women, and increasing levels of cholesterol do not have a consistent relationship to death. The relationship is simpler for risk of cardiovascular disease: High levels of cholesterol are related to increased deaths (Grundy et al., 2004). However, a puzzling finding is that very low cholesterol levels do not lower total mortality rates. Instead, very low cholesterol levels are also related to increased mortality, especially among older people (Schupf et al., 2005) but for younger people as well (Ulmer, Kelleher, Diem, & Concin, 2004). Falling cholesterol levels may be an indication of some disease process such as cancer (Song, Sung, & Kim, 2000), and people with lower cholesterol levels seem to have an increased chance of dying violent deaths such as suicide or unintentional injuries, which is a puzzling situation. Nonetheless, these findings suggest that striving for the lowest possible cholesterol level is not the best strategy for everyone.

Not all cholesterol is equally implicated in coronary heart disease; that is, total cholesterol is not the best predictor of CVD. Cholesterol circulates in the blood in several forms of **lipoproteins**, which can be distinguished by analyzing their density. The Framingham researchers found that **low-density lipoprotein (LDL)** was positively related to cardiovascular disease, whereas **high-density lipoprotein (HDL)** was negatively related. High-density lipoprotein actually seems to offer some protection against CVD, whereas LDL seems to promote atherosclerosis. For these reasons, LDL is sometimes referred to as "bad cholesterol" and HDL as "good cholesterol." Indeed, women's higher levels of HDL and greater protection from higher HDL levels may be a partial explanation for the gender gap in heart disease (Pilote et al., 2007).

Total cholesterol (TC) is determined by adding the values for HDL, LDL, and 20% of very low-density lipoprotein (VLDL), also called **triglycerides.** A low ratio of total cholesterol to HDL is more desirable than a high ratio. A ratio of less than 4.5 to 1 is healthier than a ratio of 6.0 to 1; that is, people whose HDL level is about 20% to 22% of total cholesterol have a reduced risk of CVD. Most authorities now believe that a favorable balance of total cholesterol to HDL is more critical than total cholesterol in avoiding cardiovascular disease, and much recent research has focused on lowering LDL (Grundy et al., 2004). Table 9.2 presents the desirable ranges for total cholesterol and each of the subfractions, along with a desirable and an undesirable profile.

However, cholesterol levels do not show a reliable relationship with CVD for older people. Data from a sample of older adults in the United States (Psaty et al., 2004) revealed that the blood lipid measures were not strongly related to death from heart attack or stroke. Another study (Sacco et al., 2001) indicated that cholesterol was a predictor of death from heart disease up to about age 60 but not afterward. However, another study (Strandberg et al., 2004) indicated that people who had low cholesterol levels during middle adulthood were more likely to live to be old and

to have a higher quality of life in old age. Therefore, cholesterol should be a concern through middle age, but older people can be less focused on attaining a low cholesterol level.

Research on cholesterol suggests several conclusions. First, cholesterol intake and blood cholesterol are related. Second, the relationship between dietary intake of cholesterol and blood cholesterol relates strongly to habitual diet—that is, eating habits maintained over many years. Lowering blood cholesterol level by changing diet is possible, but the process is neither quick nor easy. Third, the ratio of total cholesterol to HDL is probably more important than total cholesterol alone, but lowering LDL is an important goal.

Problems in Glucose Metabolism A third physiological risk factor for CVD comes from problems with glucose metabolism. The most obvious such problem is diabetes, a condition in which glucose cannot be taken into the cells because of problems in producing or using insulin. When this situation occurs, glucose remains in the blood at abnormally high levels. People who have juvenile onset (Type 1) diabetes are more likely to develop CVD, and longer duration problems with glucose metabolism increase the risk (Pambianco, Costacou, & Orchard, 2007). Type 2 diabetes also elevates the risk of CVD (Sobel & Schneider, 2005). (We discuss the risks of diabetes more fully in Chapter 11.)

Many people have problems with glucose metabolism that do not qualify as diabetes but may still create CVD risk. One study (Khaw et al., 2004) showed that people who have problems in glucose metabolism (but not diabetes) showed greater risks for CVD development or death than

TABLE 9.2

Desirable Ranges for Serum Cholesterol, Along With Examples of Favorable and Risky Profiles

Cholesterol Component	Desirable Range	Good Profile	Risky Profile
HDL cholesterol	>60 mg/dl	70	40
LDL cholesterol	<130 mg/dl	60	180
Triglycerides	<200 mg/dl	150	250
	(20% of VLDL)	30 (=150 × .20)	50 (= 250 × .20)
Total cholesterol	<200 mg/dl	70 + 60 + 30 = 160	40 + 180 + 50 = 270
Cholesterol/HDL ratio	<4.00	160/70 = 2.28	270/40 = 6.75

those with normal glucose metabolism. Such problems in glucose metabolism constitute one of the factors in the *metabolic syndrome*, a collection of factors proposed to elevate the risk for CVD (Johnson & Weinstock, 2006). Other components include excess abdominal fat, elevated blood pressure, and problems with the levels of two components of cholesterol. In a study testing the components of the metabolic syndrome (Anderson et al., 2004), problems in insulin metabolism were more strongly related to arterial damage than the other components.

Inflammation The body's immune system responds to a variety of invaders with inflammation, and chronic inflammation seems to raise the risk for the development of atherosclerosis (Pilote et al., 2007). The process of inflammation probably affects healing of the lining of arteries, resulting in the formation of plaques, but it can also affect the stability of plaques, making them more likely to rupture and cause a heart attack or stroke (Abi-Saleh et al., 2008). This type of inflammation need not be severe to be dangerous—the inflammation may be so minor that the person is not aware of it, but the danger is still present. Several types of inflammation have shown a relationship to CVD. For example, periodontal disease (inflammation of the gums) is positively correlated with coronary artery disease (Amabile et al., 2008). Inflammation may be related to the metabolic syndrome (Vlachopoulos, Rokkas, Ioakeimidis, & Stefanadis, 2007), suggesting that these conditions interact or have some common pathways for causing damage to the cardiovascular system. Stress and depression may also be related to inflammation (Miller & Blackwell, 2006). The findings about the risks from inflammation explain why taking anti-inflammatory drugs such as aspirin lower the risk of heart attack, and the findings about stress and depression suggest that other behavioral factors may present risks as well as ways to protect against CVD.

Behavioral Factors

Behavioral correlates of cardiovascular disease constitute a third risk category for CVD; the most important of these lifestyle factors are smoking,

diet, and physical activity. For example, women who do not smoke, eat a diet high in fiber and low in saturated fat, are not overweight, and are physically active have an 80% lower risk for coronary heart disease than other people (Stampfer, Hu, Manson, Rimm, & Willett, 2000). Each of these behaviors—smoking, food choice, weight maintenance, and physical activity—is related to CVD. Unfortunately, these behaviors are difficult to isolate and study because people who are smokers also tend to have other habits that contribute to their CVD risk, such as eating a less heart-healthy diet (Dyer et al., 2003).

Smoking Cigarette smoking is the leading behavioral risk factor for cardiovascular death in the United States, and a major contributor to deaths throughout the world (Ezzati & Lopez, 2004). In the United States, cardiovascular deaths due to smoking have begun to decline (Rodu & Cole, 2007). Between 1987 and 2002, deaths attributable to smoking declined 41% in men and 30% in women. However, such a decline has not occurred in all parts of the world—smoking continues at higher rates in many countries than in the United States. Smoking accounts for about 35% of the risk for heart attack in countries around the world (Yusuf et al., 2004), which translates into more than a million deaths per year; for example, an estimated 1,690,000 CVD deaths attributable to smoking occurred in the year 2000 (Ezzati & Lopez, 2004).

The link between smoking and heart disease has been well established for more than 35 years, since the early reports from the Framingham study (Levy & Brink, 2005). Passive smoking is not as dangerous, but exposure to environmental tobacco smoke raises the risk for cardiovascular disease by about 15% (Kaur, Cohen, Dolor, Coffman, & Bastian, 2004).

Weight and Diet The relationship between diet and cardiovascular disease has been the subject of investigations concerning the risks of overweight as well as the impact of food choices and even specific nutrients. Although the dangers of obesity seem obvious, the evaluation of obesity as an independent risk for cardiovascular disease is difficult. The main problem is that obesity is related to other risks, such as blood pressure, Type 2 diabetes, total cholesterol, LDL, and triglycerides (Ashton, Nanchahal, & Wood, 2001). All of these factors are CVD risks, so the evaluation of obesity as an independent risk factor for CVD is difficult. However, a high degree of abdominal fat is a risk factor for heart attack in men (D. A. Smith et al., 2005), in women (Iribarren, Darbinian, Lo, Fireman, & Go, 2006), and in people worldwide (Yusuf et al., 2005).

The dietary choices that people make may either increase or decrease their chances of developing cardiovascular disease, depending on the foods they eat. Results from the years of the Framingham study (Levy & Brink, 2005) have demonstrated that diets heavy in saturated fats are positively related to CVD. The foods that were considered healthy when the study started in 1948, such as red meat, whole milk, butter, and gravy, are now widely recognized as unhealthy. These high-fat foods have an obvious link to serum cholesterol levels, but other nutrients may also affect CVD risks.

For example, sodium intake has been related to blood pressure (one of the major risks for CVD; Stamler et al., 2003), and some individuals seem to be more sensitive to the effects of sodium intake than others (Brooks, Haywood, & Johnson, 2005). Potassium intake, however, seems to decrease the risk, which brings up the question: Can diet serve as protection against cardiovascular disease? A growing body of results indicates that some diets, and perhaps even some foods, offer protective effects.

For more than two decades, researchers have found that diets high in fruits and vegetables are associated with lower CVD risks. An analysis of worldwide consumption of fruits and vegetables (Lock, Pomerleau, Causer, Altmann, & McKee, 2005) led to the conclusion that consumption levels are too low for optimal health; if these levels were increased to a minimal acceptable level, the rate of heart disease could be reduced by 31% and stroke by 19%. A longitudinal study of dietary patterns (Brunner et al., 2008) confirmed the value of such a diet; people whose habitual diets were high in fruits, vegetables, whole-grain cereals, and low-fat dairy showed a decreased likelihood of experiencing coronary events or developing diabetes.

A diet high in fish seems to offer some protection against heart disease and stroke; the protective component is *omega-3 fatty acids*. Fish such as tuna, salmon, mackerel, and other high-fat fish and shellfish are high in this nutrient, but research on the benefits of fish has yielded mixed results. Not all fish meals offer the same protection (Mozaffarian et al., 2005). For example, baked or broiled fish was more beneficial than fried fish in decreasing the risk of stroke in older adults. Consuming fish seems to offer some protection against CHD (Iso et al., 2001; Torpy, 2006), and the American Heart Association has recommended two servings of fish per week (Smith & Sahyoun, 2005) based on this evidence. That advantage is balanced against the high level of mercury in some fish, which also presents risks.

Do certain vitamins or other micronutrients protect against cardiovascular disease? Many studies have indicated that people who eat diets high in antioxidants such as vitamin E, beta carotene or lycopene, selenium, and riboflavin show a number of health advantages, including lower levels of cardiovascular disease (Stanner, Hughes, Kelly, & Buttriss, 2004). These antioxidants protect LDL from oxidation and thus from its potentially damaging effects on the cardiovascular system. However, research findings have not shown that taking supplements of these nutrients is as effective as eating a diet that contains the nutrients in high levels. Such a diet may include some surprising choices (see Would You Believe . . . ? box).

Physical Activity   The benefits of physical activity in lowering cardiovascular risk are well established (see Chapter 15 for a review of this evidence). A review of the health benefits of physical activity referred to the evidence as "irrefutable" (Warburton, Nicol, & Bredin, 2006, p. 801). Unfortunately, people's jobs have become less physically strenuous, and many individuals do not engage in physical activity in their leisure time, creating large numbers of sedentary people in many industrialized societies.

WOULD YOU BELIEVE . . . ?

Chocolate May Help Prevent Heart Disease

Would you believe that chocolate—rather than being bad for you—may contain chemicals that help prevent coronary artery disease? One of the dietary components that seems to offer some protection against artery damage is a class of chemicals called *flavonoids*, which are derived primarily from fruits and vegetables (Engler & Engler, 2006). Several subcategories of flavonoids exist, each with slightly different properties. The subcategory that contains chocolate is the flavonols, which also occur in tea, red wine, grapes, and blackberries. However, all of the subcategories have been linked to health benefits, including growing evidence of the advantages of chocolate.

Not all chocolate contains the same amount of flavonoids, and thus some types of chocolate may offer more protection than others (Engler & Engler, 2006). The processing of the cacao bean, from which chocolate is made, affects the flavonoid content. Dark chocolate contains two to three times more flavonoids than milk chocolate or Dutch chocolate.

Flavonoids exert their health benefits by reducing oxidation, making them one type of antioxidant. The benefits may occur through effects on the lining of arteries (Engler & Engler, 2006). Flavonoids may be especially effective in protecting arteries against the harmful effects of low-density cholesterol and increase vascular dilation. If flavonoids protect arteries, that mechanism would explain the connection between flavonol intake and lower rates of coronary heart disease mortality (Huxley &

Neil, 2003). However, chocolate consumption has also shown cardiovascular benefits in lowering blood pressure and decreasing inflammation, both of which lower risk factors for CVD (Engler & Engler, 2006). This body of research indicates that chocolate consumption may protect against heart disease in a variety of ways.

Chocolate is not the only food that is rich in flavonols. High concentrations of this micronutrient also occurs in green and black tea, grapes, red wine, cherries, apples, blackberries, and raspberries. Thus chocolate may not offer unique health benefits, but legions of chocoholics would testify that its taste is unique. These devotees are overjoyed that a food that was once considered a sin may now offer salvation from heart disease.

The risks of inactivity are well understood and apply to the entire life span. In the United States, children have become less physically active, and their sedentary lifestyle has contributed to their increasing obesity and growing risk for cardiovascular disease (Wang, 2004). At the other end of the age spectrum, women over age 65 showed better health and lower CVD risks when they voluntarily engaged in exercise (Simonsick, Guralnik, Volpato, Balfour, & Fried, 2005). Sedentary lifestyle has also been linked to the metabolic syndrome, the pattern of CVD risks that include overweight, abdominal fat, and blood glucose metabolism problems (Ekelund et al., 2005). Thus, physical inactivity is an important behavioral risk factor for cardiovascular disease.

Psychosocial Factors

In addition to inherent factors, physiological conditions, and behaviors, researchers have identified a number of psychosocial factors that relate to heart disease (Smith & Ruiz, 2002). Although some in the biomedical field are hesitant to accept the contribution of such factors, ample evidence exists that several psychosocial factors contribute to cardiovascular disease (Krantz & McCeney, 2002). Included among these factors are education, income, marital status, social support, stress, anxiety, depression, cynical hostility, and anger.

Educational Level and Income Low educational level and low income are risk factors for cardiovascular disease. In a large-scale study of adults in Europe (Huisman et al., 2005), lower educational level appeared as a risk for all causes of death, but heart disease and stroke accounted for much of the discrepancy. The educational disparity applied to both women and men, with women at a greater disadvantage than men from low educational levels. In many countries, educational levels are related to ethnicity, but studies in the Netherlands (Bos, Kunst, Garssen, & Mackenbach, 2005) and

Israel (Manor, Eisenbach, Friedlander, & Kark, 2004) examined educational level within ethnic groups. The results showed that, independent of ethnicity, low educational level was a risk for CVD. What factors link low levels of education to high levels of heart disease? One possibility is that people with low education practice fewer health behaviors than those with higher educational levels; they eat a less healthy diet, smoke, and lead more sedentary lives, which increases their CVD risks factors (Laaksonen et al., 2008). Income level also varies along with educational level and represents another risk factor.

Income level is another risk factor for cardiovascular disease; people with lower incomes have higher rates of heart disease than people in the higher income brackets. A report from China (Yu et al., 2000) showed that socioeconomic level—defined as education, occupation, income, and marital status—related to such cardiovascular risk factors as blood pressure, body mass index, and cigarette smoking. This finding is not isolated—a body of research indicates that socioeconomic status has a relationship to health, mortality, and cardiovascular disease. A cross-national study (Kim, Kawachi, Hoorn, & Ezzati, 2008) revealed that in societies with a large discrepancy in income levels, individuals in the lower part of the income distribution had higher risk factors for CVD. The effect may occur through income level or social status; evidence exists for both. Income level relates to longevity in the form of a gradient, with higher income predicting longer life (Krantz & McCeney, 2002). Social rank and status have a variety of cardiovascular effects in many species, including humans (Sapolsky, 2004). In addition, research suggests that these socioeconomic cardiovascular risks may begin to accumulate during adolescence or even childhood (Karlamangla et al., 2005). Thus, educational level, income, and social status all show effects on the cardiovascular system and on diseases of this system.

Social Support and Marriage Prospective studies have confirmed that lacking social support is also a risk for cardiovascular disease (Krantz & McCeney, 2002). This conclusion is consistent with the wide body of research discussed in Chapter 5 that shows the value of social support and the problems that can arise from its lack. Indeed, loneliness during childhood, adolescence, and young adulthood relates to CVD risk factors (Caspi, Harrington, Moffitt, Milne, & Poulton, 2006), and these effects may become more serious with aging (Hawkley & Cacioppo, 2007). For example, older people who had experienced a heart attack were more likely to have another, fatal heart attack if they lived alone (Schmaltz et al., 2007).

Lack of social support may be a factor in the development of CVD and even more important in its progression. Studies that measured the progression of blockage of the coronary arteries in women (Wang, Mittleman, & Orth-Gomér, 2005; Wang et al., 2007) found that support at home and at work affected the progression of coronary artery blockage; high stress in either area predicted progressive blockage, whereas satisfactory support in both led to regression of arterial plaques. Another study showed that the number of people in a person's social network related to coronary mortality; CAD patients with only one to three people in their social network were nearly two and one-half times more likely to die of coronary artery disease than patients with four or more close friends (Brummett et al., 2001). Older men who were more socially involved were less likely to die of CVD than those who were more isolated (Ramsay et al., 2008).

Marriage should provide social support, and in general, married people are at decreased risk for cardiovascular disease. However, several studies have indicated that the quality of the marital relationship is a factor. In a 10-year follow-up, married men were almost half as likely to die as unmarried men (Eaker, Sullivan, Kelly-Hayes, D'Agostino, & Benjamin, 2007). For women, the benefits depended on marital communication and quality, with poor communication increasing heart disease risk. In another study (Troxel, Matthews, Gallo, & Kuller, 2005), women who reported that they were satisfied in their marriage had lower levels of several risk factors than those who were dissatisfied with their marriage. Another study (Holt-Lunstad, Birmingham, & Jones, 2008) focused specifically on marriage and also found that marital quality was important; marriage was not beneficial if the individual was dissatisfied with the relationship. However, happily married people received greater benefits in the form of lower blood pressure than single people, even those with a supportive social network.

Spouses (and other sources of social support) may reduce the risk of cardiovascular mortality by providing encouragement for compliance with a healthy lifestyle or a medical regimen or by urging a person to seek medical care. Sources of social support are usually friends, family, spouses, and even pets (Allen, 2003). Support may also affect CVD through its influence on the experience of stress and depression.

Stress, Anxiety, and Depression Stress, anxiety, and depression are related to cardiovascular disease, but they are also related to each other (Suls & Bunde, 2005). This overlap makes independent assessment of each component difficult. However, a great deal of evidence implicates these factors in cardiovascular disease. For example, the INTERHEART study (Rosengren et al., 2004) tested people from 52 countries around the world, matching people who had experienced a heart attack to similar individuals who had not in order to evaluate risk factors. The results revealed that people who had heart attacks also experienced more work and financial stress and more life events than their matched controls.

Anxiety and depression have also been implicated in CVD; the evidence for the risks from depression is especially strong. Even after controlling for other risk factors such as smoking and cholesterol, anxiety (Shen et al., 2008) and depression (Goldston & Baillie, 2008) are factors that predict the development of CVD. The risks of depression and anxiety apply not only to the development of CVD but also to its progression; however, the evidence is stronger for these two negative emotions in the development of CVD (Suls & Bunde, 2005). Indeed, evidence for the beginnings of artery damage appeared in a study of depressed adolescents (Tomfohr, Martin, & Miller, 2008), which is consistent with the long-term damage that accompanies CVD. More

evidence about the harm of negative emotions has come from the study of hostility and anger.

Hostility and Anger Researchers have also found that some types of hostility and anger are risk factors for cardiovascular disease. Much of this research grew out of work on the Type A behavior pattern, originally proposed by **cardiologists** Meyer Friedman and Ray Rosenman (1974; Rosenman et al., 1975), physicians who specialized in heart disease. Friedman and Rosenman described people with the Type A behavior pattern as hostile, competitive, concerned with numbers and the acquisition of objects, and possessed of an exaggerated sense of time urgency. During the early years of its history, the Type A behavior pattern demonstrated promise as a predictor of heart disease, but later researchers were unable to affirm a consistent link between the global Type A behavior pattern and incidence of heart disease. This situation led investigators to consider the possibility that some component of the pattern—rather than the entire pattern—might be a predictor.

In 1989, Redford Williams presented evidence that one type of hostility—cynical hostility—is especially harmful to cardiovascular health, and he contended that people who mistrust others, think the worst of humanity, and interact with others with cynical hostility are harming themselves and their hearts. Furthermore, he suggested that people who use *anger* as a response to interpersonal problems have an elevated risk for heart disease.

The research on hostility as a risk for CVD has not yielded clear evidence concerning its role, but hostility is related to heart disease for some groups of people. For example, anxiety seems to be a better predictor of CVD in women (Consedine, Magai, & Chin, 2004), whereas hostility predicts CVD better in men (Consedine et al., 2004; Player, King, Mainous, & Geesey, 2007). Another analysis (Lavie & Milani, 2005) concentrated on age and found that, among a large group of cardiac rehabilitation patients, the younger patients' hostility scores were 2.5 times as high as the older patients' scores. Hostility also appeared as a factor in long-term survival of a heart attack,

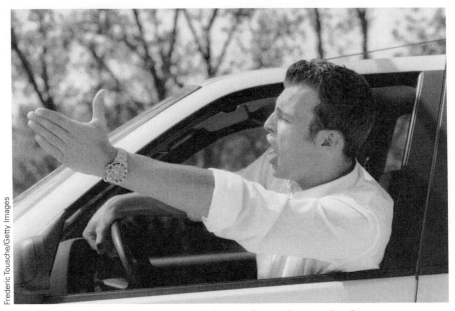

Frederic Tousche/Getty Images

Hostility and expressed anger are risk factors for cardiovascular disease.

decreasing life expectancy (Boyle et al., 2004). However, a large population study (Surtees, Wainwright, Luben, Day, & Khaw, 2005) failed to demonstrate an overall effect for hostility in the development of CVD. Thus, hostility may be a risk for some people but not others, or hostility may exert effects through some specific component, such as anger.

Hostility and anger are related, but anger can be defined as an unpleasant *emotion* accompanied by physiological arousal, whereas hostility involves a negative *attitude* toward others (Suls & Bunde, 2005). The *experience* of anger is probably unavoidable and may not present much of a risk. However, the manner in which a person deals with anger may be a factor in the development of cardiovascular disease. People may express their anger, including yelling back when someone yells at them, raising their voice when arguing, and throwing temper tantrums. Alternatively, people may suppress their anger, holding in their feelings. Some evidence suggests that either strategy may pose problems.

Anger and Cardiovascular Reactivity One way that the expression of anger might relate to coronary heart disease is through **cardiovascular reactivity (CVR)**, typically defined as increases in blood pressure and heart rate due to frustration or harassment. Most studies on CVR have been laboratory studies in which researchers present participants with various situations intended to arouse anger and monitor their physiological responses, often using a variety of cardiac measurements such as blood pressure and heart rate. The measurements may also include the persistence of such cardiac responses.

In one study using such a procedure (Suarez, Saab, Llabre, Kuhn, & Zimmerman, 2004), African American men showed a stronger blood pressure response than did European American men or women from either ethnic group. This result suggests that the higher prevalence of hypertension among African American men may relate to their tendency to higher reactivity. Another reactivity study (Merritt, Bennett, Williams, Sollers, & Thayer, 2004) focused on educational level and anger coping strategies among African American men and found that low educational level and a high effort style of coping were related to higher blood pressure reactivity. For African Americans, the experiences of racism constitute a source of anger, and one study (Clark, 2003) connected the perception of racism with blood pressure reactivity. This type of reactivity difference also appeared in a study comparing African American and European American women (Lepore et al., 2006). Thus, reactivity may relate to hypertension among African Americans.

The fairly consistent results concerning cardiovascular reactivity and ethnicity are an exception among the research on this topic; other research has shown a variety of findings. Some consistency has emerged showing gender differences in reactivity. For example, one researcher (Hughes, 2007) found that social support decreased reactivity among women but increased reactivity among men. Other research (Forcier et al., 2006) has demonstrated that physical fitness mediates reactivity, with fit individuals showing lower reactivity than those who are less fit. Yet other research (Wright, O'Donnell, Brydon, Wardle, & Steptoe, 2007) has implicated a genetic basis for reactivity. Thus, the evidence concerning cardiac reactivity suggests a role in the development of CVD, but reactions to anger and frustration constitute more of a risk for some people than for others.

Suppressed Anger If expressing anger can undermine cardiac health for some people, then would it be better to suppress anger? Results from early studies (Dembroski, MacDougall, Williams, Haney, & Blumenthal, 1985; MacDougall, Dembroski, Dimsdale, & Hackett, 1985) and more recent findings (Harburg, Julius, Kaciroti, Gleiberman, & Schork, 2003; Jorgensen & Kolodziej, 2007) suggest that suppressed anger may be more toxic than forcefully expressing anger. One version of suppressed emotion is rumination—repeated negative thoughts about an incident—which tends to increase negative feelings and depression (Hogan & Linden, 2004). Thus, people who suppress their anger but "stew" over their feelings may be using a coping style that puts them in danger. However, expressing anger (and other negative emotions) in a forceful way may act as triggers for those with CVD, precipitating a heart attack or stroke (Suls & Bunde, 2005).

Did Nancy Dorr and her colleagues (Dorr, Brosschot, Sollers, & Thayer, 2007) capture the dilemma concerning anger expression with the phrase "Damned if you do, damned if you don't" (p. 125)? How can people handle anger situations? Aron Siegman (1994) suggested that people learn to recognize their anger but to express it calmly and rationally. When people express anger in a soft, slow voice as opposed to a loud, rapid voice, they may reduce their risk of developing coronary heart disease. A study of male physicians (Eng, Fitzmaurice, Kubzansky, Rimm, & Kawachi, 2003) indicated that those who expressed moderate levels of anger experienced lower incidence of stroke and heart attacks.

Presently, evidence is lacking that any component of the Type A behavior pattern, including hostility and anger, is a strong independent risk for cardiovascular disease in the general population (Suls & Bunde, 2005). However, anger may combine with the negative emotions that accompany anxiety and depression to present a risk for the development of CVD (Bleil, Gianaros, Jennings, Flory, & Manuck, 2008). In addition, cynical hostility and anger are related to each other and may interact with other risk factors such as high blood pressure to increase a person's risk for heart disease. Figure 9.9 shows the evolution of the Type A behavior pattern to hostility, to anger, to the expression or suppression of anger, and finally to negative emotionality.

IN SUMMARY

Although the causes of cardiovascular disease are not fully understood, an accumulating body of evidence points to certain risk factors. These factors include such inherent risks as advancing age, family history of heart disease, gender, and ethnic background. Although none of these factors can be changed, people who are inherently at risk can modify other risks and thus lower their chances of developing heart disease.

Other risk factors include physiological conditions such as hypertension, problems in glucose metabolism, and high serum cholesterol levels. Other than age, hypertension is the best predictor of coronary artery disease, and a higher blood pressure equals higher risk for heart disease. Total cholesterol level is also

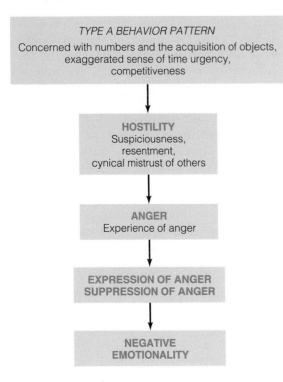

Note: **BOLDFACE** denotes components suggested by research to be the strongest link to heart disease.

FIGURE 9.9 Evolution from the Type A behavior pattern to negative emotionality.

related to coronary artery disease, but the *ratio* of total cholesterol to high-density lipoprotein (HDL) is a more critical risk factor.

Behaviors such as smoking and unwise eating also relate to heart disease. Cigarette smoking is associated with increased risk for heart disease worldwide, but nonsmokers exposed to other people's tobacco smoke probably have only a slightly increased risk. Eating foods high in saturated fat may lead to obesity, which is a risk for CVD. Also, consuming low levels of fruits and vegetables add to one's risk of heart disease.

Psychosocial risk factors related to coronary artery disease include low educational and income levels; low levels of social support and marital satisfaction; and high levels of stress, anxiety, and depression. The hostility component descended from the Type A behavior pattern is probably not an independent risk factor for heart disease. One of its dimensions—anger—may have a larger effect,

at least for some people. Both the violent expression and the suppression of anger may be related to CHD disease. Expressing anger in a soft, calm voice is a better coping strategy than violently expressing anger or timidly holding it in.

REDUCING CARDIOVASCULAR RISKS

Psychology's main contribution to cardiovascular health has focused on changing unhealthy behaviors before these behaviors lead to heart disease. In addition, psychologists may help people who have been diagnosed with heart disease; that is, they often help cardiac rehabilitation patients adhere to an exercise program, a medical regimen, a healthy diet, and smoking cessation.

Before Diagnosis: Preventing First Heart Attacks

What can people do to lower their risks for cardiovascular disease? Ideally, people should prevent CVD by modifying risk factors before the disease process causes damage. A longitudinal study by Jerry Stamler and his colleagues (1999) indicated that prevention is possible—maintaining a low level of risk factors protects against CVD. This study examined young adult and middle-aged men and women in five large cohorts to see if a low-risk profile would reduce both CVD and other causes of mortality. After dividing the participants into risk groups and screening for as long as 57 years, results indicated that low-risk participants had lower rates of death not only from CHD and stroke but also from all causes. Thus, young and middle-aged men and women who can modify CVD risks to attain low risk profiles will also lower their risk for all-cause mortality and can expect to live 6 to 10 years longer.

The factors examined by Stamler et al. (1999) included smoking, cholesterol levels, and blood pressure—three major risk factors for CVD. Modifying these behaviors can help people avoid this disease. However, the importance of maintaining a healthy lifestyle may begin as early as childhood (Beilin & Huang, 2008), when dietary and physical activity patterns become established, and definitely continues during adolescence, when most smokers begin their habit. Keeping risk factors low can pay substantial dividends in later years (Matthews, Kuller, Chang, & Edmundowicz, 2007). After people acquire high risks from behavioral factors such as smoking and unwise eating, managing those risks is more difficult. But psychologists have been concerned with changing behavior, and many of their techniques can be used to modify behaviors that place people at risk for developing cardiovascular disease.

The most serious behavioral risk factor is cigarette smoking, a behavior also implicated in a variety of other disorders, especially lung cancer. For this reason, all of Chapter 12 is devoted to a discussion of tobacco use. Although hypertension and serum cholesterol are not behaviors and thus cannot be directly modified through behavioral interventions, both can be affected indirectly through changes in behavior, making these factors candidates for intervention (Linden, 2000).

Before people will cooperate with programs to change their behavior, they must perceive that these behaviors place them in jeopardy, which may be a problem for people who have no symptoms of cardiovascular disease. These individuals may recognize established risk factors in calculating their personal risk, but they often display what Neil Weinstein (1984) called an **optimistic bias** in assessing their risk. That is, they tend to believe that they are immune from the risks that make other people vulnerable. These thoughts place such individuals in the precontemplation or contemplation stage, according to the transtheoretical model, when they are not ready to make changes (Prochaska et al., 1992, 1994; see Chapter 4 for more on this model). The technique of motivational interviewing challenges current cognitions with the goal of moving people toward making positive change; this technique was part of a successful program to increase fruit and vegetable consumption (Resnicow et al., 2001). Thus, moving people to the point of making changes in their health habits is one challenge for health psychologists involved in cardiovascular health.

Reducing Hypertension Lowering high blood pressure into the normal range is difficult because a number of physiological mechanisms act to keep blood pressure at a set point (Osborn,

2005). Many different feedback systems either raise or lower blood pressure when the body senses that blood pressure is out of the critical range. The body may even perpetuate hypertension by means of these feedback mechanisms, regulating blood pressure to the hypertensive level instead of regulating it into the normal range. Because complex feedback systems work against rather than for the maintenance of appropriate blood pressure, hypertension tends to be difficult to control.

Interventions aimed at hypertension usually try to control blood pressure through antihypertensive drugs that require a physician's prescription. The goal is typically to lower blood pressure to 130/80 mmHg or lower (USDHHS, 2003). Because hypertension presents no unpleasant symptoms and the medications may, many patients are reluctant to follow this regimen. (The factors affecting adherence to this and other medical regimens are discussed in Chapter 4.)

Several behaviors relate to both the development and the treatment of hypertension, and these behaviors have been the targets of interventions. Obesity is correlated with hypertension, and many obese people who lose weight lower their blood pressure into the normal range (Moore et al., 2005). Thus, losing weight is part of blood pressure control. (We discuss strategies for losing weight in Chapter 15.) Hypertensive individuals also typically receive recommendations to restrict sodium intake and make dietary changes (Bhatt, Luqman-Arafath, & Guleria, 2007). The Dietary Approach to Stop Hypertension (DASH) approach originated as a plan to control hypertension; it includes a diet high in fruits, vegetables, whole grain, and low-fat dairy products as well as other lifestyle changes. Not only is this diet effective in lowering blood pressure, but it also decreases the risk for stroke and CHD in women (Fung et al., 2008). A regular physical activity program has also been found effective in controlling hypertension, especially in people who have been sedentary (Murphy, Nevill, Murtagh, & Holder, 2007). (We discuss exercise in Chapter 15.) Other techniques for reducing blood pressure include stress management and relaxation training, and we discuss both in Chapter 5. Thus, a program to control hypertension may have both drug and behavioral components.

Lowering Serum Cholesterol Interventions aimed at lowering cholesterol levels can include drugs, dietary changes, increased physical activity, or a combination of these components. Eating a diet low in saturated fat and high in fruits and vegetables and maintaining a program of regular physical activity are good strategies for preventing high cholesterol levels, and dietary and exercise interventions are key components in managing high cholesterol levels (USDHHS, 2003). However, once a person develops high cholesterol levels, a prudent diet and physical activity are not likely to lower cholesterol to an acceptable level. Thus, many people with high cholesterol cannot achieve substantially lower cholesterol levels through diet and exercise.

Cholesterol-lowering drugs such as the *statin* drugs are frequently prescribed for patients with high total cholesterol levels or high LDL levels (Grundy, 2007). These drugs act by blocking an enzyme that the liver needs to manufacture cholesterol, and they are especially effective in lowering LDL. Despite their effectiveness, these drugs require a prescription, cost money, and have side effects.

The recommendations for cholesterol lowering are complex. First, relying on drugs to lower cholesterol without behavioral changes is not a good strategy. Behavioral interventions can help both men and women adhere to a regular exercise program as well as a low-fat diet. Such adherence can lower LDL and improve the ratio of total cholesterol to HDL. If lifestyle changes do not lower cholesterol, then drugs are an option, but not before, especially for people with low levels of risk. Second, the ratio of total cholesterol to HDL is more important than total cholesterol. Statins tend to lower LDL rather than raise HDL, but these drugs lower cholesterol and incidence of heart attacks and stroke, making them a good choice for people with very high or resistant cholesterol levels (Cheng, Lauder, Chu-Pak, & Kumana, 2004). Third, people with multiple risks for CVD, such as hypertension, diabetes, or smoking, should consider cholesterol

lowering more urgent than those with fewer risks (Grundy, 2007).

Modifying Psychosocial Risk Factors Earlier, we discussed research that has linked psychosocial factors such as stress, anxiety, depression, and anger with cardiovascular disease. The evidence for these risks is sufficiently compelling for some authorities to call for the development of *behavioral cardiology* (Rozanski, Blumenthal, Davidson, Saab, & Kubzansky, 2005), urging cardiologists to screen for psychological risks and to recommend psychological interventions to decrease anxiety and depression and to manage stress and anger. Consistent with this concept, research on people who received angioplasty (Helgeson, 2003) indicated that those who had a more positive outlook about themselves and their future were less likely to experience a recurrence of cardiovascular disease. These results are good news for former president Bill Clinton, whose optimistic outlook was evident even before his cardiac surgery (King & Henry, 2004).

Anger and negative emotions can be dealt with in a therapeutic manner, and clinical health psychologists have recommended a variety of strategies for coping with hostility, anger, and depression. To reduce the toxic element in anger, perpetually angry people can learn to become aware of cues from others that typically provoke angry responses. They can also remove themselves from provocative situations before they become angry, or they can do something else. In interpersonal encounters, angry people can use self-talk as a reminder that the situation will not last forever. Humor is another potentially effective means of coping with anger (Godfrey, 2004), but one must be careful with its use. Sarcastic or hostile humor can incite additional anger, but silliness or mock exaggerations often defuse potentially volatile situations. Relaxation techniques can also be effective strategies for dealing with anger. These techniques can include progressive relaxation, deep-breathing exercises, tension reduction training, relaxing to the slow repetition of the word "relax," and relaxation imagery, in which the person imagines a peaceful scene.

BECOMING HEALTHIER

1. Learn about your family risk for heart disease. Although you cannot change this risk factor, knowing that you are at high risk can motivate you to change some modifiable risk factors.

2. Have your blood pressure checked. If it's in the normal range, you can keep it that way by exercising, controlling your weight, and moderating alcohol consumption. Also try some of the relaxation techniques discussed in Chapter 8. If your blood pressure is above the normal range (even a little), consult a physician.

3. Know your cholesterol level, but be sure to ask for a complete profile, one that includes measures of both HDL and LDL as well as the ratio of total cholesterol to HDL.

4. If you are a smoker who has tried to quit but failed, keep trying. Many ex-smokers made multiple attempts before quitting successfully.

5. Keep a food diary for at least one week. Note the amount of saturated fat as well as fruits and vegetables you eat and the approximate number of calories consumed per day. A heart-healthy diet is low in saturated fat and includes five servings of fruits and vegetables per day.

6. If you are persistently angry and react to anger-arousing events with loud, sudden explosions of anger or if you "stew" over such events, try to change your reactions by expressing your frustrations in a soft, quiet voice.

Finally, angry people can lower their blood pressure by constructively discussing their feelings with other people (Davidson, MacGregor, Stuhr, Dixon, & MacLean, 2000).

Discussing their feelings with a therapist may also benefit people who are depressed, but this problem is not widely recognized. Thus, screening for depression among people at risk for CVD is an urgent need (Goldston & Baillie, 2007). Depression is also common among people who have experienced a heart attack or other CVD event. These individuals may be more willing to undertake changes to avoid another heart attack or stroke.

After Diagnosis: Rehabilitating Cardiac Patients

After people have experienced a heart attack, angina, or other symptoms of CVD, they typically receive a referral to a cardiac rehabilitation program to change their lifestyle and thereby lower their risk for a subsequent (and possibly even more serious) event. In addition to survival, the goals of cardiac rehabilitation programs are to help patients deal with psychological reactions to their diagnosis, to return to normal activities as soon as possible, and to change to a healthier lifestyle.

Patients recovering from heart disease, as well as their spouses, often experience a variety of psychological reactions that include depression, anxiety, anger, fear, guilt, and interpersonal conflict. For cardiac patients, the most common psychological reaction to a myocardial infarction is *depression*, which is related to other risk factors (Artham, Lavie, & Milani, 2008), decreases adherence to medication and lifestyle changes (Kronish et al., 2006), and increases the risk of death to 3.5 times that for nondepressed cardiac patients (Guck et al., 2001). A cardiac rehabilitation program that included a therapeutic component for depression (Schneiderman et al., 2004) demonstrated its effectiveness in lowering depression, but only European American men derived survival benefits from the treatment.

Another common psychological reaction to heart attack is *anxiety*, which is also related to depression. A follow-up study of cardiac rehabilitation patients (Michie, O'Connor, Bath, Giles, & Earll, 2005) showed that those who completed the rehabilitation program continued to make progress not only in lowering their physiological risks but also in lowering their levels of anxiety and depression and increasing their feelings of control. One common source of anxiety among heart patients and their spouses is the resumption of sexual activity. The probable source of this anxiety is concern about the elevation of heart rate during sex, especially during orgasm. However, sexual activity poses little threat to those who have experienced a heart attack. Also, male CAD patients who take Viagra do not have an elevated risk of subsequent heart problems, but this drug may interact in dangerous ways with drugs for hypertension that such patients may be taking (Jackson, 2004).

Cardiac rehabilitation programs usually include components to help patients stop smoking, eat a low-fat and low-cholesterol diet, control weight, moderate alcohol intake, learn to manage stress and hostility, and adhere to a prescribed medication regimen. Also, cardiac patients frequently participate in a graduated or structured exercise program in which they gradually increase their level of physical activity. In other words, the same lifestyle recommendations for avoiding a first cardiovascular event are also prescribed for people who have survived a myocardial infarction, coronary artery bypass graft surgery, or stroke. In addition, cardiac patients are often encouraged to join a social support group, participate in health education programs, and allow support from their primary caregiver. Some research (Clark, Whelan, Barbour, & MacIntyre, 2005) indicated that cardiac patients rated such social support and being with others who shared the same problem as the most valuable aspects of the program.

Dean Ornish and his colleagues (1998) devised a comprehensive cardiac rehabilitation program with diet, stress management, smoking cessation, and physical activity components in an effort to *reverse* heart patients' coronary artery damage. Although similar to the interventions that attempt to alter risk factors, this program was more comprehensive and imposed more stringent modifications, especially with regard to diet. The Ornish program recommends that cardiac patients reduce their consumption of fat to only 10% of their total caloric intake, which necessitates a careful vegetarian diet with no added fats from oils, eggs, butter, or nuts. An evaluation of the program included a control group that received a typical cardiac rehabilitation program along with the experimental group of participants on the Ornish program.

Early research on the benefits of the program painted a slightly more optimistic picture of its benefits than later research. After one year of the program, Ornish and his colleagues (1990) found that 82% of patients in the treatment group showed a regression of plaques in the coronary arteries. After five years, this program produced less artery blockage and fewer coronary events. More recent research (Aldana et al., 2007) failed to confirm the reversal of arterial plaque. Instead, this study showed that patients on the Ornish program decreased their risk factors to a greater extent than those in a standard cardiac rehabilitation program and decreased their symptoms of angina substantially. The benefits in decreasing angina also appeared in another study (Frattaroli, Weidner, Merritt-Worden, Frenda, & Ornish, 2008). The main disadvantage of the program is the difficulty of following such a stringent diet (Dansinger, Gleason, Griffith, Selker, & Schaefer, 2005). No cardiac rehabilitation program can be optimally effective if patients fail to adhere or drop out.

Are rehabilitation programs effective in reducing cardiac mortality? An important obstacle to the effectiveness of a cardiac rehabilitation program is adherence. Only 15% to 30% of cardiac patients complete their rehabilitation regimen (King, Humen, Smith, Phan, & Teo, 2001). Many cardiologists fail to endorse programs, which affects their patients' willingness to participate. Women are even less likely to complete a program than men (Jackson, Leclerc, Erskine, & Linden, 2005). Many different programs can be effective, including brief interventions (Fernandez et al., 2007) and at-home rehabilitation programs (Jolly, Taylor, Lip, & Stevens, 2006).

A meta-analysis of studies on the effectiveness of two components of cardiac rehabilitation programs (Dusseldrop, van Elderen, Maes, Meulman, & Kraaj, 1999) found that heart disease patients who followed a health education and stress management program had a 34% reduction in cardiac mortality and a 29% reduction in recurrence of a heart attack. Specific evaluations of the exercise component of cardiac rehabilitation programs (Blumenthal et al., 2004; R. S. Taylor et al., 2004) confirmed the value of physical activity for survival after a heart attack. Exercise may present some risks for cardiac patients, but the benefits far outweigh the risks. For example, a graded exercise program can enhance patients' self-efficacy for increasing levels of activity (Cheng & Boey, 2002) as well as increase self-esteem and physical mobility (Ng & Tam, 2000). After a diagnosis of heart problems, exercise programs have three main goals (Thompson, 2001). First, exercise can maintain or improve functional capacity; second, it can enhance a person's quality of life; and third, it can help prevent recurrent heart attacks. Thus, cardiac rehabilitation programs are an effective but underused strategy.

IN SUMMARY

Health psychologists can contribute to reducing risks for a first cardiovascular incident as well as to rehabilitating people who have already been diagnosed with CVD. Many of the risks for CVD are behaviors or relate to behaviors, such as smoking, diet, physical activity, and management of negative emotions. Combinations of lifestyle change and drugs are effective in lowering hypertension and cholesterol level, two important risks for CVD. In addition, health psychologists can help people modify negative emotions such as anxiety, depression, and anger, all of which are risks for CVD and often occur in patients after heart attacks. Health psychologists may also be involved with ways to keep cardiac patients in rehabilitation and in boosting their levels of physical activity.

ANSWERS

This chapter has addressed four basic questions:

1. **What are the structures, functions, and disorders of the cardiovascular system?**

   The cardiovascular system includes the heart and blood vessels (veins, venules, arteries, arterioles, and capillaries). The heart pumps blood throughout the body, delivering oxygen and removing wastes from body cells. Disorders of the cardiovascular system include (1) coronary artery disease (CAD), which occurs when the arteries that supply blood to the heart become clogged with plaque and restrict the blood supply to the heart muscle; (2) myocardial infarction (heart attack), which is caused by blockage of coronary arteries; (3) angina pectoris, which is a nonfatal disorder with symptoms of chest pain and difficulty in breathing; (4) stroke, which occurs when the oxygen supply to the brain is disrupted; and (5) hypertension (high blood pressure), which is a silent disorder but a good predictor of both heart attack and stroke.

   Heart attack and stroke account for more than 30% of deaths in the United States.

2. **What are the risk factors for cardiovascular disease?**

   Beginning with the Framingham study, researchers have discovered a number of cardiovascular risk factors. These factors include (1) inherent risk, (2) physiological risks, (3) behavioral and lifestyle risks, and (4) psychosocial risks. Inherent risk factors, such as advancing age, family history, gender, and ethnicity, cannot be changed, but people with inherent risk can alter their other risks to lower their chances of developing heart disease.

   The two primary physiological risk factors are hypertension and high cholesterol, and diet can play a role in controlling each of these. Behavioral factors in CVD include smoking, a diet high in saturated fat and low in fiber and antioxidant vitamins, and low physical activity level. Psychosocial risks include low educational and income levels, lack of social support, and persistently high levels of stress, anxiety, and depression. In addition, hostility and both loud, violent expressions of anger and suppression of anger elevate risk slightly.

3. How does lifestyle relate to cardiovascular health?

Lifestyle factors such as cigarette smoking, unwise eating, and a sedentary lifestyle all relate to cardiovascular health. During the past three decades, deaths from heart disease have steadily decreased in the United States; perhaps as much as 50% of that drop is a result of changes in behavior and lifestyle. During this same time period, millions of people have quit smoking, altered their diet to control weight and cholesterol, and begun an exercise program.

4. What behaviors allow people to lower their cardiovascular risks?

Both before and after a diagnosis of heart disease, people can use a variety of approaches to reduce their risks for CVD. Hypertension can be controlled by drugs, sodium restriction, and weight loss. Cholesterol levels can be lowered through drugs and, to some extent, through diet and exercise. Lowering the ratio of total cholesterol to HDL is probably a better idea, but the statin type of cholesterol-lowering drugs tends to lower LDL, which can also be beneficial. Also, people can learn to manage stress more effectively, enter therapy to improve depression, and learn to manage anger to avoid loud, quick outbursts and to express their frustrations in a soft, slow manner.

SUGGESTED READINGS

Holt-Lunstad, J., Birmingham, W., & Jones, B. Q. (2008). Is there something unique about marriage? The relative impact of marital status, relationship quality, and network social support on ambulatory blood pressure and mental health. *Annals of Behavioral Medicine, 35*, 239–244. This journal article gives a technical analysis of social support, considering the notion that good marriages provide the best type of support.

Levy, D., & Brink, S. (2005). *A change of heart: How the Framingham Heart Study helped unravel the mysteries of cardiovascular disease.* New York: Knopf. This report on the Framingham Heart Study includes not only the fascinating history of this project but also the major findings from the study and tips for maintaining heart health.

Miller, G. E., & Blackwell, E. (2006). Turning up the heat: Inflammation as a mechanism linking chronic stress, depression, and heart disease. *Current Directions in Psychological Science, 15,* 269–272. This brief article reviews the concept of inflammation and its risks while attempting to build a model that integrates stress and depression into an explanation for the development of heart disease.

Yusuf, S., Hawken, S., Ôunpuu, S., Dans, T., Avezum, A., Lanas, F., et al. (2004). Effect of potentially modifiable risk factors associated with myocardial infarction in 52 countries (the INTERHEART study): Case-control study. *Lancet, 364,* 937–952. The INTERHEART study identified nine factors that predicted most of the variance in heart attack deaths in countries throughout the world. This report details the study and presents the relative contributions of each of the nine.

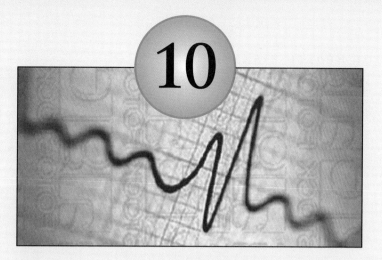

10

BEHAVIORAL FACTORS IN CANCER

QUESTIONS

This chapter focuses on five basic questions:

1. What is cancer?

2. Are cancer death rates increasing or decreasing?

3. What are the inherent and environmental risk factors for cancer?

4. What are the behavioral risk factors for cancer?

5. How can cancer patients be helped in coping with their disease?

CHECK YOUR HEALTH RISKS

Check the items that apply to you.

☐ 1. Someone in my immediate family (a parent, sibling, aunt, uncle, or grandparent) developed cancer before age 50.

☐ 2. I am African American.

☐ 3. I have never had a job where I was exposed to radiation or hazardous chemicals.

☐ 4. I have never been a cigarette smoker.

☐ 5. I am a former smoker who quit during the past five years.

☐ 6. I have used tobacco products other than cigarettes (such as chewing tobacco, a pipe, or cigars).

☐ 7. My diet is low in fat.

☐ 8. My diet includes lots of smoked, salt-cured, or pickled foods.

☐ 9. I rarely eat fruits or vegetables.

☐ 10. My diet is high in fiber.

☐ 11. I have light-colored skin, but I like to get at least one nice tan every year.

☐ 12. I have had more than 15 sexual partners during my life.

☐ 13. I have never had unprotected sex with a partner who was at high risk for HIV infection.

☐ 14. I am a woman over age 30 who has not given birth to a child.

☐ 15. I have at least two alcoholic drinks every day.

☐ 16. I exercise on a regular basis.

Each of these topics is either a known risk factor for some type of cancer or has the potential to protect against it. Items 3, 4, 7, 10, 13, and 16 describe situations that may offer some protection against cancer. If you checked none or only a few of these items and a large number of the remaining items, your risk for some type of cancer is higher than people who checked different items. Behaviors related to smoking and diet (items 4–10) place you at a greater risk than other behaviors, such as item 15 (alcohol).

REAL-WORLD PROFILE OF GWYNETH PALTROW

Actress Gwyneth Paltrow lost her father, director and producer Bruce Paltrow, to cancer in 2002. Her father was not the only family member who died of cancer; the disease also killed her two grandmothers, an aunt, and a 23-year-old cousin. Paltrow described cancer as "the curse of my family" (Metro, 2007, ¶ 5) and used the term "evil genes" to describe what she believes to be the underlying cause of her family's cases of cancer.

To combat this threat, Paltrow says that she wants to fight the genetic influence with natural means (Metro, 2007). She tries to follow a strict vegetarian diet, not only for herself but also for her young children and husband. Another of her strategies involves the use of organic soap and household cleaning products. In addition to making changes in her personal habits, Paltrow has become an activist in the battle to combat cancer.

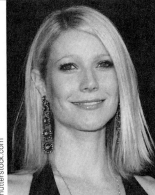

Entertainment Press, 2008/Used under license from Shutterstock.com

Gwyneth Paltrow's family has experienced several cases of cancer, sensitizing the actress to the risks for this disease.

But Gwyneth Paltrow spent years as a smoker, beginning during high school and becoming a two-pack-a-day smoker by graduation (Female Celebrity Smoking List, 2008). She has quit several times but has also relapsed, not only into smoking but also away from her vegetarian diet. She has acknowledged that she enjoys smoking and has found it difficult to quit. Paltrow seems to fail to place the same importance on quitting smoking as she does on her vegetarian diet and use of organic soap.

Are Gwyneth Paltrow's attitudes correct about the causes and strategies for prevention of cancer? To what extent do genes determine the development of this disease? Can diet and the use of natural products prevent cancer? How important is smoking in the development of cancer? We will explore these questions, but first, we need to define what cancer is.

What Is Cancer?

The first medical document to describe cancer was the *Ebers Papyrus*, written around 1500 B.C. That document did not give a detailed description of cancer, only a description of the swellings that accompany some tumors. Hippocrates gave the disorder the name *cancer*, and the Greek physician, Galen, first used the word *tumor*. These ancient physicians did not know much about cancer, however, because they did not have microscopes or use dissection, two procedures that greatly facilitated an understanding of cancer.

Cancer is a group of diseases characterized by the presence of new cells that grow and spread beyond control. During the 19th century, the great physiologist Johannes Muller discovered that tumors, like other tissues, consisted of cells and were not formless collections of material. However, their growth seemed unrestrained by the mechanisms that control other body cells.

The finding that tumors consist of cells did not shed light on what causes their growth. During the 19th century, the leading theory of cancer was that a parasite or infectious agent caused the disorder, but researchers could find no such agent. Because of this failure, the mutation theory arose, holding that cancer originates because of a change in the cell—a mutation. The cell continues to grow and reproduce in its mutated form, and the result is a tumor.

Cancer is not unique to humans; all animals get cancer, as do plants. Indeed, any cell that is capable of division can be transformed into a cancer cell. In addition to the diverse *causes* of cancer, many different *types* exist. However, different cancers share certain characteristics, the most common of which is the presence of **neoplastic** tissue cells, which are characterized by new and nearly unlimited growth that robs the host of nutrients and that yields no compensatory beneficial effects. All true cancers share this characteristic of neoplastic growth.

Neoplastic cells may be **benign** or **malignant**, although the distinction is not always easy to determine. Both types consist of altered cells that reproduce true to their altered type. However, benign growths tend to remain localized, whereas malignant tumors tend to spread and establish secondary colonies. The tendency for benign tumors to remain localized usually makes them less threatening than malignant tumors, but not all benign tumors are harmless. Malignant tumors are much more dangerous because they invade and destroy surrounding tissue and may also move, or **metastasize**, through blood or lymph and thus spread to other sites in the body.

The most dangerous characteristic of tumor cells is their autonomy—that is, their ability to grow without regard to the needs of other body cells and without being subject to the restraints of growth that govern other cells. This unrestrained tumor growth makes cancer capable of overwhelming its host, damaging other organs or physiological processes, or using nutrients essential for body functions. The tumor then becomes a parasite on its host, gaining priority over other body cells.

Malignant growths can be divided into four main groups: carcinomas, sarcomas, leukemias, and lymphomas. **Carcinomas** are cancers of the epithelial tissue, cells that line the outer and inner surfaces of the body, such as skin, stomach lining, and mucous membranes. **Sarcomas** are cancers that arise from cells in connective tissue, such as bone, muscles, and cartilage. **Leukemias** are cancers that originate in the blood or blood-forming cells, such as stem cells in the bone marrow. These three types of cancers—carcinomas, sarcomas, and leukemias—account for more than 95% of malignancies. The fourth type of cancer is **lymphoma**, a cancer of the lymphatic system, which is one of the rarer types of cancer.

Although some people may have a genetic predisposition to cancer, as Gwyneth Paltrow believes, the disease itself is almost never inherited.

Behavior and lifestyle are primary contributors to cancer, making it possible for the rates of cancer to change over relatively short periods of time.

THE CHANGING RATES OF CANCER DEATHS

For the first time since records have been kept, the death rate from cancer in the United States began to decline during the 1990s. This trend ended a century-long increase in cancer deaths that peaked in 1993, when cancer mortality was more than three times higher than in 1900. Figure 10.1 shows an increase in total cancer death rates in the United States from 1900 to 1990 and then a gradual decline. The decrease is significant— more than 18% for men and more than 10% for women since 1990 (Jemal et al., 2008).

Why have cancer death rates dropped in recent years? At least two explanations are possible. First, the decline might be due to improved treatment that prolongs the life of cancer patients. The validity of this explanation can be tested by looking at the difference between cancer incidence and cancer deaths. If incidence remained the same or even increased while deaths declined, then better treatment would account for the drop in cancer deaths. However, the evidence does not support this hypothesis. A review from the American Cancer Society (Jemal et al., 2008) reported that the incidence rate declined during the 1990s and that it has now stabilized. The death rate for cancers decreased beginning in 1992. Some of that decrease is attributable to the lower incidence of certain cancers, such as lung cancer in men, and some of it is due to improved early detection and treatment, such as the decline in deaths from prostate and breast cancer. Thus, better treatment regimens play a role in the recent decrease in cancer rates, but people are developing

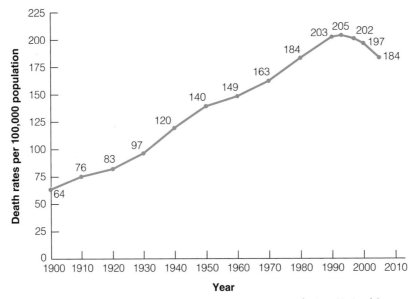

FIGURE 10.1 Death rates from cancer per 100,000 population, United States, 1900–2005.

Sources: Data from *Historical Statistics of the United States: Colonial Times to 1970, Part 1* (p. 68) by U.S. Bureau of the Census, 1975, Washington, DC: U.S. Government Printing Office; *Statistical Abstract of the United States, 2008* (127th edition), by U.S. Census Bureau, (2007). Washington, DC: U.S. Government Printing Office; Cancer statistics, 2008, by A. Jemal et al., 2008, *CA: Cancer Journal for Clinicians, 58,* 71–96.

cancer less often than they did a decade ago. An explanation for the lower incidence of cancer comes from changes in U.S. lifestyle—people are smoking much less and eating a healthier diet than they did 40 years ago. Because lifestyle factors such as smoking, diet, and physical inactivity account for about two-thirds of all cancer deaths in the United States (American Cancer Society, 2008), improvements in these areas should result in lower rates of cancer.

Cancers With Decreasing Death Rates

Cancer of the lungs, breast, prostate, and colon/rectum account for about half of all cancer deaths in the United States, and mortality rates for each of these sites are currently declining.

Lung cancer accounts for about 28% of all cancer deaths and about 15% of all cancer cases—figures that reveal the deadliness of lung cancer. Between 2002 and 2004, total lung cancer deaths in the United States declined for men but not for women (Jemal et al., 2008; see Figures 10.2 and 10.3). Figure 10.2 shows that lung cancer mortality for women rose dramatically from 1965 to 1995, but since that time death rates

have been almost level. Because cigarette smoking is the primary cause of lung cancer deaths, the current decline in women's smoking rates should eventually bring about a decrease in lung cancer mortality for women.

Other than skin cancer, *breast cancer* has the highest incidence (but not death rate) of any cancer in the United States, accounting for about 26% of cancer cases among women. Men also develop breast cancer, but women account for about 99.2% of all new cases. Although very few differences seem to exist between female and male cases of breast cancer (Weiss, Moysich, & Swede 2005), more research is clearly needed before scientists can determine those differences. The incidence of female breast cancer increased from 1980 to 2001 but then began to decline. One factor that may be involved in this decline is the decrease in the number of postmenopausal women using hormone replacement therapy, some types of which have been linked to breast cancer (Jemal et al., 2008).

Prostate cancer has the highest incidence of cancer among men in the United States, but again, it does not have the highest mortality rate—about

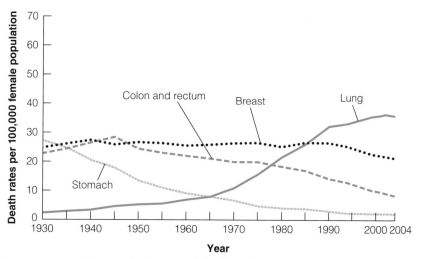

FIGURE 10.2   Cancer death rates for selected sites, women, United States, 1930–2004.

Source: Cancer Facts & Figures, 2008 (p. 3), by American Cancer Society, 2008. Atlanta: Author. Reprinted by permission of the American Cancer Society.

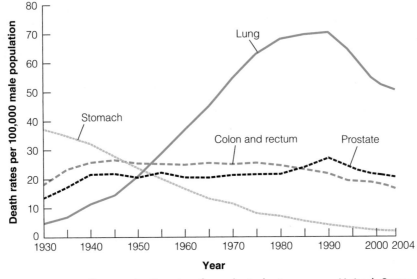

FIGURE 10.3 Cancer death rates for selected sites, men, United States, 1930–2004.

Source: Cancer Facts & Figures, 2008 (p. 2), by American Cancer Society, 2008. Atlanta: Author. Reprinted by permission of the American Cancer Society.

twice as many men die each year from lung cancer as from prostate cancer. In 2008, the number of men diagnosed with prostate cancer was estimated to be a bit higher than the number of women diagnosed with breast cancer (Jemal et al., 2008). As with breast cancer incidence, new cases of prostate cancer increased sharply during the 1980s when prostate-specific antigen (PSA) screening was first introduced (see Figure 10.3). In more recent years, however, the number of new cases—about 25% of all cancer cases in men—has declined slightly.

Colorectal cancer is the second leading cause of cancer deaths in the United States and other developed countries, exceeded only by lung cancer. However, in the United States, both the incidence and the mortality rates of colorectal cancer are going down. Incidence and morality rates vary widely by ethnic background, with African Americans much more likely to be diagnosed with colorectal cancer than either Hispanic Americans or European Americans (Jemal et al., 2008). Although the incidence of colorectal cancer increased slightly until about

1985, the mortality rate has been declining since about 1945 (see Figures 10.2 and 10.3).

Death rates from *stomach cancer* have dropped from being the leading cause of cancer deaths for both women and men to having a very low mortality rate. As we discuss later, modern refrigeration and fewer salt-cured foods probably account for most of the decrease in stomach cancer.

Cancers With Increasing Incidence and Mortality Rates

In general, incidence rates for the four leading cancers—lung, breast, prostate, and colorectal—are declining, especially for men. However, not all cancer rates are decreasing. Several cancers have increased in recent years (Jemal et al., 2008).

Liver cancer, like lung cancer, is quite lethal, with a death rate nearly twice as high as its incidence rate. This cancer is the only type that is increasing among both women and men (Jemal et al., 2008). As mentioned, lung cancer continues to show a slight increase among women but a continuing decline among men. Melanoma, a potentially fatal form of skin cancer, is increasing among men but not women. Cancer of the esophagus is increasing among men yet falling among women.

IN SUMMARY

Cancer is a group of diseases characterized by the presence of neoplastic cells that grow and spread without control. These new cells may form benign tumors, which tend to remain localized, or malignant tumors, which may metastasize and spread to other organs.

After more than a century of rising mortality rates, cancer deaths are beginning to decline. This decrease is most evident from a look at the incidence and mortality of the four cancers that contribute to about half of all cancer deaths—lung, breast, prostate, and colorectal cancers. Since 1992, incidence and death rates among men for these four cancers have declined at a slow but steady pace, whereas women have not experienced the same magnitude of decrease. The leading cause of cancer deaths for both women and men continues to be lung cancer. The incidence of breast cancer among women and prostate cancer among men is much higher than the incidence of lung cancer, but lung cancer kills far more people in the United States than does either breast cancer or prostate cancer.

CANCER RISK FACTORS BEYOND PERSONAL CONTROL

Most risk factors for cancer result from personal behavior, especially cigarette smoking. However, some factors are largely beyond personal control; these factors include both inherent and environmental risks.

Inherent Risk Factors for Cancer

Inherent risks for cancer include genetics and family history, ethnic background, and age. Like Gwyneth Paltrow, many people attribute their risk of cancer to these factors, especially genetics. A survey ("Practical Nurse," 2008) indicated that 9 out of 10 people overestimated the genetic risk,

and 60% of people named genetics as the primary risk for cancer. Does their perception agree with the research? How important are genetic and other inherent risk factors such as ethnicity and age?

Ethnic Background Compared with European Americans, African Americans fare more poorly; they have a greater incidence of most cancers, and mortality is higher in almost every category (American Cancer Society, 2008). However, Hispanic Americans, Asian Americans, and Native Americans have lower rates than either African Americans or European Americans (USCB, 2007). These discrepancies appear to be due to behavioral and psychosocial factors rather than to biology. For example, although Asian Americans generally have lower total cancer death rates than European Americans, they have a much higher mortality rate for stomach cancer, which is strongly influenced by diet (Jemal et al., 2008).

Minority status plays a greater role in survival of cancer than it does in cancer incidence. For cancer sites with a low mortality level, the discrepancy between incidence and mortality widens with ethnic background. With breast cancer, for example, European American women have a higher incidence rate than African American women, but African American women are more likely to die from this cancer (Jemal et al., 2008).

How does minority status contribute to cancer outcomes—that is, length of survival and quality of life? Although Hispanic Americans, African Americans, Native Americans, and Asian Americans develop many cancers at a lower rate than European Americans, their diagnoses tend to come at a later stage of their cancers (Jemal et al., 2008). This difference has implications for survival; later diagnoses tend to mean more advanced disease, more difficulty in treatment, and lower survival rates. An examination of survival differences between African Americans and European Americans (Du, Meyer, & Franzini, 2007) showed that controlling for socioeconomic factors erased the difference in survival rates, which suggests that social and economic factors create the disparity.

Advancing Age The strongest risk factor for cancer—and many other diseases—is advancing

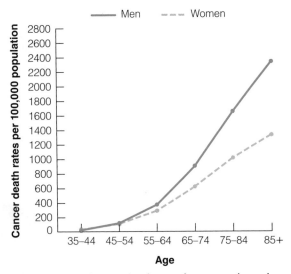

FIGURE 10.4 Cancer death rates by age and gender, United States, 2004.

Source: Data from *Health United States, 2007* (p. 207), by National Center for Health Statistics, 2007, Hyattsville, MD: U.S. Government Printing Office.

age. The older people become, the greater their chances of developing and dying of cancer; that is, 80-year-old people are more likely than 50-year-old people to die of cancer. However, the percentage of total deaths due to cancer is higher for 50-year olds than for 80-year olds. Figure 10.4 shows a steep increase in cancer mortality by age for both men and women, but especially for men.

Cancer is also the second leading cause of death among children between ages 1 and 14 (exceeded only by unintentional injuries; Jemal et al., 2008). Cancers that are most common among children include leukemia, cancers of the brain and nervous system, and non-Hodgkin's lymphoma. Testicular cancer is also an exception to the general rule concerning age: The highest risk for this cancer occurs during young adulthood. These cancers are likely to have some genetic component.

Family History and Genetics Although physicians observed that cancer seemed to "run in families," some of the early evidence of a genetic component for cancer came from the Nurses' Health Study (Colditz et al., 1993), which showed that women whose mothers had been diagnosed with

breast cancer before age 40 were more than twice as likely to develop breast cancer. A sister with breast cancer also doubled the risk, and having both a sister and a mother with breast cancer increased a woman's risk by about two and a half times. This research has progressed to the identification of specific genes involved in breast cancer, the BRCA 1 and BRCA 2 genes. These genes protect against cancer by providing the code for a protective protein (Paull, Cortez, Bowers, Elledge, & Gellert, 2001). Women who have a mutated form of BRCA 1, which does not allow that protective protein to develop, are as much as seven times more likely to develop breast cancer as women with the healthy form of this gene. Mutations in BRCA 1 and BRCA 2 have also been implicated in the development of breast cancer in men and pancreatic cancer in both women and men (Lynch et al., 2005). This gene does not create a certainty of developing cancer, but people with the mutation have a sharply increased risk.

The form of breast cancer involving BRCA 1 and BRCA 2 is responsible for no more than 10% of breast cancer, and the other cancers associated with BRCA are even less likely to be caused by a gene mutation. Thus, many genes for breast cancer remain unidentified, or most of the risk for developing breast cancer comes from other sources (Oldenburg, Meijers-Heijboer, Cornelisse, & Devilee, 2007). However, the search for single genes that underlie the development of cancer has been largely unsuccessful (Hemminki, Försti, & Bermejo, 2006). Instead, researchers have identified configurations of genes that seem to lead to vulnerabilities for specific cancers; research has also examined environmental factors that interact with genes, changing the genes' function in ways that increase vulnerability.

Another approach to understanding the genetic component of cancer is through the study of twins. Genetic factors that prompt the development of cancer should act similarly on monozygotic (identical) twins because these twin pairs have identical genes. Differences in the incidence of cancer in twin pairs must represent other influences, making twins very interesting for genetics researchers. A large-scale study of twin pairs (Baker, Lichtenstein, Kaprio, & Holm, 2005) found limited influence of genes. The strongest influence was for prostate cancer, followed by breast cancer and colorectal cancer, but the genetic component accounted for less than half of the risk. Therefore, despite the widespread publicity about genetic causes of cancer (and Gwyneth Paltrow's beliefs), genes play a fairly minor role in the development of cancer; environmental factors are much more important.

Environmental Risk Factors for Cancer

Environmental risk factors for cancer include exposure to risks such as radiation and asbestos and to pollutants such as pesticides, motor exhaust, and other chemicals (Miligi, Costantini, Veraldi, Benvenuti, & Vineis, 2006). In addition, arsenic, benzene, chromium, nickel, vinyl chloride, and various petroleum products are possible contributors to a number of cancers (Boffetta, 2004; Siemiatycki et al., 2004).

Longtime exposure to asbestos can produce risk for lung cancer, depending on the type of asbestos and the frequency and duration of exposure. A study in Sweden (Gustavsson et al., 2000) looked into the possible carcinogenic effects of asbestos as well as diesel exhaust, motor exhaust, metals, welding fumes, and other environmental conditions that some workers encounter on the job. The results showed that workers who were most exposed to environmental carcinogens had about a 9% additional chance of developing lung cancer compared with people who were not exposed to these conditions. A 25-year longitudinal study of asbestos workers in China (Yano, Wang, Wang, Wang, & Lan, 2001) reported that male asbestos workers, compared with other workers, had a relative risk of 6.6 for lung cancer and 4.3 for all cancers.

Exposure to radiation is also a risk. Nuclear power plant workers exposed to high levels of radiation showed elevated risks for leukemia and cancers of the rectum, colon, testicles, and lung (Sont et al., 2001). Living in a community with a nuclear power plant, however, seems to present no elevated risk; the observed rate of cancer in such communities is similar to that of other communities (Boice, Bigbee, Mumma, & Blot, 2003). The radioactive gas radon also presents increased risks for lung cancer, both for miners who are

exposed and for people who live in homes with high levels of this type of radiation (Krewski et al., 2006).

Some infections and chronic inflammation also present elevated risks for cancers. Infection with the bacterium *Helicobacter pylori* is widespread throughout the world and increases the risk for gastric ulcers as well as gastric cancer (McColl, Watabe, & Derakhshan, 2007). Hepatitis infection is a risk for liver cancer. Chronic inflammation is a factor in the development of bladder cancer (Michaud, 2007) and possibly in prostate cancer (De Marzo et al., 2007). However, infection and inflammation may be more attributable to behavior than to environmental exposure.

IN SUMMARY

Inherent risks for cancer include ethnic background, advancing age, and family history and genetics. African Americans have a higher cancer incidence and higher death rates than European Americans, but people from other ethnic backgrounds have a lower incidence. These differences are due not to biology but to differences in socioeconomic status, which is related both to the incidence of cancer and to five-year survival with the disease.

The strongest risk factor for cancer—as well as many other diseases—is advancing age. The older one becomes, the greater one's risk for cancer. Both men and women increase their risk for cancer as they get older, but men have an even greater increase than women.

Although cancer seldom develops as a result of a single gene, family history and genetic predisposition play a role in the development of a some cancers, especially prostate and breast cancer. A woman who has a mother or sister with breast cancer has a two- to threefold higher chance of developing the disease, and mutations of the BRCA 1 and BRCA 2 genes place people at elevated risk for breast and pancreatic cancer. However, twin studies indicate that genetic factors play a relatively small role in the development of cancer.

Environmental risks may also contribute to cancer incidence and deaths. Pollutants, pesticides, radiation exposure, and infections increase the risk for various cancers. Workers exposed to asbestos and radiation are at increased risk, as are people living in homes with high levels of radon.

BEHAVIORAL RISK FACTORS FOR CANCER

Cancer results from an interaction of genetic, environmental, and behavioral conditions, most of which are still not clearly understood. As with cardiovascular diseases, however, a number of behavioral cancer risk factors have been identified. Recall that risk factors are not necessarily *causes* of a disease, but they do predict the likelihood of a person's developing or dying from that disease. Most risk factors for cancer relate to personal behavior and lifestyle, especially smoking and diet. Other known behavioral risks include alcohol, physical inactivity, exposure to ultraviolet light, sexual behavior, and psychosocial factors.

Smoking

The vast majority of smoking-related cancer deaths are from lung cancer, but smoking is also implicated in deaths from several other cancers, including leukemia and cancers of the lip, oral cavity, pharynx, esophagus, pancreas, larynx, trachea, urinary bladder, and kidney. There is not a consistent relationship between smoking and breast cancer, but women who smoke throughout adolescence may increase their risk for this type of cancer (Ha et al., 2007). The risk of cigarette smoking also applies to other countries around the world; smoking is the single largest risk for cancer mortality worldwide (Danaei, Vander Hoorn, Lopez, Murray, & Ezzati, 2005).

What Is the Risk? Epidemiologists generally agree that sufficient research evidence exists for a causal relationship between cigarette smoking and lung cancer. Chapter 2 includes a review of that evidence and also explains how epidemiologists can infer causation from nonexperimental studies. The strong relationship between smoking and lung cancer can be seen by observing the way

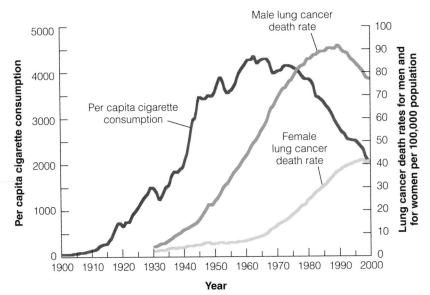

FIGURE 10.5 The parallel paths of cigarette consumption and lung cancer deaths for men and women, United States, 1900–2000.

Sources: Data on death rates from U.S. Mortality Public Use Tapes, 1900–2000, U.S. Mortality Volumes, 1930–1959, National Center for Health Statistics, Centers for Disease Control and Prevention, 2002; data on cigarette consumption from U.S. Department of Agriculture, 1900–2000.

lung cancer rates track smoking rates. About 25 to 40 years after smoking rates began to increase for men, lung cancer rates started a steep rise; about 25 to 40 years after cigarette consumption decreased for men, lung cancer death rates for men began to drop (see Figure 10.5). Women's smoking has declined more gradually, and so have their lung cancer mortality rates.

The strong relationship holds when analyzed by income. Low-income men smoke more than high-income men, and they have a higher lung cancer mortality rate; low-income women smoke a little less than high-income women, and they have a slightly lower rate of lung cancer mortality (Weir et al., 2003). The dose–response relationship between cigarette smoking and lung cancer and the close tracking of smoking rates and lung cancer rates provide compelling evidence for a causal relationship between smoking behavior and the development of lung cancer.

How high is the risk for lung cancer among cigarette smokers? The United States Department of Health and Human Services (USDHHS, 2004) estimated the relative risk of death for male smokers at about 23.3, meaning that men who smoke are 23.3 times more likely to die of lung cancer than men who have never smoked. The risk that cigarette smokers have of dying of lung cancer is the strongest link between any behavior and a major cause of death. Thus, cigarette smokers' relative risk in the vicinity of 23.3 for lung cancer clearly establishes smoking as a primary contributor to death from lung cancer—the leading cancer-related death for both men and women.

In addition to smoking, such factors as polluted air, socioeconomic level, occupation, ethnic background, and building material in one's house have all been linked to lung cancer. Each of these has an additive or possibly a **synergistic effect** with smoking, so studies of different populations may yield quite different risk factor rates, depending on the combination of risks that cigarette smokers have in addition to their risk as a smoker. For example, Chinese men who smoke have an elevated risk for lung cancer that is magnified by their exposure to smoke from burning coal, a common practice for household heating and cooking in China (Danaei et al., 2005).

What Is the Perceived Risk? Despite their heightened vulnerability to cancer, many smokers do not perceive that their behavior puts them at risk. They show what Neil Weinstein (1984) referred to as an *optimistic bias* concerning their chances of dying from cigarette-related causes. Both smokers and nonsmokers acknowledge that smoking is a health risk. Despite knowledge to the contrary, both high school smokers (Tomar & Hatsukami, 2007) and adult smokers (Peretti-Watel et al., 2007) believe that, unlike other smokers, they will somehow escape the deadly effects of cigarette smoking. The adult smokers expressed the belief that smoking is dangerous at some level—but not at the level of their consumption. Consistent with the concept of optimistic bias, these smokers have found a way to discount the risks of their behavior. Gwyneth Paltrow may be subject to a similar process; in her statements voicing concern about cancer, smoking was not a topic. She has not seemed to put as high a priority on the dangers from smoking and has focused on risks from genes and diet.

Diet

Another risk factor for cancer is an unhealthy diet. The American Cancer Society (2008) has estimated that one-third of all cancer deaths in the United States are a result of dietary choices and sedentary lifestyle. Poor dietary practices are associated with a wide variety of cancers, and good choices decrease the risks.

Foods That May Cause Cancer Some foods are suspected of being **carcinogenic**—that is, of causing cancer, almost always because of contaminants or additives (Abnet, 2007). Like Gwyneth Paltrow, many people imagine that foods without additives or preservatives are safer, but some may be less so. "Natural" foods lack preservatives, which can result in high levels of bacteria and fungi. A long list of bacteria and fungi present risks for stomach cancer. The sharp decline in this cancer is due in part to increased refrigeration during the last 75 years and to lower consumption of salt-cured foods, smoked foods, and foods stored at room temperature (see Figures 10.2 and 10.3). Aflatoxin is a fungus that grows on improperly stored grains and peanuts; exposure to this toxin increases the risk for cancer of the liver (World Cancer Research Fund/American Institute for Cancer Research [WCRF/AICR], 2007). However, food additives used as preservatives can also be carcinogenic, and toxic chemicals produced by various industries can work their way into the environment and into foods, as in the case of dioxin. Thus, both foods that lack preservatives and those with preservatives may present some risk.

In Chapter 9, we saw that dietary fat is an established risk for cardiovascular disease; a number of studies have shown that dietary fat is also a risk for cancer, especially colon cancer (Murtaugh, 2004). However, a high-fat diet is a stronger risk for cardiovascular disease than it is for cancer. Much of the research on dietary fat and cancer has centered on breast cancer, and an evaluation of this body of research (Freedman, Kipnis, Schatzkin, & Potischman, 2008) led to the conclusion that dietary fat is a modest but reliable risk factor for this cancer. A high-fat diet is also related to high cholesterol levels, which appeared as a risk factor for testicular cancer in men—raising the risk 4.5 times (Dobson, 2005).

Colorectal cancer is the second leading cause of cancer deaths in the United States and other developed countries, exceeded only by lung cancer, yet the causes of colorectal cancer are not well understood. An extensive review (Williams & Hord, 2005) indicated that consumption of preserved meat (such as ham, bacon, and hot dogs) and red meat raises the risk of this type of cancer. A possible risk associated with red meat is the method of cooking; charred, smoked, or overcooked red meats may be a factor in this risk (Alaejos, González, & Afonso, 2008), and salt-cured or heavily salted meats also raises risks for stomach cancer (WCRF/AICR, 2007).

A stronger risk for this cancer comes not from any specific dietary component but from overweight and obesity (WCRF/AICR, 2007; Williams & Hord, 2005). The link between obesity and colorectal cancer is strong. Obesity is also strongly related to cancer of the esophagus, breast (in postmenopausal women), endometrium, and kidney. Abdominal fat is a risk not only for cardiovascular disease but also for cancer of the pancreas, endometrium, and kidney. Although eating several specific types of food increases the risk for cancers, a diet that leads to overweight or obesity is more of a risk.

Foods That May Protect Against Cancer If specific foods and overall diet can increase the risk for cancer, might some dietary measures offer protection? If so, which foods should people consume to reduce their risk of cancer? One team of researchers has calculated that if people around the world were to eat an adequate amount of fruits and vegetables, as many as 2.635 million deaths per year would be eliminated (Lock et al., 2005). The same researchers estimated that this fruit and vegetable rich diet might reduce the incidence of stomach cancer by 19%, esophageal cancer by 20%, lung cancer by 12%, and colorectal cancer by 2%. Consistent with this analysis, another review (Williams & Hord, 2005) concluded that the evidence is strong for a high-fiber diet as protective for colorectal cancer.

Evidence for specific nutrients that may protect against the development or proliferation of cancer is not yet clear. This lack of clarity may have several underlying reasons that relate to the methods used to investigate dietary components. Researchers have developed hypotheses concerning which nutrients may be protective by examining large populations for the incidence of various cancers (Boyd, 2007). When differences appear between populations in the incidence of a cancer, researchers then want to examine that particular component. For example, population studies showed that people in countries with a high-fiber diet experienced lower rates of colorectal cancer than people in countries with a low-fiber diet. This result prompted research using the case–control method in which people who eat a high-fiber diet were compared to those who eat a low-fiber diet (see Chapter 2 for a description of this method). Such studies involve many fewer people than population studies, so small effects of fiber in the diet may not be clear using this approach. Alternatively, other differences between the two groups may contribute to the effect of fiber in the diet, making a clear conclusion difficult. If case–control

WOULD YOU BELIEVE . . . ?

Pizza May Prevent Cancer

Would you believe that pizza may prevent cancer? For pizza lovers everywhere, this is indeed good news. However, before you begin eating two or three pizzas a day, you should be aware of a few cautions. Pizza is not entirely healthy. The cancer-protective effects of pizza are limited to the tomato sauce, which contains a specific nutrient—lycopene. Toppings such as ground meat, pepperoni, anchovies, and cheese are high in fat, and high-fat diets have many risks, especially for cardiovascular disease. In addition, the protective value of lycopene is not large.

The lycopene in tomato sauce is a type of chemical that is inversely related to the development of cancer (Campbell et al., 2004; Giovannucci, 1999). However, as we see in this chapter, specific

nutrients, including lycopene, seldom have the ability to protect against cancer. Indeed, other phytochemicals in tomatoes may interact, resulting in a combination of effects.

What are the pathways through which lycopene and other nutrients in food may offer some protection against cancer? At the earliest stage of prevention, antioxidants can counteract carcinogens before they damage cells; that is, certain chemical components of food can prevent damage to cells, proteins, and DNA (WCRF/AICR, 2007). After entering the body, carcinogens are converted from precursors into agents that damage DNA and produce malignancies. You may be able to slow this process by eating lots of vegetables, including tomato paste and garlic.

Another possible route for protection comes from nutrients that suppress tumor growth. Like other growing cells, malignancies depend on growth factors to establish and promote growth, and suppression of these factors can thwart cancer proliferation. A chemical in red grapes, carrots, rosemary, and turmeric has the ability to block blood vessel formation, thus preventing a tumor from establishing itself. Eating these foods will not cure cancer, and most of the research on the preventive powers of nutrients has been carried out on rats. However, diet is a factor in the establishment and spread of cancer, so a cancer-healthy diet exists. This diet includes foods with specific nutrients that seem to offer protection against particular types of cancer—so have a slice of pizza.

studies indicate that the nutrient has a positive effect, which they have for fiber and colorectal cancer (WCRF/AICR, 2007), researchers then perform experimental studies.

The randomized clinical trial is an experimental method that is considered the best method for detecting differences between groups. For dietary studies, however, this method has drawbacks (Boyd, 2007). Such studies are experimental, involving the manipulation of a factor—in this case a dietary component. Half the participants are exposed to the component, and half are not, creating a clear comparison. However, the exposure is typically short term; few clinical trials last longer than a few years, and most have limited follow-ups. Eating a high-fiber diet for two years may not provide sufficient exposure to have an impact on the development of colorectal cancer, which develops over years. Or participants may need to ingest nutrients during childhood or adolescence

for maximum benefit, but most studies include only adult participants. In addition, randomized clinical trials usually isolate a nutrient and provide that nutrient through supplements rather than through broad changes to the diet. Taking supplements often fails to produce the benefits of eating a diet high in the same nutrients. Thus, the benefits of specific nutrients may be complex, and randomized clinical trials may miss some of those important benefits.

These limitations have restricted researchers from coming to conclusions about the cancer-preventive benefits of many nutrients. (See Would You Believe . . . ? box for one specific nutrient that may protect against cancer.) An extensive review of the evidence (WCRF/AICR, 2007) was able to place several nutrients into the category of *probable* (but not *convincing*) evidence for benefits. **Beta-carotene** is one of the carotenoids, a form of vitamin A found abundantly in foods such as carrots and sweet potatoes. Eating a diet rich in carotenoids probably lowers the risk of cancer of the mouth, larynx, pharynx, and lungs; high beta-carotene intake has a similar benefit for the risk of cancer of the esophagus, as does a diet rich in vitamin C. People who eat foods high in folate, one of the B vitamins, probably decrease their chances of developing pancreatic cancer. Evidence for any protective power for these nutrients is weaker for other types of cancer.

Evidence concerning selenium intake is somewhat stronger (Williams & Hord, 2005). **Selenium** is a trace element found in grain products and in meat from grain-fed animals. It enters the food chain through the soil, but not all soils throughout the world contain equal amounts of selenium. In excess, selenium is toxic, but in moderate amounts, it provides some protection against colon and prostate cancers. Foods with high levels of selenium protect against colon cancer in laboratory rats (Finley, Davis, & Feng, 2000), and selenium supplements can significantly reduce cancer incidence, but only in men (Bardia et al., 2008). Calcium has received a great deal of publicity for its benefit in preventing bone mineral loss, but it may also offer some protection against colorectal cancer (WCRF/AICR, 2007).

Thus, an evaluation of the extensive research suggests that some nutrients can protect against some cancers, but the evidence of a protective effect is stronger concerning overall diet and maintaining close to ideal body weight. A healthy diet includes lots of fruits and vegetables, whole grains, legumes, nuts, fish and seafood, and low-fat dairy products; the amount of preserved and red meat, saturated fat, salt-cured foods, and foods made of highly processed ingredients is low. This description fits with the concept of a Mediterranean-type diet, emphasizing a plant-based diet with a variety of foods that people can adopt as part of a healthy lifestyle (Williams & Hord, 2005). Another element of the Mediterranean diet is alcohol—but in limited amounts.

Alcohol

For cancers of all sites, alcohol is not as strong a risk factor as either smoking or eating an imprudent diet. Nevertheless, alcohol has been implicated in cancers

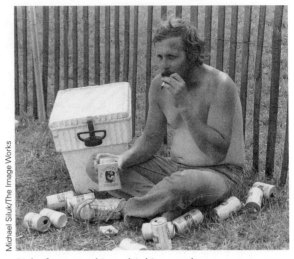

Michael Siluk/The Image Works

Risks from smoking, drinking, and sun exposure can have a synergistic effect, multiplying the chances of developing cancer.

of the mouth, esophagus, breast, and liver (Danaei et al., 2005). The liver has primary responsibility for detoxifying alcohol. Therefore, persistent and excessive drinking often leads to cirrhosis of the liver, a degenerative disease that curtails the organ's effectiveness. Cancer is more likely to occur in cirrhotic livers than in healthy ones (WCRF/AICR, 2007), but alcohol abusers are likely to die of a variety of other causes before they develop liver cancer.

Does drinking alcohol cause breast cancer? Current evaluations of the research indicate that the evidence is convincing (WCRF/AICR, 2007). The risk varies by exposure; women who consume three or more drinks per day have a moderate to strong risk for breast cancer, and women who consume as little as one to two drinks daily have some risk (Singletary & Gapstur, 2001). The risk is not equal in all countries. In the United States, about 2% of breast cancer cases can be attributed to alcohol, but in Italy, where alcohol intake is considerably higher, as many as 15% of breast cancer cases may be due to drinking. Table 10.1 summarizes the risks and benefits of specific dietary choices and alcohol consumption.

Alcohol has a synergistic effect with smoking, so people who both smoke and drink heavily have a relative risk for certain cancers exceeding that of the two independent risk factors added

Table 10.1
Diet and Its Effects on Cancer

Type of Food	Findings of Increased Risk	Studies
"Natural" foods with no preservatives	Grains and peanuts may be contaminated with aflatoxin, which is carcinogenic Spoiled food increases risk for stomach cancer	Abnet, 2007
Foods high in preservatives	Preservatives can be carcinogenic	Abnet, 2007
High-fat diet	Contributes to colon cancer Modest risk for breast cancer High cholesterol level is a strong risk for testicular cancer	Murtaugh, 2004 Freedman et al., 2008 Dobson, 2005
Consumption of preserved meats and red meat	Increases the risk for colorectal cancer, especially if meat is smoked or charred	Williams & Hord, 2005; WCRF/AICR, 2007
Overweight and obesity	Strong link to colorectal, esophageal, breast, endometrial, and kidney cancer Abdominal fat is a risk for cancer of the pancreas, endometrium, and kidney	WCRF/AICR, 2007; Williams & Hord, 2005
Alcohol	Raises the risk of cancers of the mouth, esophagus, breast, and liver, especially heavy drinking and drinking combined with smoking	Danaei et al., 2005

Type of Food	Findings of Decreased Risk	Studies
Diet rich in fruits and vegetables	Could reduce worldwide rates of stomach cancer by 19%, esophageal cancer by 20%, lung cancer by 12%, and colorectal cancer by 2%	Lock et al., 2005
Diet rich in fiber	Protects against colon cancer	Williams & Hord, 2005
Diet high in carotenoids, including beta-carotene	Probably lowers the risk of cancer of the mouth, larynx, pharynx, and lungs Diets high in beta-carotene (but not supplements) lower the risk for cancer of the esophagus	WCRF/AICR, 2007
Vitamin C	Probably lowers the risk of cancer of the esophagus	WCRF/AICR, 2007
Diet high in folate	Probably lowers the risk of pancreatic cancer	WCRF/AICR, 2007
Selenium	Protects against colon cancer in laboratory rats Reduces risk of several types of cancer in men	Finley et al., 2000 Bardia et al., 2008
Calcium	May protect against colon cancer	WCRF/AICR, 2007
Summary	Overall diet and healthy weight are more strongly related to cancer than any one dietary component	Williams & Hord, 2005; WCRF/AICR, 2007

together. People who both drink and smoke and who have a family history of esophageal, stomach, or pharynx cancers have an increased risk for cancers of the digestive tract (Garavello et al., 2005). These data suggest that people who both drink heavily and smoke could substantially reduce their chances of developing cancer by giving up either smoking or drinking. Quitting both, of course, would reduce the risk still more.

Sedentary Lifestyle

A sedentary lifestyle seems to promote some types of cancer but not others, or alternatively, physical activity seems to protect against some cancers but not others (WCRF/AICR, 2007). The cancers in question include cancers of the colon, endometrium, breast, lung and pancreas. The evidence for the beneficial effects of exercise is stronger for colon, endometrial, and breast cancer (in women after menopause); the effects are less clear for lung and pancreatic cancer and for breast cancer in premenopausal women. Some studies (Bernstein, Henderson, Hanisch, Sullivan-Halley, & Ross, 1994; Thune, Brenn, Lund, & Gaard, 1997) suggest that women who begin a physical activity program when they are young and who continue to exercise four hours a week greatly reduce their risk for breast cancer. This age-sensitive effect may make the overall benefit of exercise difficult to determine for premenopausal women.

Another indirect benefit of physical activity for cancer risk is its relationship with body weight. Physical activity is important for maintaining a healthy body weight and a favorable level of body fat, both of which are related to a number of cancers. Thus, some form of vigorous physical activity can lower cancer risk in several ways. The benefits (and potential risks) of physical activity are discussed more fully in Chapter 15.

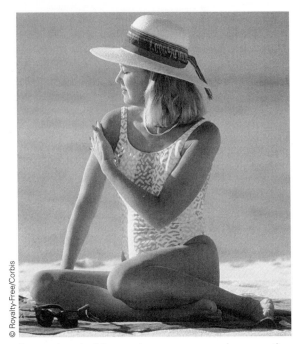

© Royalty-Free/Corbis

Protective clothing and sunscreen can decrease the risks associated with exposure to ultraviolet light.

Ultraviolet Light Exposure

Exposure to ultraviolet light, particularly from the sun, has long been recognized as a cause of skin cancer, especially for light-skinned people (WCRF/AICR, 2007). Both cumulative exposure and occasional severe sunburn seem to relate to subsequent risk of skin cancer. Since the mid-1970s, the incidence of skin cancer has risen dramatically in the United States. However, because this form of cancer has a low mortality rate, it has only slightly affected total cancer mortality statistics. Not all skin cancers, however, are harmless. One form, malignant melanoma, is often deadly. Malignant melanoma is especially prevalent among light-skinned people exposed to the sun.

Although skin cancer is associated with a behavioral risk (voluntary exposure to the sun over a long period of time), it also has a strong genetic component (Pho, Grossman, & Leachman, 2006). Light-skinned, fair-haired, blue-eyed individuals are more likely than dark-skinned people to develop skin cancer, and much of the damage occurs with sun exposure during childhood. During the past 50 years, the relationship between melanoma mortality rates and geographic latitude has gradually decreased; residence in areas of the United States with high ultraviolet radiation is no longer a risk factor for melanoma but remains a risk for other types of skin cancer (Qureshi, Laden, Colditz, & Hunter, 2008). Fair-skinned people should avoid prolonged and frequent exposure to the sun by taking protective measures, including using sunscreen lotions and wearing protective clothing.

Not all exposure to sunlight is detrimental to health. Vitamin D has been linked both to sun exposure and to lower rates of several types of cancer, including cancers of the breast, colon, prostate, ovary, lungs, and pancreas (Ingraham, Bragdon, & Nohe, 2008). However, the level of vitamin D necessary to protect against cancer is seldom attained through diet alone. Therefore, low levels of exposure to ultraviolet light can be a healthy means of supplying vitamin D. How much sun exposure is enough but not too much? In addition to the usual dietary supply of vitamin D, as little as 5 to 10 minutes of sun exposure of the arms and legs or the arms, hands, and face two or three times a week seems sufficient (Holick, 2004). Alternatively, dietary supplementation can provide vitamin D and its protective benefits (Ingraham et al., 2008).

Sexual Behavior

Some sexual behaviors also contribute to cancer deaths, especially cancers resulting from acquired immune deficiency syndrome (AIDS). Two common forms of AIDS-related cancers are Kaposi's sarcoma and non-Hodgkin's lymphoma. **Kaposi's sarcoma** is a malignancy characterized by soft, dark blue or purple nodules on the skin, often with large lesions. The lesions can be so small at first as to look like a rash but can grow to be large and disfiguring. Besides covering the skin, these lesions can spread to the lung, spleen, bladder, lymph nodes, mouth, and adrenal glands. Until the 1980s, this type of cancer was quite rare and was limited mostly to older men of Mediterranean background. However, AIDS-related Kaposi's sarcoma occurs in every age group and in both men and women. Not all people with AIDS are equally susceptible to this disease; gay men with AIDS are much more likely to develop Kaposi's sarcoma than are people who developed AIDS as a result of injection drug use or heterosexual contact (Henke-Gendo & Schulz, 2004).

Non-Hodgkin's lymphoma is characterized by rapidly growing tumors that are spread through the circulatory or lymphatic system. Like Kaposi's sarcoma, non-Hodgkin's lymphoma can occur in AIDS patients of all ages and both genders. However, most people with non-Hodgkin's lymphoma do *not* have AIDS. The greatest risk for AIDS-related cancers continues to be unprotected sex with an HIV-positive partner.

The presence of invasive cervical cancer has also become a basis for diagnosing AIDS, but again, the majority of cases of cervical cancer are unrelated to HIV infection. However, this type of cancer is related to infection with the human papillomavirus (Baseman & Koutsky, 2005; Danaei et al., 2006), a sexually transmitted virus that is a necessary condition for the development of cervical cancer. The rates of infection with this virus are high, especially for sexually active young people (Datta et al., 2008). Thus, women who have had many sex partners and those whose first sexual intercourse experience occurred early in life are most vulnerable to cervical cancer because these behaviors expose them to the virus. Cervical cancer is related not only to the sexual behavior of women but also to the sex practices of their male partners. When men have multiple sex partners, specifically with women who have had many sex partners, their female sex partners are at increased risk of cervical cancer.

Other sexual practices put both women and men at risk for cancer. For women, early age at first intercourse and a large number of sex partners are both strongly implicated in the development of cancer of the cervix, vagina, and ovary. However, some of the danger is offset by physiological changes in women's bodies resulting from pregnancy and childbirth that seem to protect against breast, ovarian, and endometrial cancers. These cancers are less common in women who have had children early in life compared with those who have had children later in life or who have no children (Lee et al., 2003). Having a first child later in the childbearing years does not confer the same protection as it does during earlier years.

For men, too, sexual practices can increase the risk of cancer, especially prostate cancer. Karin Rosenblatt and her associates (Rosenblatt, Wicklund, & Stanford, 2000) found a significant positive relationship between prostate cancer and lifetime number of female sex partners (but not male sex partners), early age of first intercourse, and prior infection with gonorrhea. However, they found no risk for prostate cancer associated with lifetime frequency of sexual intercourse.

Psychosocial Risk Factors in Cancer

Since the days of the Greek physician Galen (A.D. 131–201), people have speculated about the relationship between personality traits and certain diseases, including cancer. However, that speculation does not match the findings from scientific research. For example, a prospective study from the Swedish Twin Registry (Hansen, Floderus, Frederiksen, & Johansen, 2005) found that neither extraversion nor neuroticism—as measured by the Eysenck Personality Inventory—was related to increased risk of cancer.

This study and its findings are fairly typical of attempts to relate psychosocial factors to cancer incidence and mortality. During the past 30 or 40 years, a number of researchers have been interested in the association between a variety of psychological factors and cancer development and prognosis. Some studies have identified various personality factors that seemed to relate to the development of cancer, but large-scale studies and reviews of the topic (Aro et al., 2005; Garssen, 2004; Levin & Kissane, 2006; Stürmer, Hasselbach, & Amelang, 2006) have found only weak association between any psychosocial factor and cancer. Factors that show the strongest relationship come from negative emotionality and the tendency to repress (rather than express) emotion. However, these traits show a stronger relationship to response to a diagnosis of cancer than to the development of cancer.

IN SUMMARY

Cigarette smoking and unwise dietary choices account for a significant number of cancer cases and cancer deaths in the United States and around the world. In addition, alcohol, an inactive lifestyle, ultraviolet light, and unsafe sexual behaviors contribute to cancer risk. Psychological and social factors show only a weak relationship to cancer risk.

Cigarette smoking is the leading risk factor for lung cancer. Although not all cigarette smokers die of lung cancer and some nonsmokers develop this disease, clear evidence exists that smokers have a greatly increased chance of developing some form of cancer, particularly lung cancer. The more cigarettes per day people smoke and the more years they continue this practice, the more they are at risk.

The relationship between diet and the development of cancer is complex, with some types of food presenting dangers for the development of cancer and others offering some protection. "Natural" foods avoid the risk of preservatives but increase the likelihood of other toxins. A high-fat diet is related to colon and breast cancer, but a diet that produces overweight or obesity is a risk for a variety of cancers, including colorectal, esophageal, breast (in postmenopausal women), endometrial, and kidney cancer. Some dietary components can protect against cancer, including fruits, vegetables, and other high-fiber foods. The evidence for specific nutrients in foods is less persuasive, and taking supplements generally offers no protection.

Alcohol is probably only a weak risk factor for cancer. Nevertheless, it has a synergistic effect with cigarette smoking; when the two are combined, the total relative risk is much greater than the risks of the two factors added together. Lack of physical activity and high exposure to ultraviolet light are additional risk factors for cancer. Also, certain sexual behaviors, such as number of lifetime sex partners, relate to both cervical and prostate cancer as well as to cancers associated with AIDS.

In general, psychosocial factors show only weak relationships to cancer incidence. Negative affect and repression of emotion may contribute to the development of cancer, but the relationship is not strong.

Ⓛ LIVING WITH CANCER

Each year in the United States, more than a million people receive a diagnosis of cancer (American Cancer Society, 2008). Most of these people receive their diagnosis with feelings of fear, anxiety, and anger, partly because they fear the disease and partly because current cancer treatments produce unpleasant effects for many cancer patients. Psychologists have been involved in assisting patients in coping with their emotional reactions to a cancer diagnosis, providing social support to patients and families, and helping patients prepare for the negative side effects of some cancer treatments.

Problems With Medical Treatments for Cancer

Nearly all medical treatments for cancer have negative side effects that may add stress to the lives of cancer patients, their friends, and their families. The three most common therapies are also the three most stressful: surgery, radiation, and chemotherapy. In recent years, some **oncologists** have added hormonal treatment and immunotherapy to their arsenal of treatment regimens, but these newer treatments are generally not yet as effective as surgery, radiation, or chemotherapy.

Surgery is often recommended when cancerous growth has not yet metastasized and when physicians have some confidence that the surgical procedure will be successful in making the tumor

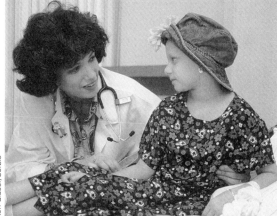

Negative side effects of chemotherapy such as hair loss add to the stress of cancer patients.

more manageable. Cancer patients who undergo surgery are likely to experience distress, rejection, and fears, and they often receive less emotional support than other surgery patients. These reactions are especially likely for patients with breast cancer (Wimberly, Carver, Laurenceau, Harris, & Antoni, 2005) and prostate cancer (Couper, 2007) because of the sexual implications of their surgery. Postsurgery stress and depression lead to lower levels of immunity, which may prolong recovery time and increase vulnerability to other disorders (Antoni & Lutgendorf, 2007).

Radiation also has severe side effects. Many patients who receive radiation therapy anticipate their treatment with fear and anxiety, dreading loss of hair, burns, nausea, vomiting, fatigue, and sterility. Most of these outcomes occur, so patients' fears are not unreasonable. However, patients are seldom adequately prepared for their radiation treatments, and thus their fears and anxieties may exaggerate the severity of these side effects.

Chemotherapy has some of the same negative side effects as radiation, and these side effects often precipitate stressful reactions in cancer patients. Cancer patients treated with chemotherapy experience some combination of nausea, vomiting, fatigue, loss of coordination, decreased ability to concentrate, depression, weight change, loss of appetite, sleep problems, and hair loss. Not only do these negative effects create

problems in adjusting to a diagnosis of cancer, but patients' expectations of the negative effects of chemotherapy (Olver, Taylor, & Whitford, 2005) and their beliefs about the nature of the disease (Thuné-Boyle, Myers, & Newman, 2006) contribute to distress and adjustment.

Adjusting to a Diagnosis of Cancer

Adjusting to a diagnosis of cancer is a challenge for everyone, but some people have more difficulties than others. One factor that predicts a poor reaction is the same as the emotional components that show some relationship to the development of cancer—negative affect and social inhibition (Verma & Khan, 2007). If negative affect is a problem for adjustment, then optimism should be an advantage, and research generally supports this hypothesis. Optimism is especially strongly related to adjusting well to a diagnosis of cancer (Carver et al., 2005), but its relationship to long-term outcome is less clear (Segerstrom, 2005, 2007). This difference may arise from the difficulty of the task of adjusting to cancer treatment or from miscalculations on the part of optimists concerning the course and outcome of their treatments (Winterling, Glimelius, & Nordin, 2008). When outcomes are disappointing, optimists may find adjustment more difficult than those who have more realistic expectations.

After diagnosis, people with cancer show a variety of responses and different trajectories in adjusting and functioning over the course of their treatment and afterward (Helgeson, Snyder, & Seltman, 2004). Most cancer survivors report improvement in their functioning over time, but some long-term survivors attributed problems with low energy, pain, and sexual functioning to their cancers (Phipps, Braitman, Stites, & Leighton, 2008). Even eight years after cancer, survivors report some problems, which are much more likely to be physical complications than psychological problems (Schroevers, Ranchor, & Sanderman, 2006).

The same emotional factors that enhance the survival of heart disease patients may not be similarly helpful to cancer patients. That is, the calm expression of emotion that may be good advice for cardiovascular patients cannot be recommended for cancer patients; expression of emotion seems to be a better strategy. For example, for children (Aldridge & Roesch, 2007) and for men coping with prostate cancer (Roesch et al., 2005), use of emotion-focused coping did not present the disadvantages that this strategy typically does (see Chapter 5 for a discussion of coping strategies). Expression of both positive and negative emotions can be beneficial (Quartana, Laubmeier, & Zakowski, 2006). However, expressing some negative emotions may do more harm than good (Lieberman & Goldstein, 2006); expressing anger seems to lead to a better adjustment, whereas expressing fear and anxiety related to lower quality of life and higher depression. Being able to express emotions and being guided to do so in the most helpful manner requires appropriate social support.

Social Support for Cancer Patients

Social support can help cancer patients adjust to their condition, but type and timing of support play a role in how helpful it is. For recently diagnosed individuals, health care providers can supply information and help with decision making, which such patients rated as supportive and useful (Arora, Rutten, Gustafson, Moser, & Hawkins, 2007). During the same time period, family and friends can be helpful by providing emotional support. Partners who are supportive without being obvious provide advantages to cancer patients; "invisible" support may be the best kind (Bolger, Zuckerman, & Kessler, 2000). That is, support that one partner provided but the other partner did not notice was better at relieving stress than support that the partner noticed. However, partners' attempts to protect their spouses from the reality of their illness were not helpful (Hagedoorn et al., 2000). Thus, social support from families may or may not provide the type of support people with cancer need. Many people with cancer turn to support groups or therapists to provide emotional support.

Support groups may be led by professionals such as psychologists, nurses, or oncologists, but often the groups consist of other individuals who are cancer survivors. Some studies have indicated that some people profit from support groups more than others. For example, women with breast cancer who lacked adequate marital support profited more from peer group support than from support

of their partners, whereas women with strong support from their partners had poorer adjustments when they participated in a peer discussion group (Helgeson, Cohen, Schulz, & Yasko, 2000). Breast and prostate cancer survivors differed in the benefits they received from support group participation, but they also varied in terms of the topics discussed in each type of group (Ullrich, Rothrock, Lutgendorf, Jochimsen, & Williams, 2008). A systematic review of the value of peer support groups for cancer survivors (Hoey, Ieropoli, White, & Jefford, 2008) indicated that such groups could be but were not always helpful. In general, face-to-face support delivered by an individual and Internet groups demonstrated the best outcomes, but all types of groups can be effective for some individuals.

Psychotherapy With Cancer Patients

Psychologists have used both individual and group techniques to help cancer patients cope with their diagnosis. To be effective, psychotherapy should accomplish at least one of two objectives: It should improve emotional well-being, increase survival time, or both. Whether psychological interventions have attained either goal is controversial. The goals of reducing psychological distress and improving patients' quality of life have come closer to success than extending the life of cancer patients.

A review of psychological interventions (Manne & Andrykowski, 2006) indicated that psychological interventions can be successful in helping cancer patients manage the distress related to their condition. Evaluating interventions is not easy; few studies include a clearly psychological intervention and no other component. In addition, most studies are not randomized, controlled trials. However, evidence for the effectiveness of cognitive behavioral interventions seems clear. Evidence for other components is less clear, but reports of programs with multiple components also indicate success. For example, a program that targeted emotional regulation (Cameron, Booth, Schlatter, Ziginskas, & Harman, 2007) indicated success. However, this emphasis may not be the best approach for everyone. Individual needs and variation are concerns that may not be adequately addressed in formulating interventions. As one research team asked,

"Does one size fit all?" (Zimmerman, Heinrichs, & Baucom, 2007, p. 225). This question highlights the need to match the characteristics and needs of people with cancer to a psychotherapy, support, educational, or multicomponent program that will be effective for each person.

The question of psychological interventions prolonging life span for people with cancer remains more controversial. This possibility arose when David Spiegel and colleagues (Spiegel, Bloom, Kraemer, & Gottheil, 1989) conducted a multicomponent intervention to help breast cancer patients adjust to the stressful aspects of their disease and their treatment. An analysis of the results indicated that not only was the intervention successful in managing pain, anxiety, and depression, but the women in the intervention group lived longer than those in the comparison group. That finding prompted researchers to examine how psychosocial and CAM interventions might prolong the life of those with cancer (see Chapter 8 for a discussion of integrative cancer treatments). Plausible mechanisms include the effect on the immune system and improvements in functioning that allow cancer patients to adhere to their medical treatment regimen (Antoni & Lutgendorf, 1007; Spiegel, 2004; Spiegel & Geise-Davis, 2003).

However, the basic finding that psychosocial interventions can prolong life has come into question. Large-scale reviews have found little evidence that psychotherapy extends survival time for breast cancer patients (Edwards, Hailey, & Maxwell, 2004; Smedslund & Ringdal, 2004). Despite a plausible mechanism for such action and despite the hope that such a benefit is possible (Coyne, Stefanek, & Palmer, 2007), little evidence exists at this point that psychological interventions prolong the life of those with cancer.

IN SUMMARY

After people have been diagnosed with cancer, they typically experience fear, anxiety, depression, and feelings of helplessness. The standard medical treatments for cancer—surgery, chemotherapy, and radiation—all have negative side effects that often produce added stress and discomfort. These side effects include loss of hair, nausea, fatigue, sterility, and other negative conditions. Receiving social support from family and friends, joining support groups, and receiving emotional support through psychological interventions probably help some people with cancer to increase psychological functioning, decrease depression and anxiety, manage pain, and enhance quality of life. Little evidence exists that psychotherapy can increase survival time.

ANSWERS

This chapter has addressed five basic questions:

1. What is cancer?

Cancer is a group of diseases characterized by the presence of new (neoplastic) cells that grow and spread beyond control. These cells may be either benign or malignant, but both types of neoplastic cells are dangerous. Malignant cells are capable of metastasizing and spreading through the blood or lymph to other organs of the body, thus making malignancies life threatening.

2. Are cancer death rates increasing or decreasing?

Cancer is the second leading cause of death in the United States, accounting for about 22% of deaths. During the first nine and a half decades of the 20th century, cancer death rates in the United States rose threefold, but since the mid-1990s, death rates have begun to decline, especially for cancers of the lung, colon and rectum, breast, and prostate—the four leading sites for cancer deaths in the United States. Currently, lung cancer death rates for women are beginning to level off and may soon begin to decline.

3. What are the inherent and environmental risk factors for cancer?

The uncontrollable risk factors for cancer include family history, ethnic background, and advancing age. Family history is a factor in many types of cancer; inheritance of a mutated form of a specific gene increases the risk of breast cancer two- to threefold. Ethnic background is also a factor; compared with European Americans, African Americans have a significantly higher rate of mortality from cancer, but other ethnic groups have lower rates. Advancing age is the single most powerful mortality risk for cancer, but age is also the leading risk for death from cardiovascular and other diseases. Environmental exposure to airborne pollutants, radiation, and infectious organisms constitute significant risks for cancer if the exposure is heavy and prolonged.

4. **What are the behavioral risk factors for cancer?**

More than half of all cancer deaths in the United States have been attributed to either smoking or unwise lifestyle choices, such as diet and exercise. Smoking cigarettes raises the risk of lung cancer by a factor of 23 times, but smoking also accounts for other cancer deaths.

The relationship between diet and cancer is complex; diet can increase or decrease the risk for cancer. Toxins and contaminants in food raise the risks, but a diet high in fruits, vegetables, whole grains, low-fat dairy products, beans, and seeds and low in fat, red meat, processed meat, and salt tends to be associated with lowered risk for a variety of cancers. A diet that leads to overweight or obesity raises the risk. Alcohol is not as strong a risk for cancer as diet, but combining alcohol with smoking sharply increases the risk. A sedentary lifestyle also presents a risk, especially for breast cancer. Exposure to ultraviolet light and sexual behaviors can increase the risks for various cancers. Research has also revealed a weak link between negative affect and depression and cancer.

5. **How can cancer patients be helped in coping with their disease?**

Cancer patients usually benefit from social support from spouse, family, and health care providers, but the type and timing of support affect its benefits. Support groups offer another type of support that is beneficial to some cancer patients, especially in allowing the expression of emotion. Therapists can use cognitive behavioral methods to assist cancer patients in coping with some of the negative aspects of cancer treatments and adjusting to their disease, thus increasing the quality of life for cancer patients, but no evidence exists that psychosocial factors can increase survival time.

SUGGESTED READINGS

American Cancer Society. (2008). *Cancer facts and figures 2008.* Atlanta: American Cancer Society. This yearly publication provides extensive, updated information about cancer in the United States with some international comparisons.

Antoni, M. H., & Lutgendorf, S. (2007). Psychosocial factors in disease progression in cancer. *Current Directions in Psychological Science, 16,* 42–46. This brief article focuses on the influence of psychosocial factors and how these factors may affect the biology of cancer.

Danaei, G., Vander Hoorn, S., Lopez, A. D., Murray, C. J. L., & Ezzati, M. (2005). Causes of cancer in the world: Comparative risk assessment of nine behavioural and environmental risk factors. *Lancet, 366,* 1784–1793. For those who want an international perspective, this article examines nine behavioral and environmental factors and traces the differing rates of cancer in countries throughout the world related to these factors.

Williams, M. T., & Hord, H. G. (2005). The role of dietary factors in cancer prevention: Beyond fruits and vegetables. *Nutrition in Clinical Practice, 20,* 451–459. This review provides not only good information about the dangers and benefits of specific dietary factors but also gives advice about eating to prevent cancer.

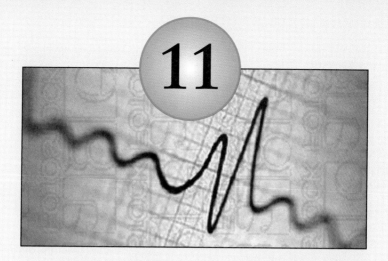

11

LIVING WITH CHRONIC ILLNESS

QUESTIONS

This chapter focuses on six basic questions:

1. What is the impact of chronic disease on patients and families?

2. What is the impact of Alzheimer's disease?

3. What is involved in adjusting to diabetes?

4. How does asthma affect the lives of people with this disease?

5. How can HIV infection be managed?

6. What adaptations do people make to dying and grieving?

REAL-WORLD PROFILE OF PRESIDENT RONALD REAGAN

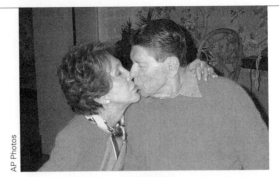

After Ronald Reagan was diagnosed with Alzheimer's disease, his wife, Nancy, learned how to cope with the consequences of living with this chronic illness.

On September 30, 1983, President Ronald Reagan declared the month of November 1983, to be National Alzheimer's Disease Month. On November 4, 1994, the former president issued a letter revealing that he had been diagnosed with Alzheimer's disease (Alzheimer's Organization, 2004). The 1983 proclamation included information on how serious and how widespread Alzheimer's disease is, and later reports about the experience of the former president and his family confirmed the devastation that Alzheimer's disease brings.

During the decade between the announcement of his Alzheimer's disease and his death on June 5, 2004, Reagan and his family experienced the same stresses and frustrations that millions of families endure when a family member is chronically ill. For daughter Maureen, her first realization that something was wrong with her father came in 1993, when he could not remember making one of his favorite movies (Ellis, 2004). Soon afterward, Reagan noticed that he sometimes felt disoriented. His wife, Nancy, however, said that she noticed no problems at all and was "dumbfounded" when her husband was diagnosed with Alzheimer's disease. Experts have commented (in Ellis, 2004) that the tendency to overlook problems is common among those closest to the

patients—it's easy to deny serious problems when they present subtle symptoms.

As Reagan's symptoms became worse, Nancy was faced with the reality of his symptoms and her increasing loneliness (Ellis, 2004). Despite their resources and fame, Nancy felt isolated, a typical experience for those who are caregivers for Alzheimer's patients. She wrote, "But no one can really know what it's like unless they've traveled this path—and there are many right now traveling the same path I am. You know that it's a progressive disease and that there's no place to go but down, no light at the end of the tunnel. You get tired and frustrated, because you have no control and you feel helpless" (Reagan, 2000, p. 184).

Unlike the other millions of cases of Alzheimer's disease, Ronald Reagan's case stirred public interest, and his family's activism spurred research initiatives. The 109th Congress of the United States passed a bill to amend the Public Health Service Act; this bill, known as the Ronald Reagan Alzheimer's Breakthrough Act of 2005, provides increased funding for Alzheimer's disease research, more help for caregivers, and greater efforts in public education and prevention. Alzheimer's disease is one of the chronic diseases that have increased in frequency and will continue to do so, unless research finds a cure or preventive.

This chapter looks at the consequences of living with chronic illnesses such as Alzheimer's disease, diabetes, asthma, and AIDS. These and other chronic illnesses share many elements. The

diseases vary in physiology, but the emotional and physical adjustments, the disruption of family dynamics, the need for continued medical care, and the necessity of self-management also apply to such chronic diseases as arthritis, heart disease, cancer, kidney disease, multiple sclerosis, head injury, and spinal cord injury.

THE IMPACT OF CHRONIC DISEASE

The diagnosis of chronic disease may be interpreted as a crisis (Moos & Schaefer, 1984), but other models provide alternative ways of conceptualizing the impact of chronic disease. Several models specify stages through which people pass in their adjustment to chronic disease, but a review (Stanton, Revenson, & Tennen, 2007) indicated little research support for stage models. Instead, adjustment seems to be a dynamic process influenced by the characteristics of the disease, such as rapidity of progress; characteristics of the individual, such as a dispositional optimism; and characteristics of the person's social environment, such as social support. More useful models may come from an acknowledgment of the variable nature of the adjustment process and an acceptance of individual factors as important moderators of that process (Parker, Schaller, & Hansmann, 2003). Any useful model must stress adaptation, emphasizing that successful adjustment to chronic disease is a process of adapting to changes that chronic disease brings, changes that affect the patient and the family.

Impact on the Patient

Adapting to chronic disease includes dealing with the symptoms of the disease, managing the stresses of treatment, living as normal a life as possible, and facing the possibility of death. Adjustment to some chronic diseases is more difficult than others because of symptom severity and the demands of coping with symptoms. However, quality of life may be affected less than healthy people imagine (Damschroder, Zikmund-Fisher, & Ubel, 2005). Research that evaluated the functioning of large groups of patients with a variety of chronic illnesses (Arnold et al., 2004; Heijmans et al., 2004) found similarities and differences among people with different chronic diseases. For some chronic diseases, such as hypertension and diabetes, people reported levels of functioning similar to those with no chronic disease. However, people with heart disease, rheumatoid arthritis, and cancer experienced more intrusive symptoms than did those with hypertension, asthma, or diabetes. Psychological functioning showed the strongest relationship to quality of life, highlighting the contribution of adaptation and coping (Arnold et al., 2004). Using a variety of coping strategies allowed people to deal with the stresses of chronic disease (Heijmans et al., 2004); however, active coping strategies tend to produce better results than avoidant strategies (Stanton et al., 2007).

Receiving treatment for chronic diseases also requires adaptation. Interactions with the health care system are likely to create frustrations and problems for people with chronic illness (Parchman, Noel, & Lee, 2005). When patients are forced to interact with the health care system, they tend to feel deprived not only of their sense of competence and mastery but also of their rights and privileges. That is, sick people begin to be treated as "nonpersons" and to experience loss of personal control and threats to self-esteem (Stanton et al., 2007).

Developing and maintaining relationships with health care providers also present challenges, for both patients and practitioners. The medical system and people's experience of illness are oriented toward acute conditions. This experience may lead sick people to believe in the power of modern medicine and to be optimistic about cures. Physicians and other health care workers usually share this attitude (Bickel-Swenson, 2007), which may play a role in creating a positive climate of trust and optimism for their treatment. Conversely, people with a chronic illness may have a hopeless and even helpless attitude toward their condition—modern medicine can offer them no cure. This attitude is often reflected in their relationship with their health care professionals, who also tend to be oriented toward providing cures. When they cannot do so, they may feel less positive about those whom they cannot cure (Bickel-Swenson, 2007; Turner & Kelly, 2000). These feelings can create a difficult climate for treatment, with patients questioning and resisting health care providers, and providers feeling frustrated and annoyed with patients who fail to follow treatment regimens and do not get better. Such negative attitudes may be diminishing among younger physicians (Lloyd-Williams, Dogra, & Petersen, 2004), which will benefit treatment and may help to counteract the growing difficulty in negotiating the U.S. health care system experienced by people with chronic conditions.

People with chronic diseases tend to adopt a number of coping strategies to deal with their illness. A variety of strategies can be successful, but some work better in certain situations. For example, avoidance-oriented coping, such as denial or ignoring the problem, is typically a less effective strategy than problem-focused strategies, such as planning and information seeking (Livneh &

Antonak, 2005; Stanton et al., 2007). However, when events are uncontrollable, avoidance coping may be effective in easing negative emotions; when events are controllable, this strategy would be a very poor choice. Attaining a sense of control was one of the themes that emerged in an analysis of individuals with a variety of chronic illnesses (Cagle, 2004). Feeling overwhelmed after receiving a diagnosis was common, and emotion-focused strategies of coping, such as joining a support group, worked for many people. A second theme involved longer-range adjustments. Successful strategies focused on self-care, including maintaining an overall healthier lifestyle and finding ways to maintain good relationships with health care providers.

Physicians often feel less than adequately prepared to help patients deal with these emotional reactions (Bickel-Swenson, 2007; Turner & Kelly, 2000). Such deficits have led to two types of supplements: psychological interventions and support groups. For many chronic illnesses, health psychologists have created interventions that emphasize the management of emotions such as anxiety and depression. Support groups have also addressed emotional needs by providing emotional support to patients or family members who must confront an illness with little chance of a cure. These services supplement conventional health care and help chronically ill patients maintain compliance with the prescribed regimen and sustain a working relationship with health care providers. A meta-analysis of studies dealing with the effectiveness of psychosocial interventions with cancer patients (Osborn, Demoncada, & Feuerstein, 2006) indicated that cognitive behavioral interventions provided effective assistance in relieving depression and anxiety. Another meta-analysis of studies dealing with the effectiveness of programs for managing chronic disease (Weingarten et al., 2002) showed that a variety of behavioral, informational, and educational methods helped patients adjust emotionally and functionally to their symptoms and their treatment. A large-scale review of studies (Barlow & Ellard, 2004) indicated that cognitive behavioral interventions are most effective for children and adolescents with chronic diseases as well as for their family members.

A major impact of chronic illness involves the changes that occur in how people think of themselves; that is, the diagnosis of a chronic disease changes self-perception. Chronic illness and treatment force many patients to reevaluate their lives, relationships, and body image (Livneh & Antonak, 2005). Being diagnosed with a chronic illness represents a loss (Murray, 2001), and people adapt to such losses through a process of grieving (Rentz, Krikorian, & Keys, 2005). Finding meaning in the experience of loss is more extensive than grieving, but developing an understanding of the meaning of the loss is an important part of coping with chronic disease. Some chronically ill people never move past the grief (Murray, 2001). Other people reconstruct the meaning of their lives in positive ways.

People with chronic diseases often find some positive aspect to their situation (Folkman & Moskowitz, 2000). Part of healthy adjustment is accepting the changes that disease brings, but some research (Fournier, de Ridder, & Bensing, 2002) found that positive expectancies and even unrealistic optimism were advantages in coping with chronic disease. As Annette Stanton and her colleagues (2007, p. 568) summarized, "A disease that disrupts life does not preclude the experience of joy." Thus, some people manage to experience personal growth through loss and grief (Hogan & Schmidt, 2002). This outcome applies not only to patients with chronic diseases but also to their families and caregivers.

Impact on the Family

Illness requires adaptation not only for people who are ill but also for their families. Families may react with grief and feel loss during the sick person's lifetime because families see the person's loss of abilities and sometimes the sense of self.

Involving family members in psychosocial interventions may have additional benefits for all (Martire, Lustig, Schulz, Miller, & Helgeson, 2004), but some emphases are more effective components than others. For example, interventions that emphasize communication and interactions—especially those affecting health—provide greater benefits for patients than interventions with other components (Martire & Schulz, 2007). People with chronic illness also benefit from a type of support that can be described as "invisible" (Bolger et al., 2000). This type of interaction may be easier to manage when a partner is not ill; a sick partner needs help, but being the obvious recipient of assistance makes that support stressful as well as helpful. Therefore, chronic illness presents difficulties even to well-intentioned, caring partners.

Although the rates of childhood diseases declined dramatically in the 20th century, a significant number of children still experience chronic diseases (Brace, Smith, McCauley, & Sherry, 2000). The majority of these illnesses are relatively minor, but many children experience severe chronic conditions such as cancer, asthma, rheumatoid arthritis, and diabetes—conditions that limit mobility and activity. These illnesses bring changes in the lives of the entire family. Parents and siblings try to "normalize" family life while coping with therapy for the sick child (Knafl & Deatrick, 2002). However, parents may experience shock, grief, and anger. For example, the parents of children newly diagnosed with Type 1 diabetes exhibited grief for the loss of their formerly healthy child (Lowes et al., 2005). Such parents face the task of providing support and care, plus the adjustments that chronically ill patients face in finding meaning in the experience of illness. Siblings also face challenges in adjusting to the illness of a family member, tending to notice the differences between their families and "normal" families and feeling some combination of sympathy for and resentment of their sick sibling (Waite-Jones & Madill, 2008a).

For adults, the changes that come with illness can alter their relationships and redefine their identity, but for children who are sick, illness can be even more distressing and disruptive. For some children, the restrictions that come with chronic illness are very difficult, leading to isolation, depression, and distress, whereas other children cope more effectively (Melamed, Kaplan, & Fogel, 2001). Younger children have cognitive difficulties in conceptualizing the nature of their disease, and older children and adolescents may resent the restrictions that their disease imposes. Health care providers and parents can help these children make adjustments by offering alternative or modified activities.

Families of sick children face problems similar to couples: They must continue their relationships and manage the problems of caregiving (Knafl & Deatrick, 2002). A child who is ill requires a great deal of emotional support, most of which is supplied by mothers. These efforts can leave mothers so drained that they have little emotional energy left for their husbands, which can leave husbands feeling abandoned and excluded from the family. Fathers tend to cope by concealing their distress and through avoidance, which is seldom an effective coping strategy (Waite-Jones & Madill, 2008b).

Recommendations for families include trying to be flexible and establishing a family routine that is as close to normal as they can manage (Knafl & Deatrick, 2002). One example of this would be to put the disease into the background and focus on the ways in which the sick child is similar to other children and other family members. Magnifying the ways that the disease makes the child different and focusing on the changes to family routine tend to lead to poorer adaptations. Families should find ways to meet sick children's needs without reinforcing their anxiety and depression (Brace et al., 2000). Like individuals with chronic illness, families tend to make a better adjustment if they focus on finding meaning and some positive aspect in their situation (Ylvén, Björck-Åkesson, & Granlund, 2006).

Another task for families is finding ways to express their negative emotions, such as anger and frustration over their situation. Families with sick children should also set aside time for themselves and not spend all their energy caring for the sick child. Many parents of sick children join support groups to help them meet their emotional needs. In addition to helping families manage their emotions, support groups also provide information about their child's condition. Both emotional support and information are useful.

IN SUMMARY

Chronic diseases bring changes that require adaptation for both the person with the disease and family members. Chronically ill patients must manage their symptoms, seek appropriate health care, and adapt to the psychological changes that occur in this situation. Their social and emotional needs may be neglected by health care professionals who attend to the patients' physical needs. Health psychologists and support groups help provide for the emotional needs associated with chronic illness. The adaptations that occur may lead to prolonged feelings of loss and grief or to changes that constitute personal growth.

LIVING WITH ALZHEIMER'S DISEASE

Alzheimer's disease, a degenerative disease of the brain, is a major source of impairment among older people (Mayeaux, 2003). This disease varies in prevalence among countries but remains a major source of cognitive disability in both industrialized and developing countries. Medical researchers identified the brain abnormalities that underlie Alzheimer's disease in the late 19th century. In 1907, a German physician, Alois Alzheimer, reported on the relationship between autopsy findings of neurological abnormalities and psychiatric symptoms before death. Shortly after his report, other researchers began to call the disorder Alzheimer's disease.

The disease can be diagnosed definitively only through autopsy, but brain imaging technology is capable of diagnosing Alzheimer's disease with close to 90% accuracy (Vemuri et al., 2008). In addition, Alzheimer's patients show behavioral symptoms of cognitive impairment and memory loss that may lead to a provisional diagnosis (Mayeaux, 2003). During autopsy, a microscopic examination of the brain reveals "plaques" and tangles of nerve fibers in the cerebral cortex and hippocampus. These tangles of nerve fibers are the physical basis for Alzheimer's disease.

The biggest risk factor for Alzheimer's disease is age; the incidence of Alzheimer's disease rises sharply with advancing age. The prevalence of Alzheimer's disease is low for those under age 75— about 9% of people in this age group (Fitzpatrick et al., 2004; Lindsay, Sykes, McDowell, Verreault, & Laurin, 2004). However, the percentage of affected individuals doubles about every five years, so that by age 85, almost 50% of individuals exhibit

signs of Alzheimer's disease. The increase seems not to continue at the same rate; people in their 90s who have not developed signs of the disease are not nearly as likely to do so as people between ages 65 and 85 (Hall et al., 2005). The high number of people over 85 years old who have symptoms of probable Alzheimer's disease presents a pessimistic picture for the aging population in many industrialized and some developing countries, where Alzheimer's seems destined to become a large public health problem (Haan & Wallace, 2004).

The underlying mechanisms in the development of the disease are not yet completely understood, but research has identified two different forms of the disease: an early onset version that occurs before age 60 and a late onset version that occurs after age 60. The early onset type is quite rare, representing fewer than 5% of all Alzheimer's patients (Bertram & Tanzi, 2005). Early onset Alzheimer's can be traced to a genetic defect, and at least three different genes on chromosomes 1, 14, and 21 contribute.

The late onset type has symptoms similar to the early onset type but begins after age 60, as President Reagan's disease did. Susceptibility to this version of the disease also has a genetic component related to apolipoprotein ε, a protein involved in cholesterol metabolism (Bertram & Tanzi, 2005; Ertekin-Taner, 2007). One form of apolipoprotein, the ε4 form, affects accumulation of the amyloid ε protein, which forms the building blocks for amyloid plaque (Selkoe, 2007). This plaque seems to constitute the underlying pathology for Alzheimer's disease. The risk increases by about three times for individuals who have one ε4 gene and about 15 times for individuals who have two. Older adults who do not have Alzheimer's disease but who carry the ε4 variant of this gene show lower levels of cognitive functioning than those with other variants of the gene (Small, Rosnick, Fratiglioni, & Bäckman, 2004). The ε2 form of the gene may actually offer some protection against Alzheimer's disease.

The genetic contribution is not straightforward inheritance but rather a susceptibility. A variety of environmental and behavioral factors play a role in the development of Alzheimer's disease, interacting with the genetics of the disease. For example, having a stroke increases the risk,

WOULD YOU BELIEVE . . . ?

Using Your Mind May Help Prevent Losing Your Mind

Although age and genetics contribute to the risk of developing Alzheimer's disease, not everyone of the same age or even with the same genes is at equal risk. Your intelligence, education, job, and even your television viewing habits also contribute to the risk.

People with more education have a lower risk of developing Alzheimer's disease. Because education and IQ are strongly related, separating the protective effect of education is not easy, but one study (Pavlik, Doody, Massman, & Chan, 2006) estimated that IQ score, not educational level, was a better predictor of the progression of Alzheimer's disease. This result suggests that being intelligent offers some protection against this

disease. Other research, however, hints that being intelligent is by no means completely protective.

What you do with your mind may be more important than how intelligent you are in combating Alzheimer's disease. For example, the complexity of people's jobs affects the risk. In a study of pairs of twins, in which one twin had been diagnosed with Alzheimer's disease and the other had not (Andel et al., 2005), a distinguishing feature was the complexity of work performed by the unaffected twins. Because the study involved twins, genetic factors could not have played a role. The results indicated that those whose work involved more complexity, in terms of tasks with people or data, were likely to be unaffected by the disorder. This

result suggests that using your mind is protective.

Work complexity is not the only type of mental activity that may offer protection. A study of leisure time activities (Lindstrom et al., 2005) found that leisure activities during middle age could be protective or risky. People who participated in intellectually stimulating leisure and social activities were at lower risk of Alzheimer's disease during their older years, whereas those who watched television were at increased risk. Indeed, each additional daily hour of television viewing raised the risk. So, using your mind during young and middle age may protect against the development of Alzheimer's disease later in life—presenting another case of "use it or lose it."

and so does head injury (Pope, Shue, & Beck, 2003). These risks may apply more strongly to people who carry the ε4 form of the gene for apolipoprotein. Type 2 diabetes increases the risk for Alzheimer's disease, but the combination of ε4 apolipoprotein and diabetes raises the risk more than five times (Peila, Rodriguez, & Launer, 2002). The process of inflammation is also a risk for Alzheimer's, as it is for cardiovascular disease (Martins et al., 2006). This risk may accrue throughout life, with increased risk for people who experience prolonged bouts of inflammation, even during young or middle adulthood (Kamer et al., 2008). Fat intake during middle adulthood also increases the risk (Laitinen et al., 2006), but high cholesterol during older age has no relationship (Reitz et al., 2008).

Research into risk factors for Alzheimer's disease has also revealed some protective factors. Cognitive activity decreases the risk, so people whose jobs demand a high level of cognitive processing

are less likely to develop Alzheimer's disease than others with less cognitively demanding jobs (see Would You Believe . . . ?). Low levels of alcohol consumption cut the risk in half in one study (Ruitenberg et al., 2002). Regular doses of nonsteroidal anti-inflammatory drugs (NSAIDs) also appear to decrease the risk. An epidemiological study (In'tVeld et al., 2001) found that people who took NSAIDs such as ibuprofen or aspirin for two years or longer showed a sharply decreased risk for Alzheimer's disease. A controlled study (Szekely et al., 2008) confirmed the benefit of NSAIDs (but not acetaminophen) for lowering the risk of Alzheimer's disease, but only for people who carry the ε4 form of the apolipoprotein gene. Therefore, it is possible to modify the genetic risk through this behavior. Many of the risks for Alzheimer's disease overlap with those for cardiovascular disease and cancer, and so do the protective factors. That is, a healthy lifestyle may offer protection for a range of disorders.

TABLE 11.1

Risks and Protective Factors for the Development of Alzheimer's Disease

Risks	Protective Factors
Age—over age 65 presents increasing risk	
Inheriting apolipoprotein ε4	Inheriting apolipoprotein ε2
Stroke, head injury, or diabetes, especially for those who carry apolipoprotein ε4	
Inflammation	Taking anti-inflammatory drugs (NSAIDs)
High-fat diet during middle adulthood	
Low levels of education	Higher levels of education
Cognitively undemanding job	Cognitively demanding job
	Low-to-moderate alcohol intake

Table 11.1 presents a summary of these risks and protective factors.

Because the symptoms of Alzheimer's include a number of behavior problems that are also symptoms of psychiatric disorders, the disease can be difficult to diagnose. These symptoms occur in a majority of people with Alzheimer's disease (Weiner, Hynan, Bret, & White, 2005). In addition to memory loss, behavioral symptoms include agitation and irritability, sleep difficulties, delusions such as suspiciousness and paranoia, inappropriate sexual behavior, and hallucinations. People with Alzheimer's disease are more likely than similar others to engage in dangerous behavior (Starkstein, Jorge, Mizrahi, Adrian, & Robinson, 2007). Even individuals with mild Alzheimer's disease show psychiatric symptoms similar to those with more severe cases (Shimabukuro, Awata, & Matsuoka, 2005). These behavioral symptoms can be the source of much distress to patients as well as to their caregivers, and more severe behavioral symptoms predict shorter survival times (Weiner et al., 2005).

The most common psychiatric problem among Alzheimer's patients is depression, with as many as 20% of patients exhibiting symptoms of clinical depression (van Reekum et al., 2005). Depression may even precede the development of Alzheimer's disease, serving as a risk factor. The experience of negative mood is especially common among people in the early phases of the disease and in early onset Alzheimer's. Those who retain awareness of their problems find their deterioration distressing and respond with feelings of helplessness and depression.

The memory loss that characterizes Alzheimer's patients may first appear in the form of small, ordinary failures of memory, which represent the early stages of the disease (Morris et al., 2001). This memory loss progresses to the point that Alzheimer's patients fail to recognize family members and forget how to perform even routine self-care; former President Reagan experienced these losses. In the early phases of the disease, patients are usually aware of their memory failures, as Reagan was, making this symptom even more distressing.

The common symptoms of paranoia and suspiciousness may also relate to cognitive impairments. Alzheimer's patients may forget where they have put belongings and, because they cannot find their possessions, accuse others of taking them. However, suspicious and accusatory behaviors are not limited to misplaced belongings. Verbal aggression was noted in about 37% of Alzheimer's patients and physical aggression in about 17% (Weiner et al., 2005).

Although difficulties in staying asleep are common among older adults, Alzheimer's patients have even more severe problems than their peers (Tractenberg, Singer, & Kaye, 2005). As a result, these patients tend to wander at all times of the day and night. This behavior can disturb those who sleep in the same house and provide opportunities for patients to injure themselves. Incontinence and sexual behaviors are acutely distressing to both patients and their caregivers, and incontinence is very common in patients with advanced cases of Alzheimer's disease. A pattern of behavioral symptoms, such as Ronald Reagan exhibited, is strong indication of Alzheimer's disease and the only means of diagnosis before autopsy.

Helping the Patient

At present, Alzheimer's disease remains without a cure. However, incurability and untreatability are two different things; the physical symptoms and other accompanying disorders of Alzheimer's disease can be treated. Although researchers have worked toward developing drugs that would prevent the disease, the primary focus of treatment has been on the use of drugs to slow its progress. Treatment approaches include drugs for delaying the progression of cognitive deficits and neuroleptic drugs for reducing agitation and aggression. Unfortunately, a systematic review (Seow & Gauthier, 2007) indicated that the drugs that target cognitive deficits offer only modest benefits. For some patients, these drugs slow the progress of the disease by months or even a few years, but they do not stop or cure it. One drug (donepezil) slows the loss of neurons in the hippocampus, the brain location critical for formation of new memories. This finding explains why this drug is effective for some Alzheimer's patients in delaying cognitive losses. Another drug (mematine) also shows benefits for cognitive measures and overall functioning. In addition, some researchers (Langa, Foster, & Larson, 2004) have found some benefits of statin drugs, typically prescribed for cardiovascular patients, in slowing the dementia associated with Alzheimer's disease.

Behavioral approaches can be helpful for people with Alzheimer's disease. These approaches include sensory stimulation and reality orientation to help Alzheimer's patients retain their cognitive abilities. A systematic review (Verkaik, Van Weert, & Francke, 2005) indicated that a few programs have demonstrated some effectiveness. Those that show the most promise are programs that provide pleasant stimulation, such as music, aromatherapy, and exposure to sunlight, and programs that concentrate on cognitive skills and

problem solving. Music therapy may be more useful than other types of sensory stimulation (Svansdottir & Snaedal, 2006). A meta-analysis of programs to develop cognitive skills (Sitzer, Twamley, & Jeste, 2006) indicated that such programs can be helpful in improving memory, verbal and visual learning, and activities of daily living. In addition, caregivers can manage behavior problems of Alzheimer's patients through improvements in communication and modification of the environment to help decrease confusion and manage problem behaviors (Yuhas, McGowan, Fontaine, Czech, & Gambrell-Jones, 2006). For example, locking exit doors may prevent wandering. For those who get lost in their own homes, labeling the doors can be helpful.

Although none of these treatments can cure Alzheimer's disease, most will help control undesirable behaviors and alleviate some of the distressing symptoms of the disease. Any treatment that can delay symptoms of Alzheimer's disease can make a significant difference in the number of cases and in the costs of management (Haan & Wallace, 2004). In the early phases of Alzheimer's disease, both patients and their families are distressed by its symptoms, but as the patient worsens and loses awareness, the stress of Alzheimer's becomes more severe for the family. The burden of caregiving is one factor in the decision to have a family member institutionalized (Mausbach et al., 2004), which adds to the cost of this disease.

Helping the Family

As with other chronic illnesses, Alzheimer's disease affects not only patients but also family members, who bear the burden of caregiving. Some of the distressing symptoms can make caregiving difficult—caring for a spouse or parent who may be abusive and no longer recognizes you is a very difficult task. Cognitive impairments lead to changes in behavior that may make the affected one no longer seem like the same person.

Caregiving affects families in industrialized and developing countries similarly: Caring for a family member with a dementing disease such as Alzheimer's creates a burden for families (Prince, 2004). This burden is emotional and practical. The problems of taking care of an Alzheimer's patient require time, demand new skills, and greatly disrupt family routine.

In the United States (Cancian & Oliker, 2000) and around the world (Prince, 2004), the caregiver role is occupied mostly by women. In a study of those providing care for older family members with memory impairments (Chumbler, Grimm, Cody, & Beck, 2003), almost 70% were women; daughters were about twice as likely as spouses to be providing such care. Unfortunately, the anger and suspiciousness that are common symptoms of Alzheimer's disease are more distressing to female than to male caregivers (Bédard et al., 2005), so that women tend to feel more burdened by providing care than men do. Their tasks may be burdensome indeed. A survey of Alzheimer's caregivers (Georges et al., 2008) indicated that these tasks may occupy more than 10 hours a day when the recipients of care are late-stage dementia patients.

The chronic stress of caregiving makes these family members of interest to psychoneuroimmunologists, who have studied how this chronic stress affects the immune system. Janice Kiecolt-Glaser and her colleagues (2002) have studied Alzheimer's caregivers and found that they experience poorer physical and psychological health and poorer immunological function than people of similar age who are not caregivers. Also, the level of impairment of the Alzheimer's patient is directly related to the level of distress in the caregiver (Robinson-Whelen et al., 2001); that is, the more impaired the patient, the more distressed the caregiver. Furthermore, their distress does not decrease when their caregiving ends (Aneshensel, Botticello, & Yamamoto-Mitani, 2004). Thus, caregiving imposes severe burdens, extending even after the death of the Alzheimer's patient.

Recognition of the burdens of caregiving has prompted increased attention to and assistance for these individuals. For example, programs now exist to help people develop the skills they will need to be effective caregivers for someone with Alzheimer's disease (Paun, Farran, Perraud, & Loukissa, 2004). Caregivers do not feel so overwhelmed when they have the knowledge and skills to perform the necessary tasks. A review of such interventions (Gallagher-Thompson & Coon, 2007) indicated that this approach is

successful. Support groups can also be sources of information about caring for patients and about community resources that provide respite care. Many support groups exist to provide information and emotional support for caregivers. In addition, the Internet can be a source of support. An online and telephone-based service provides support to caregivers who have not received assistance from other sources (Glueckauf, Ketterson, Loomis, & Dages, 2004).

Alzheimer's caregivers frequently experience feelings of loss for the relationship that they once shared with the patient; these feelings of loss may begin with a partner's diagnosis (Robinson, Clare, & Evans, 2005). Making sense of dementia and adjusting to the loss is a strain for partner and family. However, only 19% of those caring for someone with Alzheimer's disease reported only strains (Sanders, 2005); most found positive aspects to their caregiving, such as feelings of mastery and personal and spiritual growth. In most ways, Nancy Reagan was more fortunate than the typical caregiver. She was able to hire others to help her provide care for her husband, but she and the Reagan family felt helpless and frustrated as they saw the former president progressively losing abilities (Ellis, 2004). Nancy said that she needed and appreciated the support of the many people who sent letters. Nancy's feelings of isolation and frustration were typical of caregivers for Alzheimer's patients, but Nancy and the Reagan family struggled to find meaning in their experience. One way that they did so was to become activists in the effort to find a cure or prevention for Alzheimer's disease.

IN SUMMARY

Alzheimer's disease is a progressive, degenerative disease of the brain that affects cognitive functioning, especially memory. Other symptoms include agitation and irritability, paranoia and other delusions, sleep disorders, wandering, depression, and incontinence. These symptoms are also indicative of some psychiatric disorders, making Alzheimer's disease difficult to diagnose and distressing to both patients and caregivers.

Increasing age is a risk factor for Alzheimer's disease, with as many as half the people over 85 exhibiting symptoms. Both genetics and environment seem to play a role in development of the disease; both early and late onset varieties exist.

At this point, treatment is largely oriented toward slowing the progress of the disease, managing the negative symptoms, and helping family caregivers cope with the stress. Drug treatments intended to slow the progress of the disease have limited effectiveness, but help some people. Management of symptoms can include providing sensory and cognitive stimulation to slow cognitive loss and changing the environment to make care less difficult. Training and support are also desirable for those who provide care to Alzheimer's patients, because caregivers are burdened by the demands of caring for someone with this disease.

ADJUSTING TO DIABETES

In 1989, actress Halle Berry had a role in a television sitcom and was working longer, harder hours than she ever had (Siegler, 2003). She had no opportunity to rest when she was tired or to eat a candy bar when she felt that her blood glucose level was low. Berry has **diabetes mellitus**, and her failure to take care of herself caused her to go into a coma that lasted seven days. Despite that terrifying experience, Berry says that she left the hospital feeling better than she had in years. She sees the experience as a "wake-up call" that forced her to attend to her health. Now she is very careful about her diet, exercise, and stress. She regulated her blood glucose level by taking insulin, but in October 2007, Berry announced that she had cured herself of diabetes through a healthy diet and no longer took insulin (Goldman, 2007). Her remarks caused a furor because Berry had been diagnosed with Type 1 diabetes, for which there is no cure; if she no longer requires insulin injections, then her diabetes was really Type 2 all along. Her diagnosis, behavior, and even her misunderstanding of her disease illustrate some of the challenges presented by diabetes.

Gregg DeGuire/WireImage/Getty Images

Actress Halle Berry has followed a diet and exercise regimen to control her diabetes and managed to have a healthy pregnancy.

The Physiology of Diabetes

Before examining the psychological issues in the management of diabetes, let's look more closely at the physiology of the disorder. The **pancreas**, located below the stomach, produces different types of secretions. The **islet cells** of the pancreas produce several hormones, two of which, glucagon and insulin, are critically important in metabolism. **Glucagon** stimulates the release of glucose and therefore acts to elevate blood sugar levels. The action of **insulin** is the opposite. Insulin decreases the level of glucose in the blood by causing tissue cell membranes to open so glucose can enter the cells more freely. Disorders of the islet cells result in difficulties in sugar metabolism. Diabetes mellitus is a disorder caused by insulin deficiency. If the islet cells do not produce adequate insulin, sugar cannot be moved from the blood to the cells for use. Lack of insulin prevents the blood sugar level from being regulated by the body's control mechanisms. Excessive sugar accumulates in the blood and also appears in abnormally high levels in the urine. When Halle Berry went into a coma in 1989, she thought she was going to die, and she might have. Both coma and death are possibilities for uncontrolled diabetes.

The two types of diabetes mellitus are (1) insulin-dependent diabetes mellitus (IDDM), also known as Type 1 diabetes, and (2) non-insulin-dependent diabetes mellitus (NIDDM), also known as Type 2 diabetes. Type 1 diabetes is an autoimmune disease that occurs when the person's immune system attacks the insulin-making cells in the pancreas, destroying them (Permutt, Wasson, & Cox, 2005). This process usually occurs before age 30 and leaves the person without the capability to produce insulin and thus dependent on insulin injections. Type 1 diabetes was Halle Berry's diagnosis when she fell into a coma; her age and symptoms were consistent with Type 1 diabetes, but that diagnosis may have been incorrect. People with Type 1 diabetes do not recover from this disease.

Halle Berry was diagnosed with Type 1 diabetes and followed the demands and restrictions of that regimen for years, including insulin injections, daily exercise with a personal trainer, and a low-fat/low-carbohydrate diet with lots of vegetables, fish, and chicken but few fruits and sweets. In 2007, Berry announced that she had "weaned" herself off insulin and now considered herself to have Type 2 diabetes (Goldman, 2007). Medical experts said that she was mistaken; no one can make a transition from Type 1 to Type 2 diabetes. It is likely that her initial diagnosis was mistaken and that she always had Type 2 diabetes.

Until a few years ago, Type 2 diabetes was called adult onset diabetes because it typically developed in people past the age of 30. However, Type 2 diabetes has begun to appear among children and adolescents, accounting for at least 33% of diabetes cases among this age group (Ludwig & Ebbeling, 2001). This trend appears not only in the United States but also in developed countries throughout the world (Malecka-Tendera & Mazur, 2006). For both children and adults, Type 2 diabetes affects ethnic minorities disproportionately, and those who develop this disease are often overweight, sedentary, and poor. The characteristics of both types of diabetes are shown in Table 11.2. A third type of diabetes is *gestational diabetes*, which develops in some women during pregnancy. Gestational diabetes ends when the pregnancy is completed, but the disorder complicates pregnancy and presents a risk for the development of Type 2 diabetes in the future (Reader, 2007).

The management of all types of diabetes requires lifestyle changes in order for the person to adjust to the disease and to minimize health complications. Diabetes requires daily monitoring of blood sugar levels and relatively strict compliance with both medical and lifestyle regimens to

TABLE 11.2

Characteristics of Type 1 and Type 2 Diabetes Mellitus

Type 1	Type 2
Onset occurs before age 30	Onset may occur during childhood or adulthood
Patients are underweight	Patients are overweight
Patients experience frequent thirst and urination	Patients may or may not experience frequent thirst and urination
Affects equal numbers of men and women	Affects more women than men
Has no socioeconomic correlates	Affects more poor than middle-class people
Requires insulin injections	Requires no insulin injections
Carries risk of kidney damage	Carries risk of cardiovascular damage
Accounts for 10% of diabetics	Accounts for 90% of diabetics

regulate blood sugar. Like other chronic diseases, diabetes can be controlled but not cured.

In addition to the danger of coma, the inability to regulate blood sugar often causes people with diabetes to have a host of other health problems. Oral or injected insulin can control the most severe symptoms of insulin deficiency but does not mimic the normal production of insulin. People with diabetes still experience elevated levels of blood sugar, which seem to be involved in the development of (1) damage to the blood vessels, leaving diabetics prone to cardiovascular disease (diabetics are twice as likely as other people to have hypertension and to develop heart disease); (2) damage to the retina, leaving diabetics at risk for blindness (diabetics are 17 times as likely to go blind as nondiabetics); and (3) kidney diseases, leaving diabetics prone to renal failure. In addition, diabetics, compared with nondiabetics, have double the risk of cancer of the pancreas (Huxley, Ansary-Moghaddam, de González, Barzi, & Woodward, 2005).

The Impact of Diabetes

The diagnosis of any chronic disease produces an impact on patients for two reasons: first, the emotional reaction to having a lifelong incurable disease, and second, the lifestyle adjustments required by the disease. For diabetes that begins during childhood, both children and their parents must come to terms with the child's loss of health (Lowes, Gregory, & Lyne, 2005) and the management of the disorder, which includes careful restrictions in diet, insulin injections, and recommendations for regular exercise. Dietary restrictions include careful scheduling of meals and snacks as well as adherence to a set of allowed and disallowed foods.

Diabetics must test their blood sugar levels at least once (and possibly several times) a day, drawing a blood sample and using the testing equipment correctly. The results guide diabetics to appropriate levels of insulin. Injections are the standard mode of administration for Type 1 diabetics, and the daily (or more frequent) injections can be a source of fear and stress. Alternative modes of testing and insulin administration are desirable because drawing blood samples and

taking injections are painful, and diabetics tend to perform less testing and fewer injections than would be optimal in managing their blood sugar.

Alternatives to finger-prick testing are available, but their accuracy is not as good as that of standard testing. Other modes of insulin administration have been developed, including external or implanted insulin pumps and inhaled insulin. Pumps are appropriate for some individuals, including children and adolescents, providing more stable blood glucose levels (Pickup & Renard, 2008). An inhaled form of insulin was available for several years, but its manufacturer withdrew it from the market because of safety concerns ("Exubera Lung Cancer Warning," 2008). Although blood glucose testing and insulin administration are critically important, these aspects of diabetes care present difficulties for most diabetics.

Non-insulin-dependent (Type 2) diabetes often does not require insulin injections, but this type of diabetes does require lifestyle changes and oral medication. African Americans, Hispanic Americans, and Native Americans are at higher risk for Type 2 diabetes than are European Americans (Peek, Cargill, & Huang, 2007), and being overweight is a risk for all groups. Indeed, gaining weight increases, and losing weight decreases, the risk for Type 2 diabetes (Black et al., 2005). Therefore, frequent components of treatment are weight loss and a healthy diet.

Type 2 diabetics must deal with dietary restrictions and attend to their schedule of oral medication. Diabetes often affects sexual functioning in both men and women, and diabetic women who become pregnant often have problem pregnancies. Halle Berry announced that she was pregnant in 2007 (Bonilla, 2007). Although Halle Berry said that she felt some fear in connection with her pregnancy, she expressed a great deal more optimism and joy. Her fame and wealth allowed her to obtain excellent medical care, and her faithful adherence to her diabetes care helped minimize the potential complications; she gave birth to a healthy baby girl in 2008.

Type 2 diabetes is more likely to cause circulatory problems, leaving these individuals prone to cardiovascular problems, which is their leading cause of death. Both women (Hu et al., 2000)

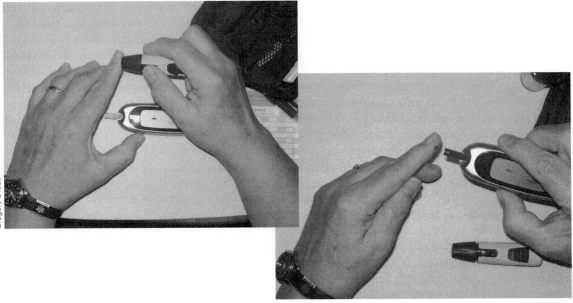

Gregory Draus

Learning to test blood sugar is one of the skills that people with diabetes must master and practice regularly.

and men (Lotufo et al., 2001) with Type 2 diabetes are at dramatically increased risk for death from all causes, but especially from cardiovascular disease.

Some diabetics deny the seriousness of their condition and ignore the need to restrict diet and take medication. Others acknowledge the seriousness of their problems but believe that the recommended regimen will be ineffective (Skinner, Hampson, & Fife-Schaw, 2002). Others become aggressive; they either direct their aggression outward and refuse to comply with their treatment regimen or turn their aggression inward and become depressed. Finally, many diabetics become dependent and rely on others to take care of them, thus taking no active part in their own care. All these reactions can interfere with the management of blood sugar levels and lead to serious health complications, including death.

Health Psychology's Involvement With Diabetes

Health psychologists are involved in both researching and treating diabetes (Gonder-Frederick, Cox, & Ritterband, 2002). Psychologist Richard Rubin became head of the American Diabetes Association in 2006, and he emphasized the role of psychology: "I want more and more people to understand that behavior and emotion play a part in diabetes and how that affects human and economic outcomes" (quoted in Dittmann, 2005, p. 35).

Research efforts have concentrated on the effect of stress on glucose metabolism, the ways that diabetics understand and conceptualize their illness, the dynamics of families with diabetic children, and the factors that influence patient compliance with medical regimens. Health psychologists orient their efforts toward improving adherence to medical regimens so diabetics can control their blood glucose levels and minimize health complications.

Stress has been hypothesized to play two roles in diabetes: as a possible cause of diabetes and as a factor in the regulation of blood sugar in diabetics. To examine the role of family stress in the development of diabetes, a team of researchers (Sepa et al., 2005) followed a large group of infants for the first year of their lives, measuring family stress and taking blood samples to test for signs of the autoimmune response that underlies Type 1 diabetes. The results revealed that stress may be involved in the development of diabetes. However, a prospective study with Native Americans (Daniels, Goldberg, Jacobsen, & Welty, 2006) found no relationship between stress during adulthood and subsequent development of Type 2 diabetes.

Several studies indicate that stress affects glucose metabolism and control. Two studies examined the role of stress in metabolic control of adolescents (Farrell et al., 2004) and adults (Weisli et al., 2005) with Type 1 diabetes. Both found that stressful negative events predicted poorer metabolic control after a meal. A study of people with Type 2 diabetes (Surwit et al., 2002) showed that adding a stress management component to diabetes education has a small but significant effect on blood sugar levels. Depression is another factor that affects diabetics and worsens blood glucose control (Lustman & Clouse, 2005). Thus, negative emotions can adversely affect diabetes, and interventions to manage stress and depression can be a worthwhile (and cost-effective) component for diabetes management programs.

Health psychologists also research diabetic patients' understanding of their illness and how that understanding affects their behavior. Both patients and health care workers assume that patients understand the disease and recognize the symptoms of high and low blood glucose levels. These assumptions are not always true. For example, people's perception of the risk of developing diabetes is neither accurate nor based on their existing risk factors, even for physicians (Walker, Mertz, Kalten, & Flynn, 2003). Rather, having a close friend or family member with diabetes was a circumstance that raised the perception of vulnerability (Montgomery, Erblich, DiLorenzo, & Bovbjerg, 2003). Perceptions also affect how people with diabetes care for themselves. Their conceptualizations of diabetes affect their coping behavior (Searle, Norman, Thompson, & Vedhara, 2007). For example, belief in the consequences of diabetes predicted the use of problem-focused coping strategies, and those who believed they were able to control their diabetes were more likely to use their medication.

Inaccurate beliefs can have a significant impact on self-care. In a study of the interrelationships among beliefs, personality characteristics, and self-care behavior among diabetics (Skinner et al., 2002), beliefs emerged as the most important component. The perceived effectiveness of the treatment regimen predicted all aspects of diabetes self-care. This finding emphasizes the importance of diabetes education in building adherence to the diet, exercise, and medication regimen that is necessary to control blood glucose levels.

Complete adherence to the medication and lifestyle regimen is rare (Cramer, 2004). As Chapter 4 explored, a number of factors are related to poor adherence, and diabetes combines several of these factors. First, complexity makes adherence more difficult, and second, making lifestyle changes is more difficult than taking medication. Diabetics must do both. Third, they must also perform blood sugar testing several times a day, even when they feel well. Fourth, their adherence will not cure the disease, and serious complications may be years away. Thus, poor adherence is common, and improving adherence is of primary concern to psychologists involved in providing care for diabetics.

The role of health psychology in diabetes management is likely to expand, because behavioral components are important in controlling blood glucose levels. Indeed, lifestyle changes can prevent the development of diabetes in individuals who exhibit blood glucose tolerance problems (Gillies et al., 2007). A behavioral component can add to the effectiveness of educational programs for diabetic patients. Education alone is not adequate in helping diabetics follow their regimen (Rutten, 2005). Because situational factors such as stress and social pressure to eat the wrong foods affect adherence, programs with a behavioral skills training component might be a valuable addition to diabetes management training. A program that fostered feelings of control (Macrodimitris & Endler, 2001) improved diabetics' adherence to diet, exercise, and blood glucose testing, and another program (Rosal et al., 2005) used a cognitive behavioral framework to increase self-management skills in low-income Spanish-speaking diabetics.

Although behavior-based strategies can improve patients' control, some authorities (Glasgow & Anderson, 1999; Rutten, 2005) have argued that diabetes management needs to change its emphasis from patient compliance to patient responsibility and self-management. They have urged health care professionals to make changes in their approach to dealing with patients to form cooperative alliances and to help diabetics develop the responsibility and skills they need to manage their disease. People who are diabetic are totally responsible for their own care; health care professionals should help them do a good job.

IN SUMMARY

Diabetes mellitus is a chronic disease that results from failure of the islet cells of the pancreas to manufacture sufficient insulin, affecting blood glucose levels and producing effects in many organ systems. Type 1 diabetes is an autoimmune disease that typically appears during childhood; Type 2 diabetes also affects children but is more typical of people over age 30. People with diabetes must maintain a strict regimen of diet, exercise, and insulin supplements to avoid the serious cardiovascular, neurological, and renal complications of the disorder.

As with other chronic diseases, a diagnosis of diabetes mellitus produces distress for both patients and their families. Health psychologists have studied adjustment to the disorder and compliance with the necessary lifestyle changes. Few people with diabetes adhere to all aspects of blood glucose testing, medication, diet, and exercise that minimize the risks of health complications. Skills training programs have shown some success in helping diabetics manage their disorder, but health care professionals need to find ways to encourage the development of responsibility and self-management in order to put diabetics in charge of their own health.

THE IMPACT OF ASTHMA

Seeing Jackie Joyner-Kersee out of breath was not unusual for those who followed women's track and field events in the 1980s and 1990s. Joyner-Kersee won six Olympic gold medals performing in events such as the long jump and the heptathlon (which includes seven events), so she struggled frequently to get her breath. What she hid for years from most people, including her coaches and teammates, was that she also experienced asthma attacks (Moran, 2002). Her asthma attacks brought her to the emergency room on several occasions, but she persisted in ignoring and denying her problem. She says that doing so nearly cost her life—she had a nearly fatal attack. Similar to Halle Berry and her diabetic coma, Jackie Joyner-Kersee took this health crisis as a wake-up call. She became careful about her health, and she now participates in a program to bring the message about the dangers of asthma to children across the United States.

The number of people with asthma grew throughout the 1980s and into the 1990s in the United States but began to decrease by the late 1990s (American Lung Association, 2007). About 18 million adults in the United States have asthma (8.5%), but the rate is highest for children and adolescents between 5 and 17 years old. For all age groups, the rates are higher for African Americans than for other ethnic groups. The death rate from asthma is not high, and that mortality rate has decreased in recent years, but asthma is the largest cause of disability among children and the leading cause of missed school days, making it a serious health problem in the United States.

The Disease of Asthma

Asthma is a chronic inflammatory disease that causes constriction of the bronchial tubes, preventing air from passing freely. People experiencing an asthma attack will wheeze, cough, and have trouble breathing; such an attack can be fatal. At other times they appear to be fine, but the underlying inflammation remains (Cohn et al., 2004).

Asthma shares some features with chronic obstructive lung diseases (COLD) such as chronic bronchitis and emphysema, but asthma also differs in some ways (Barnes, 2008). All of these conditions involve inflammation, though not to the same extent or through the same immune system mechanisms. But the most important difference is that people with COLD experience constant problems, whereas people with asthma may go for long periods of time without any problems in breathing.

The cause of asthma is not understood. Indeed, asthma may not be one disease but rather a number of diseases that share symptoms yet have differences in underlying pathologies (Wenzel, 2006). Until recently, experts believed that asthma was an allergic reaction to substances in the environment, but several newer explanations involve more complex reactions of the immune system (Cohn et al., 2004; Renz, Blümer, Verna, Sel, & Garn, 2006). One view holds that a genetic vulnerability makes some infants' immune systems respond with an allergic reaction to substances in the environment that other infants' immune systems encounter without problems. This *diathesis–stress model* is a variation on the traditional view that asthma is an allergic reaction triggered by environmental allergens. These allergens include an assortment of common substances such as tobacco smoke, household dust (along with dust mites), cockroaches, animal dander, and environmental pollutants. People with the vulnerability who are exposed to the substance to which they are sensitive develop asthma; those who are not exposed fail to develop asthma or show such mild symptoms that they are not diagnosed.

Another view, called the *hygiene hypothesis*, holds that asthma is a result of the cleanliness that has become common in modern societies (von Hertzen & Haahtela, 2004). Infants have undeveloped immune systems, and in hygienic environments they encounter too little dirt and too few bacteria, leaving their immune systems underprepared to deal with these substances. Exposure then leads to overresponsiveness, which produces inflammation; this inflammation forms the basis for asthma. A refinement of the hygiene hypothesis (Martinez, 2001) combines elements of genetic vulnerability and early exposure to substances in the environment that influence immune system development to either sensitize or protect children from asthma and allergic conditions.

Both of these views (and the combination) are consistent with some of the evidence about asthma. Support for the genetic vulnerability view is found in a study of the Hutterites, a religious group that immigrated to the United States from Europe in the 1870s (Shell, 2000). Symptoms of asthma are very uncommon among the Hutterites, who nevertheless show high rates of the type of inflammation that characterizes asthma. The rural, farming lifestyle of these people puts them into contact with few of the triggers for asthma attacks, leaving these vulnerable individuals without serious symptoms. However, the children of parents from underdeveloped countries who immigrate to industrialized countries tend to have asthma at rates similar to those of other children in the industrialized country (von Hertzen & Haahtela, 2004). That is, the combination of genetic vulnerability, underdevelopment of the immune system, and exposure to triggers results in asthma.

As the hygiene hypothesis suggests, asthma is more common in developed countries that emphasize cleanliness and a hygienic environment for infants. For example, asthma is less common in rural China than in the United States, Sweden, Australia, and New Zealand (von Hertzen & Haahtela, 2004). However, within the United States, asthma is more common in the urban inner city, where air pollution is more common, and research has confirmed the risk of high levels of air pollution for the development of asthma (Islam et al., 2007). In addition, asthma varies with ethnicity, and African Americans, such as Jackie Joyner-Kersee, are more vulnerable than people from other ethnic groups (American Lung Association, 2007).

Other risk factors for asthma include sedentary lifestyle and obesity (Gold & Wright, 2005). People take few deep breaths when they are sedentary, which may be the link between lack of exercise and asthma. In addition, staying indoors exposes people to some of the allergens that provoke asthma attacks. The link between asthma and obesity is significant: Obese people are two to three times more likely to have asthma than nonobese people. Psychological factors also show a relationship with the development of asthma (Chida, Hamer, & Steptoe, 2008), serving as predictors of its development and appearing as a result of living with the disease. Depression is a specific psychological factor that is related to asthma (Strine, Mokdad, Balluz, Berry, & Gonzalez, 2008). Although the factors related to the development of asthma are complex and not completely understood, the triggers for attacks are better known.

Triggers are substances or circumstances that cause the development of symptoms, provoking the narrowing of the airways that cause difficulty in breathing. The substances include allergens such as mold, pollen, dust and dust mites, cockroaches, and animal dander; infections of the respiratory tract; tobacco or wood smoke; and irritants such as air pollutants, chemical sprays, or other environmental pollution (Harder, 2004). The circumstances include exercise and emotional reactions such as stress or fear. Any of these substances and experiences may provoke an attack, but most people with asthma are sensitive to only a few. Identifying an individual's triggers is part of managing asthma.

Managing Asthma

Managing asthma shows some similarities (and similar problems) to managing diabetes. Both disorders require frequent contact with the health care system, can be life threatening, affect children and adolescents, impose restrictions on lifestyle, and pose substantial adherence problems (Elliott, 2006). People with diabetes may manage their blood sugar levels so that they have no symptoms, but even with careful management, people with asthma have attacks. The underlying inflammation of the bronchial tract is always present, but a person with asthma may go for weeks or months without an attack. Minimizing attacks is the primary goal of managing asthma. Daily attention to symptoms and status improves the chances of avoiding attacks, and behaviors are critical.

Managing asthma requires a variety of medications as well as learning personal triggers and avoiding them (Courtney, McCarter, & Pollart, 2005). To decrease the chances of an attack, people with asthma must take medication, which is usually an anti-inflammatory corticosteroid or some other medication that decreases the respiratory inflammation that underlies asthma. These drugs require daily attention and have unpleasant side effects, such as weight gain and lack of energy. The schedule may be very complicated, and as Chapter 4 detailed, complexity decreases compliance with medical regimens. The side effects also contribute to problems

in adherence. Thus, adherence to their preventive medication is a major problem for people with asthma, especially for children and adolescents (Asthma Action America, 2004; Elliott, 2006).

When people with asthma have an attack, they have trouble breathing or cannot breathe. Gasping for breath, they either use a bronchodilator to inhale medication that relieves the symptoms or go to a hospital emergency room for treatment (Asthma Action America, 2004). If used improperly, bronchodilators produce a type of "high," and asthma experts believe that most people with asthma rely on bronchodilators too much and on preventive medication too little. More than 20% of people with asthma use their inhalers improperly, decreasing the effectiveness of this important device (Molimard & Le Gros, 2008). Relying on emergency rooms for managing asthma is an expensive choice and contributes to rising medical costs.

A large-scale survey (Asthma Action America, 2004) revealed widespread misunderstandings and misperceptions concerning asthma among parents and other caregivers. Misunderstandings included what underlies the condition and what constitutes adequate management; misperceptions included the frequency of children's symptoms. People with asthma also hold incorrect beliefs about the disease (Elliott, 2006). For example, they may believe that asthma is not a serious disease or that it is an intermittent disease that does not require daily care. All of these misperceptions may affect appropriate care.

Boosting self-care and increasing adherence to medication regimens are major goals for improving asthma care. A number of interventions have targeted these goals, with some success. Many of these interventions have been oriented toward education for people with asthma, assuming that when people understand the severity of the disease and the steps that are necessary to manage it, they will adhere. Research has not supported those assumptions; interventions that are basically educational may increase knowledge but are not very successful in changing behavior (Bussey-Smith & Rossen, 2007; Coffman, Cabana, Halpin, & Yelin, 2008). Interventions with a behavioral component, such as developing self-care (Guevara, Wolf, Grum, &

Clark, 2003) or providing a written action plan (Bhogal, Zemek, & Ducharme, 2006), tend to be more successful. Adhering to the medication and behavioral regimen to control this disorder is a challenge for people with asthma, but behavioral interventions represent a promising strategy for helping them take their medication and avoid situations that precipitate attacks.

IN SUMMARY

Asthma is a chronic disease that involves inflammation of the bronchial tubes, which leads to difficulties in breathing. Substances such as smoke or allergens and situations such as fear can trigger attacks that have symptoms of coughing, wheezing, and choking. The cause for the inflammation that underlies asthma remains unknown, but theories include a genetic component and an overreaction of the immune system that occurs in hygienic environments.

Asthma usually develops during childhood, and children and adolescents experience problems in coping with their disease. People with asthma need to take medication to decrease the chances of attacks and identify their triggers so as to avoid them. The complex schedule of medications and their unpleasant side effects contribute to adherence problems. A major goal of treatment is to help people with asthma take medication to prevent attacks rather than rely on inhaled medications to stop symptoms or use hospital emergency room assistance. Behavioral strategies to increase compliance and self-management skills have shown some success.

DEALING WITH HIV AND AIDS

Earvin "Magic" Johnson was the best basketball player in the world when he retired in 1991 ("Then and Now," 2005). That retirement came as a surprise, but his announcement that he was HIV positive was more so. A routine physical examination by a team physician had revealed that he was infected with the human immunodeficiency virus (HIV). Until that announcement, HIV infection was considered a disease of gay

European Americans, and Johnson was neither. Johnson's openness about his HIV status helped to change public opinion about this disease, and his celebrity status enabled him to raise money for HIV research and education. More than 17 years after his diagnosis, Johnson remains healthy and has become an advocate for increasing minority participation in clinical trials. He attributes his continued health to someone who participated in a clinical trial for the many drugs that were developed to treat HIV infection (Gambrill, 2008).

AIDS is a disorder in which the immune system loses its effectiveness, leaving the body defenseless against bacterial, viral, fungal, parasitic, cancerous, and other opportunistic diseases. Without the immune system, the body cannot protect itself against the many organisms that can invade it and cause damage. (For a more complete discussion of the immune system and its function, see Chapter 6.) The danger from AIDS comes from the opportunistic infections that start when the immune system no longer functions effectively. In this way, AIDS is similar to the immune deficiency in children who have been born without immune system organs and are susceptible to a variety of infections.

AIDS is the result of exposure to a contagious virus, the **human immunodeficiency virus (HIV)**. So far, two variants of the human immunodeficiency virus have been discovered: HIV-1, which causes most AIDS cases in the United States; and HIV-2, which is responsible for most AIDS cases in Africa, although some HIV-2 cases have appeared in the United States. The progression from HIV infection to AIDS varies, and people such as Magic Johnson who are HIV positive may remain free of AIDS symptoms for many years.

Incidence and Mortality Rates for HIV/AIDS

AIDS appears to be a relatively new disease, first recognized in 1981 and identified in 1983. The disease originated in Africa in a virus that affects monkeys (Moore, 2004). How and when that virus was transmitted to humans remains the subject of controversy. The first confirmed case of AIDS appeared in the Congo in 1959, but the disease was very limited. During the 1960s, the disease spread

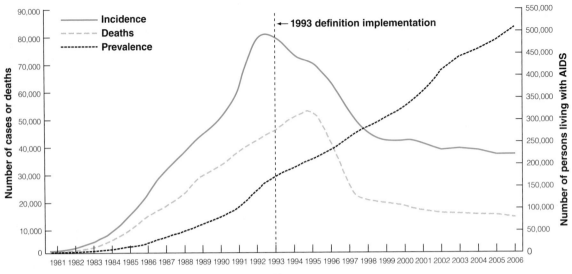

FIGURE 11.1 Incidence, prevalence, and deaths from AIDS cases by year, United States, 1981–2005.

Sources: "Update, AIDS—United States, 2000," by R. M. Klevens & J. J. Neal, 2002, *Morbidity and Mortality Weekly Report*, vol. 51, no. 27, p. 593; *HIV/AIDS Surveillance Report, 2002*, by Centers for Disease Control and Prevention, 2004, vol. 14; *HIV/AIDS Surveillance Report, 2006*, by Centers for Disease Control and Prevention, 2008, vol. 18.

to Haiti and from there to other places in North America and the world (Gilbert et al., 2007). Both the number of new cases and the number of deaths from AIDS spread during in the 1980s.

In the mid-1990s, death rates from AIDS declined sharply in the United States, but only recently has the rate begun to level worldwide (UNAIDS, 2007). AIDS remains among the leading causes of death in the world, and the leading cause of death in Africa. According to one estimate (Lamptey, 2002), AIDS is the deadliest plague in history. Almost 40 million people were infected by 2001; when those people die, HIV will surpass the number of people killed by the bubonic plague in the 14th century. About 2.5 million people acquire HIV infection each year, which represents a decline in the rate of infection, but also poses a number that extends this plague (UNAIDS, 2007). Despite intensive efforts to find a vaccine that would prevent the disorder, no successful vaccine yet exists (Sahloff, 2005), but drugs have been successful in extending the life of people who are infected (UNAIDS, 2008).

In 1992, the Centers for Disease Control and Prevention (CDC, 1992) revised its definition of HIV infection so that incidence figures from 1992

and subsequent years are not directly comparable to earlier figures. The number of cases in 1992 appears to rise sharply (see Figure 11.1), but this count includes a large backlog of people who in previous years would not have been classified as having AIDS. As Figure 11.1 shows, AIDS cases reported each year (incidence) began a steady decline after 1992.

Incidence has declined, but mortality from this disease has dropped even more. In the United States, deaths in 2004 were 27% of what they had been in 1995, a decrease far greater than for any other leading cause of death (USCB, 2007). One reason the number of deaths from AIDS has declined is that HIV-infected individuals are living longer. People diagnosed with AIDS in 1984 had an average survival time of 11 months (Lee, Karon, Selik, Neal, & Fleming, 2001), whereas 84% of people diagnosed in 2002 were alive more than three years later (CDC, 2008). Magic Johnson is an example of this increased life expectancy for HIV-positive individuals; Johnson has lived more than 17 years since his diagnosis.

The number of people living with AIDS (prevalence) continues to increase, as Figure 11.1 shows, but combinations of antiretroviral drugs have changed the course of HIV infection, drastically slowing the progression of infection and prolonging lives (UNAIDS, 2008). This increased survival time is a result of more effective drug therapies, early detection, and lifestyle changes. Giving up unhealthy habits such as smoking, drinking alcohol, and taking illicit drugs; becoming more vigilant about their health; and exercising more control over their treatment can help infected persons live longer and healthier lives (Chou, Holzemer, Portillo, & Slaughter, 2004). An optimistic attitude also contributes to longevity (Moskowitz, 2003).

The HIV and AIDS Epidemics

In the United States and Europe, HIV infection was first associated with gay men, but an analysis of people infected with HIV reveals at least four distinct epidemics of the infection. These four epidemics exist around the world, but the proportion of people infected by each differs a great deal. For example, men who have sex with men accounted for many of the first U.S. and European cases of AIDS, but in Africa and some parts of Asia, heterosexual sex is the most common method of transmission, and in some parts of Asia, Thailand, and India, injection drug use fuels the epidemic (UNAIDS, 2007). Male–male sexual contact is still the leading source of HIV infection in the United States. This mode of transmission declined during the 1990s, but has increased slightly during the past few years; it now accounts for less than half of HIV transmissions in the United States (CDC, 2008).

A second epidemic affects injection drug users, with the percentage of these cases declining in the United States but growing in parts of Central Europe and Asia (UNAIDS, 2007). A third epidemic involves transmission through heterosexual contact; this number is decreasing slowly in the United States and Western Europe but remains the main mode of infection in Africa. A fourth epidemic occurs through transmission from women to their children during the birth process. This mode of transmission has decreased sharply with the availability of antiretroviral medication for pregnant women who are HIV positive. Throughout the countries in Africa with

the highest prevalence of AIDS, young pregnant women were less likely to be HIV positive in 2007 than in 2001 (UNAIDS, 2007), which predicts a decrease in this mode of transmission.

In the United States and Europe, HIV infection affects men much more often than women (see Figure 11.2). As of 2006, women accounted for about 23% of AIDS cases in the United States (CDC, 2008). Women in the United States are exposed to HIV infection primarily through two routes of transmission: heterosexual contact (about 66% of cases) and injection drug use (about 32% of cases). Worldwide, the situation differs from that in the United States: Women account for 50% of the AIDS cases, and most are exposed through heterosexual contact (UNAIDS, 2007).

Minority ethnic groups in the United States have been affected disproportionately, especially by the epidemics affecting heterosexuals and injection drug users. As Magic Johnson has pointed out ("Then and Now," 2005), African Americans have become the largest segment of the U.S. population with HIV; by 2006, they accounted for 44% of people living with AIDS (CDC, 2008). European Americans accounted for 35% of the cases, Hispanic Americans 19%, and Asian Americans about 1%. The trend toward declining rates of HIV infection has not occurred for minorities as rapidly as for European Americans, creating a disproportionate number of ethnic minorities with HIV. As of 2006, African American women made up 60% of women diagnosed with HIV (CDC, 2008). Figure 11.3 shows the percentages of men and women of different ethnic backgrounds infected with HIV.

Age is also a factor in HIV infection. The birth process is one mode of transmission, so some infants and children are HIV infected, but only about 1% of AIDS cases are in people younger than 13 (CDC, 2008). Young adults are more likely to be infected than other age groups, largely due to their risky behaviors, lack of information about HIV, and lack of power to protect themselves from unsafe sex (Mantell, Stein, & Susser, 2008). Recent analyses have indicated that this situation is improving, at least in Africa. People over age 50 are less likely to be infected than younger adults, but when infected, they tend

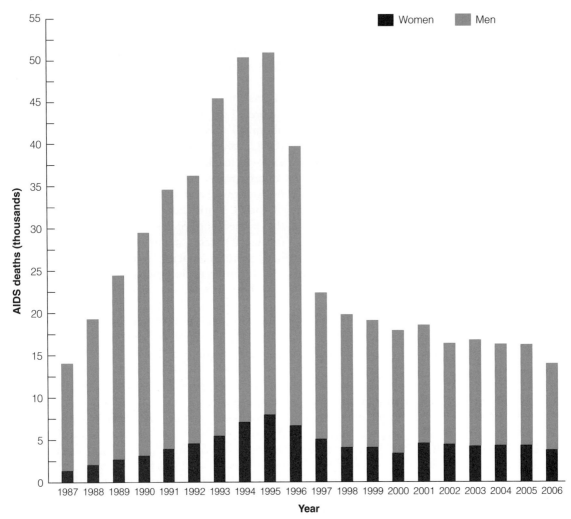

FIGURE 11.2   Deaths from AIDS by gender, United States, 1987–2006.

Sources: HIV/AIDS Surveillance Reports, 1989 (Table 13), *1991* (Table 13), *1993* (Table 14), and *2003* (Table 7), by Centers for Disease Control and Prevention, retrieved July 31, 2002, and July 10, 2005, from www.cdc.gov/hiv/stats.htm; *HIV/AIDS Surveillance Report, 2006*, by Centers for Disease Control and Prevention, 2008, vol. 18 (Table 7).

to develop AIDS more rapidly and to get more opportunistic infections (CDC, 2008).

Symptoms of HIV and AIDS

Typically, HIV progresses over a decade or more from infection to AIDS, but the progression varies. During the first phase of HIV infection, symptoms are not easily distinguishable from those of other diseases. Within a week or so of infection, people may (or may not) experience symptoms consisting of fever, sore throat, skin rash, headache, and other symptoms that resemble the flu (Cibulka, 2006). This phase lasts from a few days to four weeks and is typically followed by a period that may last as long as 10 years during which infected people are asymptomatic or experience only minimal symptoms. The immune systems of infected people are being destroyed during this time, even though the infected individuals may remain unaware of their HIV status.

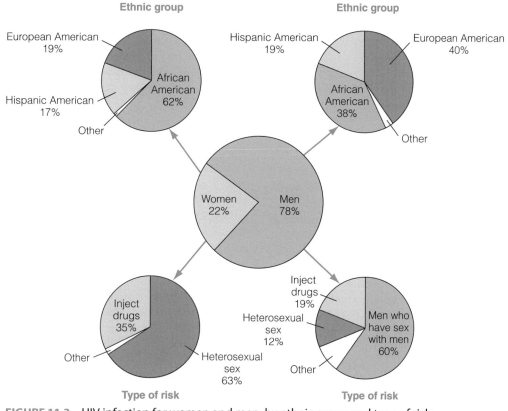

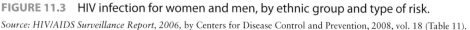

FIGURE 11.3   HIV infection for women and men, by ethnic group and type of risk.

Source: HIV/AIDS Surveillance Report, 2006, by Centers for Disease Control and Prevention, 2008, vol. 18 (Table 11).

People who go untreated usually progress to symptoms, which is the beginning of HIV disease (Cibulka, 2006). Early symptomatic HIV disease occurs when a person's CD4+ T-lymphocyte cell count drops and the person's immune system becomes less able to fight infections. When the CD4+ count falls to 200 or less per cubic millimeter of blood (healthy people have a CD4+ count of 1,000), the person has AIDS. As their immune system begins to lose its defensive capacities, people with early symptomatic HIV disease become susceptible to various opportunistic infections that a healthy immune system would resist. They may experience weight loss, persistent diarrhea, white spots in the mouth, painful skin rash, fever, and persistent fatigue.

As the supply of CD4+ T-lymphocytes is depleted, the immune system loses an important mechanism for fighting infections within cells. The diseases associated with HIV are caused by a variety of agents, including viruses, bacteria, fungi, and parasites. The HIV virus damages or kills the part of the immune system that fights *viral* infections, leaving no way for the body to fight HIV. But HIV does not destroy the antibodies that the immune system has already manufactured, so the immune system response that occurs through antibodies circulating in the blood remains intact. Therefore, HIV disease does not often cause a person to develop, for example, infections with the bacterium that causes strep throat or the virus that causes influenza. Most HIV-infected people have antibodies to fight against these common agents.

As their CD4+ count falls to the level defining AIDS, people are subject to lung, gastrointestinal, nervous system, liver, bones, and brain damage from infections from otherwise rare organisms, which leads to such diseases as *Pneumocystis carinii* pneumonia, Kaposi's sarcoma, tuberculosis, and toxoplasmic encephalitis. Symptoms include greater weight loss, general fatigue, fever, shortness of breath, dry cough, purplish bumps on the skin, and AIDS-related dementia.

The Transmission of HIV

Although HIV is an infectious organism with a high fatality rate, the virus is not easily transmitted from person to person. The main routes of infection are from person to person during sex, from direct contact with blood or blood products, and from mother to child during pregnancy, birth, or breastfeeding (UNAIDS, 2007). Concentrations of HIV are especially high in the semen and blood of infected people. Therefore, contact with infected semen or blood is a risk. Other body fluids do not contain such a high concentration of HIV, making contact with saliva, urine, or tears much less of a risk. No evidence exists that any sort of casual contact spreads the infection. Eating with the same utensils or plates or drinking from the same cup as someone who is infected does not transmit HIV, nor does touching or even kissing someone who is infected. Insect bites do not spread the virus, and even being bitten by someone who is infected is not likely to infect the person who is bitten.

People most at risk for HIV infection are those affected by causes of the four epidemics: male–male sexual contact, injection drug use, heterosexual contact, and transmission from mother to baby. Each of the groups reflected by these four epidemics experiences somewhat different risks.

Male–Male Sexual Contact In the early years of AIDS, men who had sex with men made up the majority of AIDS cases in North America and Western Europe. HIV infection rates have decreased among gay and bisexual men, but this group still remains the largest risk group in these countries (CDC, 2008). Among gay and bisexual men, unprotected anal intercourse is an especially risky behavior, particularly for the receptive partner. Because the delicate lining of the rectum is often damaged during anal intercourse, the receptive person is at high risk if his partner is infected with HIV. The damaged rectum makes an excellent route for the virus to enter the body, and infected semen has a high concentration of HIV. Unprotected oral sex with an infected partner is also a risky practice because HIV can enter the body through any tiny cut or other lesion in the mouth.

Condom use became common among gay men, but as treatment became more effective, gay men became less concerned with contracting HIV (Kalichman et al., 2007), and a subculture of gay men are attracted to unprotected anal intercourse, despite their knowledge of its dangers (Shernoff, 2006). Using alcohol or other drugs contributes to the decision to have unprotected sex (Celentano et al., 2006). In addition, the Internet has become a meeting place for men who want to have casual sex with other men, and these encounters are less likely to include condoms than other types of meetings (Garofalo, Herrick, Mustanski, & Donenberg, 2007). Thus, risky sexual behaviors continue to put men who have sex with men in danger of HIV exposure.

Injection Drug Use Another high-risk behavior is the sharing of unsterilized needles by injection drug users, a practice that allows the direct transmission of blood from one person to another. Injection drug use is the second most frequent source of HIV infection in the United States (CDC, 2008). Some injection drug users engage in this behavior in certain situations—for example, when intoxicated or when there is no immediate access to sterile drug equipment. Some evidence (Heimer, 2008) indicates that relatively small-scale needle exchange programs can be effective in controlling HIV infection in a variety of communities.

Transmission through injection drug use accounts for a greater percentage of infected African Americans and Hispanic Americans than European Americans (CDC, 2008). Also, a higher percentage of infected women than men are exposed to the virus through this route. Several behavioral factors are related to HIV infection for women who inject drugs, including the number of sex partners and whether they have traded sex for money or drugs. These behaviors increase the chances for transmission through heterosexual sex.

Heterosexual Contact Heterosexual contact is the leading source of HIV infection in Africa (UNAIDS, 2007), but in the United States, heterosexual sex accounts for about 30% of cases (CDC, 2008). African Americans and Hispanic Americans are disproportionately represented among those infected through heterosexual contact, and women from these two ethnic backgrounds are in greater danger than men from heterosexual contact.

This gender asymmetry comes from ease of transmission during sexual intercourse. Although men are susceptible to HIV through sexual contact with women, male-to-female transmission is eight times more likely than female-to-male transmission. Despite women's greater likelihood of being infected through heterosexual sex, they tend to see their sexual partners as safer than men do (Crowell & Emmers-Sommers, 2001).

Trust and confidence in one's partner in a heterosexual relationship may be unfounded and result in HIV infection. One study (Crowell & Emmers-Sommers, 2001) questioned HIV-positive individuals, who looked back at their sexual attitudes, beliefs, and behaviors and assessed a high level of trust in their partners and a low level of perceived risk for themselves. Another study (Klein, Elifson, & Sterk, 2003) found that women who perceived themselves to be at some risk behaved in ways that raised their risks, but half of women who felt no risk still engaged in at least some risky behaviors. Thus, people's overly trusting view of partners and failure to accept the possibility of risks lead to unprotected sex. Regular use of condoms may provide a high level of safety for heterosexual men and women, but many young heterosexual couples use condoms more as a means of preventing pregnancy than of preventing HIV (Bird, Harvey, Beckman, & Johnson, 2000).

Transmission During the Birth Process Another group at risk for HIV infection is children born to HIV-positive women. This transmission tends to occur during the birth process. Breastfeeding can also transmit the virus (Steinbrook, 2004). Children infected with HIV during the birth process suffer a variety of developmental disabilities, including intellectual and academic impairment, psychomotor dysfunction, and emotional and behavioral difficulties (Mitchell, 2001). In addition, many of these children are born to mothers who ingested drugs during pregnancy and thus are put at further risk for developmental difficulties.

Most individuals who are HIV positive are within their reproductive years, and knowledge of HIV-positive status does not necessarily deter people from reproduction (Delvaux & Nostlinger, 2007). Both HIV-positive women and men may wish to have children, and the family traditions of some Asian cultures push couples toward decisions to reproduce (Ko & Muecke, 2005). With people who are HIV positive, reproduction is a risk for the child. Semen carries HIV that may be transmitted to the fetus, and transmission during the birth process is likely unless the HIV-positive mother undergoes antiretroviral therapy. Therefore, seeking prenatal counseling and care are critically important for HIV-positive women and men who wish to start a pregnancy. Early prenatal care can reduce the risk of transmission from mother to child to about 1%.

Psychologists' Role in the HIV Epidemic

From the beginning of the AIDS epidemic, psychologists have had an important role in combating the spread of infection (Kelly & Kalichman, 2002). During the early years of the epidemic, psychologists were involved in both primary and secondary prevention efforts. Primary prevention includes changing behavior to decrease HIV transmission. Secondary prevention includes helping people who are HIV positive to live with the infection, counseling people about being tested for HIV, helping patients deal with social and interpersonal aspects of the disease, and helping patients adhere to their complex treatment program. Much of the improvement in length of survival of HIV-infected patients rests with the effectiveness of drug treatments, highly active antiviral therapy (HAART). This treatment consists of a combination of pills that must be taken on a strict schedule, making adherence a challenge. Psychologists' knowledge concerning adherence to medical regimens is now relevant to managing HIV infection.

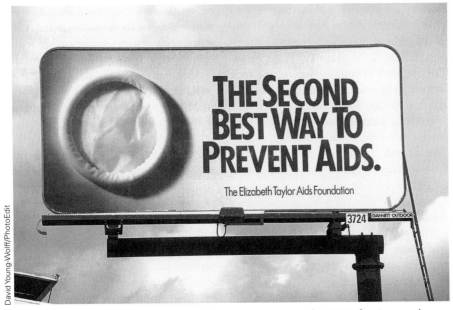

Psychologists have been involved in primary prevention for HIV infection, such as promoting condom use.

Encouraging Protective Measures Except for infants born to HIV-infected mothers, most people have some control in protecting themselves from the human immunodeficiency virus. Fortunately, HIV is not easily transmitted from person to person, making casual contact with infected persons a low risk. Health care workers who participate in surgery, emergency care, or other procedures that bring them into contact with blood should be careful to prevent infected blood from entering their body through an open wound. For example, dentists and dental hygienists wear protective gloves, and health care workers are taught to adhere to a set of standard protective measures.

Although some risks are specific to certain professions, most people who are infected with HIV were exposed through sexual behavior or by sharing contaminated needles. People can protect themselves against infection with HIV by changing those behaviors that are high risks for acquiring the infection—namely, having unprotected sexual contact or sharing needles with an infected person. Limiting the number of sex partners, using condoms, and avoiding shared needles are three behaviors that will protect the largest

number of people from HIV infection. However, these behaviors have proven difficult to change. A variety of factors contribute to this difficulty.

One factor that makes behavior change difficult is perception of risk. Most people in the United States do not perceive that they are at risk for HIV infection, and they are correct (Holtzman, Bland, Lansky, & Mack, 2001). That is, most adults do not engage in the behaviors that are primary HIV risks. However, some people are at risk and fail to perceive that risk accurately. For example, young men who have sex with men reported overly optimistic beliefs about their risk (MacKellar et al., 2007), as did college students in Nigeria (Ijadunola, Abiona, Odu, & Ijadunola, 2007). Their misperceptions play a role in their continued risky behavior, and culture is an important influence in sexual risk behaviors.

Cultures in which male dominance is supported by social custom or religion and in which women have little access to economic resources also have high rates of heterosexually transmitted HIV, such as countries in sub-Saharan Africa, the Caribbean, and Latin America (UNAIDS, 2007). When women are financially dependent on men and have limited access to economic resources, they may have little control over sexual encounters or even be vulnerable to forced or coerced sex. Thus, they may be unable to negotiate condom use, which increases their risk for infection. These dangers also apply to women in the United States. A study of HIV-positive African American women (Lichtenstein, 2005) confirmed the presence of abuse and dominance as factors in these women's HIV infection, and a large study of young adults confirmed the contribution of alcohol use and violence to HIV transmission (Collins, Orlando, & Klein, 2005).

Taking a cautionary lesson from the worldwide epidemic, authorities in North America and Western Europe understand that containing the heterosexual transmission of HIV is an important goal. Changing sexual behavior is a difficult process that occurs within a complex personal and cultural context, but interventions that consider cultural context and target individuals' social networks may be more effective than those that attempt to change individual behavior (Latkin & Knowlton, 2005).

Helping People With HIV Infection People who believe they may be infected with HIV, as well as those who know that they are, can benefit from various psychological interventions. People who engage in high-risk behaviors may have difficulty deciding whether to be tested for HIV, and psychologists can provide both information and support for these people. Individuals from several high-risk groups have not been tested for HIV, including (1) a significant minority of gay and bisexual men, (2) a significant minority of injection drug users, and (3) a larger proportion of heterosexual men and women with multiple partners and inconsistent use of condoms (Awad, Sagrestano, Kittleson, & Sarvela, 2004). Indeed, many people who are HIV positive have not been tested and thus do not know their HIV status.

The decision to be tested for HIV has both benefits and costs to the individual, but testing is considered essential to the control of HIV infection (Janssen et al., 2003). Far too many people undergo testing after their disease has progressed and treatment options are less effective; a prominent part of Magic Johnson's campaign has tar-

geted early testing and services for people whose tests indicate infection. Early testing for those who are HIV positive allows early treatment, which will prolong their lives and will permit them to find ways to reduce or eliminate behaviors that place others at risk.

The costs of being tested include all the problems of arranging a health care visit, plus the distress that comes with the potential for bad news. Currently, HIV testing is not part of routine health examinations, and individuals must seek testing (Clark, 2006). At least 25% of those with HIV infection are unaware of their status because they have not sought testing. In addition, many people who agree to testing never take steps to learn the results. Alternatives to the standard testing procedure, such as rapid results testing and at-home testing, increase receiving results (Hutchinson, Branson, Kim, & Farnham, 2006).

Learning of HIV-positive status is a traumatic event; people learning of a positive result typically react with increased anxiety, depression, anger, and distress. Using avoidance coping, such as denying reality or clinging to illusory hope, is associated with high levels of psychological distress and with lower levels of CD4+ cells (Mulder, van Griensven, Sandfort, de Vroome, & Antoni, 1999). Using active coping, including problem solving and seeking social support, is related to better adjustment. Receiving support both from health care professionals and from family and friends also leads to better adjustments (Reilly & Woo, 2004). Interventions tailored to the person's specific situation and needs have advantages over less personalized programs (Moskowitz & Wrubel, 2005). Cognitive behavioral interventions can reduce the anxiety, depression, and anger of those who are HIV positive (Crepaz et al., 2008).

Psychologists can also help HIV patients adhere to the complex medical regimens designed to control HIV infection (Kelly & Kalichman, 2002). HAART consists of a combination of antiretroviral medications; patients often take other drugs to combat side effects of the antiretroviral drugs as well as drugs to fight opportunistic infections. These regimens may include as many as a dozen drugs, all of which must be timed precisely. When patients do not follow the schedule,

BECOMING HEALTHIER

1. If you have a chronic illness, understand your condition and form a cooperative relationship with health care professionals. However, take charge of its management yourself; you are the person most affected by your condition.

2. If you are the primary caregiver for someone who is chronically ill, don't ignore your own health—both physical and psychological. Regularly schedule some time for yourself.

3. If you have Type 1 diabetes, don't try to hide your illness from your friends. Although you have a chronic disease, you can live a long and productive life, but you must adhere faithfully to a lifelong regimen that includes diet,

insulin injection, and regular exercise. If you live with someone with diabetes, offer social and emotional support, and encourage that person to stick with required health practices.

4. Know your blood sugar level. Type 2 diabetes can develop at any age, and this disorder may have few symptoms.

5. If you have asthma, try to minimize attacks and use of dilators. Concentrate on taking preventive medication and knowing your triggers to avoid attacks.

6. Protect yourself against HIV infection. The most common mode of transmission is sexual, and condoms make sex safer.

7. If you are the primary caregiver for someone with a

terminal chronic disease such as AIDS or Alzheimer's disease, seek social and emotional support through groups specifically convened to offer such support. Take breaks from caregiving, allowing others to assume those responsibilities for a while.

8. If you have a chronic disease or if you are the caregiver for someone with such a disease, use the Internet to gain information and support. A wide variety of websites offer information, and online support groups are available for all disorders. Do not use these websites as a substitute for health care, but allow these resources to supplement your knowledge and support.

the effectiveness diminishes. Psychologists can help patients adhere to this schedule as well as facilitate their self-management skills. For example, the technique of motivational interviewing appeared to be successful in helping with the scheduling aspect of HAART adherence (DiIorio et al., 2008).

Another aspect of adjustment to HIV infection is finding meaning in the experience and developing the potential for growth and positive experiences. People with AIDS and their caregivers often succeed in finding positive experiences in their lives. In one study (Milam, 2004), 59% of individuals with HIV or AIDS had experienced positive changes, and in another study (Folkman & Moskowitz, 2000), more than 99% of AIDS patients and caregivers were able to recall a positive experience. The search for positive meaning

and other positive cognitions may even influence the course of HIV infection by affecting CD4 count (Ickovics et al., 2006). This quest for positive meaning is common to the experience of many people with chronic illness, and this attitude may also appear in those who are dying.

IN SUMMARY

Acquired immune deficiency syndrome (AIDS) is the result of depletion of the immune system after infection with the human immunodeficiency virus (HIV). When the immune system fails to defend the body, a number of diseases may develop, including bacterial, viral, fungal, and parasitic infections that are uncommon in people who have functioning immune systems.

The modes of transmission of HIV are behavioral, with receptive anal intercourse and the sharing of needles for intravenous drug injection the two behaviors that have spread the infection to the most people in the United States. Unprotected heterosexual contact with an infected partner accounts for a larger proportion of people with HIV worldwide. The number of babies infected with HIV has decreased because antiretroviral drug therapies sharply decrease transmission from an infected mother during the birth process.

Psychologists use a variety of interventions to help patients reduce high-risk behaviors, cope with their illness, manage their symptoms, and adhere to the complex drug regimens that improve survival. In addition, psychologists have provided counseling services for those seeking to be tested and for those whose tests reveal infection. These programs not only encourage protective behaviors but also emphasize the role of positive health in combating AIDS.

FACING DEATH

The increase in life expectancy has affected perceptions of death. People do not necessarily expect a long life, but they prefer it, saying that a life of about 85 years is about right (Lang, Baltes, & Wagner, 2007). However, they also want to have control over the end of their lives, including when and how they die. This desire is consistent with the concept of "the good death," which consists of physical comfort, social support, appropriate medical care, and attempts to minimize psychological distress for the dying person and the family (Carr, 2003). Thus, end-of-life issues encompass those who are dying and those who grieve for them before and after they die.

Adjusting to Terminal Illness

The experience of a "good death" is possible for many. Most of the leading causes of death in the United States and other industrialized countries are associated with chronic diseases such as cardiovascular disease, cancer, chronic lower respiratory disease, Alzheimer's disease, kidney disease, chronic liver disease, and HIV infection. These diseases are often fatal, but death is not sudden,

giving people and their families an opportunity to adjust. Even if the chronic disease does not signal terminal illness, the diagnosis entails loss and thus the need to adapt (Murray, 2001).

The processes of adapting to a chronic condition or a terminal illness should be similar. The notion of stages of adapting to terminal illness was popularized by Elizabeth Kübler-Ross (1969). Kübler-Ross's stages included denial, anger, bargaining, depression, and acceptance. Denial is a failure to accept the validity or the severity of the diagnosis; people use this defense mechanism to deal with the anxiety they experience when they learn of their condition (Livneh & Antonak, 2005). Anger is another emotional reaction, and bargaining often takes the form of trying to negotiate a better outcome, either with God or with health care personnel. Depression is a common response of those who come to understand the progression of their disease, followed by acceptance of the situation.

Although Kübler-Ross hypothesized that these reactions follow a sequence, research has failed to confirm that view (Schulz & Aderman, 1974). Instead, researchers have found that these reactions occur—but not in any set pattern. Therefore, people diagnosed with chronic diseases and people with terminal illness usually exhibit a range of negative reactions, but they may also experience positive responses oriented around growth and finding meaning in their situation.

A more useful conceptualization of adaptation to terminal illness is the notion of the dying role (Emanuel, Bennett, & Richardson, 2007). This role is proposed as an extension of the sick role, which we described in Chapter 3. Like the sick role, the dying role includes certain privileges and responsibilities and can take many forms, both healthy and unhealthy. Three key elements are involved: practical, relational, and personal. The practical element includes the tasks that people need to arrange at the end of their lives, such as arranging financial matters and making plans for medical care as the disease progresses. The relational element involves reconciling the dying role with other roles, such as caregiver, spouse, and parent. This reconciliation may be difficult: the dying role is not automatically compatible with these other roles, so the dying person must work to find ways to integrate these roles. The personal element involves "finishing one's life story" (Emanuel et al., 2007, p. 159). This element may prompt people to reexamine their life while thinking about its end and to derive new meaning from it. This new meaning may constitute a reintegration (Knight & Emanuel, 2007), or some less healthy outcome may occur.

Barriers to a good adjustment include institutional impediments and lack of access to palliative care. Institutional barriers occur when people are not allowed to assume the dying role because health care professionals keep them in the sick role, even through it is inappropriate (Emanuel et al., 2007). Medical care is so oriented toward cures that accepting death may be difficult for medical practitioners. Appropriate care, such as hospice care or support for home care, may be unavailable, forcing people to stay in a hospital that may not serve their needs. Concentrating on the physical aspects of dying does not allow people to work toward the social and personal tasks from which they may derive a feeling of completion and reintegration.

Entry into the dying role is typically accompanied by loss and grief (Emanuel et al., 2007). The person faces the loss of physical abilities, social relationships, and the experiences of continued life. People imagine that those in this situation are frightened of dying, but research involving people with terminal illnesses indicated otherwise (McKechnie, Macleod, & Keeling, 2007). Instead, their concerns revolved around anxiety—over their condition, whether they would be able to complete planned activities, and provisions for managing their comfort during the last stages of their disease. Because their disease imposed physical limitations on their activities, they felt unable to "live until they died" (McKechnie et al., 2007, p. 367).

Grieving

Loss and grief are also common to bereavement, making the reactions and processes of adaptation applicable to family and friends after the death of a loved one (Murray, 2001). Thus, a diagnosis of chronic illness, awareness of a terminal condition, and loss of a loved one provoke similar reactions, with similar possibilities for outcomes. That is, bereavement may result in caregivers' experiencing worsened symptoms or improvements (Aneshensel et al., 2004) and, eventually, growth (Hogan & Schmidt, 2002).

The similarities between those who are dying and those who are bereaved have led to similar theories of adaptation, including a stage theory of bereavement with stages of disbelief, yearning, anger, depression, and then acceptance. As with Kubler-Ross's stage theory of adaptation to dying, there is little evidence to support a stage theory of bereavement (Maciejewski, Zhang, Block, Prigerson, 2007). People exhibited all reactions, but not as stages, and the reactions overlapped in time.

The good death that is possible for the dying is beneficial for those whom they leave behind (Carr, 2003). That is, the quality of the death affects the bereaved. Spouses of those who died a good death reported stronger feelings of yearning but reduced feelings of anger. On the other hand, spouses of those who died a difficult, painful death experienced greater lingering anger.

Bereavement inevitably includes negative emotions, and people have difficulty accepting such emotions as normal. Even among health care professionals, the grieving process may be interpreted as abnormal when people exhibit strong negative reactions or their feelings persist for a time considered too lengthy. Research has indicated that thoughts of lost loved ones and longings for their company persist for many years (Camelley, Wortman, Bolger, & Burke, 2006).

Even the terminology used by mental health professionals carries negative connotations. People who are adapting to the loss of a loved one are referred to as *recovering*, which implies that these individuals will go back to "normal" and that their grief reactions signal psychological problems. This tendency to "pathologize" the bereavement process should be avoided (Tedeschi & Calhoun, 2008). Some grief responses may present problems for adaptation, but like the process of adapting to chronic and terminal illness, grieving offers the promise of transformative and spiritual growth (Tedeschi & Calhoun, 2006). Thus, all three processes share essential elements.

IN SUMMARY

Facing death requires adjustment for the person who is dying and for the family. Although the process of stages of acceptance has gained popular appeal, no research supports this view. Instead, people who are dying experience a variety of negative reactions that may be better conceptualized as a role with practical, relationship, and personal elements. Some people are able to work through challenges and have access to the facilities to experience a "good death," allowing them to die without pain but with

social support, appropriate medical care, and minimal psychological distress. Their adaptation may leave them with a sense of completion and even transcendence. Growth is also a possibility for those who grieve for loved ones, but the bereaved also face a process of adjustment that includes negative emotions. This process has also been conceptualized as a series of stages, but research also fails to confirm this stage approach. The negative emotions that are involved in grieving should not be seen as abnormal; resolving grief may take years, but this process also offers the promise of positive change.

ANSWERS

This chapter has addressed six basic questions:

1. **What is the impact of chronic disease on patients and families?**

   Long-term chronic illnesses bring about a transition in people's lives, requiring adaptations to live with symptoms and receive medical care, changing relationships, and pushing people toward a reevaluation of themselves. Support groups and programs designed by health psychologists help people cope with the emotional problems associated with chronic illness, problems that traditional medical care often overlooks. Chronic diseases may be terminal, which forces people to consider their impending death.

2. **What is the impact of Alzheimer's disease?**

   Alzheimer's disease damages the brain and produces memory loss, language problems, agitation and irritability, sleep disorders, suspiciousness, wandering, incontinence, and loss of ability to perform routine care. The most common form of Alzheimer's disease occurs through a genetic vulnerability combined with environmental risks. Age is the main risk, with the prevalence doubling for every decade after age 65. Lifestyle factors relate to the development of Alzheimer's disease, making prevention a possibility. Medical treatments are being developed, but the main management strategies consist of interventions to allow patients

longer periods of functioning and counseling and support groups for family members, who frequently experience more stress than the patient.

3. **What is involved in adjusting to diabetes?**

   Diabetes, both insulin-dependent (Type 1) and non-insulin-dependent (Type 2), requires changes in lifestyle that include monitoring and adherence to a treatment regimen. Treatments include insulin injections for Type 1 diabetics and adherence to careful dietary restrictions, scheduling of meals, avoidance of certain foods, regular medical visits, and routine exercise for all diabetics. Health psychologists are involved in helping diabetics learn self-care to control the dangerous effects of their condition.

4. **How does asthma affect the lives of people with this disease?**

   Inflammation of the bronchial tubes is the underlying basis for asthma. Combined with this inflammation, triggering stimuli or events cause bronchial constriction that produces difficulty in breathing. Asthma may be fatal, and it is the leading cause of disability among children. The origin of this process is not understood, but medication can control the inflammation and decrease the risk of attacks. People with asthma are faced with a complex medication regimen that they must follow to decrease the risk of attacks.

5. How can HIV infection be managed?

Infection with the human immunodeficiency virus (HIV) depletes the immune system, leaving the body vulnerable to acquired immune deficiency syndrome (AIDS) and a variety of opportunistic infections. Four different populations in the United States have been affected by HIV epidemics: (1) men who have sex with men, (2) injection drug users, (3) heterosexuals, and (4) children born to HIV-positive mothers. Psychologists are involved in the HIV epidemic by encouraging protective behaviors, counseling infected people to help them cope with living with a chronic disease, and helping patients adhere to complex medical regimens that have changed HIV infection to a manageable chronic disease.

6. What adaptations do people make to dying and grieving?

People tend to react to the knowledge that they have a terminal illness with a variety of negative emotions, and the process of grieving also includes negative emotions. Contrary to popular conceptualizations, however, these reactions do not progress through a pattern of stages. Instead, dying may be conceptualized as a role that includes practical, relational, and personal elements that people encounter in their process of adaptation. Grieving can also be conceptualized as a process with negative emotions but also with the possibility of growth.

SUGGESTED READINGS

Asthma Action America. (2004). *Children and asthma in America*. Retrieved August 29, 2008, from http://www.asthmainamerica. com/frequency.html. This comprehensive survey details the impact of asthma on the lives of children and their caregivers, examining the misperceptions about the disease, the available treatments, and recommendations for more effective strategies to deal with this disease.

DeBaggio, T. (2002). *Losing my mind: An intimate look at life with Alzheimer's.* New York: Free Press. When former newspaper writer Thomas DeBaggio began to recognize symptoms of Alzheimer's disease at age 57, he decided to write about his experience of "losing his mind." The result is a moving account of Alzheimer's disease from an insider's point of view.

Kalichman, S. C. (2003). *The inside story on AIDS*. Washington, DC: American Psychological Association. Seth Kalichman uses a question-and-answer format to provide a variety of information on AIDS, based on the most common questions asked on AIDS hotlines.

Stanton, A. L., Revenson, T. A., & Tennen, H. (2007). Health psychology: Psychological adjustment to chronic disease. *Annual Review of Psychology, 58*, 565–592. This article examines the growing body of longitudinal research on adjustment to chronic illness, exploring the important environmental and personal influences that affect the process.

UNAIDS. (2007). *AIDS epidemic update, 2007*. Geneva: Joint United Nations Programme on HIV/AIDS. This comprehensive report details the status of HIV infection worldwide and in each geographic area, analyzing the nature of the epidemic in each region and the progress that has been made in controlling the disease.

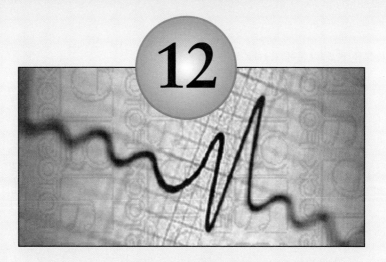

12

SMOKING TOBACCO

QUESTIONS

This chapter focuses on five basic questions:

1. How does smoking affect the respiratory system?

2. Who chooses to smoke and why?

3. What are the health consequences of tobacco use?

4. How can smoking rates be reduced?

5. What are the effects of quitting?

CHECK YOUR HEALTH RISKS

Check the items that apply to you.

☐ 1. I have not smoked more than 100 cigarettes in my life.

☐ 2. I have probably smoked between 100 and 200 cigarettes in my life, but I have not smoked at all in more than 5 years and have no desire to do so.

☐ 3. I currently smoke more than 10 cigarettes a day.

☐ 4. I currently smoke more than two packs of cigarettes a day.

☐ 5. I am a smoker who believes that the health risks of smoking have been exaggerated.

☐ 6. I am a smoker who believes that smoking is probably harmful, but I plan to stop smoking before those effects can harm me.

☐ 7. I don't smoke cigarettes, but I do smoke at least one cigar a day.

☐ 8. I don't smoke cigarettes, but I do smoke my pipe at least once a day.

☐ 9. I smoke cigars because I believe that they carry a very low risk for heart disease and cancer.

☐ 10. I smoke a pipe because I believe that pipe smoking is safer than cigarettes.

☐ 11. I live with someone who is a heavy smoker.

☐ 12. I use smokeless tobacco (chewing tobacco) on a daily basis.

Except for the first two statements, each of these items represents a health risk from tobacco products, which account for about 438,000 deaths a year in the United States, mostly from heart disease, cancer, and chronic lower respiratory disease. Count your check marks for the last 10 items to evaluate your risks. As you read this chapter, you will see that some of these items are riskier than others.

REAL-WORLD PROFILE OF CHRISTY TURLINGTON

Supermodel Christy Turlington began sneaking cigarettes from her father when she was 12 or 13 years old (Smoking List, 2004). By the time she started modeling at 14, she was smoking occasionally, and by 16, her smoking escalated to more than a pack a day. But Christy fit into the world of high fashion modeling, where most of the models smoked.

At age 19, Christy tried to quit smoking because she believed that she was harming her body. She tried hypnosis and acupuncture and quit for 2 years, but she relapsed. After trying to quit by using the nicotine patch and other methods, she finally succeeded when she decided to "just put the pack down and not pick it up again" (Smoking List, 2004). Her father also tried to quit and finally succeeded, but he had smoked for 50 years and already had lung cancer. He died of the disease six months later. His death prompted Christy to become an antismoking activist.

Christy Turlington has a website and a video that promote smoking prevention. She is also a spokesperson for the Centers for Disease Control and Prevention

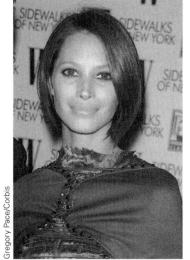

Gregory Pace/Corbis

Christy Turlington became an antismoking activist after her father died of lung cancer.

and its efforts to deter teens from smoking (Smoking List, 2004). As part of her advocacy, she underwent a lung scan while filming a documentary on women and smoking. From that scan, Turlington learned that she has early-stage **emphysema**, a chronic lung disease in which scar tissue and mucus obstruct the respiratory passages.

Although she quit smoking five years before her diagnosis, the years of smoking had already damaged her lungs permanently.

Smoking is the most preventable cause of death in the United States. Every year 438,000 people die in the United States from tobacco use (American Cancer Society, 2008). It's quite easy to read through the number 438,000, but let's see if we can personalize it. *Each year*, smoking kills enough people to wipe out half the population of Montana. More people die every year from smoking than live within the city limits of Atlanta. The number who die from smoking-related causes is nearly 75% of the population of Boston. Stated differently, an average of 1,205 people die *every day* in the United States from tobacco-related causes. Cigarettes kill more U.S. citizens than alcohol, car crashes, suicide, homicide, AIDS, and illegal drugs—combined (American Cancer Society, 2008). Later, we summarize the various risks from cigarette, cigar, and pipe smoking, as well as from other tobacco products, including the dangers of passive smoking and smokeless tobacco. This chapter also includes information on the prevalence of smoking in the United States, the reasons why people smoke, and some methods of preventing and reducing smoking. First, however, we briefly review the effects of smoking on the respiratory system, the body system most immediately affected by smoking.

SMOKING AND THE RESPIRATORY SYSTEM

Respiration takes oxygen into the body and expels carbon dioxide. This process draws air deep into the lungs, and with the air can come other particles that may damage the lungs. Smoking routinely introduces a variety of particles into the lungs, and several diseases are associated with smoking.

Functioning of the Respiratory System

The exchange of oxygen and carbon dioxide occurs deep in the lungs. To get air into the lungs, the **diaphragm** and the muscles between the ribs (intercostal muscles) contract, increasing the volume within the chest. As the space inside the chest increases, the pressure within the chest falls below atmospheric pressure, and air is forced into the lungs by that pressure.

Figure 12.1 illustrates where air goes on its way to the lungs. The nasal passages, pharynx, larynx, trachea, bronchi, and bronchioles conduct air into the lungs. These passages have little ability to absorb oxygen, but in the process of inhalation, the air is warmed, humidified, and cleansed. Millions of alveoli, located at the ends of the bronchioles, are the site of oxygen and carbon dioxide exchange. Each tiny alveolus in the lungs is like a bubble, giving the lungs a spongy appearance. The alveoli have thin walls (only one cell in thickness) that allow the easy exchange of gases.

Air rich in oxygen is drawn into the lungs and reaches the alveoli. Blood that has circulated through the body travels back to the heart and then back to the lungs. This blood has a high carbon dioxide content and a low oxygen content. In the lungs, the blood circulates to the capillaries that surround each alveolus, where an exchange of carbon dioxide and oxygen occurs based on differences in diffusion pressures. The blood, now oxygen rich, travels back to the heart and is pumped out to all areas of the body.

During exhalation, the diaphragm and the muscles between the ribs relax. The air in the alveoli is compressed, and the increased pressure forces the air out of the lungs by the same route through which it entered. The expelled air contains a great deal of carbon dioxide and little oxygen. Not all air leaves the lungs during exhalation, and each breath mixes new air with air that remains in the lungs.

Air is an excellent medium for the introduction of foreign matter into the body. Airborne particles potentially move into the lungs with every breath. Protective mechanisms in the respiratory system, such as sneezing and coughing, expel some dangerous particles. Noxious stimulation in the nasal passages may activate the sneeze reflex, whereas stimulation in the lower respiratory system promotes the cough reflex.

Another protective mechanism in the respiratory system is called the **mucociliary escalator**. Diffusion of gases requires a moist environment, and the respiratory system is kept moist by its mucous membrane lining. In the nasal cavity, pharynx, and bronchi, the lining of the respiratory system contains **cilia**, tiny hairlike structures. The cilia and mucous membranes form the

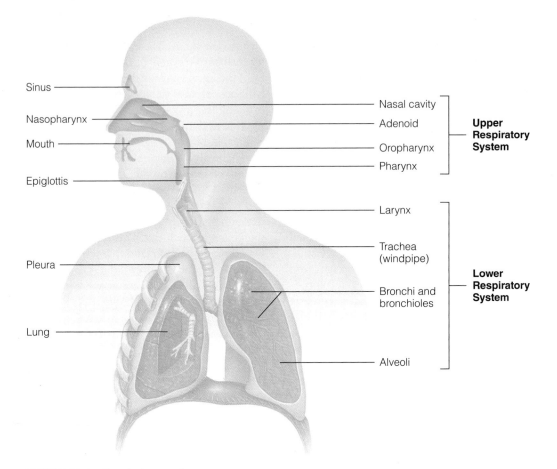

FIGURE 12.1   Respiratory system.

Source: Introduction to Microbiology (p. 525), by J. L. Ingraham & C. A. Ingraham, 1995, Belmont, CA: Wadsworth. Copyright 1995 by Wadsworth Publishing Company. Reprinted by permission.

mucociliary escalator. Mucus is secreted in the respiratory system, and the beating of the cilia moves the mucus toward the pharynx, where it is usually swallowed or coughed out. This transport mechanism cleanses the system of inhaled particles, providing an important defense against dangerous ones.

Several respiratory disorders are of interest to health psychologists. All kinds of smoke, as well as other types of air pollution, increase mucus secretion in the respiratory system but decrease the activity of the cilia, thus decreasing the efficiency of the mucociliary escalator. As mucus builds up, people cough to get rid of the mucus, but

coughing may also irritate the bronchial walls. Irritation and infection of the bronchial walls may damage the cilia and destroy tissue in the bronchi. The formation of scar tissue in the bronchi, irritation or infection of bronchial tissue, and coughing are characteristics of **bronchitis**, one of several *chronic lower respiratory diseases* (previously called chronic obstructive pulmonary disease or COPD) that are the third leading cause of death in the United States.

Acute bronchitis is caused by infection and usually responds quickly to antibiotics. When the irritation persists and the mechanism underlying the illness continues, it can become a chronic problem. Cigarette smoke is the major cause of chronic bronchitis, but environmental air pollution and occupational hazards may also underlie chronic bronchitis.

The most common of the chronic lower respiratory diseases is *emphysema*, the disorder that Christy Turlington developed because of her smoking. This disorder occurs when scar tissue and mucus obstruct the respiratory passages, bronchi lose their elasticity and collapse, and air is trapped in the alveoli. The trapped air breaks down the alveolar walls, and the remaining alveoli become enlarged. Both damaged and enlarged alveoli have reduced surface area for the exchange of oxygen and carbon dioxide. Damage also obstructs blood flow to the undamaged alveoli, and so the respiratory system becomes

restricted. The loss of efficiency in the respiratory system means that respiration delivers a limited amount of oxygen. People with emphysema usually cannot exercise strenuously, and even normal breathing can become impossible for them.

Chronic bronchitis, emphysema, and lung cancer are all diseases of the respiratory system associated with the inhalation of irritating, damaging particles such as smoke. Figure 12.2 shows how smoke can damage the lungs, producing bronchitis and emphysema. Cigarette smoking is of particular interest to health psychologists because it is a voluntary behavior that can be avoided, whereas air pollution and occupational hazards are social problems not under direct personal control. Thus, smoking is the target for much negative publicity and for interventions

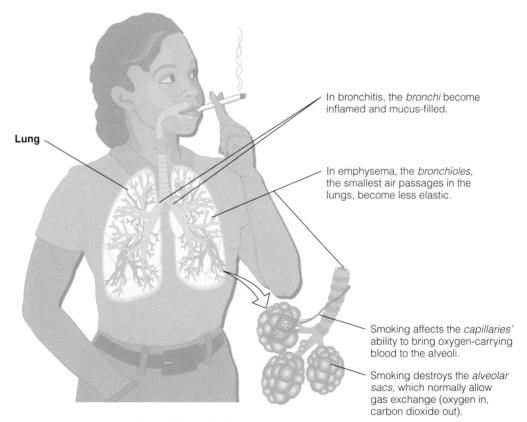

Lung

In bronchitis, the *bronchi* become inflamed and mucus-filled.

In emphysema, the *bronchioles,* the smallest air passages in the lungs, become less elastic.

Smoking affects the *capillaries'* ability to bring oxygen-carrying blood to the alveoli.

Smoking destroys the *alveolar sacs,* which normally allow gas exchange (oxygen in, carbon dioxide out).

FIGURE 12.2   How smoking affects the lungs.

Source: An Invitation to Health (7th ed., p. 493) by D. Hales, 1997, Pacific Grove, CA: Brooks/Cole. Copyright 1997 by Brooks/Cole Publishing Company. Reprinted by permission.

for change. But what specifically makes inhaled smoke dangerous?

What Components in Smoke Are Dangerous?

The processed tobacco in cigarettes contains at least 4,000 compounds, and at least 60 of these are known carcinogens—substances that are capable of causing cancer (American Cancer Society, 2008). But which of these components in cigarette smoke might be dangerous? Nicotine is the pharmacological agent that underlies addiction to cigarette smoking, but is nicotine the main culprit responsible for the adverse health effects of smoking? Can nicotine cause coronary heart disease, cancer, bronchitis, and emphysema? What does this drug do in the body?

Nicotine is a stimulant drug, an "upper." It affects both the central and peripheral nervous systems. Certain central nervous system receptor sites are specific for nicotine; that is, the brain responds to nicotine, as it does to many drugs. But smoking is a particularly effective means of delivering drugs to the brain. Nicotine, for example, can be found in the brain 7 seconds after having been ingested by smoking—twice as fast as via intravenous injection. The half-life of nicotine, the time it takes to lose half its strength, is 30 to 40 minutes. Addicted smokers rarely go more than this length of time between "fixes."

When nicotine is delivered to the brain, catecholamines, neurotransmitters that include epinephrine and norepinephrine, are released. These substances act as stimulants, increasing cortical arousal, which can be measured by an electroencephalograph (EEG). In addition, smoking releases beta-endorphins; the pleasurable effects of smoking may be due to the release of these natural opiates produced by the body. Nicotine also increases the metabolic level, which explains the tendency for smokers to be thinner than nonsmokers.

The term *tars* describes the water-soluble residue of tobacco smoke condensate, which is known to contain a number of compounds identified or suspected as carcinogens. Although tobacco companies have recently reduced the level of tars in cigarettes, no level is safe. Nevertheless, as tar levels go down, death rates from smoking-related diseases also go down. However, experienced smokers who smoke low-nicotine cigarettes tend to increase their rate of smoking and to inhale more deeply, thus exposing themselves to more of the dangerous tars.

Several other by-products of tobacco smoke are suspected of being health risks. **Acrolein** and **formaldehyde** belong to a class of irritating compounds called **aldehydes**. Formaldehyde, a demonstrated carcinogen, disrupts tissue proteins and causes cell damage. **Nitric oxide** and **hydrocyanic acid** are gases generated in smoking tobacco that affect oxygen metabolism and therefore could be dangerous. Because tobacco companies do not provide the public with specific information about the content of cigarettes, consumers cannot accurately know their level of health risk (American Cancer Society, 2008).

IN SUMMARY

The respiratory system allows oxygen to be taken into the lungs where an exchange with carbon dioxide occurs at the level of the alveoli. Along with air, other particles can enter the lungs; some of these particles can be harmful. Cigarette smoke can cause damage to the lungs, and smokers are prone to bronchitis, an inflammation of the bronchi. Cigarette smoke contributes heavily to the development of chronic lower respiratory diseases, such as chronic bronchitis and emphysema.

Several chemicals, either within the tobacco itself or produced as a by-product of smoking, can cause organic damage. Although nicotine in large doses is extremely toxic, its precise harmful effects on the average smoker are difficult to assess. This difficulty exists because the level of nicotine in commercial cigarettes varies with the level of tars, another class of potentially hazardous substances. Thus, determining what specific components of smoke connect to which sources of illness and death is difficult.

A BRIEF HISTORY OF TOBACCO USE

When Christopher Columbus and other early European explorers arrived in the Western hemisphere, they found that the Native Americans had a custom considered odd by European standards: The natives carried rolls of dried leaves, which they set afire, and then "drank" the smoke. The leaves were, of course, tobacco. Those early European sailors tried smoking, liked it, and soon became quite dependent on it. Although Columbus disapproved of his sailors' using tobacco, he quickly recognized that "it was not within their power to refrain from indulging in the habit" (Kluger, 1996, p. 9). Within a century, smoking and the cultivation of tobacco spread around the world, and no country where people have learned to use tobacco has ever successfully barred the habit (Brecher, 1972).

Smoking was a habit that grew rapidly in popularity among Europeans, but it was not without its detractors. Elizabethan England adopted the use of tobacco, although Elizabeth I disapproved, as did her successor, James I. Another prominent Elizabethan, Sir Francis Bacon, spoke against tobacco and the hold it exerted over its users. Many objections to tobacco were of a similar nature—namely, that people who became addicted to it often spent money on tobacco even though they could not afford it. Because of its scarcity, tobacco was expensive; in London in 1610, it sold for an equal weight of silver.

In 1633, the Turkish Sultan Murad IV decreed the death penalty for subjects who were caught smoking. He then conducted "sting" operations on the streets of his empire and beheaded those vulnerable people who were seduced to use tobacco (Kluger, 1996). From the early Romanoff Empire in Russia to 17th-century Japan, the penalties for tobacco use were also severe. Still the habit spread. In the Spanish colonies, smoking by priests during Mass became so prevalent that the Catholic Church forbade it. In 1642 and again in 1650, tobacco was the subject of two formal papal bulls, but in 1725, Pope Benedict XIII annulled all edicts against tobacco—he liked to use snuff, which is ground tobacco.

Over the centuries, tobacco has been used in a variety of forms, including snuff, pipes, cigars, and cigarettes. Cigarettes (shredded tobacco rolled in paper) were not popular until the 20th century, although some soldiers smoked them during the U.S. Civil War. However, cigarette smoking was not widespread during the last half of the 19th century because many men considered it rather effeminate. Ironically, cigarette smoking was not socially acceptable for women either, and few women smoked during this period. Cigarette smoking became more popular during the 1880s, when ready-made cigarettes came on the market. Gradually, people came to prefer factory-made cigarettes to those they had to roll themselves.

The widespread adoption of cigarette smoking was aided in 1913 by the development of the "blended" cigarette, a mixture of air-cured Burley and Turkish varieties of tobacco with flue-cured Virginia tobacco. This blend provided a cigarette with a pleasing flavor and aroma that was also easy to inhale. Cigarette smoking became increasingly popular during World War I, and during the 1920s, the age of the "flapper," cigarette smoking started to gain popularity among women.

From the time of Columbus until the mid-19th century, tobacco did not lack enemies, but no one tried to ban it for scientific or medical reasons. Historically, the assault on tobacco came from people who damned it on moral, social, xenophobic, or economic grounds (Kluger, 1996). The tobacco industry continued to grow despite (or perhaps because of) the fact that many in authority condemned the use of tobacco for one or more of these reasons. It was not until the mid-1960s that the scientific evidence on the dangerous consequences of smoking became widely recognized.

During the 1940s and 1950s, it was not uncommon for physicians to smoke and to recommend the practice to their patients as a method of relaxation and stress reduction. Tobacco companies, of course, used a variety of techniques to increase smoking rates. Besides multiple advertising approaches, they provided free cigarettes to soldiers during World War II and continued to give away free samples after the war. At that time, only a few people suspected that smoking might have negative health consequences, so the choice to smoke was a common one.

Sixty years after tobacco companies convinced people that cigarette smoking was chic, sexy, and stylish, their approach to advertising continues to pay dividends, as the Would You Believe . . . ? box discusses.

WOULD YOU BELIEVE . . . ?

Tobacco Sales Are Doing Fine

Would you believe that tobacco companies continue to prosper despite heavy financial blows to their industry? The first blow came during the late 1990s, when tobacco companies were forced to pay individual states billions of dollars as part of a legal settlement. This settlement resulted from lawsuits that accused the major tobacco companies of knowingly distributing and selling a lethal substance that they knew causes death—namely, cigarettes.

Revenues from this settlement were designated for medical expenses incurred by smokers and former smokers, but individual states were free to use the money as they wished. To offset expenses, the major tobacco companies raised the price of cigarettes, a maneuver that kept these established tobacco companies in business. Some enterprising individuals began their own small tobacco companies on the assumption that they were exempt from heavy fines because no studies had ever been conducted showing that cigarettes manufactured by these new companies had ever killed anyone!

A second financial setback resulted from the steady decline in domestic sales of cigarettes, forcing tobacco companies to look elsewhere for revenue. Tobacco companies have attempted to solve this problem by promoting cigarettes to adolescents. John Pierce and his associates (Pierce, Choi, Gilpin, Farkas, & Berry, 1998) surveyed adolescents who had no susceptibility to smoking when first interviewed. Three years later, more than half of these young people could name a favorite cigarette advertisement, and having a favorite commercial was a good predictor

of who would begin smoking. Pierce et al. estimated that 34% of experimentation with cigarettes was due to advertising, a figure that would translate to more than 700,000 new smokers each year, or a quarter of a million *more* than the number of people who die each year of smoking-related causes.

Despite these financial challenges, tobacco companies remain optimistic. Reason for this optimism lies in the expanding markets in Africa, Eastern Europe, and Asia. Richard Kluger (1996) has remarked that in those areas of the world, the cigarette is regarded as a sign of being up-to-date, "an emblem of advancement, fashion, savoir faire, and adventure as projected in images beamed and plastered everywhere by its makers" (p. xii). To Kluger, the situation is ironic in that "the more evidence accumulated by science on the ravaging effects of tobacco, the more lucrative the business has become and the wider the margin of profit" (p. xii). In Kluger's interesting and informative book, *Ashes to Ashes,* he notes that many governments in emerging nations have themselves become addicted to cigarettes because of the taxes they receive from cigarette sales.

Russia and other nations of the former Soviet Union present an alluring potential market to American and British tobacco companies. Although Russians have been longtime smokers, their consumption was traditionally limited to inferior-tasting cigarettes manufactured in outmoded domestic factories that could not keep up with a growing demand. Despite a shortage of creature comforts, Russians have continued their strong appetite for tobacco products.

Into this potentially lucrative market rode the Marlboro man, dispatched by his parent, Philip Morris. This prominent U.S. tobacco company proceeded to renovate old factories, build new ones, and spend a total of $1.5 billion during the first four years after the Soviet breakup (Kluger, 1996). Their investment, of course, has reaped dividends. Thanks to Russia and the other former Soviet countries, Philip Morris's international sales have increased by 10% a year, easily compensating for any erosion of the U.S. market (Kluger, 1996).

As appealing as the countries of Eastern Europe appear, China presents an even larger prize to Western tobacco companies. The number of current smokers in China is not precisely known, but Kluger (1996) estimated the number at 300 million—about one-quarter of the population and about 30% of the world's smoking population. However, unlike governments of the former communist countries of Eastern Europe, the Chinese government has been more reluctant to open its doors to foreign tobacco and has actively sought to reduce smoking among its people by restricting cigarette advertising and putting health warnings on cigarette packs. Undaunted, Philip Morris has taken a patient course of action. It has sponsored a national soccer league, presented U.S.-style television shows, and displayed other forms of advertising, even "though the Chinese couldn't get near the product" (Kluger, 1996, p. 721). Only time will tell if these tactics will be successful, but given the history of tobacco companies, it seems safe to predict that these efforts will eventually pay off.

CHOOSING TO SMOKE

Unlike many health hazards, smoking is a voluntary behavior, with each person choosing to smoke or not to smoke. What factors have influenced this choice?

Several historical and social events in the United States have accompanied the increasingly popular choice not to smoke. First was the 1964 report of the Surgeon General of the United States that spelled out the adverse effects of smoking on health (U.S. Public Health Service [USPHS], 1964). Other events included placing a warning of the potential danger of cigarettes on each cigarette package, banning cigarette advertising on television, designating public buildings as smoke free, increasing the price of cigarettes, removing cigarette machines from public places, and designing and implementing programs aimed at inoculating students to turn down offers of cigarettes. Coincidental with these and other programs, smoking rates in the United States declined. The highest rate of per capita cigarette

consumption was in 1966, two years after the first Surgeon General's report on the dangers of smoking. Figure 12.3 shows a significant decrease in the per capita consumption of cigarettes in the United States since the Surgeon General's report; it also shows historical events that may have increased or decreased the per capita consumption of cigarettes.

Who Smokes and Who Does Not?

Currently, slightly fewer than 21% of adults in the United States are classified as smokers, a percentage less than half of the 44% who smoked in 1966 (USCB, 2007). Currently, there are more former smokers than current smokers in the United States (see Figure 12.4).

How Do Smokers Differ From Nonsmokers?
Smokers differ from nonsmokers in gender, ethnicity, age, occupation, educational level, and a variety of other factors. By gender, about 23.4% of adult men and 18.4% of adult women in the

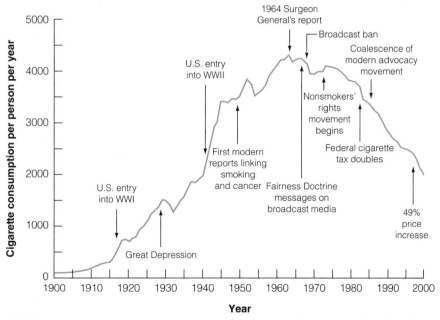

FIGURE 12.3   Cigarette consumption per person 18 and over, United States, 1900–2000.

Sources: "Surveillance for Selected Tobacco Use Behaviors—United States, 1900–1994," by G. A. Givovino et al., 1994, *Morbidity and Mortality Weekly Report, 43,* No. SS-3, pp. 6–7; National Center for Health Statistics, 2001, *Health, United States 2001,* Hyattsville, MD: U.S. Government Printing Office.

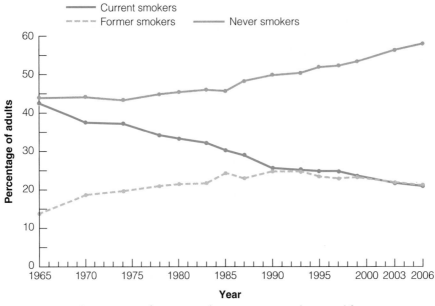

FIGURE 12.4 Percentage of never smokers, current smokers, and former smokers among adults, United States, 1965–2006.

Sources: Centers for Disease Control and Prevention (CDC), 2007, "Percentage of Young Adults Who Were Current, Former or Never Smokers, Overall and by Sex, Race, and Education," *National Health Interview Surveys—United States, 1965–2006.* Retrieved July 21, 2008, from http://www.cdc.gov/tobacco/data_statistics/tables/adult/table_12.htm.

United States are defined as current smokers. From 1965 to about 1985, the quit rate for men was higher than it was for women, thus producing a sharper decline in the number of men who smoked and suggesting that women might eventually have higher smoking rates than men. However, this trend has not continued (see Figure 12.5). During the past 20 years, the quit rates for women and men have been nearly identical, with both genders showing a very slight decline in smoking rates and no indication that women's smoking rate will "catch up" to men's.

As for ethnic groups, American Indians (including Alaska Natives) have the highest rate of cigarette consumption (about 33%), and Asian Americans have the lowest percentage of smokers (fewer than 6%) (NCHS, 2007). Perhaps because many longtime smokers die of cigarette-related causes, smoking prevalence is lowest for people age 65 and older, with about 8% of older people classified as smokers. Despite the high cost of cigarettes, people living below the poverty level have higher smoking rates (31%) than those at or above the poverty level (20%) (Rock et al., 2007). Even for those who are not poor, smoking is inversely related to personal net wealth—smokers are poorer than nonsmokers (Zagorsky, 2004).

Finally, level of education is a reasonably accurate predictor of smoking rates: the higher the level of education, the lower the rate of smoking (Rock et al., 2007; Wetter et al., 2005). In the United States, for example, only 7.3% of people with a graduate (master's or doctoral) degree are current smokers, whereas more than 51% of people with a General Education Diploma (GED) are current smokers (Rock et al., 2007). Figure 12.6 shows the inverse relationship between level of smoking and level of education in the United States.

The inverse relationship between level of education and level of smoking holds true for most, but not all, segments of European society. A similar pattern appeared in a large sample of people in Germany (Schulze & Mons, 2006). For

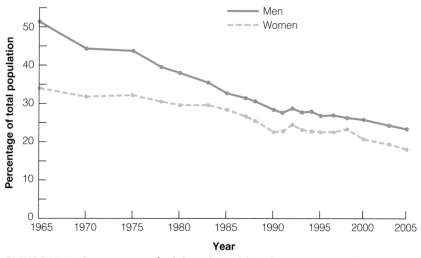
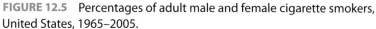

FIGURE 12.5   Percentages of adult male and female cigarette smokers, United States, 1965–2005.

Source: Statistical Abstract of the United States: 2008 (127th edition), by U.S. Census Bureau, 2007. Washington, DC: U.S. Government Printing Office.

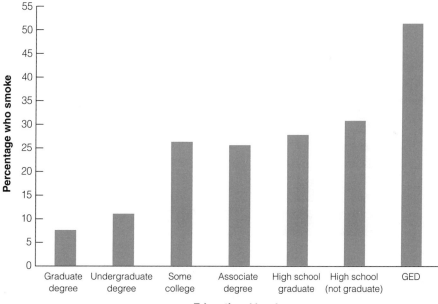

FIGURE 12.6   Percentage of persons 18 and older who are smokers, by educational level, United States, 2006.

Source: "Cigarette Smoking Among Adults—United States, 2006," by V. J. Rock, A. Malarcher, J. W. Kahende, K. Asman, C. Husten, & R. Caraballo, *Morbidity & Mortality Weekly Report, 56*, p. 1159.

Italian men and British men and women, however, tobacco consumption is positively related to educational level; that is, the lower the level of education, the lower the rate of smoking (Giskes et al., 2005).

Smoking Rates Among Young People In 1994 the National Center for Health Statistics changed its definition of what constitutes a current smoker, making it easier to be classified as a current smoker but also making the earlier statistics about smoking rates not comparable to those afterward. Using these newer definitions, about 12% of ninth-grade boys and 16% of ninth-grade girls are classified as current smokers who have smoked at least once during the month before the survey (Eaton et al., 2008). By this age,

Christy Turlington was a smoker. Figure 12.7 shows slightly different patterns of smoking for female and male students, with male students increasing their levels of smoking throughout high school. By the time students reach 12th grade, about 13% of the boys and 11% of the girls are frequent smokers.

Many adolescents begin to experiment with smoking during middle school and high school, but adolescence is probably not the time that young people adopt a consistent pattern of smoking. This pattern is usually established after age 18 and may consist of being a nonsmoker, a light smoker, an occasional smoker, or a heavy smoker. Christy Turlington did not fit this pattern. By the time she was 16, she smoked about a pack and a half of cigarettes a day.

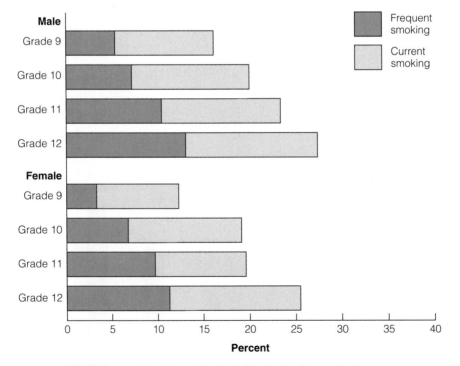

NOTE: Current cigarette smoking is defined as having smoked cigarettes on 1 or more days of the 30 days preceding the survey; frequent cigarette smoking is defined as having smoked cigarettes on 20 or more of the 30 days preceding the survey.

FIGURE 12.7 Current cigarette smoking among high school students by gender, frequency, and grade level, United States, 2006.

Source: "Youth Behavior Risk Surveillance—United States, 2007," by D. K. Eaton, L. Kann, S. Kinchen, S. Shanklin, J. Ross, J. Hawkins, et al., *Morbidity and Mortality Weekly Report*, 2008, vol. 57, p. 63.

Compared to school students, much less attention has been given to young adults 18 to 24. A study from Canada (Hammond, 2005) found that the highest rate of smoking in that country was among young adults—a finding that supports data from the United States. Smoking rates for each age group in the United States except 18–24 have declined by about 5 percentage points during the past 15 years, but the rates for young adults have remained about the same—about 27% (Eaton et al., 2008). Figure 12.8 shows the percentage of young adults who were never smokers, current smokers, and former smokers.

Why Do People Smoke?

Despite widespread publicity linking cigarette smoking to a variety of health problems, millions of people continue to smoke. That situation is puzzling because many smokers themselves acknowledge the potential dangers of their habit. The question of why people smoke can be divided into two separate ones: Why do people begin to smoke, and why do they continue?

Answers to the first question are difficult because most young people are aware of the hazards of smoking, and many of them become ill from their first attempt at smoking. The best answer to the second question seems to be that different people smoke for different reasons, and the same person may smoke for different reasons in different situations.

Why Do People Start Smoking? Most young people are aware of the hazards of smoking (Waltenbaugh & Zagummy, 2004), yet thousands of them begin to smoke each year. Many of these young people have an optimistic bias, believing that the dangers do not apply to them. In addition to this optimistic bias, researchers have examined at least four explanations for why people begin smoking despite being aware of the dangers: genetic predisposition, peer pressure, advertising, and weight control.

Genetics The first evidence that smoking has some genetic component appeared in the 1950s from studies on twins (Pomerleau & Kardia,

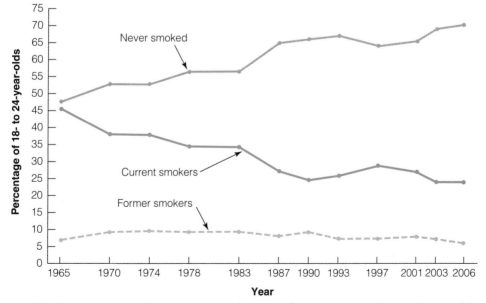

FIGURE 12.8 Never smokers, current smokers, and former smokers, 18- to 24-year-olds, 1965–2006.

Source: "Percentage of Young Adults Who Were Current, Former or Never Smokers, Overall and by Sex, Race, and Education," *National Health Interview Surveys, Selected Years—United States, 1965–2006,* retrieved July 21, 2008, from http://www.cdc.gov/tobacco/data_statistics/tables/adult/table_12.htm.

1999). These studies indicated that identical twins tended to be more similar than fraternal twins in their choice to smoke or not. More recent research has implicated genetic factors for both smoking initiation and nicotine dependence (Li, Ma, & Beuten, 2004). Twin and adoption studies have revealed a genetic component in smoking, but attempts to locate specific genes have not yet been successful (Munaf & Johnstone, 2008).

Research evidence for one genetic mechanism is stronger than others, and that mechanism involves the reception and transport of the neurotransmitter dopamine (Erblich, Lerman, Self, Diaz, & Bovbjerg, 2005; Laucht et al., 2008; Li et al., 2004). This neurotransmitter is important in the brain's reward system. Variations in genes involved in one of the dopamine receptors and another involved in dopamine transport seem to increase the likelihood that a person will become and remain a smoker (Ling, Niu, Feng, Xing, & Xu, 2004) or be successful in quitting (Stapleton, Sutherland, & O'Gara, 2007).

Thus, a great deal of evidence indicates that smoking has heritable components, but evidence for location of specific genes has not appeared. Instead, the likelihood is that genes and environmental influences combine to influence smoking (Munaf & Johnstone, 2008). In a longitudinal study of smoking initiation that controlled for genetic relatedness (Slomkowski, Rende, Novak, Lloyd-Richardson, & Niaura, 2005), both genetics and social environment contributed to smoking initiation: Adolescents who reported a closer connection to smoking siblings were more likely to become smokers. These results highlight the interaction between social and genetic factors in the initiation of smoking.

Social Pressure Many teenagers are sensitive to social pressure, and having friends, parents, or siblings who smoke increases the chances that a teen will smoke (Milton et al., 2004). Teenagers may be encouraged to smoke and to continue smoking by peers who offer them cigarettes, but overt pressure is not necessary—young people may begin to smoke to fit in with a social group (Stewart-Knox et al., 2005). However, the behavior of friends is important; having a close childhood friend who smokes increases the chances

that an adolescent will try smoking (Bricker et al, 2006). Parents and siblings who smoke may not encourage a teenager to start, but they furnish a model that is influential. Thus, teens in families in which parents or siblings smoke are more likely to do so than teens in nonsmoking families (Hoving, Reubsaet, & de Vries, 2007; Slomkowski et al., 2005). Some evidence (Mercken, Candel, Willems, & de Vries, 2007) indicates that siblings are more influential than parents in starting to smoke. But parents may be more influential in their children's decision not to smoke; middle and high school students were less likely to smoke when neither parent smoked and when parents were very concerned that their teenagers not smoke (Kalesan, Stine, & Alberg, 2006).

People are not the only source of model for smoking; movies can be a source of social pressure. Movies aimed at adolescent audiences contain more positive messages about cigarette smoking than R-rated movies (Escamilla, Cradock, & Kawachi, 2000). A growing body of evidence implicates movies as a source of influence to begin smoking. John Pierce and his colleagues (Distefan, Pierce, & Gilpin, 2004; Pierce, 2005) have examined the influence that movies have on young adolescents and have found that they are highly influenced by viewing their favorite movie stars smoking on film. In a series of studies, Pierce and his colleagues asked adolescents to list their favorite movie star. Next, they reviewed popular films to count the number of times favorite stars smoked on film. The researchers found that viewing a popular movie star smoking on screen created a powerful incentive for girls to begin smoking, but the influence was not as strong for boys. In a longitudinal study with a representative sample of adolescents in the United States (Wills, Sargent, Stoolmiller, Gibbons, & Gerard, 2008), viewing smoking in movies appeared to influence positive attitudes about smoking and to prompt affiliating with friends who smoked. Both attitudes and friends who smoke relate to smoking initiation.

The influence of smoking in movies extends to young people in countries other than the United States (although the movies that portray smoking are mostly from the United States). In a study of German children between ages 10 and 17 (Hanewinkel & Sargent, 2007), viewing movies

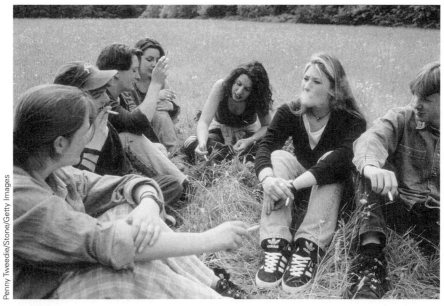

Penny Tweedie/Stone/Getty Images

Acceptance into a social group can be a powerful source of reinforcement for adolescents, increasing the pressure to begin smoking.

with portrayals of smoking influenced the initiation and continuation of smoking. Thus, the social environment provides many sources that may influence young people to smoke or to decline, and advertising is part of that environment.

Advertising In addition to social pressure, tobacco companies have used advertising as a means of getting teenagers interested in smoking. John Pierce and associates (Pierce, Distefan, Kaplan, & Gilpin, 2005) studied how adolescents may become susceptible to advertising by dividing 12- to 15-year-old adolescents who had never smoked into two groups: committed never smokers who showed no interest in smoking, and susceptible never smokers who reported some interest in smoking. An important difference between the two groups was curiosity. Committed never smokers who lacked curiosity tended to pay little attention to tobacco ads and were unlikely to begin smoking. The conclusion from this study is that curiosity may be a critical ingredient in adolescents' decision to smoke or not to smoke. Advertising that arouses curiosity can be an effective means of marketing any product, including cigarettes.

During the late 1990s, tobacco companies argued that their marketing campaigns were

directed at influencing people to switch brands and not aimed at getting young people to begin smoking. Research (Biener & Siegel, 2000) has repudiated these arguments. By establishing a baseline of adolescents who had smoked no more than one cigarette and then interviewing these participants four years later, the researchers found that advertising had an impact. Young people who owned a tobacco promotional item and who could name a brand whose advertisements attracted their attention were nearly three times more likely to smoke. Another longitudinal study (Gilpin, White, Messer, & Pierce, 2007) showed that adolescents who had a favorite cigarette advertisement or were willing to use cigarette promotional items were more likely to be smokers three and six years later. Thus, cigarette advertisements are not simply designed to get people to change brands but have the effect of influencing adolescents to begin smoking.

If prosmoking advertising is effective, can antismoking advertising be effective as well? Antismoking media campaigns can be effective, but possibly not as effective as advertising to promote smoking. One study found that antismoking media campaigns are effective with young adolescents, ages 12 to 13, but not with older adolescents 14 to 15 years old (Siegel & Biener, 2000). Another study found that both antismoking and prosmoking advertising is effective, but the antismoking messages were not strong enough to counteract the prosmoking appeals (Weiss et al., 2006). Thus, both types of advertising can be effective but not equally so.

Weight Control Many girls and some boys begin smoking because they believe it will help them control their weight. Weight control appeared as a reason for starting smoking in a survey of adolescents, but only among young women who were European American (Paxton, Valois, & Drane, 2004). Smoking also appeared as a weight control strategy in another study (Fulkerson & French, 2003), but this study showed a more widespread effect—only young African American women were immune from this tactic. This study also showed that young men were willing to use smoking for weight control, with Native American and Asian American men adopting this strategy more often than young men from other ethnic groups.

Young women who were dieting reported that they used smoking as a strategy to lose weight (Jenks & Higgs, 2007). Adolescent smokers who wanted to lose weight were likely not only to use smoking as a strategy but also to use other unhealthy dieting strategies, such as diet pills or laxatives (Delnevo, Hrywna, Abatemarco, & Lewis, 2003). Thus, smoking is a choice for losing weight among young people, and this risky practice is associated with other risky weight control behaviors.

Why Do People Continue to Smoke? Different people smoke for different reasons, including being addicted to nicotine, receiving positive and negative reinforcement, having an optimistic bias, and fearing weight gain.

Addiction Once people begin to smoke, they quickly become dependent on the habit. The Centers for Disease Control and Prevention (CDC, 1994) surveyed smokers 10 to 22 years old and found that nearly two-thirds of those who had smoked at least 100 cigarettes during their lifetime reported that "It's really hard to quit," but only a small number of those who had smoked

fewer than 100 lifetime cigarettes gave this response. In addition, nearly 90% of participants who smoked more than 15 cigarettes a day found quitting to be very hard. These results suggest that people will become dependent on smoking and have great difficulty quitting once they have smoked about 100 cigarettes or have increased their cigarette consumption to more than 15 per day. These results are consistent with Christy Turlington's smoking—her smoking escalated rapidly, and she became an addicted smoker who had a great deal of difficulty quitting.

When addicted smokers are restricted to low-nicotine cigarettes, they will smoke more cigarettes to compensate for the scarcity of nicotine they are receiving. An early study by Stanley Schachter (1980) manipulated the amount of nicotine in cigarettes supplied to heavy, long-duration smokers. The participants smoked 25% more low-nicotine than high-nicotine cigarettes and took more puffs from low-nicotine cigarettes. A recent laboratory study (Strasser, Lerman, Sandborn, Pickworth, & Feldman, 2007) performed a similar manipulation and obtained similar results—smokers compensate when they smoke lower-nicotine cigarettes.

Addicted smokers are not only aware of smoking but are also keenly conscious of the fact when they are *not* smoking. They usually know how long it has been since their last cigarette and how long it will be before their next one. Addicted smokers never leave home or office without first checking their supply of cigarettes. They often keep several extra packs available in case of emergency. These smokers will be willing to smoke bad-tasting cigarettes, whereas smokers whose focus is pleasure or relaxation will not (Leventhal & Avis, 1976).

Nicotine addiction, however, does not explain why some people are light smokers and others smoke heavily. In addition, if nicotine were the only reason for smoking, then other modes of nicotine delivery should substitute fully for smoking. Evidence, however, indicates that other delivery methods are not entirely satisfactory to smokers. Researchers (Hughes, 2003; Sweeney, Fant, Fagerstrom, McGovern, & Henningfield, 2001) have examined a variety of nicotine delivery systems, including the patch, gum, nasal spray inhaler, and lozenges, and found that although smokers may decrease smoking when nicotine is available through other modes, they still find it difficult to stop smoking. Although nicotine may play a role in the reason people continue to smoke, this research indicates that something other than nicotine is involved.

Positive and Negative Reinforcement A second reason why people continue to smoke is that they receive either positive or negative reinforcement, or both. Behaviors are positively reinforced when they are followed immediately by a pleasant or pleasurable event. The smoking habit is strengthened by such positive reinforcers as pleasure from the smell of tobacco smoke, feelings of relaxation, and satisfaction of manual needs.

Negative reinforcement may also account for why some people continue to smoke. Behaviors are negatively reinforced when they are followed immediately by the removal of or lessening of an unpleasant condition. After smokers become addicted, they must continue to smoke to avoid the aversive effects of withdrawal; that is, when addicted smokers begin to feel tense, anxious, or depressed after not smoking for some period of time, they can remove these unpleasant symptoms by smoking another cigarette (Stevens, Colwell, Smith, Robinson, & McMillan, 2005).

Examinations of smokers' motivations are consistent with both types of reinforcement. Smokers attending a cessation clinic (McEwen, West, & McRobbie, 2008) rated relief from stress and boredom as their top two reasons for smoking, and these reasons were similar among deployed military personnel (Poston et al., 2008). Relief from an unpleasant emotion meets the definition of negative reinforcement. Smokers also reported pleasure and enjoyment as reasons for smoking (McEwen et al., 2008), which fit into the category of positive reinforcement.

Optimistic Bias In addition to addiction and reinforcement, many people continue to smoke because they have an **optimistic bias** that leads them to believe that they personally have a lower risk of disease and death than do other smokers (Weinstein, 1980). For example, when asked about their chances of living to be 75 years old,

people who had never smoked and those who were former and light smokers estimated fairly accurately (Schoenbaum, 1997). Heavy smokers, on the other hand, greatly overestimated their chances of living to age 75.

Neil Weinstein (2001) reviewed research on smokers' recognition of their vulnerability to harm and found strong support for the hypothesis that smokers tend to have an optimistic bias. That is, smokers do not perceive that they are at the same level of risk as other smokers. This effect appeared in a study in which smokers were asked to rate their risk of cardiovascular disease, lung cancer, and emphysema (Waltenbaugh & Zagummy, 2004); the results indicated that smokers perceive the risk of these diseases but do not apply that risk to themselves as much as they do to other smokers. Thus, smokers tend to retain an optimistic bias concerning their vulnerability to smoking-related dangers, which allows them to keep on smoking.

Fear of Weight Gain Adolescents are not the only age group using cigarette smoking as a means of weight control. Adults, too, often continue to smoke for fear of weight gain. In a later section, we examine the validity of those concerns, but here we look at the magnitude of fears concerning weight gain.

Concern about weight gain extends to a wide range of smokers but occurs more in younger than in older smokers and more often in women than in men. Young adults are more likely than older adults to use cigarette smoking as a means of weight control. Christina Wee and colleagues (Wee, Rigotti, Davis, & Phillips, 2001) looked at adults trying to lose weight and found that weight-conscious people 30 years old and younger were more likely than other young people to be current smokers, whereas older adults trying to control weight were no more likely than other older adults to be current smokers.

Gender is an even stronger predictor of using smoking for weight control. For example, college-age women with body image problems were more likely to be smokers than women without such body image problems (Stickney & Black, 2008). A study of German adults (Twardella et al., 2006) indicated that weight plays a role in successful quitting—heavier people were more successful.

Overweight men were more successful at quitting than thinner men, perhaps because they feared the health consequences of smoking, whereas the thin women were more likely to drop out, perhaps because they feared weight gain. A study of women with strong weight concerns (King, Saules, & Irish, 2007) indicated that such women were much more likely to smoke (37.5%) compared to women without strong weight concerns (22%). Should women with high weight concerns quit smoking, their concerns may increase; normal weight women who were ex-smokers expressed higher concerns over their weight than normal weight women who had never smoked (Pisinger & Jorgenson, 2007). These results point to a factor of weight concern, which some people attempt to manage through choosing to smoke and to whom quitting presents a threat.

IN SUMMARY

The rate of smoking in the United States has slowly declined since the mid-1960s. Presently, about 18% of adult women and 23% of adult men in the United States meet the definition of smoker. Ethnic background is a factor in smoking for both adolescents and adults, with Native Americans having the highest smoking rate, followed by African American, European Americans, Hispanic Americans, and Asian Americans. Currently, educational level is a better predictor of smoking status than gender, with highly educated people smoking at a much lower rate than those with less education.

Reasons for smoking can be divided into questions concerning why people begin to smoke and why they continue to smoke. Most smokers begin as teenagers, at a time when peer pressure is especially strong. Genetics may play a role in beginning to smoke, but social factors such as friends, siblings, and parents who smoke; advertising; and weight concerns also influence smoking initiation. The question about why people continue is a difficult one because people smoke for a variety of reasons. Nearly every smoker in the United States is familiar with the potential dangers of smoking,

but many do not relate those hazards to themselves; that is, their knowledge of the dangers of smoking is attenuated by an optimistic bias. For many people, smoking reduces stress, anxiety, and depression and therefore provides negative reinforcement. Some people smoke because they are addicted to the nicotine in tobacco products, and others continue to smoke because they are concerned about weight gain.

HEALTH CONSEQUENCES OF TOBACCO USE

Tobacco use is responsible for more than 438,000 deaths yearly in the United States, or more than 1,000 deaths a day (Rock et al., 2007), and more than 5 million per year worldwide (Poupard, 2007). All forms of tobacco use have health consequences, but smoking cigarettes is the most common and thus the most hazardous. Those hazards include cardiovascular disease, cancer, chronic lower respiratory disease, and a variety of other disorders.

Cigarette Smoking

Cigarette smoking is the single deadliest behavior in the history of the United States, and it is the largest preventable cause of death and disability. In Chapter 2, we discussed how scientists have found evidence to support the criteria for establishing a cause-and-effect relationship between smoking and several diseases, even though experimental research is not possible with human participants. Evidence for the harmful effects of tobacco use began to emerge as early as the 1930s, and by the 1950s, the relationship between cigarette smoking and cardiovascular disease, cancer, and chronic lower respiratory disease was well established (USDHHS, 2004). These diseases remain the three leading causes of death in the United States, and cigarette smoking contributes to all three.

Smoking and Cardiovascular Disease Cardiovascular disease (including both heart disease and stroke) is the leading cause of death in the

United States. Until the mid-1990s, the largest number of smoking-related deaths was from cardiovascular disease, but these deaths have begun to decline, whereas those from cancer have not declined so rapidly. Now, CVD is the second largest cause of tobacco-related deaths.

What is the level of risk for cardiovascular disease among people who smoke? In general, research suggests that the relative risk is about 2.0 (CDC, 1993), which means that people who smoke cigarettes are twice as likely as people who do not smoke to die of cardiovascular disease. The risk is slightly higher for men than for women, but both male and female smokers have a significantly increased chance of both fatal and nonfatal heart attack and stroke.

What biological mechanism might explain the association between smoking and cardiovascular disease? Research during the 1990s began to reveal that relationship (USDHHS, 2004). Smoking damages the inner wall of arteries and speeds the formation of plaque within the arteries. Smoking is also related to formation of blood clots along the walls of arteries, which is a dangerous complication to artery damage. In addition, smoking is related to inflammation, not only in the lungs but also within the entire body; growing evidence implicates the role of inflammation in the development of artery disease. Smoking has also been implicated in harmful changes in lipid metabolism, so smoking may be linked to unfavorable cholesterol levels. Smoking also decreases the availability of oxygen to the heart muscle while at the same time increasing demand for oxygen by the heart. The exact mechanisms through which these reactions occur remain poorly understood, but nicotine itself has been implicated, and carbon monoxide is also a suspect. However, smoking produces a variety of physiological reactions that increase the risks for CVD.

Smoking and Cancer Cancer is the second leading cause of death in the United States, and smoking plays a role in the development of a long list of cancers, especially lung cancer. Sufficient evidence exists to conclude that smoking is a causal factor in cancers of the lip, pharynx, esophagus, pancreas, larynx, trachea, urinary bladder, kidney,

cervix, and stomach (USDHHS, 2004). Both female and male smokers have an extremely high risk of dying from cancer, with men's relative risk being about 23.3. This risk is the strongest link established to date between any behavior and a major cause of death.

From 1950 to 1989, lung cancer deaths rose sharply, a trend that lagged about 20 to 25 years behind the rapid rise in cigarette consumption. During the mid-1960s, cigarette consumption began to drop sharply, and then about 25 to 30 years later, lung cancer deaths among men began to decline. Figure 10.5 (see Chapter 10) shows the close tracking of men's and women's deaths from lung cancer and the rise and fall of cigarette consumption in the United States. This is strong circumstantial evidence for a causal link between smoking and lung cancer.

Could other factors, including environmental pollutants, be responsible for the rapid rise in lung cancer deaths before 1990? Evidence from a prospective study (Thun, Day-Lally, Calle, Flanders, & Heath, 1995) strongly suggested that neither pollution nor any other nonsmoking factor was responsible for the increase in lung cancer deaths from 1959 to 1988. Another piece of evidence against smoking is data showing that lung cancer deaths for smokers rose significantly during this period, whereas lung cancer deaths among nonsmokers remained about the same (USDHHS, 1990), indicating that indoor/outdoor pollution, radon, and other suspected carcinogens had little or no effect on increases in lung cancer mortality. These results, along with those from earlier epidemiological studies, strongly suggest that cigarette smoking is the primary contributor to lung cancer deaths.

Smoking and Chronic Lower Respiratory Disease
Chronic lower respiratory disease includes a number of respiratory and lung diseases; the two most deadly are emphysema and chronic bronchitis. These diseases are relatively rare among nonsmokers. Only 4% of male nonsmokers and 5% of female nonsmokers receive a diagnosis of chronic lower respiratory disease, and a small portion of these have been exposed to passive smoking, mostly from a spouse who smokes.

In summary, the three leading causes of death in the United States are also the three principal smoking-related causes of death. The U.S. Public Health Service has estimated that about half of all cigarette smokers eventually die from their habit (USDHHS, 1995).

Other Effects of Smoking In addition to cancer, cardiovascular disease, and chronic lower respiratory disease, a number of other problems have been linked to smoking. For example, as many as 1,000 people die each year from fires begun by cigarettes (USDHHS, 2004). The people most likely to die in a house fire are those whose income is below the poverty level and who have not finished high school (Ahrens, 2004). Smoking cigarettes while drinking alcohol produces a number of fatal and nonfatal burns every year, but smoking by itself contributed more to those fires than drinking by itself.

People who smoke are two to four times more likely to have been diagnosed with psychiatric disorders and substance abuse disorders (Kalman, Morissette, & George, 2005). People who both are nicotine dependent and have psychiatric disorders smoke 70% of all cigarettes consumed in the United States (Grant, Hasin, Chou, Stinson, & Dawson, 2004). Smoking also has an interactive effect with depression; that is, smokers have more than their share of depressive symptoms, and depressed people do more than their share of smoking (Windle & Windle, 2001). This relationship may exist because nicotine apparently helps people prone to depression attain a more positive mood; depression-prone smokers exposed to a positive mood induction experienced better mood when they smoked a cigarette with nicotine compared to one without nicotine (Spring et al., 2008).

Smoking also relates to diseases of the mouth, pharynx, larynx, esophagus, pancreas, kidney, bladder, and cervix (USDHHS, 2004). Smokers also have more than their share of periodontal disease (Bánóczy & Squier, 2004), multiple sclerosis (Hernán et al., 2005), diminished physical strength, poorer balance, impaired neuromuscular performance (Nelson, Nevitt, Scott, Stone, & Cummings, 1994), and a variety of injuries,

including motor vehicle crashes (Wen et al., 2005). Smokers are also more likely than nonsmokers to commit suicide (Miller, Hemenway, & Rimm, 2000), to develop acute respiratory disease such as pneumonia (USDHHS, 2004), to experience problems with cognitive functioning (Sabia, Marmont, Dufouil, & Singh-Manoux, 2008), and to suffer from macular degeneration (Jager, Mieler, & Miller, 2008).

Women who smoke experience risks specific to their gender. Smoking at least one pack of cigarettes a day places women at double the risk for cardiovascular disease and a tenfold risk of dying from chronic lower respiratory disease. Female smokers have an increased risk of infertility, preterm delivery, stillbirth, low-birth-weight infants, and sudden infant death syndrome (USDHHS, 2004). Pregnant women who smoke double their chances of delivering a stillborn infant, and they also double their risk of having an infant die during the first year of life (Wisborg, Kesmodel, Henriksen, Olsen, & Secher, 2001). Children and adolescents who smoke have slower growth of lung function and begin to lose lung function at earlier ages than those who do not smoke (USDHHS, 2004).

Male smokers also experience some specific risks from their habit. Smoking not only may make men look older and less attractive (Ernster et al., 1995), but it also increases their chances of experiencing erectile dysfunction (USDHHS, 2004).

In any given year, at least 14% of smokers and former smokers will experience a chronic disease (Kahende, Woollery, & Lee, 2007). The negative effects are not limited to individual smokers. Society, too, pays a price. Smoking-related illnesses and economic losses cost the people of the United States $167 billion annually (USDHHS, 2004). These costs, of course, are not limited to smokers—they affect everyone who pays health insurance premiums and everyone who pays for lost worker productivity. Smokers obviously cannot legitimately argue that their smoking habit affects only themselves. They may pay $3.00 to $4.00 for a pack of cigarettes, but the cost to society is an additional $3.00 to $4.00 per pack (USDHHS, 2004).

Cigar and Pipe Smoking

Are cigar and pipe smoking as hazardous as cigarette smoking? People from Australia, Canada, the United Kingdom, and the United States responded that smoking cigars or pipes was less hazardous than smoking cigarettes (O'Connor et al., 2007). The tobacco used in pipes and cigars differs somewhat from the tobacco used to make cigarettes, but pipe and cigar tobacco is similarly carcinogenic. Whereas cigarette-only smokers have a risk for lung cancer of about 23 times that of nonsmokers (USDHHS, 2004), cigar and pipe smokers have a much lower risk, so the opinions of lower risk for cigar and pipe smokers is correct. However, pipe and cigar smokers continue to have a substantial risk for lung cancer as well as many other cancers.

Cigar and pipe smoking reduces life expectancy but not as drastically as cigarette smoking (Streppel, Boshuizen,Ocké, Kok, & Kromhout, 2007). Heavy cigarette smoking produced a reduction in life expectancy of 8.8 years, whereas cigar or pipe smoking decreased life expectancy by 4.7 years. The diseases that kill cigar and pipe smokers are the same as those that increase the mortality of cigarette smokers—heart disease, chronic lower respiratory disease, and a variety of cancers.

A study of middle-aged British men who smoked both cigars and pipes (Shaper, Wannamethee, & Walker, 2003) found a relative risk for lung cancer of 4.35, which was nearly identical to the risk that light cigarette smokers have for lung cancer. Men who are exclusive pipe smokers also have a relative risk for lung cancer of about 5.0 (Henley, Thun, Chao, & Calle, 2004). In general terms, pipe and cigar smokers have about a 1.5 additional risk for coronary heart disease and death, 3.0 for chronic lower respiratory disease, and 5.0 for lung cancer morbidity or mortality. Heavy cigar smokers who inhale have the same risk for death as cigarette smokers (Baker et al., 2000), but those who do not inhale have about the same risk for diseases as passive smokers. These findings suggest that cigar and pipe smoking may be less hazardous than cigarettes, but they are not safe.

Passive Smoking

Many nonsmokers find the smoke of others to be a nuisance and even irritating to their eyes and nose. Exposure to the smoke of others is common among nonsmokers; 43% of nonsmokers show evidence of such exposure (USDHHS, 2006). But is **passive smoking**, also known as **environmental tobacco smoke** (ETS) or secondhand smoke, harmful to the health of nonsmokers? In the 1980s, some evidence began to accrue that passive smoking might be a health hazard. Specifically, passive smoking has been linked to lung cancer, breast cancer, heart disease, and a variety of respiratory problems in children.

Passive Smoking and Cancer The effect of passive smoking on lung and other cancers is difficult to determine because of the amount and duration of exposure. In general, the more environmental tobacco smoke people are exposed to and the longer the exposure, the higher the risk for cancer.

People whose jobs expose them to high levels of passive smoking may have an increased risk of lung cancer mortality. What are the occupations with high levels of exposure to nicotine? One review (Siegel & Skeer, 2003) looked specifically at the "5 B's"—bars, bowling alleys, billiard halls, betting establishments, and bingo parlors. Longtime employees of these establishments had up to 18 times higher nicotine concentrations than people who worked in restaurants, residences, and offices. The authors estimated that workers in the "5 B's" would have a higher rate of lung cancer mortality than people who were not exposed to secondhand smoke, but causal evidence is still lacking. Results from a later study (Vineis, 2005) confirmed these findings; that is, passive smoking is related to lung cancer. The increased risk is 20–30% (USDHHS, 2006).

Although evidence suggests that passive smoking may contribute to some additional risk for lung cancer, relative risks should be interpreted with reference to the prevalence of the disease within the comparison group—in this case, nonsmokers who are not exposed to cigarette smoke. Because lung cancer in this comparison group is quite rare, an elevated risk of 20% or 30% for nonsmokers exposed to environmental tobacco smoke does not add a great number of nonsmokers to the lung cancer mortality rates. However, no level of exposure to smoke is safe (USDHHS, 2006).

Passive Smoking and Cardiovascular Disease Although the effect of environmental tobacco smoke on cancer is not large, its effects on cardiovascular disease are substantial. Exposure to smoke prompts some of the same physiological reactions as smoking—inflammation, formation of blood clots, and changes to the lining of arteries—which increases the risks for heart disease (Venn & Britton, 2007). A meta-analysis of studies (He et al., 1999) showed that the excess risk of heart disease for passive smokers is about 25%, a little less than the risk for stroke (You, Thrift, McNeil, Davis, & Donnan, 1999). However, even this small elevation of risk for heart disease translates into thousands of deaths each year from passive smoking. Although environmental tobacco smoke kills thousands of people each year, the risk from passive smoking is only about one-tenth the risk from active smoking.

Passive Smoking and the Health of Children Infants and young children are especially vulnerable to exposure to tobacco smoke, which can affect their development and health even before they are born (USDHHS, 2006). Typically, those effects are not fatal, but they can be; the risks include sudden infant death syndrome (SIDS). Other health problems include chronic lower respiratory disease, low birth weight, and provocation of asthma attacks (USDHHS, 2006) as well as increases in childhood cancers (John, Savitz, & Sandler, 1991). In general, the negative effects of environmental tobacco smoke diminish as children age, but school-age children exposed to passive smoking have more than their share of wheezing, missed school days, and weaker lung function volume (Mannino, Moorman, Kingsley, Rose, & Repace, 2001).

In summary, passive smoking is a health risk for lung cancer, cardiovascular disease, and many health problems of children. In general, the greater the exposure, the greater is the risk.

Smokeless Tobacco

Smokeless tobacco includes snuff and chewing tobacco, forms of tobacco that were more popular during the 19th century than at present. Currently, Hispanic American and European American male adolescents use smokeless tobacco more than any other segment of the U.S. population (Eaton et al., 2008), but smokeless forms of tobacco use are common among adolescents and young men in some areas of the world, especially in the eastern Mediterranean region (Warren et al., 2008). Although many of the young people who use smokeless forms of tobacco acknowledge that it carries risks, they tend to believe that it is safer than smoking.

The use of smokeless tobacco has increased throughout North America and parts of Europe and become controversial because some advocate its use as a safer substitute for smoking (Tomar, 2007). In some sense, these advocates are correct; smokeless tobacco does not carry as high a risk for some forms of cancer as smoking does, but tobacco is still a toxin and a carcinogen, regardless of the form of its use. Evidence from Norway showed that regular users of smokeless tobacco were more likely to die from pancreatic cancer than from pharyngeal, esophageal, or any other cancer associated with the oral cavity (Boffetta, Aagnes, Weiderpass, & Andersen, 2005). Smokeless tobacco users who had never smoked showed no increase in risk for heart attack, but those who had smoked and had used smokeless tobacco showed an increased risk (Wennberg et al., 2007). In addition, its use as a substitute for smoking is questionable; adolescents who begin to use smokeless tobacco are more likely to begin smoking than those who do not try this form of tobacco (Severson, Forrester, & Biglan, 2007). The risks of using smokeless tobacco are not as great as those associated with smoking cigarettes; nevertheless, chewing tobacco presents significant health hazards.

IN SUMMARY

The health consequences of tobacco use are multiple and serious. Smoking is the number one cause of preventable mortality in the United

States, causing about 438,000 deaths a year, mostly from cancer, cardiovascular disease, and chronic lower respiratory disease. But smoking also carries a risk for nonfatal diseases and disorders such as periodontal disease, loss of physical strength, infertility among women, respiratory disorders, cognitive dysfunction, erectile dysfunction, and macular degeneration.

Many nonsmokers are bothered by the smoking of others, but many of these nonsmokers also have an excess risk of respiratory disease from passive smoking, especially infants and young children. Research suggests that environmental tobacco smoke does not contribute substantially to death from lung cancer, but it may be responsible for several thousand deaths a year from cardiovascular disease.

Like cigars and pipes, smokeless tobacco is not as dangerous as cigarette smoking. Teenagers who use smokeless tobacco tend to believe that this form of tobacco is much safer than cigarette smoking, and some advocates argue that smokeless tobacco may be a safer substitute for smoking. However, no use of tobacco is safe.

INTERVENTIONS FOR REDUCING SMOKING RATES

Although smoking rates are declining in many industrialized, wealthy nations, smoking rates are increasing in developing nations, which will prompt an increase in smoking-related diseases throughout the world (World Health Organization, 2008a). Thus, the need to reduce smoking rates has become a worldwide goal. Interventions designed to reduce smoking rates can be divided into those that deter people (usually adolescents) from beginning and those that encourage current smokers to stop.

Deterring Smoking

Information alone is not an effective way to change behavior, which applies to deterring smoking. Nearly every teenager in the United States (and many other parts of the world) knows that smoking is dangerous to health, yet about 20% of high school students in the United States smoke at least once a month (Eaton et al., 2008).

Choosing to smoke does not occur because children or adolescents lack information about the dangers of tobacco; they receive many messages about the dangers of smoking through antismoking media messages (Weiss et al, 2006), health officials, and concerned parents. By the time adolescents are 14 years old, they pay little attention to health warnings, making such warnings worthless (Siegel & Biener, 2000). Thus, information about the health dangers of smoking does not create successful prevention programs. Deterring smoking is a challenge that requires more and different types of interventions.

The most common approach to preventing children from beginning to smoke is through school-based programs, which vary in terms of who delivers the antismoking message, length of intervention, and age of the target students. The most common such program is Project D.A.R.E., which is oriented to drug use but also includes tobacco. This intervention includes antidrug use messages delivered by police officers, typically once a week for a school semester. Evaluations of this program (West & O'Neal, 2004) have revealed that it is not effective in deterring smoking or other drug use. However, other programs have shown more success (Dobbins, DeCorby, Manske, & Goldblatt, 2008). The elements of more successful school-based programs include integrating smoking prevention into a comprehensive health education program, providing booster sessions over several years, and reinforcing prevention messages in the community as well as by parents and through media messages (La Torre, Chiaradia, & Ricciardi, 2005). The evidence is more impressive for short-term effectiveness (Dobbins et al., 2008) than for long-term effectiveness (Wiehe, Garrison, Christakis, Ebel, & Rivara, 2005). These results indicate that deterring children and adolescents from smoking is not an easy task, and successful efforts are likely to involve programs with multiple components. The evidence concerning quitting smoking shows some similarities to the results for deterring smoking.

Quitting Smoking

A second method of reducing smoking rates is for current smokers to quit. Although quitting smoking is not easy, millions of Americans have done so during the past 50 years. As a result, there are now more former smokers in the United States than there are current smokers—about 23% are former smokers and about 21% are current smokers. Figure 12.4 indicates that the decline in smoking rates is due not merely to fewer people starting to smoke but in large part to increased cessation rates.

Nevertheless, many barriers to quitting exist. One barrier to quitting smoking is its addictive quality. Most people who both smoke and drink alcohol consider smoking to be the more difficult habit to break. People seeking treatment for alcohol or drug dependence who also smoked were asked which would be more difficult to quit—their problem substance or tobacco (Kozlowski et al., 1989). A majority of these people reported that cigarettes would be more difficult to quit.

Despite the difficulties of quitting, many smokers have quit on their own, and others have done so with the assistance of nicotine replacement therapy, psychological interventions, and communitywide antismoking campaigns.

Quitting Without Therapy

Most people who have quit smoking have done so just as Christy Turlington did—on their own, without the aid of formal cessation programs. In the United States, about 44% of smokers try to quit each year, and about 64% of those people used no cessation treatment (Shiffman, Brockwell, Pillitteri, & Gitchell, 2008). Who are the smokers most likely to quit on their own?

In an important study on unaided quitting, Stanley Schachter (1982) surveyed two populations: the psychology department at Columbia University and the resident population of Amaganset, New York. Schachter found a success rate of more than 60% for both groups, with an average abstinence length of more than seven years. Surprisingly, nearly a third of the heavy smokers who quit said they had no problems in quitting. Schachter interpreted the high success rate, even for heavy smokers, as evidence that quitting may be easier than the clinic evaluations indicate. He suggested that people who attend clinic programs are, for the most part, those who have failed in attempts to quit on their own, and

research on the use of smoking cessation treatment (Shiffman et al., 2008) confirms this reasoning. In addition, Schachter hypothesized that the clinic success rates of 20% to 30% represent success for each program, with those who fail in one program going on to another, in which they may also have about a 20% to 30% quit rate. Smokers who try to quit on their own largely succeed and never attend a clinic. Thus, people who attend clinics are an atypical group, self-selected on the basis of previous failure. These people, therefore, do not represent the general population of smokers, and failure rates based on clinic populations may be too high.

Using Nicotine Replacement Therapy

People who have not been able to quit on their own often seek help from outside sources, including nicotine replacement therapy. Currently, a variety of nicotine replacements techniques are available to people trying to quit smoking. These include nicotine gum, nicotine inhalers, nicotine lozenges (tablets), nicotine patches, and nicotine spray. Nicotine replacement techniques work by releasing a small, continuous dose of nicotine into the body. Smokers move from a larger dose to a smaller one until they are no longer dependent on nicotine.

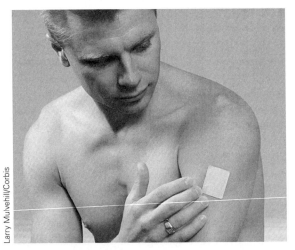

Larry Mulvehill/Corbis

Nicotine replacement can help smokers with symptoms of withdrawal, but the effectiveness is higher when combined with behavioral techniques.

How effective are these nicotine replacement therapies? A recent large-scale analysis of more than 100 well-designed studies (Silagy, Lancaster, Stead, Mant, & Fowler, 2005) and a systematic review (Stead, Perera, Bullen, Mant, & Lancaster, 2008) examined studies with various types of nicotine replacement therapy and concluded that this form of treatment is successful, with higher quit rates for nicotine replacement than for no treatment or placebos. Adding other components may boost effectiveness, but nicotine replacement alone is helpful in quitting.

Each of the nicotine replacement techniques has potential side effects. None should be used by pregnant women, unless the beneficial effects of quitting clearly outweigh the potential risk of nicotine replacement. Also, people with a recently diagnosed heart attack should not use nicotine replacement therapy. Other possible side effects include nausea, light-headedness, and sleep disturbances.

Nicotine replacement is an important component in a pharmacologically based program with the assumption that nicotine withdrawal may produce depressive symptoms or a major depressive episode (Hughes, 2003; Hughes, Stead, & Lancaster, 2004). If the various nicotine replacements can lessen or eliminate depression, then the smoker has a better chance of successful cessation.

Receiving a Psychological Intervention Psychological approaches aimed at smoking cessation typically include a combination of strategies, such as behavior modification, cognitive behavioral approaches, contracts made by smoker and therapist in which the smoker agrees to stop smoking, group therapy, social support, relaxation training, stress management, "booster" sessions to prevent relapse, and other treatment approaches.

Most psychologists working with smoking cessation problems begin with some implicit or explicit theory, such as one or more of the models we discussed in Chapters 3 and 4. For example, they may use the stages of change model of James Prochaska. In this model, smokers at the *precontemplation* stage have no intention to quit and, therefore, are not yet good candidates for

psychological interventions. When smokers are at this level, a technique such as motivational interviewing may help them move to the *contemplation* stage, at which they are aware of the problem and may consider quitting sometime in the future (Colby et al., 2005). However, a study that matched smokers' stage to an appropriate intervention manual (Velicer et al., 2006) failed to find an advantage for this approach.

Both individual and group counseling can be successful in helping some people quit smoking. Psychologists, physicians, and nurses can be effective providers, but effectiveness is positively related to the amount of contact between client and therapist. For example, receiving advice from a physician to quit produces only small increases in cessation (Stead, Bergson, & Lancaster, 2008). The increased costs of intensive interventions are offset by their improved effectiveness. Programs that include more sessions tend to be more effective than programs with fewer sessions. For example, counseling and behavioral programs of smoking cessation are successful for individuals who have experienced heart attacks when these programs are of sufficient duration (Barth, Critchley, & Bengel, 2008). The most effective programs include both a counseling component and a nicotine replacement component. Each of these elements is effective, and the combination of the two improves outcomes (Carpenter, Hughes, & Solomon, 2005; Stead, Perera, et al., 2008).

Participating in a Community Campaign Many people stop smoking as a result of their participation in a communitywide health campaign. Such health campaigns are not new, dating back to Cotton Mather more than two centuries before anyone suspected the dangers of cigarette smoking. Mather used pamphlets and oratory to persuade the people of Boston to accept smallpox inoculations (Faden, 1987). Today, several hundred large community programs exist throughout the world (Secker-Walker et al., 2000). Such campaigns are typically sponsored by government agencies or by large corporations as an intervention designed to improve the health of large numbers of people. One effective form is the restriction of places in which people are allowed to smoke. A systematic review of studies on smoke-free workplaces (Fichtenberg & Glantz, 2002) indicated that this strategy not only reduces the number of cigarettes that workers smoke but also decreases the prevalence of smoking, creating a low-cost approach to reducing smoking rates. Another effective community or national strategy to decrease smoking is raising the price of cigarettes, which affects young smokers' willingness to purchase cigarettes.

The percentage of people who change behavior as a result of a community or media health campaign is usually quite small, but if the message reaches millions of people, then the approach is successful. For example, an intervention in Vermont and New Hampshire (Secker-Walker et al., 2000) used random-digit dialing to contact female smokers and to encourage them to quit. After four years, the quit rate was higher in the two intervention counties than in two matched comparison counties—24% versus 21%. This difference may seem small, but it represents hundreds of women who might not have quit otherwise. A systematic review of media campaigns (Bala, Strzeszynski, & Cahill, 2008) indicated that such campaigns have been successful in decreasing smoking rates, increasing quitting, and on other measures of cessation success. Thus, attempting to reach large numbers of people through media campaigns can be a successful strategy.

Who Quits and Who Does Not?

Who is successful at quitting, and who is not? Investigators have examined several factors that may answer this question, including age, gender, educational level, quitting other drugs, and weight concern (which we discuss in a later section). Age shows a relation to quitting. In general, younger smokers, especially those who smoke at a high level, are more likely to continue smoking than older smokers (Ferguson, Bauld, Chesterman, & Judge, 2005; Nordstrom et al., 2000).

Are men more likely than women to quit smoking? Because men have had higher quit rates than women over the past 50 years, many observers assumed that women have more difficulty quitting than men. Although some evidence exists to support this idea (Vastag, 2001), the reason

may be that female smokers who try to quit have more obstacles to overcome. Women may feel less motivated to quit and less confident that they can succeed (Schnoll, Patterson, & Lerman, 2007). In addition, women tend to use smoking to manage stress, anxiety, and depression. Losing a coping strategy presents difficulties; people who use smoking as a coping strategy are less likely to quit than those who smoke for pleasure (Ferguson et al., 2005). It has been proposed that women experience more severe symptoms of cessation, but some research has indicated no gender differences in severity of symptoms (Weinberger, Krishnan-Sarin, Mazure, & McKee, 2008) or in success at quitting (Ferguson et al., 2005). However, people who experience severe symptoms tend to be less successful at quitting, as are those who live with a smoker.

A supportive social network may also help people quit smoking, but only about 24% of smokers in the United States who tried to quit reported that they experienced social support (Shiffman et al., 2008). Cessation programs are more effective in maintaining abstinence when spouses of participants are trained to offer support to the partner who is trying to quit. Also, pregnant women who smoke are more likely to quit if their partners are nonsmokers or if they receive support from their partners (McBride et al., 1998).

Do difficulties in quitting smoking explain the inverse relationship between educational level and rate of smoking—that is, does educational level relate to quitting? Some research (Droomers, Schrijvers, & Mackenbach, 2002) suggests an affirmative answer. This longitudinal study of Dutch participants found that people with low educational levels at baseline were more than twice as likely to remain smokers. More important, smokers with lower levels of education (1) began smoking earlier, (2) had higher scores on neuroticism (anxiety, depression, guilt, and low self-esteem), (3) had lower scores on emotional support, and (4) had low levels of perceived personal control. These factors, rather than level of knowledge about the hazards of smoking, may be important reasons why lower educational level is associated with higher smoking rates.

Finally, do smokers who abuse alcohol and other drugs find it harder to give up cigarettes? Clinical psychologists have long recognized the strong relationship between smoking and drinking, but until recently there has been little research on how quitting one substance affects quitting the other. Some evidence now suggests that problem drinkers who are able to stop drinking are also able to quit smoking (Burling, Burling, & Latini, 2001)—that is, some people can stop two addictive behaviors simultaneously.

Relapse Prevention

The problem of relapse is not unique to smoking. Relapse rates are quite similar among people who have quit smoking, given up alcohol, and stopped using heroin (Hunt, Barnett, & Branch, 1971). For those who endeavor to quit, some do succeed in quitting or cutting down, but 22% go back to smoking at a higher rate than before their quit attempt (Yong, Borland, Hyland, & Siahpush, 2008). The high rate of relapse after smoking cessation treatment prompted G. Alan Marlatt and Judith Gordon (1980) to examine the relapse process itself. For some people who have been successful in quitting, one cigarette precipitates a full relapse, complete with feelings of total failure. Marlatt and Gordon termed this phenomenon the *abstinence violation effect*. They incorporated strategies into their treatment to cope with patients' despair when they violate their intention to remain abstinent. By training patients that one "slip" does not constitute a relapse, Marlatt and Gordon buffer them against a full-blown relapse. Slips are common even among people who will eventually quit. One-fourth of successful self-quitters slip at one time or another (Hughes et al., 1992). Thus, a single slip should not discourage people from continuing their efforts to stop smoking.

Self-quitters have very high relapse rates, with two-thirds of smokers who quit on their own having relapsed after only two days (Hughes et al., 1992), and 75% resuming smoking within six months (Ferguson et al., 2005). Smoking cessation programs that include relapse prevention may be more successful for some people, but a systematic review of the research on relapse prevention (Lancaster, Hajek, Stead, West, & Jarvis, 2006) failed to find much benefit for such interventions.

Effective relapse prevention is a critical component of successful cessation programs. If current efforts are not successful, then new, innovative approaches are necessary. One suggestion is not new (Fiore et al., 1996), but its implementation may be: tailor relapse prevention to each ex-smoker's "triggers." This approach would require therapists to review reasons for relapse, such as fear of weight gain, unpleasant withdrawal symptoms, negative mood or depression, and lack of social support for cessation. Once these factors have been identified, therapists can work to reduce or eliminate them. Another possibility appeared in a study (R. A. Brown et al., 2008) that conceptualized relapse prevention as developing a tolerance for distress, which will be an inevitable experience for smokers who quit.

IN SUMMARY

Smoking rates can be reduced either by prevention or by quitting. Providing young people with information on the dangers of smoking is not an effective strategy, and many of the school-based prevention programs have limited effects. Some of the programs that are lengthy and well-integrated into the school health curriculum can provide short-term deterrence. Research indicates that long-term prevention is much more difficult.

How can people quit smoking? Most people who attempt to quit do so without seeking any type of program to help, but some try nicotine replacement or psychological interventions, and others are exposed to media and community campaigns to decrease smoking. Because giving up nicotine may result in withdrawal symptoms, many successful cessation programs include some form of nicotine replacement, such as a patch or gum. Both are more effective than a placebo or no treatment. A second approach to quitting is psychological counseling, which can be effective. Another approach to reducing smoking rates involves large-scale community programs, which usually include anti-tobacco

BECOMING HEALTHIER

1. If you do not smoke, don't start. College students are still susceptible to the pressure to smoke if their friends are smokers. The easiest way to be a nonsmoker is to stay a nonsmoker.

2. If you smoke, don't fool yourself into believing that the risks of smoking do not apply to you. Examine your own optimistic biases regarding smoking. Do not imagine that smoking low-tar and low-nicotine cigarettes makes smoking safe. Research indicates that these cigarettes are about as risky as any others.

3. If you smoke, try to quit. Even if you feel that quitting will be difficult, make an attempt to quit. If your first attempt is not successful, try again. Keep trying until you quit. Research indicates that people who

keep trying are very likely to succeed.

4. If you have tried to quit on your own and have failed, look for a program to help you. Remember that not all programs are equally successful. Research indicates that the most effective programs combine some psychological techniques with nicotine replacement therapy.

5. The best cessation programs allow for some individual tailoring to meet personal needs. Try different techniques until you find one that works for you.

6. If you are trying to quit smoking, find a supportive network of friends and acquaintances to help you stop and to boost your motivation to quit. Avoid people who try to sabotage your attempts to quit, and be cautious in going to places or engaging in

activities that have a high association with smoking.

7. Cigar smoking has undergone a resurgence in popularity. Cigar and pipe smoking are not as dangerous as cigarette smoking, but remember that no level of smoking is safe.

8. Even if you do not smoke, remember that no level of tobacco exposure is safe. Exposure to environmental tobacco smoke is not nearly as dangerous as smoking, but it is not safe either. Smokeless tobacco use carries a number of health risks.

9. If you smoke, do not expose others to your smoke. Young children are especially vulnerable, and smoking parents can minimize the risks of respiratory disease in their children by keeping smoke away from them.

mass media campaigns. If even a small percentage of people exposed to such campaigns stop smoking, this change can translate into thousands of people giving up tobacco. Some studies have found that men are more likely to be successful at quitting than women, but other studies find no gender difference. Many people are able to quit for six months to a year, but the problem of relapse remains serious. Programs aimed at this relapse problem have not demonstrated the degree of success that is needed; relapse is a serious problem for those who quit smoking.

EFFECTS OF QUITTING

When smokers quit, they experience a number of effects, almost all of which are positive. However, one possible negative effect is weight gain.

Quitting and Weight Gain

Many smokers fear weight gain if they give up smoking; this fear applies to men (M. M. Clark et al., 2004) as well as women (King, Matacin, White, & Marcus, 2005). Are such concerns justified? Several factors need to be examined when considering the health benefits of quitting smoking and adding weight.

The weight gain associated with quitting is quite modest for most people who have stopped smoking, but that weight gain may make a difference in the health benefits associated with quitting. A study on the overall benefits of smoking cessation (Chinn et al., 2005) found that some of the respiratory benefits of quitting were offset by weight gain.

When people quit smoking, the variation in weight gain is large. Some people experience increased appetite as a symptom of nicotine withdrawal (John, Meyer, Rumpf, Hapke, & Schumann, 2006) and gain a great deal of weight (Filozof, Fernández Pinilla, & Fernández-Cruz, 2004). One study (O'Hara et al., 1998) found that the average weight gain was a little more than 11 pounds for women and a little less than 11 pounds for men one year after quitting. Another study (John, Hanke, Rumpf, & Thyrian, 2005) found that men gained weight after quitting, but women did not. Thus, weight gain is not assured. In addition, weight gain following smoking cessation can be temporary; for female ex-smokers, both body mass index and body weight tend to decrease with years of smoking cessation (Kawada, 2004). Former smokers were heavier one year after quitting than two to four years afterward. Therefore, even former smokers who gain weight tend to lose the weight they have gained.

Physical activity for ex-smokers can curtail weight gain. For example, research on female smokers (Prapavessis et al., 2007) revealed that women who increased their level of exercise and used nicotine replacement after quitting smoking gained less weight than women who quit but did not become more physically active. Similarly, a study with men (Froom et al., 1999) found that those who stopped smoking had a slight increase in body mass index, but men who were active in sports gained less than sedentary ex-smokers. Although maintaining close to ideal weight and quitting smoking are both desirable, the extra weight gained by former smokers does not negate the health benefits of quitting smoking. Quitting smoking is much more beneficial to health than maintaining a lower weight (Taylor, Hasselblad, Henley, Thun, & Sloan, 2002).

Health Benefits of Quitting

Can smokers reduce their all-cause mortality by quitting smoking? An extensive review of existing studies (Critchley & Capewell, 2003) compared a large group of smokers who continued to smoke with another large group who were able to stop smoking and found that smokers who quit reduced their all-cause mortality by 36%. The authors saw this reduction in mortality as solid evidence that quitting smoking can decrease rate of mortality. To receive these health benefits, however, smokers must quit and not just cut down the number of cigarettes smoked (Pisinger & Godtfredsen, 2007).

Two important questions for smokers considering quitting are: (1) Can smokers regain some of their life expectancy by quitting? (2) How long must ex-smokers remain abstinent before they reverse the detrimental effects of smoking? The 1990 report of the Surgeon General (USDHHS, 1990) summarized studies on the health benefits of quitting for different levels and durations of smoking, and the International Agency for Research on Cancer (Dresler, Leon, Straif, Baan, & Secretan, 2006) conducted a similar review. The results of both reviews were consistent: quitting improves a range of risks for health problems produced by smoking. The earlier analysis indicated that former light smokers (fewer than 20 cigarettes a day) who were able to abstain for 16 years had about the same rate of mortality as people who had never smoked. Figure 12.9 shows that after more than 15 years of abstinence, women's mortality risk decreased substantially. Figure 12.10 shows that men's mortality risk reduces steadily for up to 16 years.

Longtime smokers who quit reduce their chances of dying from heart disease much more rapidly than they lower their risk of death from lung cancer (Dresler et al., 2006; USDHHS, 1990). Their risk of some cancers remains elevated for 15 years or longer. Thus, men who quit smoking for 30 years reduce their risk of both cardiovascular disease and lung cancer, but their risk for lung cancer remains substantially higher than that of men who have never smoked. Women also reduce their risks by quitting, and the younger they are when they quit, the less likely they will be to die of lung cancer (Zhang et al., 2005).

These studies suggest that by quitting smoking, both male and female smokers can reduce their risk of cardiovascular disease to that of nonsmokers, although they may never completely erase their elevated risk of lung and other cancers. Thus, never starting to smoke is healthier than quitting, but quitting, though seldom easy, can pay off.

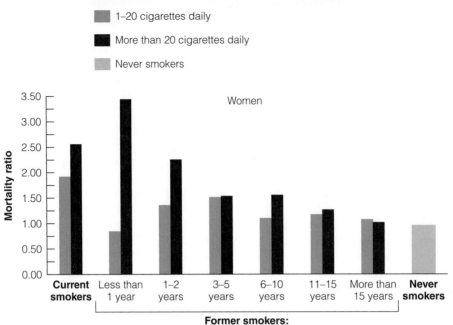

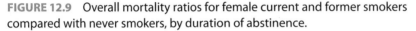

FIGURE 12.9 Overall mortality ratios for female current and former smokers compared with never smokers, by duration of abstinence.

Source: The Health Benefits of Smoking Cessation: A Report of the Surgeon General (p. 78), by U.S. Department of Health and Human Services, 1990, DHHS Publication No. CDC 90–8416, Washington, DC: U.S. Government Printing Office.

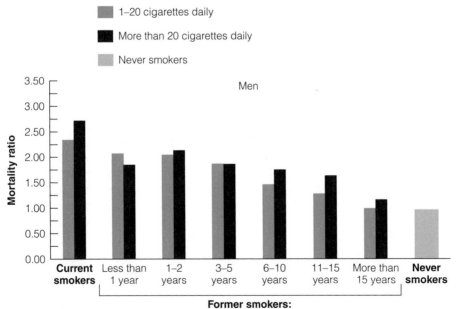

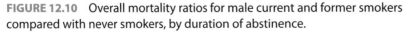

FIGURE 12.10 Overall mortality ratios for male current and former smokers compared with never smokers, by duration of abstinence.

Source: The Health Benefits of Smoking Cessation: A Report of the Surgeon General (p. 78), by U.S. Department of Health and Human Services, 1990, DHHS Publication No. CDC 90–8416, Washington, DC: U.S. Government Printing Office.

These findings suggest that the overall health of smokers is enhanced by quitting. For the average male and female smokers who are free of heart disease, eating a diet with no more than 10% of calories from saturated fat would extend their lives somewhere between 3 days and 3 months (Grover, Gray-Donald, Joseph, Abrahamowicz, & Coupal, 1994). By contrast, quitting smoking at age 35 would add 7 to 8 years to life expectancy. Smokers who quit earlier realize even greater extension of life expectancy, but even men who quit at age 65 gain, on average, 1.5 to 2.0 years of extra life.

IN SUMMARY

Many smokers fear that if they stop smoking, they will gain weight, but the evidence shows that most people do not gain a lot of weight. Even excessive weight gain is less risky than continuing to smoke. On a more positive note, stopping smoking improves health and extends life expectancy. Some evidence suggests that after smokers have quit for 16 years, their all-cause mortality rate may return to that of nonsmokers, although they may continue to have an excess risk for cancer mortality.

ANSWERS

This chapter has addressed five basic questions:

1. **How does smoking affect the respiratory system?**
   The respiratory system allows for the intake of oxygen and the elimination of carbon dioxide. Cigarette smoke drawn into the lungs eventually damages the lungs. Chronic bronchitis and emphysema are two chronic pulmonary diseases related to smoking. Tobacco contains several thousand compounds, including nicotine, and smoke exposes smokers to tars and other compounds that contribute to heart disease and cancer.

2. **Who chooses to smoke and why?**
   About 20% of all U.S. adults smoke, slightly more are former smokers, and a little more than half have never smoked. Slightly more men than women smoke, but gender is not as important as educational level as a predictor of smoking—higher education is associated with lower smoking rates. Most smokers start as adolescents, and genes contribute to both initiation and nicotine dependence. Additional motivation comes from peers, parents, siblings, positive media images, and advertising. Smoking is part of a risk-taking, rebellious style that is consistent with the way some adolescents

want to see themselves. No conclusive answer exists for why people continue to smoke, but the addictive properties of nicotine play a role, especially for some smokers. Smokers may derive positive reinforcement such as relaxation or stress reduction from smoking, or they may receive negative reinforcement from relief of withdrawal symptoms. Other smokers, especially young women, may use smoking as a weight control technique.

3. **What are the health consequences of tobacco use?**
   Smoking is the number one cause of preventable death in the United States, causing about 438,000 deaths a year, mostly from cancer, cardiovascular disease, and chronic lower respiratory disease. Smoking also carries a risk of nonfatal diseases and disorders such as periodontal disease, loss of physical strength and bone density, respiratory disorders, cognitive dysfunction, erectile dysfunction, and macular degeneration. Passive smoking does not contribute substantially to death from lung or breast cancer but does contribute to cardiovascular deaths. Environmental tobacco smoke also raises young children's risk of respiratory disease and even death. Cigar and pipe smoking is less risky than cigarette smoking, but these forms of smoking are not safe. Smokeless

tobacco is probably somewhat safer than cigarette smoking, but the use of smokeless tobacco
is associated with increased rates of oral cancer
and periodontal disease and may be related to
coronary heart disease.

4. How can smoking rates be reduced?

One way to reduce smoking rates is to prevent
people from starting. Such programs are often part of school health programs, but many
such programs have only small or temporary
effects. Most people who quit do so on their
own without any formal cessation program,
but relapse is a problem for these smokers.
Nicotine replacement in the form of a nicotine
patch or nicotine gum can be a useful component in smoking cessation, but use of nicotine
replacement can be even more successful when
combined with behavioral interventions. Psychological counseling can also be effective in
helping people quit. Mass media or community-
based campaigns that reach thousands or even
millions of smokers are successful in helping
some smokers quit.

5. What are the effects of quitting?

Many smokers fear weight gain upon quitting,
and a modest gain (9 to 11 pounds) is common.
Nevertheless, gaining weight is not as hazardous to a person's health as continuing to smoke.
Quitting improves health and extends life, but
returning to the risk level of nonsmokers for
cardiovascular mortality can take 16 years or
longer, and most ex-smokers will retain some
elevated risk for lung cancer unless they quit
smoking when they were young.

SUGGESTED READINGS

Corrigan, P. W. (2004). Marlboro man and the
stigma of smoking. In S. Gilman & Z. Xun
(Eds.), *Smoke: A global history of smoking*
(pp. 344–354). London: Reaktion Books.
More than 50 years ago, the Marlboro man
was introduced to the smoking world as a vir-
ile yet cool cowboy. The image was unmistak-
ably masculine, and advertising was oriented
around that image. In this article, Patrick
Corrigan writes about the social stigma of
smoking and why Marlboro country is not the
place to be.

Jamieson, P., & Romer, D. (2001). What do
young people think they know about the risks
of smoking? In P. Slovic (Ed.), *Smoking: Risk,
perception & policy* (pp. 51–63). Thousand
Oaks, CA: Sage. In this chapter, Patrick
Jamieson and Daniel Romer review research
on a variety of topics about young people's
knowledge of the risks of smoking. In some
areas, the beliefs of young people were reasonably accurate, but in other areas, their beliefs
did not agree with the research. In general,
however, these youth did not adequately understand the dangers of smoking.

Parascandola, M. (2001). Cigarettes and the US
Public Health Service in the 1950s. *American
Journal of Public Health, 91*, 196–205. Public
concern about the hazards of smoking began
mostly with the 1964 Surgeon General's
report. As shown in this article by Mark
Parascandola, most scientists within the
National Institutes of Health knew about the
dangers of smoking by the mid-1950s, but
they did not view their role as one of fighting
against the tobacco industry. Thus, nearly a
decade was lost before they began to battle
against cigarette smoking.

World Health Organization (WHO). (2008). *The
WHO report on the global tobacco epidemic,
2008.* Geneva: World Health Organization.
This extensive report details tobacco use
around the world and offers interesting contrasts between smoking in the United States
and other countries.

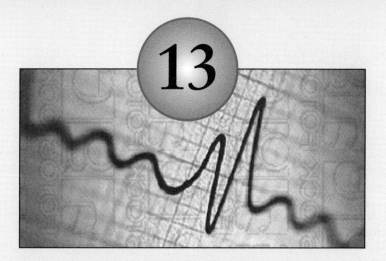

USING ALCOHOL AND OTHER DRUGS

QUESTIONS

This chapter focuses on six basic questions:

1. What are the major trends in alcohol consumption?

2. What are the health effects of drinking alcohol?

3. Why do people drink?

4. How can people change problem drinking?

5. What problems are associated with relapse?

6. What are the health effects of other drugs?

CHECK YOUR HEALTH RISKS

Check the items that apply to you.

☐ 1. I have had five or more alcoholic drinks in one day at least once during the past month.

☐ 2. I have had five or more alcoholic drinks on the same occasion on at least five different days during the past month.

☐ 3. When I drink too much, I sometimes don't remember a lot of the things that happened.

☐ 4. I sometimes ride with a driver who has been drinking.

☐ 5. On at least one occasion during the past year, I drove a motor vehicle after having an alcoholic drink.

☐ 6. I rarely have more than two drinks in one day.

☐ 7. I do not drive when I am intoxicated, but I have driven an automobile after drinking.

☐ 8. I sometimes play sports or go swimming after drinking.

☐ 9. Some of my friends or family have told me that I drink too much.

☐ 10. I have tried to cut down on my drinking, but I never seem to succeed.

☐ 11. At least once in my life, I tried to completely quit drinking, but I was not successful.

☐ 12. I believe that the best way to enjoy many activities (such as a dance or a

football game) is to drink alcohol.

☐ 13. After waking up with a hangover, I sometimes have a drink to feel better.

☐ 14. There are some activities that I perform better after drinking.

☐ 15. I have drunk fewer than 10 alcoholic drinks in my lifetime.

Most of these items represent a health risk related to using alcohol by increasing risk for diseases and unintentional injuries. However, item 6 probably reflects a healthy pattern of consumption for most people, but 15 is not necessarily as healthy as many people believe. As you read this chapter, you will learn that some of these items are riskier than others.

REAL-WORLD PROFILE OF DREW BARRYMORE

Drew Barrymore became a movie star at age 6, when she appeared in the movie *E.T.* Other film and television appearances followed, and Drew experienced problems dealing with the pressure. She began drinking at age 9, used marijuana at age 10, and began cocaine at age 12. She said, "I loved cocaine, period. Just thinking about it caused my palms to sweat. By then, I didn't drink for fun, I drank to get drunk. As soon as people forgot I was the little girl in *E.T.*, they got to know me as Hollywood's youngest alcoholic" (in Townley, 2004). By age 13, her life was out of control.

Drew's mother admitted her to ASAP Drug and Family Treatment Center, but she escaped from

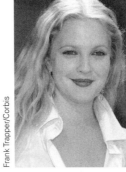

Frank Trapper/Corbis

Drew Barrymore experienced alcohol and drug problems during her early teens.

the facility and stole her mother's credit card (Acme Celebs, 2002). She was captured by authorities and returned to treatment. After being released from treatment, Drew made a film warning teens about drug abuse. But she relapsed, attempted suicide, and returned to treatment. After similar episodes, she stopped drinking, quit drugs, and now is reluctant to use drugs (Bipolar–Lives .com, 2007–2008). Her acting career has been successful, and she has also produced several movies, becoming a Hollywood success story.

Certainly, Drew Barrymore is not typical in most ways. Few children are movie stars by age 6. Most 9-year-olds do not use alcohol. Indeed, fewer than 40% of all eighth-grade students in the United States (who are between 12 and 14) have ever tried alcohol, only about 14% have tried marijuana, and only about 3% have tried cocaine (Johnston et al., 2007). By the time Drew was that age, she was in treatment for drug abuse. However, her wealth and fame were risks for drug abuse; children of wealthy families are at higher risk for drug use and abuse than children from middle-class families (Luthar & Latendresse, 2005). Like Drew Barrymore, most individuals use alcohol before any other drug, but her use of illicit drugs was far from typical.

ALCOHOL CONSUMPTION— YESTERDAY AND TODAY

Alcohol is more widely consumed than other drugs, not only in the United States but in many other countries (Edwards, 2000), and its use both presents problems and raises questions. Drew Barrymore's drinking caused serious problems, but is all alcohol consumption dangerous? What does alcohol do in the body, and what are its risks? What drinking patterns present problems? This chapter includes answers to these questions, but first we examine the history of drinking, which reveals different attitudes about children's alcohol use in the past. Alcohol use among children was once a well-accepted practice rather than a sign of serious problems.

A Brief History of Alcohol Consumption

The use of alcohol is not something that can easily be traced; it was discovered worldwide and repeatedly, dating back before recorded history. Producing beverage alcohol requires no sophisticated technology: The yeast that is responsible for producing alcohol is airborne, and fermentation occurs naturally in fruits, fruit juices, and grain mixtures. There is evidence that most ancient cultures used beverage alcohol (Anderson, 2006). Ancient Babylonians discovered both wine (fermented grape juice) and beer (fermented grain), as did the ancient Egyptians, Greeks, Romans, Chinese, and Indians. Pre-Columbian tribes in the Americas also used fermented products.

Ancient civilizations also discovered drunkenness, of course. In several of those countries, such as Greece, drunkenness was not only allowed but also practically required on certain occasions, but these occasions were limited to festivals. This pattern resembles present-day practices in the United States, where drunkenness is condoned at some parties and celebrations. Most societies condone drinking alcohol but restrict drunkenness to certain occasions.

Distillation was discovered in ancient China and refined in 8th-century Arabia. Because the process is somewhat complex, the use of distilled spirits did not become widespread until they were commercially manufactured. In England, fermented beverages were by far the most common form of alcohol consumption until the 18th century, when England encouraged the proliferation of distilleries to stimulate commerce. Along with cheap gin came widespread consumption and widespread drunkenness. However, intoxication from distilled spirits was confined mostly to the lower and working classes; the rich drank wine, which was imported and thus expensive.

In colonial America, drinking was much more prevalent than it is today. Men, women, and children all drank, and it was considered acceptable for all to do so. This practice may not be consistent with our present-day image of the Puritans, but nevertheless, the Puritans did not object to drinking. Rather, they considered alcohol one of God's gifts. Indeed, in those years, alcohol was often safer than unpurified water or milk, so the Puritans had a legitimate reason to condone the consumption of alcoholic beverages. Drunkenness, however, was not acceptable. The Puritans believed that alcohol, like all things, should be used in moderation. Therefore, the Puritans established severe prohibitions against drunkenness but not against drinking.

The 50 years following U.S. independence marked a transition in the way early Americans thought about alcohol (Edwards, 2000). An adamant and vocal minority came to consider liquor a "demon" and to argue for total abstention from its use. A similar movement arose in Britain. Initially, this attitude was limited to the upper and upper-middle classes, but later, abstention came to be an accepted doctrine of the middle class and people who aspired to join the middle class. Intemperance in drinking alcohol thus became associated with the lower classes, and "respectable" people, especially women, were expected not to be heavy drinkers.

Temperance societies proliferated throughout the United States during the mid-1800s. However, the term is a misnomer. The societies did not promote *temperance*—that is, the moderate use of alcohol. Rather, they advocated *prohibition*, the total abstinence from alcohol. Temperance societies held that liquor weakens inhibitions; loosens desires and passions; causes a large percentage of crime, poverty, and broken homes; and is powerfully addicting, so much so that even an occasional drink would put one in danger. Figure 13.1 shows a dramatic decrease in per capita alcohol consumption in the United States after 1830, a decrease due directly to the spread of the

temperance (prohibition) movement. Note also the more recent decline in consumption since about 1980.

In response to the growing temperance movement, both the demographics and the location of drinking changed. Rather than being consumed in a family setting or a respectable tavern, alcohol became increasingly confined to saloons, which were patronized largely by urban industrial workers (Popham, 1978). Portrayed by the temperance movement as the personification of evil and moral degeneracy, saloons served as a focus for growing prohibitionist sentiment. Drinking became associated with the lower and working classes.

Prohibitionists were finally victorious in 1919 with the ratification of the 18th Amendment to the Constitution of the United States. This amendment outlawed the manufacture, sale, or transportation of alcoholic beverages, and per capita consumption fell drastically (as shown in Figure 13.1). The amendment was not popular and created a large illegal market for alcohol;

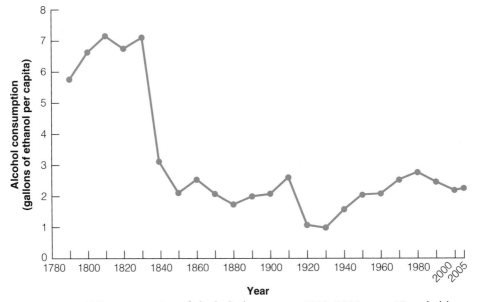

Year

FIGURE 13.1   U.S. consumption of alcoholic beverages, 1790–2005, ages 15 and older.

Sources: The Alcoholic Republic: An American Tradition (p. 9), by W. J. Rorabaugh, 1979, New York: Oxford University Press. Copyright 1979 by Oxford University Press. Also *Apparent Per Capita Ethanol Consumption for the United States, 1850–2005*, retrieved July 21, 2008, from http://www.niaaa.nih.gov/Resources/DatabaseResources/ QuickFacts/AlcoholSales/consum01.html

in 1934, the 21st Amendment repealed the 18th Amendment, and Prohibition ended. Figure 13.1 shows that after the repeal of Prohibition, alcohol consumption rose sharply. Although the current per capita consumption of alcohol is considerably higher than during Prohibition, it is less than half the rate reached during the first three decades of the 19th century.

The Prevalence of Alcohol Consumption Today

About two-thirds of adults in the United States are classified as current drinkers (defined as having had at least 12 drinks during one's lifetime and 1 drink during the past year), about half are regular drinkers, about 20% engage in binge drinking (5 or more drinks on the same occasion at least once per month), and a little less than 5% are heavy drinkers (more than 14 drinks per week for men or 7 per week for women) (NCHS, 2007). The drinking rates shown in Figure 13.2 reflect a leveling of a 20-year decline in alcohol consumption in the United States. Worldwide, about 2 billion people are current drinkers, which represent about half of the adult population (Anderson, 2006).

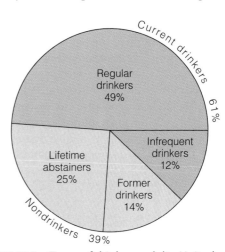

FIGURE 13.2   Types of drinkers, adults, United States, 2005.

Source: Health, United States, 2007 (Table 68), 2007, by National Center for Health Statistics, Hyattsville, MD: U.S. Government Printing Office.

The frequency of drinking and the prevalence of heavy drinking are not equal for all demographic groups in the United States. As Figure 13.3 shows, drinking varies by ethnicity. European Americans tend to have higher rates of drinking than other ethnic groups (NCHS, 2007). Rates of

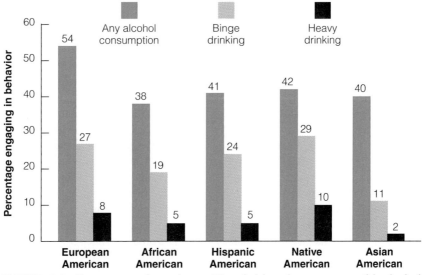

FIGURE 13.3   Percentage of people age 12 and older who report monthly alcohol use, binge drinking, and heavy drinking, by ethnic group, United States, 2003.

Source: SAMHSA, 2004, *Summary of Findings From the 2003 National Survey on Drug Use and Health* (HHS Publication No. SMA 04–3964), Rockville, MD: National Clearinghouse for Alcohol and Drug Information.

binge and heavy drinking also vary with ethnicity. Native Americans have the highest rates of these drinking patterns, and Asian Americans have the lowest.

Age is another factor in drinking. Adults 25 to 44 have the highest rates of drinking, but young adults 18 to 24 have the highest rates of binge drinking and heavy drinking. Slightly more than half of drinkers 18 to 24 are binge drinkers (NCHS, 2007), but they may later become more moderate drinkers. This increasing and then decreasing frequency of binge drinking among young people is one pattern that appeared in a study on adolescent binge drinkers (Tucker, Orlando, & Ellickson, 2003). However, many other patterns occur for binge drinking, including adolescents who accelerate their binge drinking beginning in their early teens and others who retain a stable pattern of binge drinking about once a month. Drew Barrymore was not typical, because she began to drink at a very early age and accelerated her drinking at a rapid rate.

Binge drinking can lead to a variety of hazards (especially for inexperienced drinkers), resulting in intoxication, poor judgment, and impaired coordination. Certain situations promote binge drinking, and college students are at particular risk, not only in the United States but also in Australia, Europe, and South America (Karam, Kypri, & Salamoun, 2007). College students in fraternities and sororities drink more heavily than those not in these organizations (DeSimone, 2007), partly due to students' selection of such organizations for the drinking opportunities they offer and partly due to the socialization of drinking in fraternities and sororities (Park, Sher, & Krull, 2008). However, drinking patterns tend to change when individuals are no longer affiliated. Thus, college drinking habits do not predict drinking problems after graduation (Jackson, Sher, Gotham, & Wood, 2001). During the college years, however, binge drinking is a persistent problem that creates many hazards (Wechsler et al., 2002).

Among adolescents 12 to 17, current use of alcohol dropped dramatically after the legal age for buying alcohol was raised to 21. In 1985, more than 40% of the adolescents in this age group were current users, but by 1992, only 20% were current drinkers, a rate that has remained relatively stable (Johnston et al., 2007). Although binge drinking is still common among college and high school students, the percentage of students who engage in this drinking pattern declined during the 1990s and has remained stable. Among male high school students, for example, binge drinking has declined from more than 50% during the early 1980s to about 28% in 2007 (Eaton et al., 2008). For female high school students, binge drinking decreased to 24%. One important exception to the decline in binge drinking is 21st birthday celebrations. A drinking binge on that occasion has become a rite of passage and often prompts the highest level of binge drinking in which the celebrant has ever engaged (Rutledge, Park, & Sher, 2008).

Why are young people drinking less? One possibility is that they are replacing alcohol with illicit drugs. However, the evidence for this hypothesis is not clear. A report by Lloyd Johnston and his colleagues (Johnston et al., 2007) showed an increase followed by a decrease in high school students' use of most illicit drugs from 1991 to 2007. During the early 1990s, use of marijuana among high school students rose sharply but then leveled off. Thus, alcohol use has declined, and other drug use has not risen to compensate.

Alcohol consumption rates are lowest among older adults (Substance Abuse and Mental Health Services Administration [SAMHSA], 2007). Some people decrease their alcohol consumption as they leave college with its social situations and pressures to drink. In general, alcohol intake is inversely related to age—older ages are associated with lower levels of drinking. The general trend toward decreased alcohol consumption with increasing age may be a result of people quitting or of drinkers reducing the amount they drink.

Gender and educational level are also related to alcohol consumption. Men are more likely than women to be current drinkers (68% to 55%), binge drinkers (29% to 12%), and heavy drinkers (6% to 4%) (NCHS, 2007). These percentages suggest that men have more problems with binge and heavy drinking than do women. Educational level is another predictor of drinking behavior. In Chapter 12, we saw that the more education people have, the less likely they are to smoke cigarettes. With alcohol, however, the reverse is true: the more years of schooling, the greater the likelihood that people will drink alcohol. In 2006, about 67% of college students were defined as current drinkers, compared to only 36% of people who failed to graduate from high school (SAMHSA, 2007). College graduates were less likely to be binge or heavy drinkers than any other educational group (SAMHSA, 2007), and high school dropouts were more likely to be heavy drinkers and to develop drinking problems when they reach their 30s (Muthen & Muthen, 2000).

These patterns of alcohol consumption are not unique to the United States, but countries vary in amount and patterns of alcohol consumption. Across the world, between 18% and 90% of men drink, and between 1% and 81% of women drink (Anderson, 2006). Some countries, such as the United States, Canada, and the Scandinavian countries, associate alcohol with a restricted number of occasions, whereas other countries, such as France, Italy, and Greece, integrate alcohol into daily life (Bloomfield, Stockwell, Gmel, & Rehn, 2003). Drinking is more common in the latter countries, but intoxication is more common in the former. Although binge drinking varies from country to country, it shows no clear pattern among countries.

IN SUMMARY

People have been consuming alcohol since before recorded history, and people have probably abused alcohol for almost as long. In most ancient societies—as well as modern societies—alcohol in moderation was condoned, but alcohol abuse and drunkenness were condemned.

Alcohol consumption per capita reached a peak in the United States during the first three decades of the 19th century. From about 1830 to 1850, consumption dropped dramatically due to the efforts of early prohibitionists. Presently, alcohol consumption in the United States is stable, after having decreased during the 1990s. About 50% of adults are current regular drinkers, 20% are binge drinkers, and

5% are heavy drinkers. European Americans have higher rates of alcohol consumption than Hispanic Americans and African Americans; adults 21 to 44 consume more than other age groups; and college graduates are much more likely to be drinkers than high school dropouts, who nevertheless are more likely to be heavy drinkers later in their lives. Drinking attitudes and patterns also vary among countries.

THE EFFECTS OF ALCOHOL

Essentially the same thing happens to alcohol when you drink it as when you do not—it turns to vinegar (Goodwin, 1976). In the body, two enzymes turn alcohol into vinegar, or acetic acid. The first enzyme, **alcohol dehydrogenase**, is located in the liver and has no other known function except to metabolize alcohol. Alcohol dehydrogenase breaks down alcohol into aldehyde, which is a very toxic chemical. The second enzyme, **aldehyde dehydrogenase**, converts aldehyde to acetic acid.

The process of metabolizing alcohol produces at least three health-related outcomes: (1) an increase in lactic acid, which correlates with anxiety attacks; (2) an increase in uric acid, which causes gout; and (3) an increase of fat in the liver and in the blood.

The specific alcohol used in beverages is called **ethanol**. Like other alcohols, ethanol is a poison. But cases of alcohol poisoning are rare and almost always involve inexperienced drinkers who have drunk very large amounts of distilled liquor in a very short time, often on a "dare." Otherwise, ingesting beverage alcohol is self-limiting: Intoxication usually yields to unconsciousness, preventing lethal poisoning.

Men and women are not equally affected by drinking alcohol. One factor is the difference in body weight; a 120-pound person will be more strongly affected by 3 ounces of alcohol than a 220-pound person. But body weight is not the only factor. Given the same blood alcohol level, men's brains are more strongly affected than women's brains (Wang et al., 2003). However, women's stomachs tend to absorb alcohol more efficiently, producing higher blood alcohol levels with less drinking (Bode & Bode, 1997). Thus, women and men have different physiological responses to alcohol, some of which may make women more vulnerable to the effects of alcohol.

Among the problems associated with drinking are alcohol's ability to produce tolerance, dependence, withdrawal, and addiction. Although these concepts apply to many drugs, their application to alcohol is necessary in evaluating alcohol's potential hazards.

Tolerance is a term applied to the effects of a drug when, with continued use, more and more of the drug is required to produce the same effect. Drugs with high tolerance potential are dangerous because people who build up tolerance need to take more of the drug to produce the effect they want and expect. If this amount is progressively larger, any dangerous effects or side effects of the drug will become more of a hazard. Alcohol is a drug with generally moderate tolerance potential, but it seems to affect people differentially. For some, heavy use of alcohol for an extended period is required before noticeable tolerance begins to develop. For others, tolerance can develop within a week of moderate daily consumption. With increased tolerance comes an increased risk of the physical damage that alcohol can cause.

Dependence is separate from tolerance, and it too is a term that can be applied to many drugs. Dependence occurs when a drug becomes so incorporated into the functioning of the body's cells that it becomes necessary for "normal" functioning. If the drug is discontinued, the body's dependence on that drug becomes apparent and **withdrawal** symptoms develop. These symptoms are the body's signs that it is adjusting to functioning without the drug. Dependence and withdrawal are physical symptoms connected to drug use. Generally, withdrawal symptoms are the opposite of the drug's effects. Because alcohol produces mostly depressant effects, withdrawal from it produces symptoms of restlessness, irritability, and agitation.

Many drugs produce notoriously unpleasant withdrawal, and alcohol is one of the worst. How difficult the process will be depends on many factors, including the length of use and the degree of dependence. In some cases, withdrawal from alcohol can be life threatening, and requires careful management (Mayo-Smith et al., 2004). Usually the first symptom to appear is tremor—the "shakes." Sleep difficulties are also common. In those severely addicted, **delirium tremens** occurs, with hallucinations, disorientation, and possibly convulsions. The withdrawal process usually lasts between two days and a week. The physical dangers are so severe that the process is often completed in a special facility devoted to alcohol treatment.

Tolerance and dependence are independent properties. A drug may produce tolerance but not dependence; also, a person can develop dependence on a drug that has little or no tolerance potential. However, some drugs have both a tolerance and a dependence potential. Some research even indicates that tolerance and dependence are not inevitable consequences of taking drugs (Zinberg, 1984). Not everyone who drinks alcohol does so with sufficient frequency and in sufficient quantity to develop a tolerance, and most drinkers do not become dependent.

The combination of dependence and withdrawal is sometimes described as **addiction**, but both laypeople (Chassin, Presson, Rose, & Sherman, 2007) and experts (Pouletty, 2002) use different definitions. All include some element of craving for the substance and compulsive use as part of their definition, but adolescents emphasize the cravings in their conceptualization, whereas adults focus on the compulsive use of the substance in their view of addiction (Chassin et al., 2007). More consistent with adults' definitions, experts distinguish addiction from dependence by considering the compulsive behavior and damage done to people's life through this behavior—"loss of control of drug use or the compulsive seeking and taking of drugs despite adverse consequences" (Pouletty, 2002, p. 731). Some experts even differentiate drug abuse from addiction, defining abuse as excessive and harmful use, even if the person is not dependent or addicted. Thus, considering the properties of a drug such as alcohol includes tolerance, dependence, addiction, and abuse, each of which is separable from the others.

Some people speak of "psychological" dependence or addiction, but this term is not equivalent to dependence on a drug such as alcohol. Many behaviors become part of one's habitual manner of responding. Giving up the activity is accomplished only through much difficulty because the person has become habituated to it. Psychological dependence could be extended to many behaviors that are difficult to change, such as gambling, overeating, jogging, or even watching television, some of which may seem to meet the criterion of compulsive behavior that signals addiction. Whether this conceptualization is valid remains controversial, so the term should be used with caution.

Hazards of Alcohol

Alcohol produces a variety of hazards, both direct and indirect. *Direct hazards* are the harmful physical effects of alcohol itself, exclusive of any psychological, social, or economic consequences. *Indirect hazards* are the harmful consequences that result from psychological and physiological impairments produced by alcohol. Both direct and indirect hazards contribute to an increased mortality rate for heavy drinkers (Standridge, Zylstra, & Adams, 2004).

Direct Hazards Alcohol affects many organ systems in the body, but the liver is mainly in charge of detoxifying alcohol. Thus, liver damage is the main health consideration for long-term heavy drinkers. The oxidation that occurs during alcohol metabolism may be toxic, destroying cell membranes and causing liver damage (Reuben, 2008). With prolonged heavy drinking, scarring occurs, and this scarring is typically followed by **cirrhosis**, or the accumulation of nonfunctional scar tissue in the liver. Cirrhosis is an irreversible condition and a major cause of death among alcoholics. Not all alcoholics develop liver cirrhosis, and people with no history of alcohol abuse may also develop the condition, but cirrhosis has a significant association with heavy alcohol use in countries around the world (Mandayam, 2004) and is one of the leading causes of death in the United States. For reasons not yet clearly understood, mortality from cirrhosis declined beginning in the early 1970s in the United States and some other countries but has recently begun to increase.

Chronic alcohol abuse is also a factor in developing several other disorders, including respiratory illness and severe neurological damage. Chronic alcohol abusers have an increased vulnerability to respiratory problems and lung injury (Guidot & Roman, 2002). Prolonged heavy drinking is also implicated in the development of a neurological dysfunction called Korsakoff syndrome (also known as Wernicke-Korsakoff syndrome). Korsakoff syndrome is characterized by chronic cognitive impairment, severe memory problems for recent events, disorientation, and an inability to learn new information. Alcohol is related to the development of this syndrome through its interference with the absorption of thiamin, one of the B vitamins. Heavy drinkers can experience thiamin deficiency, which is worsened by their typically poor nutrition (Stacey & Sullivan, 2004). Alcohol accelerates the progression of thiamin-related brain damage, and when this process has started, vitamin supplements do not reverse the progression. Moreover, most alcoholics do not receive treatment until the process is at an irreversible stage. Heavy, prolonged drinking is a risk factor for neurological damage (Harper & Matsumoto, 2005), but light to moderate consumption does not seem to lead to cognitive impairment. Indeed, research suggests that light to moderate drinkers are less likely to develop dementia, including Alzheimer's disease (Collins, 2008).

Does alcohol contribute to the development of cancer? A link between alcohol and cancer is not easy to establish because many other factors, such as smoking, co-occur, making it difficult to separate the effects of alcohol. However, a meta-analysis of more than 150 studies (Corrao, Bagnardi, Zambon, & La Vecchia, 2004) showed that drinking poses the strongest risk for cancer of the oral cavity, esophagus, and larynx. In addition, alcohol also significantly raised the risk for cancers of the colon, rectum, liver, and breast. For most sites, a dose–response relationship existed: Heavier drinking meant higher risk. When drinkers also smoke cigarettes, their risk is compounded for cancers of the lung and upper digestive tract.

This meta-analysis confirmed the relationship between alcohol and breast cancer in women and also showed a strong dose–response relationship

(Corrao et al., 2004). These results confirmed other large-scale studies (Seitz & Maurer, 2007; Singletary & Gapstur, 2001), which showed that even moderate levels of drinking present some risk of breast cancer, and higher levels of drinking are related to higher risk.

Alcohol also affects the cardiovascular system, but the effects may not all be negative. (The next section looks at the possible positive effects of moderate alcohol consumption on cardiovascular functioning.) Heavy chronic drinking, however, does have a direct and harmful effect on the cardiovascular system (Corrao et al., 2004; Standridge et al., 2004). In large doses, alcohol reduces oxidation of fatty acids (the heart's primary fuel source) in the myocardium. The heart directly metabolizes ethanol, producing fatty acid ethyl esters that impair functioning of the energy-producing structures of the heart. Alcohol can also depress the myocardium's ability to contract, which can lead to abnormal cardiac functioning. In addition, alcohol consumption is related to hypertension among African American women and men, although this association may be due to high levels of stress that contribute both to alcohol consumption and to increased blood pressure (Steffens et al., 2006).

Alcohol has a direct and hazardous effect on pregnancy and the developing fetus in two basic ways. First, alcohol consumption reduces fertility; women who are heavy drinkers are at increased risk for infertility (Eggert, Theobald, & Engfeldt, 2004). Women who are chronic heavy users of alcohol experience amenorrhea, cessation of the menstrual cycle, which may be caused either by cirrhosis or by a direct effect of alcohol on the pituitary or the hypothalamus. Other possibilities include alcohol's effects on hormone production and regulation and interference with ovulation.

The second direct, hazardous effect of excessive drinking during pregnancy is the increased risk of developmental problems for the fetus, such as congenital malformations of the respiratory and musculoskeletal systems (Baumann, Schild, Hume, & Sokol, 2006). The most severe form is **fetal alcohol syndrome (FAS)**, which affects many infants of mothers who drank excessively during pregnancy. Some tissues in the

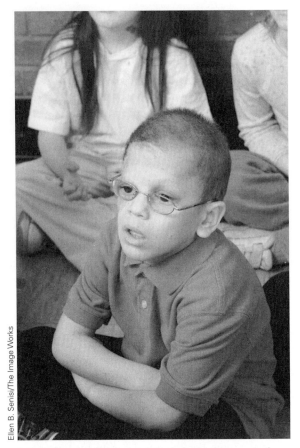

Ellen B. Senisi/The Image Works

Facial abnormalities, growth deficiencies, central nervous system disorders, and mental retardation are symptoms of fetal alcohol syndrome.

embryo, such as neurons, are especially sensitive to alcohol, and exposure causes problems in the developing embryo (Farber & Olney, 2003; Goldsmith, 2004). These problems in development produce specific facial abnormalities, growth deficiencies, central nervous system disorders, and mental retardation. The disorder has increased during recent years, climbing from an incidence of 0.1 per 1,000 births in 1979 to between 0.5 and 2.0 per 1,000 births during the 1990s (May & Gossage, 2001). Although heavy drinking is the main contributor to fetal alcohol syndrome, heavy smoking, stress, and poor nutrition are also involved, and combinations of these factors are not unusual in heavy drinkers.

What about moderate and even light drinking during pregnancy? Light to moderate drinking is not likely to cause fetal alcohol syndrome unless binge drinking is involved, but any level of alcohol exposure affects developing embryos. Even light drinking increases the risk for miscarriages and stillbirths (Kesmodel, Wisborg, Olsen, Henriksen, & Secher, 2002). Significant decreases in cognitive functioning appeared in children of mothers who reported episodes of binge drinking (Bailey et al., 2004), and fathers who abuse alcohol before conception may also contribute to cognitive and behavioral problems in their children (Abel, 2004). Even low levels of alcohol consumption by pregnant women can lead to other health problems for the fetus. For example, children born to women who average two drinks a day have a lower average birth weight, and this condition, although not itself a danger, is related to many risks for newborns. Even small amounts of alcohol, especially during the early months of pregnancy, may have direct and hazardous effects on the developing fetus (Baumann et al., 2006; Goldsmith, 2004). Unfortunately, as many as 30% of women of childbearing age in the United States fit the pattern of risky drinking (Nayak & Kaskutas, 2004).

Indirect Hazards In addition to direct physiological damage, alcohol consumption is associated with several indirect hazards. Most of the indirect dangers arise from alcohol's effects on aggression, judgment, and attention. Alcohol also affects coordination and alters cognitive functioning in ways that contribute to increased chances of unintentional injury not only to the drinker but also to others (Gmel & Rehm, 2003).

The most frequent and serious indirect hazard of alcohol consumption is the increased likelihood of unintentional injuries, the fourth leading cause of death in the United States, the leading cause of death for people under age 45, and a leading cause of death and injury worldwide (Rehm et al., 2003). A dose–response relationship exists between alcohol consumption and unintentional fatal injuries; that is, the greater the number of drinks consumed per occasion, the greater the incidence of fatalities from unintentional injuries.

As many as 32% of fatal unintentional injuries throughout the world involve alcohol.

Motor vehicle crashes account for the largest number of alcohol-related fatalities. In the United States, more than 44,000 people die each year from injuries resulting from motor vehicle crashes, and about 40% of those deaths (about 17,000 per year) are related to alcohol-impaired driving (Yi, Chen, & Williams, 2006). The National Survey on Drug Use and Health (SAMHSA, 2007) found that alcohol-impaired driving was most frequent among young people 21 to 25 years old, with 27% reporting this behavior. However, 20% of 18- to 20-year-olds, who are not yet old enough to purchase alcohol legally, also said they had driven after drinking. European Americans are more likely to drive after drinking than other ethnic groups, and men are about twice as likely as women to do so. These impaired drivers are not necessarily heavy or binge drinkers; half of the drivers involved in crashes who had used alcohol were nonproblem drinkers—who became

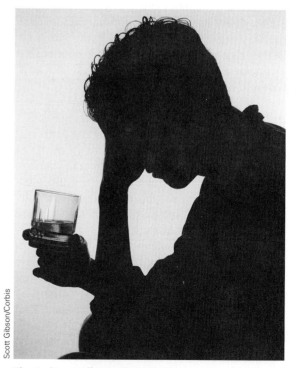

Scott Gibson/Corbis

The indirect effects of alcohol pose more dangers than the direct physiological effects.

problems when they drove after drinking (Voas, Roman, Tippetts, & Durr-Holden, 2006).

For some drinkers, alcohol consumption can also lead to more aggressive behavior. Both laboratory experiments and crime statistics have shown a relationship between alcohol and aggression, but the effect does not apply to everyone. Trait anger (the disposition to experience and respond with anger) is an important factor. Not surprisingly, men with moderate or high trait anger behaved more aggressively than men with lower levels of anger (Parrott & Zeichner, 2002). However, trait anger combined with alcohol prompted these men to administer longer and higher levels of shock than their sober counterparts and provoked both women and men to engage in more aggressive verbal exchanges (Eckhardt & Crane, 2008). Jealousy combined with alcohol predicted intimate partner violence (Foran & O'Leary, 2008). Thus, some people are more likely than others to become aggressive under the influence of alcohol.

Alcohol is also related to suicidal ideation and suicide attempts (Schaffer, Jeglic, & Stanley, 2008). Drew Barrymore attempted suicide while she was drinking and using drugs. Research indicates that alcohol use has a higher relationship to suicide attempts than other drug use (Rossow, Grøholt, & Wichstrøm, 2005).

Similarly, alcohol is related to crime. Two early studies (Mayfield, 1976; Wolfgang, 1957) indicated that either the victim or the perpetrator, or both, had been drinking in two-thirds of the homicides studied. Later research (Martin, 2001) confirmed this relationship and extended the findings to assaults, including sexual assaults and incidents of domestic violence. Not only are people who commit homicides likely to be drinking, but consuming alcohol also relates to increased chances of being a crime victim. These relationships, however, do not demonstrate that alcohol causes crime. Most crimes are committed by people who are not alcohol dependent, and the majority of alcohol abusers do not commit violent crimes. Thus, the relationship between alcohol and crime is complex (Dingwall, 2005).

Finally, drinking alcohol can influence people's decision making. A study of group decision making (Sayette, Kirchner, Moreland, Levine, & Travis, 2004) showed that when group members had been drinking, the decision was riskier than when the group was completely sober. Alterations also appear on the individual level and in nonproblem drinkers, who experienced problems in factoring several variables into a decision-making situation after drinking (George, Rogers, & Duka, 2005). In addition, drinkers who drank to the extent that their decision making and motor responses were impaired showed more hesitation in recognizing their impairment than individuals who had drunk less (Brumback, Cao, & King, 2007).

Impairment and risky decisions can be dangerous in sexual situations. For example, college-age men who were both intoxicated and sexually aroused reported more favorable attitudes toward and greater intention of having unprotected sex than did men who were sober (MacDonald, MacDonald, Zanna, & Fong, 2000). Other research indicates that people who have been drinking are more likely than others to be involved in forced sexual experiences, either as victim or as perpetrator (Testa, Vazile-Tamsen, & Livingston, 2004).

Benefits of Alcohol

Is it possible that drinking might be good for you? This question was raised as a result of several early studies (Room & Day, 1974; Stason, Neff, Miettinen, & Jick, 1976) that reported a U-shaped or J-shaped relationship between alcohol consumption and mortality. In other words, light to moderate drinkers (one to five drinks per day) seemed to have the best prospects for good health, whereas heavy drinkers and nondrinkers had the greatest risk. Later evidence from several longitudinal studies supported the findings that light or moderate drinking was positively related to both reduced mortality and lower risk of disease. These early studies prompted further research, which has consistently found some health benefits for light to moderate levels of alcohol consumption (Standridge et al., 2004). The benefits of drinking do not appear among young people but appear to begin during middle age (Klatsky & Udaltsova, 2007), which is consistent with the effects coming largely from reduced cardiovascular mortality.

Reduced Cardiovascular Mortality When researchers initially investigated the benefits of drinking, they discovered overall lower mortality for people who drank at light to moderate levels (Klatsky, 2003, 2008; Klatsky & Udaltsova, 2007). This advantage appeared first among men, but women who were light drinkers also showed lower mortality rates (Standridge et al., 2004). This reduction in mortality is due mostly to lower heart disease deaths and applies to people in cultures around the world. A meta-analysis of studies (Rimm, Williams, Fosher, Criqui, & Stampfer, 1999) concluded that people who have two drinks per day experience 25% lower heart attack risk. A large-scale study on men (Mukamal et al., 2003) found that men who drank alcohol between three and seven times a week had a 30% lower risk of heart attack than men who drank less than once a week.

The research evidence does not show as strong a protection against stroke as it does against heart disease (Ashley, Rehm, Bondy, Single, & Rankin, 2000; Klatsky, 2003). Indeed, some studies show an increased risk of stroke for people who drink. This discrepancy may be due to the different types of strokes. Similar to heart disease, people who drink at light to moderate levels derive some protection against ischemic strokes, those strokes caused by restriction of blood supply to the brain. On the other hand, drinking may pose a danger for hemorrhagic strokes, those strokes caused by rupture of a blood vessel that bleeds into the brain. Ischemic strokes are more common than hemorrhagic strokes; thus, the protection offered by drinking lowers the rate of death due to strokes. Another cardiovascular disorder, peripheral vascular disease, is also lower among drinkers.

The health benefits of drinking have been controversial, mostly because drinking carries unquestionable hazards. People who provide treatment for those with drinking problems find it difficult to recommend drinking to anyone. Researchers have also questioned the multitude of studies that find benefits in drinking, pointing out that errors may have occurred in the classification of people into categories of drinking (Fillmore, Stockwell, Chikritzhs, Bostrom, & Kerr, 2007), in the failure to account for participants who drop out of studies (Thygesen, Johansen, Keiding, Giovannucci, & Grønbæk, 2008), or in accepting that drinking is protective, whereas other factors are actually responsible for the apparent advantage (Naimi et al., 2005). During the time that some researchers were questioning the validity of the benefits, others were working toward understanding the physiology of a protective effect.

That search has resulted in findings that alcohol produces changes in the course of atherosclerosis, the disease condition that underlies most CVD (Klatsky, 2003; Standridge et al., 2004). Alcohol alters cholesterol, raising specific subfractions of high-density lipoprotein that are beneficial and reducing the tendency to form blood clots. In addition, alcohol affects insulin sensitivity and inflammation (Mukamal et al., 2005; Rimm & Moats, 2007). All of these actions may work toward reducing CVD, thus offering the beginnings of a plausible mechanism through which drinking could decrease heart disease.

Other Benefits of Alcohol Cardiovascular disease is not the only condition that is lower among those who drink. Chances of developing Type 2 diabetes are lower among light to moderate drinkers than among those who abstain (Hendriks, 2007). Alcohol affects glucose tolerance and insulin resistance, which makes this effect comprehensible. The role of alcohol in cholesterol metabolism and its effect on bile acids suggest that drinkers may be at lowered risk for gallstones (Ashley et al., 2000). Epidemiological research bears out this conjecture: Moderate drinkers experienced gallstones at about half the rate of those who did not drink.

Alcohol also has some effect on *H. pylori*, a bacterium that infects the gastrointestinal system and is involved in gastritis, ulcer development, and possibly gastric cancers. People who drink have lower concentrations of this bacterium in their digestive tracts (Ashley et al., 2000; Kuepper-Nybelen, Rothenbacher, & Brenner, 2005). (See Chapter 6 for a discussion of *H. pylori* and ulcer formation.) Reductions in the levels of this infection may decrease risk for ulcer formation and digestive tract cancers.

Some surprising evidence (Collins, 2008; Ruitenberg et al., 2002) suggests that drinking may protect against cognitive deficits. This effect is unexpected because heavy drinking is associated with Korsakoff syndrome, which produces memory problems and other cognitive deficits. However, drinking seems to relate to decreased risk for Alzheimer's disease, the most common form of dementia associated with advancing age. As Chapter 11 explained, Alzheimer's disease is a devastating degenerative brain disorder, and few protective measures have been identified. This intriguing finding offers hope of a way to combat this disease in an aging population.

For all of the diseases for which alcohol has shown some protective effect, the amount of alcohol and the pattern of drinking are important factors (Klatsky, 2003). At high levels of drinking, alcohol becomes a risk for these disorders. Binge drinking, even occasionally, fails to convey the protections of light to moderate drinking and produces several of the risks. For example, eight or more drinks at one sitting is a pattern of drinking that causes both men and women to lose their protection against heart disease and increases the risk of hypertension for men (Murray et al., 2002). Individual differences are important in calculating who may benefit from drinking how much. Women gain the protective effects of alcohol at lower levels of drinking than men and feel the hazards at lower levels. For example, women who drink more than six drinks on weekends or more than one drink per weekday experience an increased risk of dying, but those who drink one to three drinks per week have a lower mortality rate (Mørch, Johansen, Løkkegaard, Hundrup, & Grønbæk, 2008). In addition, the benefits of drinking do not appear among young people but appear to begin during middle age (Klatsky & Udaltsova, 2007).

Drinking offers more health benefits than hazards for some people. However, those people who do not drink probably should not start, and those who do drink regularly (about half the people in the United States) should strive to keep their drinking at low levels of consumption and avoid binge drinking in order to experience the health benefits.

IN SUMMARY

Alcohol consumption has both harmful and beneficial effects on health. In addition, it has some negative indirect effects on society that reach beyond an individual's physical health. The direct hazards of prolonged and heavy drinking include cirrhosis of the liver, an increased risk for some cancers, and a brain dysfunction called Korsakoff syndrome. In addition, heavy drinking during pregnancy increases the risk of fetal alcohol syndrome, a serious disorder that often includes growth deficiencies and severe mental retardation. Alcohol is also a risk factor for many types of violence, both intentional and unintentional. The level of alcohol consumption necessary to increase the risk is not as high as the level necessary to produce legal intoxication, but the more heavily people drink, the more likely it is that they will be involved in accidents and violent crimes. Finally, alcohol consumption may also lead to poor decisions.

The principal positive aspect of alcohol consumption is its buffering effect against mortality and morbidity from cardiovascular disease, including heart disease and peripheral vascular disease. Other health benefits may include lowered risks for diabetes, gallstones, *H. pylori* infection, and Alzheimer's disease, but heavy or binge drinking increases these risks.

WHY DO PEOPLE DRINK?

Investigators trying to understand drinking and alcohol abuse have proposed several models to explain behavior related to alcohol consumption. These models go beyond the pharmacological effects of alcohol and even beyond the research findings to integrate and explain drinking. To be useful, a model for drinking behavior must address at least three questions. First, why do people start drinking? Second, why do most people maintain moderate rather than excessive drinking levels? Third, why do some people drink so much that they develop serious problems?

Until the 19th century, drinking was well accepted in the United States and Europe, but drunkenness was unacceptable under most circumstances.

This attitude makes drinking the norm, thus requiring no explanation for it, but leaves drunkenness unexplained. Two models have been proposed to explain drunkenness: the moral model and the medical model (Rotskoff, 2002).

The moral model appeared first, holding that people have free will to choose their behaviors, including excessive drinking. Thus, those who do so are either sinful or morally lacking in the self-discipline necessary to moderate their drinking. The moral model of alcoholism began to fade among professionals in the late 19th century, when the medical model started to gain prominence. Unacceptable behaviors that were formerly seen as moral problems became medical problems and, thus, subject to scientific explanation and medical treatment. However, many people and even some alcoholism treatment staff still take a moralistic view of excessive drinking (Palm, 2004).

The medical model of alcoholism conceptualized problem drinking as symptomatic of underlying physical problems, and the notion that alcoholism is hereditary grew from this view. The first form of this hypothesis took the view that a "constitutional weakness" ran in families and that this weakness produced alcoholics.

Problem drinking does run in families, but the relative contributions of heredity and environment remain the subject of heated debates. Most authorities agree that both genetic and environmental influences play a role in shaping alcohol abuse (Ball, 2008). Children of problem drinkers are more likely than children of non–problem drinkers to abuse alcohol as well as other drugs. Both Drew Barrymore and her father experienced serious drinking problems. Such children often grow up in an environment marked by marital discord, tolerance for early initiation into alcohol use, and lack of parental warmth and communication, just as Drew did. Such an environment, combined with an inherited vulnerability to alcohol abuse, greatly increases a child's likelihood of becoming a problem drinker, but even in such circumstances, most do not.

How can investigators learn about the relative effects of environment and heredity on the development of problem drinking? Researchers have taken several approaches, including the degree of agreement in drinking behavior between twins or between adopted children and parents (Ball, 2008). Twin studies ordinarily involve measuring the degree of agreement between pairs of identical twins compared with the amount of agreement between pairs of fraternal twins. If identical twins are more similar to each other than fraternal twins are, the difference is assumed to be due to genetics. Indeed, research generally shows a closer concordance of problem drinking for identical twins than for fraternal twins. This greater concordance between identical twins supports the idea of at least some genetic component in alcohol abuse.

A second test of a hereditary factor in alcohol abuse is the study of adopted children (Ball, 2008). Adoption studies investigate the frequency of alcohol abuse in adoptees whose biological parent was alcoholic. Results from several large-scale studies using this approach also indicate a genetic component in problem drinking. Both types of studies indicate a stronger role for genetics in the problem drinking of men than of women.

Genes do not determine drinking. Indeed, genes do not produce any behavior. Genes govern protein synthesis, and a number of steps intervene between genes and behavior. Research has begun to explore the molecular basis of how genes affect drinking.

One effect of genes on alcohol metabolism is fairly well understood, but this type of inheritance protects against rather than creates a vulnerability for problem drinking. When individuals inherit a gene variant that results in deficient activity of aldehyde dehydrogenase (one of the enzymes that metabolizes alcohol), they experience an unpleasant "flushing" reaction when they drink (Zakhari, 2006). This gene configuration is more common among people of Asian ancestry than other ethnic groups, and people with this pattern develop problem drinking far less often than others do.

Alcohol metabolism offers various possibilities for creating a vulnerability to problem drinking. The functioning of neurotransmitters in the brain, such as dopamine, GABA, and serotonin, is affected by genetics and has also been linked to alcohol's effects (Köhnke, 2008). A specific genetic susceptibility to problem drinking may lie in a variant of the genes that are involved with alcohol dehydrogenase, which is the other enzyme involved in alcohol metabolism (Tolstrup, Nordestgaard, Rasmussen, Tybjærg-Hansen, & Grønbæk, 2008). According to this view, the speed of alcohol metabolism is related to drinking more and drinking more heavily, and variants of this gene affect that speed. However, problem drinking is unlikely to be traceable to one gene pair (Preuss et al., 2004). Considering the complexity of alcohol's effects on brain neurochemistry, researchers now expect their search to yield multiple gene locations that underlie a vulnerability to problem drinking rather than a genetic determination of alcoholism. That is, researchers are looking for genetic, biological, and environmental factors that contribute to problem drinking.

The Disease Model

The disease concept of alcoholism is a variation of the medical model, holding that people with problem drinking have the disease of alcoholism. Throughout history, isolated attempts have been made to describe alcohol intoxication as a disease brought about by the physical properties of alcohol. This view became increasingly popular beginning in the late 1930s and early 1940s. It was accepted by the American Medical Association in 1956 and remains the dominant view in psychiatric and other medically oriented treatment programs in the United States (Quinn, Bodenhamer-Davis, & Koch, 2004). The disease model is less influential in psychologically based treatment programs and in treatment programs in Europe and Australia.

The disease model of alcoholism was elevated to scientific respectability by the pioneering work of E. M. Jellinek (1960), who identified several different types of alcoholism and described various characteristics of these types. The two most common types are **gamma alcoholism**, or loss of control once drinking begins, and **delta alcoholism**, or the inability to abstain. Any model that conceptualizes alcoholism as an incurable unitary disorder is too simplistic, even if it includes different varieties of alcoholism.

The Alcohol Dependency Syndrome Dissatisfaction with Jellinek's disease model led Griffith Edwards and his colleagues (Edwards, 1977; Edwards & Gross, 1976; Edwards, Gross, Keller, Moser, & Room, 1977) to advocate the alcohol dependency syndrome, which rejects the term *alcoholism* and the notion that problem drinking is a disease. The word *syndrome* adds flexibility to the disease model by suggesting a group of concurrent behaviors that accompany alcohol dependence. Edwards and his colleagues modified several of Jellinek's concepts, including the notion that alcoholics experience loss of control. Rather, the alcohol dependency syndrome holds that those who are alcohol dependent have *impaired control*, suggesting that people drink heavily because, at certain times and for a variety of reasons, they do not exercise control over their drinking. The seven elements of the alcohol dependency syndrome appear in Table 13.1. This concept is currently the "official" one that forms the basis for a diagnosis of substance abuse dependency, based on the *Diagnostic and Statistical Manual of Mental Disorders* (American Psychiatric Association, 2000) and suggested for the revision of that manual (Li, Hewitt, & Grant, 2007).

Evaluation of the Disease Model Despite the continuing popularity of the disease model of alcoholism, the concept has only limited research support—the basis for the disease of alcoholism has not been identified. This model fails to address our first question: Why do people begin to drink? Its answer to the second question about why some people continue to drink at moderate levels is hardly adequate: People who are not alcoholic can drink with impunity.

One key concept in the disease model is loss of control or impaired control—the inability to stop or moderate alcohol intake once drinking begins. This concept has been defined in many ways, and research is less than consistent concerning its influence (Martin, Fillmore, Chung, Easdon, & Miczek, 2006). G. Alan Marlatt and his colleagues (Marlatt, Demming, & Reid, 1973; Marlatt & Rohsenow, 1980) have conducted experiments suggesting that many effects of alcohol, including impaired control, are due more to expectancy than

TABLE 13.1

Elements of the Alcohol Dependency Syndrome

Element	Behaviors Associated With This Element
Narrowing of drinking repertoire	Drinking the same beverage at the same time of day
Salience of drink-seeking behavior	Drinking begins to take precedence over other behaviors
Increased tolerance for alcohol	Drinkers become accustomed to performing daily tasks with high blood alcohol levels
Withdrawal symptoms	Restless, irritability, and agitation
Avoiding withdrawal symptoms	Additional drinking
Personal awareness of the need to drink	Drinkers acknowledge their need to drink
Reinstatement of dependence after abstinence	Drinkers who have quit become dependent more rapidly when they begin to drink again; the development of dependence is inversely related to severity of prior dependence

Source: "Alcohol Dependence: Provisional Description of a Clinical Syndrome" by G. Edwards & M. M. Gross, 1976, *British Medical Journal, i,* 1058–1061.

to any pharmacological effect of alcohol. Their experimental design, called the balanced placebo design, included four groups, two of which expected to be given alcohol and two of which did not. Two groups actually received alcohol, and two did not. Figure 13.4 shows all four combinations.

Using the balanced placebo design, several studies (Marlatt et al., 1973; Marlatt & Rohsenow, 1980) showed that people who think they have received alcohol behave as though they

have (whether they have or not). Even for those who had been in treatment for problem drinking, expectancy appeared to be the controlling factor in the craving for alcohol and in the amount consumed. These findings suggest that expectancy plays an important role in loss of control and craving for alcohol. A meta-analysis of studies on alcohol expectancy (McKay & Schare, 1999) confirmed that expectancy plays an important role in alcohol's effects.

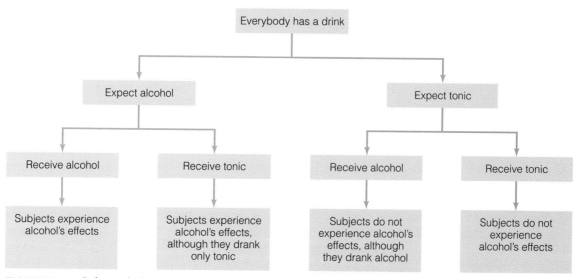

FIGURE 13.4 Balanced placebo design used in experiments on expectancy and alcohol effects.

Some investigators (Peele, 2002; Quinn et al., 2004) have criticized the disease model of alcohol, arguing that it does not adequately consider environmental, cognitive, and affective determinants of abusive drinking; that is, in its emphasis on the physical properties of alcohol, the disease model neglects the cognitive and social learning aspects of drinking.

Cognitive-Physiological Theories

Of the various alternatives to the disease model, several emphasize the combination of physiological and cognitive changes that occur with alcohol use. Rather than hypothesizing that alcohol use and misuse are based only on the chemical properties of alcohol, these models contend that alcohol use also depends on the cognitive changes experienced by drinkers.

The Tension Reduction Hypothesis As the name suggests, the tension reduction hypothesis (Conger, 1956) holds that people drink alcohol because of its tension-reducing effects. This hypothesis has much intuitive appeal because alcohol is a sedative drug that leads to relaxation and slowed reactions.

Despite its consistency with popular belief, experimental studies have furnished only limited support for the tension reduction hypothesis. Studies that have manipulated tension or anxiety to observe their effects on participants' readiness to consume alcohol have yielded contradictory results; some participants experience tension reduction, whereas others do not (Kambouropoulos, 2003). In more naturalistic settings (Frone, 2008; Moore, Sikora, Grunberg, & Greenberg, 2007), factors other than stress and tension have been found to relate to drinking. One factor that complicates assessment of the tension reduction hypothesis is expectancy. When people expect to experience tension reduction, they tend to get what they expect. Thus, tension reduction is one of many effects that may occur as a result of drinking, but expectancy may be more important than alcohol in these effects.

The realization that alcohol's effects on physiological processes are not simple led to a reformulation of the tension reduction hypothesis.

A group of researchers at Indiana University (Levenson, Sher, Grossman, Newman, & Newlin, 1980; Sher, 1987; Sher & Levenson, 1982) discovered that high levels of alcohol consumption decrease the strength of responses to stress. They labeled this decrease the *stress response dampening (SRD) effect*. People who had been drinking did not respond as strongly as nondrinking participants to either physiological or psychological stressors. People whose personality profile suggested a high risk of developing problem drinking showed the strongest SRD effect, and those whose profile indicated a low risk showed a weaker effect (Sher & Levenson, 1982). This stress response dampening effect appears in some drinkers but not in others (Zack, Poulos, Aramakis, Khamba, & MacLeod, 2007) and more strongly at higher levels of intoxication (Donohue, Curtin, Patrick, & Lang, 2007). In addition, stress response dampening tends to occur in social drinking situations, suggesting that some drinkers may use alcohol as a way to manage their stress responses (Armeli et al., 2003). However, neither the original tension reduction hypothesis nor stress response dampening provides a general explanation for drinking, especially for initiating drinking.

Alcohol Myopia Claude Steele and his colleagues (Steele & Josephs, 1990) have developed a model of alcohol use and abuse based on alcohol's psychological and physical properties. This model hypothesizes that alcohol use creates effects on social behaviors that they term *alcohol myopia*, "a state of shortsightedness in which superficially understood, immediate aspects of experience have a disproportionate influence on behavior and emotion, a state in which we can see the tree, albeit more dimly, but miss the forest altogether" (Steele & Josephs, 1990, p. 923). According to this view, alcohol blocks out insightful cognitive processing and alters thoughts related to the self, stress, and social anxiety.

Part of alcohol myopia is drunken excess, the tendency for those who drink to behave more excessively. This tendency appears as increased aggression, friendliness, sexiness, and many other exaggerated behaviors. Tendencies to behave in such extreme ways are usually inhibited, but when people drink, they experience less inhibition, and their behavior becomes more extreme.

Another aspect of alcohol myopia is self-inflation, a tendency to inflate self-evaluations. When asked to rate the importance of 35 trait dimensions for their real and ideal selves, drunken participants rated themselves higher on traits that were important to them and on which they had rated themselves low when sober (Banaji & Steele, 1989). Thus, drinking allowed participants to see themselves as better than they did when they were not drinking, confirming the ability of alcohol to inflate a person's self-evaluation.

A third aspect of alcohol myopia is drunken relief (Steele & Josephs, 1990, p. 928); that is, people who drink tend to worry less and pay less attention to their worries. When consumed in large quantities, alcohol alone may produce drunken relief, but it can also affect behavior in smaller quantities. For example, women with low self-esteem who drank alcohol interacted more with a flirtatious man after drinking than did similar women who had not been drinking and more than women with high self-esteem (Monahan & Lannutti, 2000). This finding suggests that drunken relief is not an effect entirely of alcohol but of alcohol in combination with other factors.

Several pieces of research have supported the alcohol myopia model. Intoxicated people tend to analyze information at a more superficial level and are more susceptible to distraction than people who have not been drinking (Ortner, MacDonald, & Olmstead, 2003). For example, people playing an online gambling game became less focused on suggestions concerning how to maximize their winnings after they started drinking (Phillips & Ogeil, 2007). In addition, alcohol myopia has offered a framework for interpreting a number of changes in sexual behavior that occur after drinking (George & Stoner, 2000). Several studies (Davis, Hendershot, George, Norris, & Heiman, 2007; MacDonald, MacDonald, et al., 2000) have indicated that college students' sexual decision making is affected by intoxication and that focusing on specific cues in the environment can lead to either more or less risky decisions.

When college men who were intoxicated focused on their sexual arousal, they reported more positive feelings about having unprotected sex than did men who had not been drinking (MacDonald, MacDonald, et al., 2000), but receiving strong cues concerning risky sex prompted higher intentions to use condoms among those who were intoxicated than among their sober counterparts (MacDonald, Fong, Zanna, & Martineau, 2000). That is, drinkers' tendency to process information in a limited way is influenced by what cues are present rather than by a general tendency for disinhibition. These studies demonstrate growing research support for this model.

The Social Learning Model

The social learning model provides an explanation for why people begin to drink, why they continue to drink in moderation, and why some people drink in a harmful manner. This model conceptualizes drinking as learned behavior, acquired in the same manner as other behaviors.

According to social learning theory, people begin to drink for at least three reasons. First, the taste of alcohol and its immediate effects may bring pleasure (positive reinforcement); second, drinking may allow a person to escape from an unpleasant situation (negative reinforcement); and third, the person may learn to drink through observing others (modeling). Research offers support for each of these possibilities.

First, research on the reasons for drinking among college students supported the role of positive reinforcement by revealing that interpersonal factors, such as social interaction, and mood enhancement were key reasons for drinking. These reasons applied to students in both the United States (Read, Wood, & Capone, 2005) and the United Kingdom (Orford, Krishnan, Balaam, Everitt, & van der Graaf, 2004).

Second, modeling and social pressure were related to increases in drinking during college, and students who were heavier drinkers put themselves in situations to receive different pressures than did students who drank less (Orford et al., 2004), which relates to the influence of modeling. Modeling is also consistent with one of the explanations proposed by social learning theory

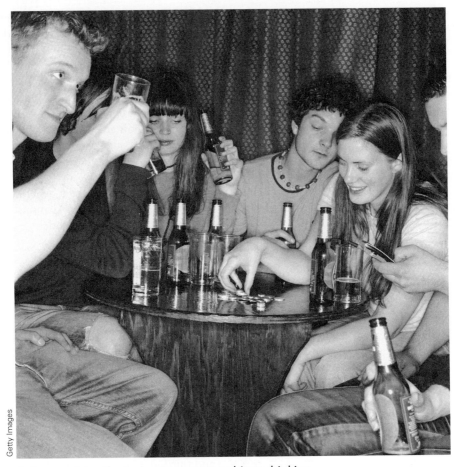

Getty Images

College social gatherings may encourage binge drinking.

for why people drink too much: Drinkers tend to adjust their level of alcohol according to the amount they see others consuming. People who are heavy drinkers tend to associate with other people who have similar drinking patterns. Thus, modeling can explain both the initiation of drinking and the tendency of some people to drink to excess.

A third explanation for excessive drinking offered by the social learning model is based on the principles of negative reinforcement. Most heavy drinkers have learned that they can avoid or reduce the painful effects of withdrawal symptoms by maintaining blood alcohol concentrations at a particular level. As this level begins to drop, the dependent drinker feels the discomfort of withdrawal. These symptoms can be avoided by

ingesting more alcohol; thus, negative reinforcement is one explanation for continuing to drink (Lowman, Hunt, Litten, & Drummond, 2000).

Excessive drinking may serve as a coping response; that is, drinkers may interpret the initial effect of small doses as enhancement of their ability to cope. This response can give drinkers a sense of power and also a feeling of avoiding responsibility or minimizing stress, which also fits with the concept of negative reinforcement. People will then continue to drink as long as they perceive that alcohol has desirable effects. Research support for this explanation comes from a study on individuals who experienced social anxiety (Lewis et al., 2008), who tended to use drinking as a coping strategy and a way of fitting in—drinking relieved them of anxiety.

Social learning theory provides an explanation for why people start drinking, why some continue to drink in moderation, and why others become problem drinkers. In addition, social learning theory suggests a variety of treatment techniques to help people overcome excessive drinking habits. Because drinking behavior is learned, it can be unlearned or relearned, with either abstinence or moderation as a goal of therapy.

IN SUMMARY

The question of why people drink has three components: (1) Why do people begin drinking? (2) Why do some people drink in moderation? (3) Why do others drink to excess? Theories of drinking behavior should be able to offer explanations in response to each of these questions. This section discussed three theories or models, each of which has some potential explanatory ability. The disease model assumes that people drink excessively because they have the disease of alcoholism. One variation of the disease model—the alcohol dependency syndrome—assumes that alcohol dependent people have impaired control and drink heavily for a variety of reasons. Cognitive-physiological models, including the tension reduction hypothesis and alcohol myopia, propose that people drink because alcohol produces alterations in cognitive function that allow them to escape tension or process information differently. Social learning theory hypothesizes that people acquire drinking behavior the same way that they learn other behaviors—that is, through positive or negative reinforcement and modeling. All three models offer some explanation of why some people continue to drink, but only social learning theory addresses all three components of drinking.

CHANGING PROBLEM DRINKING

Despite a decline in the percentage of drinkers in the United States, an increasing number of people seek help for problem drinking, with more than a million and a half people receiving treatment in recent years (SAMHSA, 2007). Men outnumber women by a ratio of 2 to 1. Women are more reluctant than men to seek treatment, and they may also seek treatment from sources that specialize in mental health treatment rather than alcohol treatment (Walter et al., 2003). Outpatient treatment is more common than inpatient treatment, but the most common form of treatment is attendance at a self-help group (SAMHSA, 2007). Private, for-profit facilities emphasize inpatient treatment, but these programs may have benefits that are limited to people with the most serious problems, and the costs are much higher. Cost is a factor in treatment, because almost half of those who receive treatment receive no insurance or other assistance in paying (SAMHSA, 2007). In addition to the various treatment settings, many alcoholics are able to quit drinking without formal treatment (Dawson et al., 2005; Scarscelli, 2006; Walters, 2000).

Change Without Therapy

Some problems (and even some diseases) disappear without formal treatment, and problem drinking is no exception. When a disease disappears without treatment, the term **spontaneous remission** is used to describe the cure. Many authorities in the field of problem drinking prefer the term *unassisted change* or *natural recovery* to describe a switch from problem to nonproblem drinking. Even these terms may be somewhat misleading because people who change their drinking patterns may have the help and support of many people, including family members, employers, and friends. However, changes of this type do occur (Scarscelli, 2006). In a study of individuals diagnosed as alcohol dependent (Dawson et al., 2005), only 25% were still in that category one year later; 18% were abstinent, and another 18% had moderated their drinking to nonproblem levels. Heavy drinkers who change their drinking behavior may be those who are less dependent (Cunningham, Blomqvist, Koski-Jännes, & Cordingley, 2005); others may need professional help or the assistance of traditional groups such as Alcoholics Anonymous.

Presently, nearly all treatment programs in the United States are oriented toward abstinence, but programs in other countries may be oriented toward harm reduction rather than abstinence and allow for the possibility that some problem drinkers can moderate their alcohol intake.

Treatments Oriented Toward Abstinence

All formal treatments—even those that permit the possibility of resuming drinking—seek immediate abstinence as their goal. This section examines several treatment programs aimed at total and permanent abstinence.

Alcoholics Anonymous Alcoholics Anonymous (AA) is one of the most widely used alcohol treatment programs, and it is often a component in other treatment programs. Founded in 1935 by two former alcoholics, AA has become the best known of all approaches to problem drinking. The organization follows a very strict version of the disease model and combines it with an emphasis on spirituality that is designed to bring the problem drinker into the group to receive support and mentoring from others who have experienced similar problems.

To adhere to the AA doctrine, a person must maintain total abstinence from alcohol. Part of the AA philosophy is that those who are in need of joining AA can never drink again; problem drinkers are addicted to alcohol and have no power to resist it. According to AA, alcoholics never recover but are always in the process of recovering. They will be alcoholics for life, even if they never take another drink.

AA and other 12-step programs have become increasingly popular, attracting large numbers of people. Each year, more than 2 million people in the United States attend a self-help program such as AA for drinking problems (SAMSHA, 2007). A majority of those individuals—perhaps as many as 75%—attend AA meetings (Magura, 2007).

The anonymity offered to those who attend AA meetings presents barriers to researchers wishing to conduct studies on the effectiveness of this program. A systematic evaluation (Ferri, Amato, & Davoli, 2006) found no experimental evidence showing that attending AA is an effective treatment for drinking problems. Experimentation would involve randomly assigning participants to attend AA or some other option, which is not how most treatment occurs. Instead, people choose to attend a program, and for some people with drinking problems, choosing AA may be helpful (Gossop, Stewart, & Marsden, 2008; Kelly, 2003). For others, the AA 12-step program with its "one-size-fits-all approach" is not helpful (Buddie, 2004, p. 61), and many drop out of AA. Alternative self-help organizations predate the development of AA and continue to proliferate around the world (White, 2004). Organizations such as Secular Organization for Sobriety, Women for Sobriety, SMARTRecovery, Rational Recovery, and Moderation Management offer the value of support and group discussions without the inflexible philosophy and religious orientation of AA. Online groups available through the Internet offer easier access than face-to-face support.

Psychotherapy Nearly as many psychotherapeutic techniques have been used to treat alcohol abuse as there are psychotherapies. Research has demonstrated that many approaches are not very effective in helping problem drinkers, whereas other techniques are much more so (Kaner et al., 2007; Miller, Wilbourne, & Hettema, 2003). Education about alcohol, alcoholism counseling, confrontational counseling, Alcoholics Anonymous, and 12-step programs were among the least effective; behavioral self-control training, social skills training, behavioral contracting, and cognitive therapy have demonstrated much higher levels of effectiveness (Miller et al., 2003). Brief interventions and techniques oriented toward changing motivation were rated as even more effective.

An example of both a brief intervention and one oriented toward changing motivation is motivational interviewing (Miller & Rollnick, 2002). Therapists using motivational interviewing convey their empathy with the client's situation and help clients resolve their ambivalence about their problem behavior. This process is designed to move clients toward change, making this approach a directive type of psychological intervention. Linking motivational interviewing to the transtheoretical model (see Chapter 4) provides a framework for understanding and promoting behavioral change. Reviews of motivational interviewing (Britt, Blampied, & Hudson, 2003; Rubak, Sanboek, Lauritzen, & Christensen, 2005) found that this type of brief intervention was effective in decreasing problem drinking. In addition to the behavioral approaches that can be effective, some chemical treatments can also be useful in controlling problem drinking.

Chemical Treatments Many treatment programs for problem drinking include administering drugs that interact with alcohol to produce a range of unpleasant effects. **Disulfiram** (Antabuse) is one such drug. Taken alone, this drug produces a few unpleasant effects, but in combination with alcohol, the unpleasant effects are severe, including flushing of the face, chest pains, a pounding heart, nausea and vomiting, sweating, headache, dizziness, weakness, difficulty in breathing, and a rapid decrease in blood pressure. The rationale behind the use of these drugs is to produce an aversion to drinking by building up an association between drinking and the unpleasant consequences. This process, called **aversion therapy**, applies to the use of disulfiram as well as other methods that involve aversive conditioning. Aversion therapy was once a common approach to the treatment of drinking problems, but its use has declined, partly because of problems in getting people to take a drug that will make them sick if they drink and partly because of its lack of effectiveness (Mann, 2004; Miller et al., 2003).

An alternative drug treatment is naltrexone, a drug that attaches to opiate receptors in the brain and prevents their activation. Its action for drinkers may be to decrease the reward that comes from drinking (Mann, 2004). Several studies have shown that patients who received naltrexone as part of their treatment were better able to maintain abstinence and experienced reduced craving for alcohol compared to patients who received a placebo. Systematic reviews (Carmen, Angeles, Ana, & María, 2004; Snyder & Bowers, 2008) indicate that naltrexone may be more useful in preventing relapse than in maintaining abstinence, and the effects may be short-term rather than longer.

Another drug that shows even more promise is acamprosate, which acts to affect GABA, one of the brain's neurotransmitters. Its action may decrease craving (Mann, 2004) and increase the chances of achieving abstinence (Carmen et al., 2004). Several reviews of treatment effectiveness (Carmen et al., 2004; Snyder & Bowers, 2008) concluded that acamprosate is a useful component in treating drinking problems.

Controlled Drinking

Until the late 1960s, all treatments for problem drinking were aimed at total abstinence. Then something quite unexpected happened. In 1962 in London, D. L. Davies found that 7 of the 93 recovered alcoholics whom he studied were able to drink "normally" (defined as consumption of up to three pints of beer or its equivalent per day) for at least a seven-year period following treatment. These moderate drinkers represented fewer than 8% of those Davies studied, but this finding was still remarkable because it opened up the possibility that diagnosed alcoholics could successfully return to nonproblem drinking. This finding provoked a controversy that continues today.

Prompted by Davies's results, several studies conducted in the United States (Armor, Polich, & Stambul, 1976; Polich, Armor, & Braiker, 1980) showed that controlled drinking occurred in a small percentage of patients who received treatment oriented toward abstinence. Publicity about this study produced a wave of criticism from those holding the position that alcoholics can never drink again, and this controversy became more heated when researchers began to design treatment programs with controlled drinking as the goal.

Problem drinkers can become moderate drinkers. Some problem drinkers in abstinence-oriented treatment programs become moderate drinkers (Sobell, Cunningham, & Sobell, 1996; Miller, Walters, & Bennett, 2001), and some who quit on their own moderate their drinking (Dawson et al., 2005). Despite the evidence concerning controlled drinking, most treatment centers in the United States have resisted the possibility that former problem drinkers can learn to moderate their use of alcohol. Many of the people who provide treatment services are people who have experienced problems themselves, received indoctrination into the disease model, and become committed to the programs that helped them (Quinn et al., 2004; Shavelson, 2001). This attitude does not extend to other countries; in England, Wales, and Scotland, nearly all treatment centers accept continued drinking among those who have experienced drinking problems. The goal is to reduce the harm that often accompanies drinking rather than eliminate drinking itself (Heather, 2006; Rosenberg & Melville, 2005).

The thought of being able to continue drinking is appealing to most drinkers, including those whose drinking is problematic. Thus, controlled drinking appeals to many with drinking problems (Kosok, 2006). This appeal is one reason for the creation of a self-help group oriented toward moderating drinking, called Moderation Management. This group includes face-to-face and online meetings, and 90% of members live in the United States. Many of those who are affiliated with Moderation Management have not sought other assistance for their drinking problems, perhaps because the available treatment is abstinence oriented.

The Problem of Relapse

Problem drinkers who successfully complete either an abstinence-oriented or a moderation-oriented treatment program do not necessarily maintain their goals. As we saw with smoking, people who complete a treatment program usually improve quite a bit, but the problem of relapse is substantial. Interestingly, the time course and rate of relapse are similar for those who complete treatment programs for smoking, alcohol abuse, or opiate abuse (Hunt et al., 1971). Most relapses occur within 90 days after the end of the program. At 12 months after the end of treatment, only about 35% of those completing the programs are still abstinent. These similarities may be attributable to the underlying brain mechanisms involved in habitual drug use, which share some similarities regardless of differences in the pharmacological properties of the drug (Camí & Farré, 2003).

Improved treatment programs lead to lower relapse rates. One factor in this improvement is the knowledge that relapse is so frequent; many programs now include relapse prevention (Witkiewitz & Marlatt, 2004). Another factor is the definition of relapse. Holding to the standard that any drinking constitutes a relapse, the success rate for treatment programs is only 25% to 35% (Miller et al., 2001). However, if the standard is improvement and a lower level of problems caused by drinking, then relapse is not as common; as many as 60% of people who complete a treatment program achieve this level of success.

Most behavior-based treatment regimens include training for relapse prevention, taking the view that a relapse offers an opportunity for learning and that behavior change is not quick (Witkiewitz & Marlatt, 2004). As discussed in Chapter 12, relapse prevention training is aimed at changing cognitions so that the addict comes to believe that one slip does *not* equal total relapse. Programs that focus on long-term goals and incorporate relapse prevention into their regimen tend to have the highest rates of success (McLellan, Lewis, O'Brien, & Kleber, 2000), but many relapse prevention programs do not have a high rate of success (Miller et al., 2003).

IN SUMMARY

Despite a decline in the percentage of drinkers in the United States, the number of people seeking help for their drinking problems has continued to grow. Many problem drinkers are able to quit without therapy; others seek formal treatment programs. Traditional alcohol treatment programs—such as Alcoholics Anonymous, the most widely sought treatment—have been oriented toward abstinence. Many problem drinkers are not able to achieve this goal; only about 25% of problem drinkers are abstinent one year after treatment. Drinking levels typically drop substantially, however, and so do alcohol-related problems.

Some behavioral programs are successful, especially brief interventions such as motivational interviewing, which are becoming more common. Chemical treatments such as the drugs disulfiram, naltrexone, and acamprosate have been used to curb alcohol consumption, and the latter two seem to be useful.

Controlled drinking may be a reasonable goal for some problem drinkers. However, this goal is very controversial, and many abstinence-oriented therapists do not consider controlled drinking a viable alternative, which may keep some problem drinkers from seeking therapy.

With all alcohol treatment approaches, relapse has been a persistent problem. Most relapses occur within 3 months after the end of treatment, and after 12 months, only 25% of those who complete programs are still abstinent. Relapse training has become a common component of behaviorally oriented programs, but the goal of sustained abstinence is a difficult one.

OTHER DRUGS

Illicit drugs have created many serious problems in the United States, but these problems are mainly social and not related to physical health. Compared with the effects of smoking cigarettes, drinking alcohol, eating unwisely, and failing to exercise, relatively few people die from the effects of illegal drugs. For example, cocaine, the deadliest of the illicit drugs, kills only 1 person for every

1,000 killed by tobacco products (Rouse, 1998). Even one death from illicit drugs, of course, is too many, and this section addresses some of the negative health consequences of both legal and illegal drugs. Table 13.2 shows the rates of use of various drugs, including alcohol and nicotine.

Researchers are beginning to understand how drugs function in the brain to alter mood and behavior. Alcohol and other drugs produce effects on neurotransmitters, the chemical basis of neural transmission. Several neurotransmitters are involved in drug actions, including GABA, glutamate, serotonin, and norepinephrine (López-Moreno, González-Cuevas, Moreno, & Navarro, 2008), but the neurotransmitter **dopamine** is especially important (Nestler & Malenka, 2004). Dopamine may be the most important neurotransmitter in a brain subsystem that relays messages from the ventral tegmental area in the midbrain to the nucleus accumbens in the forebrain. Researchers have known for years that this area is involved in the brain's experience of reward and pleasure. However, the actions of many drugs seem to be common to the same system, including these two brain structures as well as the hippocampus, amygdala, and forebrain

TABLE 13.2

Lifetime, Past Year, and Past Month Use of Various Drugs, Including Nonmedical Use of Legal Drugs, Persons Aged 12 Years and Older, United States, 2006

Drug	Lifetime Use	Use During Past Year	Use During Past Month
Alcohol	83.1%	65.0%	50.9%
Cigarettes	66.3	29.1	25.0
Smokeless tobacco	19.4	4.4	3.3
Sedatives	3.6	0.4	0.2
Tranquilizers	8.7	2.1	0.7
Heroin	1.5	0.2	0.1
Pain relievers	13.6	5.1	2.1
Stimulants	8.2	1.2	0.5
Cocaine	14.3	2.5	1.0
Crack cocaine	3.5	0.6	0.3
Marijuana	45.4	10.3	6.0
LSD	9.5	0.3	0.1
Ecstasy	5.0	0.9	0.2

Source: Results from the 2006 National Survey on Drug Use and Health: National Findings, by Substance Abuse and Mental Health Services Administration, 2007 (DHHS Publication No. SMA 07–4293). Rockville, MD: Department of Health and Human Services. Tables G.2, G.4, G.6, G.15.

WOULD YOU BELIEVE . . . ?

Brain Damage Is Not a Common Risk of Drug Use

Despite the vivid media images of a brain "fried" by drug use, most psychoactive drugs do not cause damage to the nervous system. Indeed, some of the drugs that can most wreck a person's life are among the *least* likely to damage the brain. For example, opiate drugs such as heroin, morphine, and oxycodone produce both tolerance and dependence. Repeated use of these drugs results in compulsive drug taking and a pattern of use in which social relationships and responsibilities become unimportant. People who are dependent on opiate drugs usually experience major problems, but brain damage is not among them.

Like other psychoactive drugs, opiates cross the blood–brain barrier, where they occupy receptors for endorphins, the body's own analgesics (Julien, 2008). Thus, these drugs are compatible with the brain's existing neurochemistry, so they occupy these receptors without causing damage. Their repeated use produces a host of physiological effects, some of which can be dangerous, but damage to the nervous system is unlikely.

Marijuana also acts by occupying brain receptors for neurochemicals called endocannabinoids (Nicoll & Alger, 2004). The discovery of these neurochemicals suggested that the brain makes its own marijuana-like chemicals and also explained some of the actions that marijuana takes in the brain. Marijuana also produces a wide variety of physiological and behavioral effects, some of which may be dangerous. However, those effects do not include damage to neurons in the brain (Kalant, 2004).

Both publicity and public service announcements have decried the dangers of the drug Ecstasy, but the research that formed the basis for these claims was withdrawn by the researcher because of inaccuracies (Holden, 2003). Prolonged use of Ecstasy may pose dangers (Morton, 2005), but the only evidence that implicates this drug in neural damage comes from combinations with alcohol or stimulants, and then only as a possibility (Gouzoulis-Mayfrank & Daumann, 2006).

However, some drugs do carry risks of damage to the nervous system. Those risks typically occur with heavy, long-term use to those who fit into the category of abusers. For example, the potential for brain damage as a result of extended alcohol abuse is well known (Harper & Matsumoto, 2005). Some evidence is also developing that demonstrates the toxic neurological effects of the abuse of stimulants such as cocaine (Rosenberg, Grigsby, Dreisbach, Busenbark, & Grigsby, 2002) and amphetamines (Chang et al., 2002). The evidence for brain damage from the use of household solvents is strong (Rosenberg et al., 2002). These chemicals act to alter consciousness not through changes to neurotransmitters but through oxygen restriction to the brain, so of course these substances cause brain damage.

The greatest risks from drug use are not neurological damage but rather the ability of these drugs to alter perception, decision making, and coordination. These effects increase the risk for unintentional injuries, which are a far more likely result than brain damage.

(López-Moreno et al., 2008). That is, drugs seem to activate the brain circuits that underlie reward. Indeed, experiences such as gambling may activate the same brain mechanisms (Martin & Petry, 2005).

Psychoactive drugs do not all act in the same way in this subsystem, but all increase the availability of neurotransmitters, especially dopamine. Alterations of these neurotransmitters produce temporary changes in brain chemistry but rarely damage neurons. Changing the brain's chemistry carries risks, but brain damage is not a health

effect associated with most drugs (see Would You Believe . . . ? box).

Health Effects

Even though they do not damage neurons, both legal and illegal drugs pose potential health hazards. However, illegal drugs present certain risks not found with legal drugs, regardless of pharmacological effects. Illegal drugs may be sold as one drug when they are actually another; buyers have no assurance as to dosage; and illegally manufactured drugs may have impurities that can be dangerous chemicals themselves. In addition, the sources of illegal drugs can be dangerous people. Legal drugs are free from these risks, but they are not always safe or harmless.

All drugs have potential hazards, but drugs termed *safe* are tested by the federal Food and Drug Administration (FDA) and defined as safe. The FDA considers a drug safe if its potential benefits outweigh its potential hazards. Many drugs, such as antibiotics, have been approved although they produce severe side effects in some people. The more potentially beneficial a drug, the more likely it is to be labeled safe despite unpleasant side effects.

The FDA classifies drugs into five categories, based on their potential for abuse and their potential medical benefits. Table 13.3 summarizes this schedule, presents the restrictions on availability, and gives examples of drugs in each category. This classification has evolved somewhat haphazardly over the past 100 years and represents legislative and social convention rather than scientific findings.

Sedatives **Sedatives** are drugs that induce relaxation and sometimes intoxication by lowering the activity of the brain, the neurons, the muscles, and the heart, and even by slowing the metabolic rate (Julien, 2008). In low doses, these drugs tend to make people feel relaxed and even euphoric. In high doses, they cause loss of consciousness and

can result in coma and death as a result of their inhibitory effect on the brain center that controls respiration. Sedatives include barbiturates, tranquilizers, opiates, and methadone, but the most commonly used drug in this category is alcohol.

Depressant effects are a major problem with sedative drugs, and these effects are additive when sedatives are taken in combination. The effect of mixing two or more of these drugs can be depression of the respiratory system to a dangerously low level. Some people mix alcohol with tranquilizers or other depressants, providing a potentially lethal combination. Sedatives and stimulants have opposite effects, but these effects do not cancel each other; instead, both sets of effects occur. For example, caffeine (the stimulant drug in coffee) will not sober a person intoxicated on alcohol (a sedative). Rather, caffeine merely makes a drunken person more alert and less sleepy—not less drunk.

Barbiturates are synthetic drugs used medically to induce sleep. Taken recreationally, barbiturates produce effects similar to alcohol: relaxation and intoxication in small doses, drunkenness and unconsciousness in larger doses. Because they are ingested in pill form, which does not produce immediate effects, barbiturate overdoses are more common than alcohol overdoses. Barbiturates produce both tolerance and dependence. Many people can take barbiturates in the form of sleeping pills over an extended

TABLE 13.3

FDA Drug Schedules, Restrictions, and Examples of Drugs in Each Category

Schedule	Description	Restriction on Availability	Examples
I	High abuse potential; no medical uses	Not legally available	LSD, marijuana, heroin
II	High abuse potential; medical uses	Prescription only	Morphine, oxycontin, barbiturates, amphetamines, cocaine
III	Moderate or low dependence; medical uses	Prescription only	Codeine, some tranquilizers
IV	Low dependence, low abuse potential; medical uses	Prescription only	Phenobarbital, most tranquilizers
V	Less abuse potential than drugs in Schedule IV	Over the counter	Aspirin, antacids, antihistamines, and others

BECOMING HEALTHIER

1. Avoid binge drinking—that is, drinking five or more drinks on any one occasion. There are no health benefits associated with binge drinking, and there are many risks.

2. Avoiding alcohol may not be the healthiest choice, but if you do not drink and are comfortable with that choice, do not start drinking. If you have a drink occasionally, you may receive some of the benefits of alcohol; if you don't, lead a healthy lifestyle in other ways.

3. Occasional drinking—either light or heavy—presents some risks but does not convey many benefits. The pattern that confers the most benefits is daily (or almost daily) light drinking.

4. One or two drinks per day can impair judgment and coordination. These dangers are the biggest risk of alcohol consumption, and people who drink should find ways to manage this risk.

5. Do not drive, operate machinery, or swim after drinking.

6. Do not escalate your drinking; keep to one or two drinks per day (not an average of one or two).

7. The safest level of alcohol for pregnant women is none.

8. If one or both of your parents experienced drinking problems, you may be at elevated risk. Manage this risk by moderating your drinking.

9. If you have an extremely pleasant experience with any drug (including alcohol) the first time you try it, be aware that future use of this drug may present problems for you.

10. Don't combine drugs; drugs in combination are more dangerous than taking one drug.

11. Drugs that produce dependence are more dangerous than those that do not. Be aware and cautious about using such drugs, including alcohol and nicotine as well as opiates, barbiturates, and amphetamines.

12. Illegal drugs, even those without tolerance or dependence potential, can be dangerous because they are illegal.

---

time without increasing the dose, whereas others rapidly escalate their dosage to dangerous levels. People who use barbiturates as sleeping pills on a regular basis are not able to sleep without them, and they manifest withdrawal symptoms when they stop taking them—two definite indications of dependence. Withdrawal is similar to that from alcohol, lasting up to a week and including tremor, nausea, vomiting, sweating, sleep disturbances, and sometimes hallucinations and delirium.

Tranquilizers are relatively recent, dating only to the 1960s. The most prominent variety of these chemical compositions is the *benzodiazepine* group. Like barbiturates, tranquilizers induce sedation, but they are less likely to produce sleep and more likely to suppress anxiety. Thus, tranquilizers are used to treat anxiety. Recognition of the dangers of this class of drug has led to decreased prescriptions and fewer health problems.

Benzodiazepines produce both tolerance and dependence, but only over an extended period. Neither tolerance nor dependence is particularly severe if the drug is taken in small or even moderate amounts. In large amounts, however, these drugs not only produce tolerance and dependence but also cause disorientation, confusion, and even rage, a paradoxical effect for a tranquilizer.

Another category of depressants is the **opiates**, drugs derived from the opium poppy. Opium can also be refined into *morphine*, which can be further chemically treated to produce *heroin*. Synthetic and semisynthetic compounds, including *meperidine, methadone*, oxycodone (OxyContin), and hydrocodone (Vicodin), are chemically similar to the opiates and produce similar effects.

Opium has been used for centuries for both medical and recreational purposes (Julien, 2008). It can be ingested by swallowing, sniffing, smoking, or injecting under the skin, into a muscle, or intravenously, making it one of the most versatile drugs for transmission into the body. In the 19th century in the United States, physicians prescribed opiates frequently and for a variety of conditions. Today, the principal medical use of opiates is to relieve pain. Because they act on the central nervous system and the digestive system, opiate drugs are also prescribed for cough and for diarrhea. Opiates cross the blood–brain barrier and attach to receptors in the brain, altering the interpretation of pain messages. The physical condition responsible for the pain is not halted, of course, but the person's subjective experience of pain diminishes. Opiate drugs, therefore, have important medical uses.

Opiates produce both tolerance and dependence after only a brief time, sometimes as little as 24 hours, making opiates such as heroin easily abused. However, heroin use is not common in the United States (see Table 13.4). The annual use of heroin and other opiates increased among high school students (Johnston, O'Malley, Bachman, & Schulenberg, 2008) and young adults (Johnston et al., 2007) during the 1990s, but their use has since stabilized. An important part of that increase was the growing popularity of oxycodone and hydrocodone, which continued through 2007. The trend toward increased use of opiates is thus more prominent among young people and is attributable to the use of oxycodone and hydrocodone rather than heroin, morphine, or codeine (SAMHSA, 2007).

Stimulants Stimulant drugs make some people feel more alert and energetic, more able to concentrate, and more able to work long hours. They make other users feel jittery, anxious, and unable to sit still. More specifically, stimulants tend to produce alertness, reduce feelings of fatigue, elevate mood, and decrease appetite. They are synthetic but are similar in chemical structure to norepinephrine, the neurotransmitter identified as the brain's main excitatory chemical. After a decline in the nonmedical use of stimulants from 1975 to the early 1990s, there was an increase in the use of illegal stimulants in the United States by high school seniors (Johnston et al., 2008) and young adults (Johnston et al., 2007). That

increase seems to have reversed, beginning in 2007.

Amphetamines are stimulant drugs that are often abused because of their mood-altering effects. In addition, amphetamines produce such physical symptoms as increased blood pressure, slower heart rate, increased respiration, relaxation of bronchial muscles, dilation of pupils, increased EEG activity, and increased blood supply to the muscles (Julien, 2008). These effects can be dangerous to the cardiovascular system, especially for people who have heart problems or other cardiovascular diseases, but even healthy young people are more likely to experience fatal heart attacks if they use amphetamines (Westover, Nakonezny, & Haley, 2008). Amphetamines can also produce psychological effects, including hallucinations and paranoid delusions. High energy levels combined with paranoid delusions can make amphetamine users dangerous to society. In addition to these physical, psychological, and social effects, amphetamines produce both tolerance and dependence. Thus, they are undesirable as diet pills, despite their appetite suppressant effects.

Another stimulant drug, **cocaine**, is extracted from the coca plant, which grows in the Andes Mountains in South America. In the 1880s, several European physicians, including Sigmund Freud, discovered that cocaine was capable of blocking neural transmission at the site of application and therefore was useful for **anesthesia**. For a time, cocaine was used as an anesthetic for surgery, especially eye surgery. In the 1890s, it became a popular drug in America and was widely available in tonics, wines, and soft drinks. Soon, however, people began to recognize the dangers of cocaine, and U.S. federal drug laws restricted its use. Today the medical uses of cocaine are quite limited because more effective anesthetics have been developed.

Cocaine acts as a stimulant to the nervous system. The strength and duration of its action depend not only on dose but also on mode of administration. Although South American Indians take cocaine orally by chewing the coca leaves, this method is seldom used elsewhere. Instead, cocaine is snorted through the nasal passages, smoked

TABLE 13.4

Summary of Characteristics of Psychoactive Drugs

Name	Source	Medical Use	Mode of Ingestion	Effects	Duration of Effects	Tolerance	Dependence
Stimulants							
Caffeine	Natural (tea, coffee)	Anti-depressant	Swallowed	Increases alertness, reduces fatigue	1–2 hrs	Yes	Yes
Cocaine	Natural (coca plant)	Local anesthetic	Swallowed, injected, sniffed	Produces euphoria suppresses appetite	15–30 min	Yes	Yes
Amphetamines	Synthetic	Appetite suppressant	Swallowed, injected	Produces alertness, reduces fatigue	4 hrs	Yes	Yes
Nicotine	Natural (tobacco plant)	None	Smoked, sniffed, chewed	Elevates blood pressure	30 min	Yes	Yes
Depressants							
Barbiturates	Synthetic	Sedative	Swallowed	Relaxes, intoxicates	Varies, depending on type	Yes	Yes
Tranquilizers	Synthetic	Anxiety reduction	Swallowed	Relaxes, intoxicates	3–4 hrs	Yes	Yes
Opiates	Natural (opium poppy), semisynthetic	Analgesic	Swallowed, sniffed, smoked injected	Produces euphoria, sedates	4–6 hrs	Yes	Yes
Methadone	Synthetic	Treatment for heroin addiction	Swallowed	Prevents heroin euphoria	12–24 hrs	Yes	Yes
Alcohol	Natural (fruits, grains)	External antiseptic	Swallowed	Relaxes, intoxicates	2–3 hrs	Yes	Yes
Marijuana	Natural (cannabis)	Treatment for glaucoma, antiemetic, increases appetite	Smoked	Relaxes, intoxicates	2–3 hrs	No	Yes
LSD	Synthetic	None	Swallowed	Alters perception, intoxicates	5–8 hrs	No	No
Ecstasy	Synthetic	None	Swallowed	Produces feelings of peace	2–4 hrs	No	No
Steroids							
Anabolic steroids	Natural, synthetic	Restores erectile functioning in men	Swallowed, injected	Builds muscles, increases blood pressure, reduces immune system functioning	7–14 days	Yes	No

(in the "freebase" or crack form), or injected intravenously. The stimulant effects of cocaine are short, lasting only 15 to 30 minutes. During this time, the user often feels a powerful euphoria, a strong sense of well-being, and heightened attention. But when the effects wear off, the user frequently feels fatigued, sluggish, and anxious and is left with a strong craving to repeat the experience. Frequently the user will increase the dose in a futile effort to make the euphoria last longer the next time. Cocaine was one of the drugs that Drew Barrymore used, and her behavior while intoxicated produced problems for her life. She experienced no obvious health problems as a result of her cocaine use, but others have.

The stimulant effects of increased doses of cocaine can endanger the cardiovascular system, increasing the risk of heart attack (Kloner & Rezkalla, 2003). The greatest risk occurs within a few hours of ingestion but may persist for as long as several days. The risks may be cumulative; cocaine users showed a higher degree of cardiovascular disease than nonusers (Darke, Kaye, & Duflou, 2006), but even first-time users may experience dangerous cardiac symptoms.

During the early 1990s, a group of neuropharmacology researchers (Hearn et al., 1991) discovered that cocaine and alcohol interact in the body to form a third chemical, *cocaethylene*, which produces or enhances the euphoria that cocaine users experience. However, cocaethylene is a hazardous chemical (Huq, 2007) and may boost the user's risk for cardiac problems (Tacker & Okorodudu, 2004). The mixture of these two drugs may produce a higher death rate and a greater rate of emergency room admissions than either drug alone.

Crack cocaine became a serious social problem in the United States in the 1980s, when this form of cocaine became cheap and widely available. Crack, a form of freebase cocaine, is ingested by smoking. The use of crack among high school seniors declined during the mid-1980s, increased slightly during the 1990s, and decreased slightly after 2000 (Johnston et al., 2008). For adults, the rates of current use fell from the mid-1980s through 2000 and remained low (about 0.6%) in 2006 (SAMHSA, 2007).

The annual use of both cocaine and crack cocaine is quite low in the general population (see Table 13.2).

Methylenedioxymethamphetamine (MDMA)—Ecstasy—is a derivative of methamphetamine, but people use it for its mild hallucinogenic effects, including feelings of peace, joy, and empathy with others. These feelings come from a massive release of the neurotransmitter *serotonin*, which depletes the brain of serotonin, resulting in a deficient amount for normal functioning and possibly long-lasting problems with serotonin regulation in the brain. However, the contention that this drug produces damage to neurons remains controversial (Baumann, Xiaoying, & Rothman, 2007). Other dangers include problems in regulating body temperature and negative effects on the immune system (Connor, 2004).

Ecstasy showed increasing popularity worldwide in dance clubs and "raves," beginning in the 1990s (Hunt & Evans, 2003). In the United States, use of Ecstasy rose more rapidly than any other illicit drug during the late 1990s, continued to increase until 2001, and then fell (Johnston et al., 2008). Ecstasy use remains higher among high school students than young adults. About 6.5% of high school seniors have tried Ecstasy, and about 2% of high school seniors use this drug at least monthly, whereas less than 1% of young adults do (Johnston et al., 2007).

Marijuana The most commonly used illegal drug in the United States is *marijuana* (see Table 13.2). Marijuana is composed of the leaves, flowers, and small branches of *Cannabis sativa*, a plant that flourishes in almost every climate in the world. The intoxicating ingredient in marijuana, delta-9-tetrahydrocannabinol (THC), comes from the resin of the male plants and especially the female plants. The brain contains receptors for cannabinoids in many locations, which results in a variety of effects from ingesting marijuana, including altered thought processes, memory impairment, feelings of relaxation and euphoria, increased appetite, and coordination impairment (Nicoll & Alger, 2004). Its potential for serious health consequences is still debated, but few authorities regard it as a major health risk.

The most reliable physiological effect of THC is increased heart rate, which occurs with the consumption of heavy doses. Although a rapid heartbeat may present health hazards to users with coronary problems, no evidence exists that marijuana in small or moderate doses causes any cardiac damage. Nevertheless, marijuana use poses health risks, the most prominent of which is its increased risk of injury (Kalant, 2004). Under the influence of marijuana, people tend to make riskier decisions (Lane, Cherek, Tcheremissine, Lieving, & Pietras, 2005). Considering this cognitive effect plus marijuana's effect on coordination, it is not surprising that habitual use is related to vehicle crashes (Blows et al.,

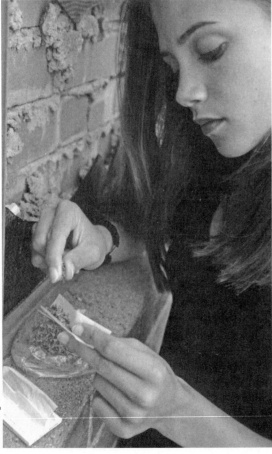

David Young-Wolff/PhotoEdit

Marijuana is the most commonly used illicit drug, particularly among adolescents and young adults.

2005). In addition, those who smoke marijuana face increased risks for respiratory problems and lung cancer (Kalant, 2004). As with many drugs, marijuana use has negative effects on the immune system (Connor, 2004).

Marijuana also has beneficial effects (Nicoll & Alger, 2004). THC and the cannabinoids that are the active ingredients in marijuana can reduce nausea and vomiting in cancer patients treated with chemotherapy (Tramer et al., 2001). Marijuana's antinausea and analgesic properties make it useful in treating people with HIV infection who are taking antiretroviral medication, which produces unpleasant symptoms (Woolridge et al., 2005). In the 1970s, researchers noticed that healthy young marijuana smokers experienced a lessening of pressure within their eyes, decreasing glaucoma (Hepler & Frank, 1971). Nevertheless, the U.S. Drug Enforcement Administration continues to reject all pleas for reclassifying marijuana to Schedule II to make it available for medical use. However, researchers are working toward understanding the various physical responses to marijuana in order to develop nonintoxicating drugs with similar benefits (Nicoll & Alger, 2004).

People involved in providing treatment to long-term heavy marijuana users have contended that marijuana is capable of producing dependence and withdrawal (Kalant, 2004). Research has confirmed that withdrawal symptoms occur in such users (Budney, 2006). However, relatively few users experience these symptoms; most people who have tried or used marijuana do not continue to use this drug (Johnston et al., 2007). For example, more than 75% of 40- to 45-year-olds have used marijuana but only 12% of that age group have used marijuana within the past year.

Recreational use of marijuana in the United States is a relatively recent phenomenon. Only 2% of people born between 1930 and 1940 used marijuana before age 21, but more than half the people born during the 1970s used this drug before their 21st birthday (Johnson & Gerstein, 1998). Marijuana use among high school students in the United States has declined slightly since the late 1990s (Johnston et al., 2008). Lifetime use among adolescents and adults is more than 50%, making marijuana by far the most commonly used illicit drug.

Anabolic Steroids In recent years, media reports have covered repeated scandals involving athletes who have used **anabolic steroids** (AS) to enhance athletic performance (King & Pace, 2005). This practice applies not only to professional and Olympic athletes but also to a range of individuals as young as junior high school. What are anabolic steroids, and do they pose health hazards?

Steroids can be either endogenous (manufactured by the body) or synthetic. Endogenous steroids are produced by the adrenal glands, which secrete cortisone, and by the ovaries and testes, which secrete estrogen and testosterone. The effects of anabolic steroids include thickening of the vocal cords, enlargement of the larynx, increase of muscle bulk, and decrease of body fat. These last two properties make AS attractive to athletes, bodybuilders, and people who wish to alter their appearance. Anabolic steroids have some medical uses, including reduction of inflammation and control of some allergic reactions.

On the other hand, anabolic steroids are potentially dangerous. They can upset the chemical balance in the body, produce toxicity, and shut off the body's production of its own steroids, leaving the person more susceptible to stress and infection and altering reproductive functioning. Other hazards include increased coronary risk factors, heart attack, abnormal liver function, stunted height, and breast development in men (Julien, 2008). Some authorities (Keane, 2003) contend that the use of steroids leads to dependence in some circumstances and produces behavioral problems in many more. These behavioral problems include aggression, euphoria, mood swings, distractibility, and confusion.

Monthly use of steroids is 1.1% for high school seniors (Johnston et al., 2008), but only 0.1% for young adults (Johnston et al., 2007). These overall percentages do not reflect the much higher rate of use among selected groups. Young men are two to five times more likely than young women to use anabolic steroid. Use among athletes is much higher, as the frequent scandals reflect.

Drug Misuse and Abuse

Most people believe that some drugs are acceptable and even desirable because of the medical benefits they confer. But all *psychoactive* drugs—drugs that cross the blood–brain barrier and alter mental functioning—pose potential health risks. Most have the capacity for tolerance or dependence (see Table 13.4). Even drugs that are not psychoactive have the potential for unpleasant side effects. For example, penicillin can cause nausea, vomiting, diarrhea, swelling, and skin eruptions. In addition, people who have allergies to penicillin can die from ingesting it. Caffeine, a drug commonly found in coffee and cola drinks, can produce effects that meet the *DSM-IV* criteria of substance dependence. A review of studies on caffeine withdrawal (Juliano & Griffiths, 2004) confirmed this diagnosis—people who habitually consume caffeine experience withdrawal symptoms that include headache, difficulty concentrating, and depressed mood. Thus, all drugs carry some risks.

Almost all drugs that have potential medical or health benefits also have the potential for misuse and abuse. The moderate use of alcohol, for instance, is related to decreased cardiovascular mortality. The *misuse* of alcohol—defined as inappropriate but not health-threatening levels of consumption—can result in social embarrassment, violent acts, and injury. And abuse of alcohol—defined as frequent, heavy consumption to the point of addiction—can lead to cirrhosis, brain damage, heart attack, and fetal alcohol syndrome.

Not all individuals who use drugs or alcohol are equally likely to become abusers. Genetic and situational factors contribute to the risks of substance abuse, but another major risk is the presence of psychopathology. Individuals with some psychiatric disorder, such as depression, schizophrenia, or posttraumatic stress disorder, are more likely than others to develop substance abuse disorders and to have greater difficulty recovering (Tate, Brown, Unrod, & Ramo, 2004).

Treatment for Drug Abuse

Treatment for the use and abuse of illegal drugs is similar to the treatment of alcohol abuse, both in the philosophy and in the administration of treatment (Schuckit, 2000). In the United States and many other countries, the goal of treatment for all types of illegal drug use is total abstinence. In many cases, the programs that treat drug abusers coexist physically with treatment programs for alcohol abuse, and patients who are receiving treatment for their drug problems participate in the same therapy as those who are receiving therapy for their alcohol problems. The philosophy that guides Alcoholics Anonymous led to the development of Narcotics Anonymous, an organization devoted to helping drug users abstain from using drugs. Self-help groups are as common in treating drug abuse as they are in dealing with alcohol abuse (Kelly, 2003).

The reasons for entering drug abuse treatment programs are often similar to those for entering treatment for alcohol abuse, and those reasons are primarily social. The abuse of illegal drugs leads to legal, financial, and interpersonal problems, just as alcohol abuse does. Like alcohol, most illegal drugs produce impairments of judgment that lead to unintentional injury and death, making such injury the leading health risk from drug abuse. The abuse of most illegal drugs does not produce as many direct health hazards as alcohol abuse. However, when health problems occur, they are likely to be major and life threatening. Such crises may precipitate a person's decision to seek treatment or lead family members to enforce treatment. Drew Barrymore did not decide to seek treatment, but her mother checked her into an inpatient treatment program that is typical of such facilities in the United States—its goal is complete abstinence, and its philosophy is the same as AA's.

Inpatient treatment programs for drug abuse are strikingly similar to those designed to treat alcohol abuse but differ from programs for alcohol abuse in several minor ways. The detoxification phase of inpatient hospitalization is typically shorter and less severe for most types of drug use than it is for alcohol, for which withdrawal can be life threatening. Alcohol is a depressant drug, as are barbiturates, tranquilizers, and opiates. Therefore, all these drugs have similar symptoms during withdrawal, including agitation, tremor, gastric distress, and possibly perceptual distortions (Julien, 2008). Stimulants such as amphetamines and cocaine produce different withdrawal symptoms—namely, lethargy and depression. These differences necessitate different medical care during detoxification.

After detoxification, additional care is important for success. Frequently, this continued care comes from joining a support group such as Narcotics Anonymous. Getting substance abusers to attend such groups is a challenge, and the low rate of success for such interventions is a problem. Other interventions show better results. A meta-analysis of psychosocial interventions (Dutra et al., 2008) identified several types as effective, including contingency management and cognitive behavioral therapy. Such interventions were most effective for marijuana use and least effective with those who abused several substances. Unfortunately, relapse prevention interventions were not among the more effective programs.

One similarity between drug and alcohol abuse treatment is the high rate of relapse. As noted earlier, alcohol, smoking, and opiate treatment all share a high rate of relapse (Hunt et al., 1971), and the first six months after treatment are critical. To ameliorate this problem, drug treatment programs, like alcohol treatment interventions, typically include some aftercare or "booster" sessions, which may consist only of attendance in a support group such as Narcotics Anonymous. A one-size-fits-all approach may not be successful for relapse prevention because people relapse for different reasons (Zywiak et al., 2006). Some people are provoked to relapse by negative feelings, others cannot withstand cravings, whereas others succumb to social pressure from their drug-using friends. Addressing individual concerns and weaknesses through interventions that are specific to individuals may improve the situation.

Drew Barrymore provides an excellent example of the problem of relapse. She had trouble staying in treatment. She escaped from her inpatient treatment center but was soon apprehended by authorities and brought back to treatment. After completing the program, she relapsed several times and received additional treatment before controlling her drug taking.

Preventing and Controlling Drug Use

Chapter 12 presented information on attempts to decrease smoking in children and adolescents by various interventions aimed at discouraging their experimentation with cigarettes and smokeless tobacco. Similar efforts have been applied to the use of other drugs (Pentz, Mares, Schinke, & Rohrbach, 2004; Roe & Becker, 2005). The prevention attempts aimed at keeping children and adolescents from experimenting with drugs are intended to delay or inhibit the initiation of drug use. As with efforts to prevent smoking (see Chapter 12), those aimed at preventing drug use do not have an impressive success rate. Programs that rely on scare tactics, moral training, factual information about drug risks, and boosting self-esteem are generally ineffective. For example, the popular Drug Abuse Resistance Education (DARE) program has minimal effects (West & O'Neal, 2004).

However, some types of prevention programs are more effective than others. The Life Skills Training program (Botvin & Griffin, 2004) has demonstrated both short-term and longer-term effectiveness. This program teaches social skills, both to resist social pressure in favor of using drugs and to enhance social and personal competence. In addition, some evidence (Springer et al., 2004) indicates that prevention programs that are tailored to be culturally compatible with the targeted groups are more effective than more general programs. A systematic review of programs (Roe & Becker, 2005) indicated that school programs that focus on life skills are more effective than programs with other components, and community programs need to have multiple components and be intensive to be effective (such as the Children at Risk program). Aiming prevention efforts at children between 11 and 13 is most effective, but programs aimed at children and adolescents are not the only approach to controlling drug use.

A more common control technique is to limit availability. This strategy is common in all Western countries through laws that limit legal access to drugs. However, legal restriction of drugs has a number of side effects, some of which create other social problems (Robins, 1995). For example, when the United States legally prohibited the manufacture and sale of alcohol, illegal manufacture and distribution flourished, creating a large criminal enterprise, huge profits, loss of tax revenue, and corruption among law enforcement agencies. Thus, limiting availability has negative as well as positive consequences, and the extent to which this approach should be enacted remains controversial.

Another strategy is control of the harm of drug use. This strategy assumes that people will use psychoactive drugs, sometimes unwisely, but that reducing the health consequences of drug use should be the first priority (Peele, 2002; Heather, 2006; O'Hare, 2007). Rather than taking a moralistic stand on drug use, this strategy takes a practical approach to minimizing the dangers of drug use. An example of the *harm reduction strategy* is helping injection drug users exchange used needles for sterile ones, thus slowing the spread of HIV infection, or encouraging the designated driver approach to avoiding vehicle injuries. The controversy surrounding such programs is representative of the debate over the harm reduction strategy, but a systematic review of harm reduction (Ritter & Cameron, 2006) concluded that the evidence indicates that this approach should be adopted as a policy for illicit drugs.

IN SUMMARY

Abuse of alcohol is a serious health problem in most developed nations, but other drugs—including depressants, stimulants, cocaine, marijuana, Ecstasy, and anabolic steroids—are also potentially harmful to health. At one time or another, many of these drugs have been available over the counter or through a physician's prescription. Although abuse of these drugs often leads to a number of personal and social problems, their health risks are much less than those associated with cigarettes or alcohol. Treatments for drug abuse are similar to those for alcohol abuse, and programs aimed at prevention are similar to those aimed at preventing smoking. A new strategy called *harm reduction* aims at decreasing the social and health risks of taking drugs by changing drug policies.

ANSWERS

This chapter has addressed six basic questions:

1. What are the major trends in alcohol consumption?

People have consumed alcohol worldwide since before recorded history. Alcohol consumption in the United States reached a peak during the first three decades of the 19th century, dropped sharply during the mid-1800s as a result of the "temperance" movement, and continued at a steady rate until it declined even more during Prohibition. Currently, rates of alcohol consumption in the United States are holding steady after a period of slow decline. About two-thirds of adults drink; half are classified as current, regular drinkers, including 20% as binge drinkers and 5% as heavy drinkers. Adult European Americans have higher rates of drinking than members of other ethnic groups, but the patterns of alcohol consumption vary in countries around the world.

2. What are the health effects of drinking alcohol?

Drinking has both positive and negative health effects. Prolonged heavy drinking of alcohol often leads to cirrhosis of the liver and other serious health problems, such as heart disease and brain dysfunction. Moderate drinking may have certain long-range health benefits, including reduced heart disease and lowered probability of developing gallstones, Type 2 diabetes, and Alzheimer's disease.

3. Why do people drink?

Models for drinking behavior should be able to explain why people begin drinking, why some can drink in moderation, and why others drink to excess. The disease model assumes that people drink excessively because they have the disease of alcoholism. Cognitive-physiological models, including the tension reduction hypothesis and alcohol myopia, propose that people drink because alcohol allows them to escape tension and negative self-evaluations. Social learning theory assumes that people acquire drinking behavior through positive or negative reinforcement, modeling, and cognitive mediation.

4. How can people change problem drinking?

Many problem drinkers seem to be able to quit without therapy, and treatment programs are moderately effective in helping people who do not succeed in quitting on their own. About 25% of treated alcoholics are abstinent at the end of one year, but many others have decreased their drinking to a level that is no longer a problem. In the United States, most treatment programs are oriented toward abstinence, and those drinkers who do not quit are often considered treatment failures. Alcoholics Anonymous is the most popular treatment program, but despite its prominence, research has not confirmed its effectiveness. Brief interventions oriented toward enhancing motivation, such as motivational interviewing, show the highest effectiveness. Chemical treatments such as disulfiram to curb drinking have been of limited usefulness, but naltrexone and acamprosate are more effective. Controlled drinking remains controversial as a treatment goal, although some problem drinkers are capable of attaining this type of drinking.

5. What problems are associated with relapse?

Relapse is common among heavy drinkers who have quit, although many are able to maintain abstinence or to drink in a controlled manner. Most relapses occur during the first three months. After a year, about 65% of all successful quitters have resumed drinking, some in a harmful manner. The knowledge of frequent relapse has led to the creation of follow-up relapse prevention treatment.

6. What are the health effects of other drugs?

Other drugs—including depressants, stimulants, Ecstasy, cocaine, marijuana, and anabolic steroids—have had some medical use, but they are also potentially harmful to health. The principal problems from most of these drugs are social, but the use of any drug brings physical risks such as stroke and heart attacks. Treatments for drug abuse are similar to those for alcohol abuse, and programs aimed at prevention are similar to those aimed at preventing smoking.

SUGGESTED READINGS

Heather, N. (2006). Controlled drinking, harm reduction and their roles in the response to alcohol-related problems. *Addiction Research and Theory, 14*, 7–18. Heather discusses the controlled drinking controversy, presenting the difference between the harm reduction approach that is common in Europe and the strategy of decreasing drug/alcohol use to a controlled level.

Klatsky, A. L. (2003, February). Drink to your health? *Scientific American, 288*, 75–82. Klatsky reviews the evidence about the health benefits of drinking and offers cautious advice about drinking that will help achieve these benefits.

Nestler, E. J., & Malenka, R. C. (2004, March). The addicted brain. *Scientific American, 290*, 78–85. This article details the brain mechanisms that underlie reward and addiction, pointing out the commonalities among all compulsive drug use.

Witkiewitz, K., & Marlatt, G. A. (2004). Relapse prevention for alcohol and drug problems. *American Psychologist, 59*, 224–235. Witkiewitz and Marlatt present a revised model for understanding the complexities of the relapse process and suggest more effective ways to combat this too common problem.

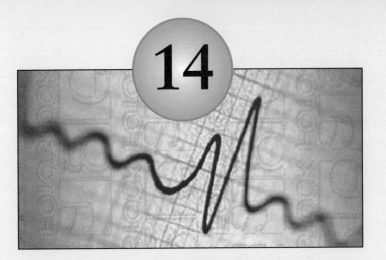

14

EATING AND WEIGHT

QUESTIONS

This chapter focuses on six basic questions:

1. How does the digestive system function?

2. What factors are involved in weight maintenance?

3. What is obesity, and how does it affect health?

4. Is dieting a good way to lose weight?

5. What is anorexia nervosa, and how can it be treated?

6. What is bulimia, and how does it differ from binge eating?

CHECK YOUR HEALTH RISKS

Check the items that apply to you.

☐ 1. I feel comfortable with my present weight.

☐ 2. Although I don't eat much, I stay heavier than I would like.

☐ 3. I have lost 15 pounds or more over the past two years.

☐ 4. I have gained 15 pounds or more over the past two years.

☐ 5. I am more than 30 pounds overweight.

☐ 6. My weight has fluctuated about 5 or 10 pounds during the past two years, but I'm not concerned about it.

☐ 7. If I were thinner, I would be happier.

☐ 8. My waist is as big as or bigger than my hips.

☐ 9. I have been on at least 10 different diet programs in my life.

☐ 10. I have fasted, used laxatives, or used diet drugs to lose weight.

☐ 11. My family has been concerned that I am too thin, but I disagree.

☐ 12. A coach, instructor, or trainer has suggested that weighing less could improve my athletic performance.

☐ 13. I sometimes lose control over eating and eat far more than I planned.

☐ 14. I would like to have liposuction or gastric bypass surgery to lose weight.

☐ 15. I have vomited after eating as a way to control my weight.

☐ 16. Food is a danger that can be managed by careful thought and mental preparation in order not to eat too much.

Items 1 and 6 reflect a healthy attitude toward weight, but each of the other items represents a health risk from improper eating or unhealthy attitudes concerning eating. Unhealthy eating not only relates to the development of several diseases, but preoccupation with weight and frequent dieting can also be unhealthy.

REAL-WORLD PROFILE OF MARY-KATE OLSEN

The gossip columns carried stories and photos about how emaciated Mary-Kate Olsen looked during the early months of 2004, when she and her twin sister Ashley received their star on the Hollywood Walk of Fame and again when they celebrated their 18th birthday (Soriano, 2004). Mary-Kate was much thinner than Ashley, and rumors of drug use and anorexia started. The Olsen family denied those rumors, but Mary-Kate checked into a treatment facility in June 2004, and her publicist admitted that she was receiving treatment for a health-related problem.

According to the rumors, Mary-Kate was suffering from **anorexia nervosa**, an eating disorder that includes intentional starvation and a distorted body image. Her emaciated appearance was consistent with this diagnosis, and her father later stated that Mary-Kate had been battling anorexia for two years. She had received treatment on an outpatient basis, but that treatment was unsuccessful, and the family came to a decision that Mary-Kate would enter the Cirque Lodge,

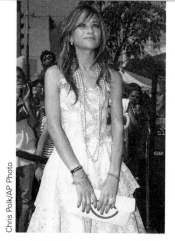

Chris Polk/AP Photo

Mary-Kate Olsen received treatment for the eating disorder anorexia nervosa.

an exclusive treatment facility in Utah ("Inside Mary-Kate's Two Year Ordeal," 2004). At Cirque Lodge, her treatment team consisted of counselors, a psychologist, and a nutritionist. She had the full support of her family, especially her twin sister, Ashley.

After six weeks at the Cirque Lodge, Mary-Kate left the treatment facility. She had gained 5 pounds but planned to continue working with her treatment team so that she could attain a healthy weight. She and Ashley moved to New York and entered NYU as they had planned. However, rumors soon began about a relapse ("Mary-Kate Olsen

Reportedly Suffers Anorexia Relapse," 2004). Mary-Kate appeared to have lost some of the weight she had gained, and concerns arose over how well she was managing her eating disorder. Those concerns arose again in 2007, when she appeared to be thinner than in the past months ("Is Mary-Kate Olsen Anorexic," 2007), but in mid-2008, she appeared healthier. Mary-Kate finally made a statement concerning her eating disorder, saying that anorexia had nearly killed her (Barbarich, 2008).

Like millions of people, Mary-Kate Olsen suffers from an **eating disorder**, a serious and habitual disturbance in eating behavior that produces unhealthy consequences. This definition of eating disorders excludes starvation resulting from the inability to find suitable food supplies and also unhealthy eating resulting from inadequate information about nutrition. Also excluded are disturbances in eating behavior such as pica, or the eating of nonnutritive substances such as plastic and wood, and the rumination disorder of infancy—that is, regurgitation of food without nausea or gastrointestinal illness. Neither of these disorders presents serious health problems to adults, and they are of relatively minor importance in health psychology.

This chapter examines in detail the four major problems of eating—overeating and dieting, anorexia nervosa (the disorder Mary-Kate Olsen has), bulimia, and binge eating—each related to difficulties in weight maintenance. To put these in context, we first consider the organs and functions of the digestive system.

THE DIGESTIVE SYSTEM

The human body can digest a wide variety of plant and animal tissues, converting these foods into usable proteins, fats, carbohydrates, vitamins, and minerals. The digestive system takes in food, processes it into particles that can be absorbed, and excretes the undigested wastes. The particles that are absorbed through the digestive system are transported through the bloodstream so as to be available to all body cells. These molecules nourish the body by providing the energy for activity as well as the materials for body growth, maintenance, and repair.

The digestive tract is a modified tube, consisting of a number of specialized structures. Also included in the digestive system are several accessory structures connected to the digestive tract by ducts. These ducted glands produce substances that are essential for digestion, and the ducts provide a way for these substances to enter the digestive system. Figure 14.1 shows the digestive system.

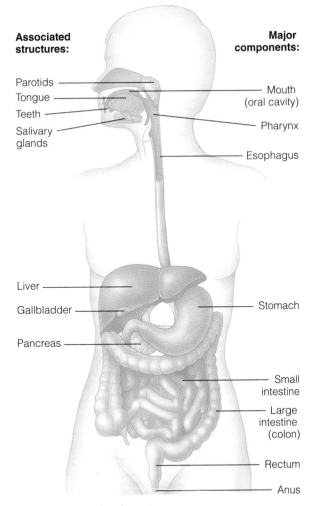

Associated structures:
Parotids
Tongue
Teeth
Salivary glands
Liver
Gallbladder
Pancreas

Major components:
Mouth (oral cavity)
Pharynx
Esophagus
Stomach
Small intestine
Large intestine (colon)
Rectum
Anus

FIGURE 14.1 The digestive system.

Source: Introduction to Microbiology (p. 556), by J. L. Ingraham & C. A. Ingraham, 1995, Belmont, CA: Wadsworth. Copyright 1995 by Wadsworth Publishing Company. Reprinted by permission.

In humans and other mammals, some digestion begins in the mouth. The teeth tear and grind food, mixing it with saliva. Several **salivary glands** furnish the moisture that allows the food to be tasted. Without such moisture, the taste buds on the tongue do not function. Saliva also contains an enzyme that digests starch, so some digestion actively begins before food particles leave the mouth.

Swallowing is a voluntary action, but once food is swallowed, its progress through the **pharynx** and **esophagus** is largely involuntary. **Peristalsis** propels food through the digestive system, beginning with the esophagus. Peristaltic movement is the rhythmic contraction and relaxation of the circular muscles of structures in the digestive system. In the stomach, rhythmic contractions mix the food with **gastric juices** secreted by the stomach and the glands that empty into the stomach. The major digestive activity of the stomach is protein digestion, initiated by the action of the enzyme **pepsin**. Little absorption of nutrients occurs in the stomach; only alcohol, aspirin, and some fat-soluble drugs are absorbed through the stomach lining. The major function of the stomach is to mix food particles with gastric juices, preparing the mixture for absorption in the small intestine.

The mixture of food particles and gastric juices moves into the small intestine a little at a time. The high acidity of the gastric juices results in a very acidic mixture, and the small intestine cannot function in high acidity. To reduce the level of acidity, the pancreas secretes several acid-reducing enzymes into the small intestine. These **pancreatic juices** are also essential for digesting carbohydrates and fats.

The digestion of starch that begins in the mouth is completed in the small intestine. The upper third of the small intestine absorbs starch and other carbohydrates. Protein digestion, initiated in the stomach, is also completed when proteins are absorbed in the upper portion of the small intestine. Fats, however, enter the small intestine almost entirely undigested. **Bile salts** produced in the **liver** and stored in the **gall bladder** break down fat molecules into a form that is acted on by a pancreatic enzyme. Absorption of fats occurs in the middle third of the small intestine. The bile salts that aid the process are reabsorbed later in the lower third of the small intestine.

Large quantities of water pass through the small intestine. In addition to the water that people drink, digestive juices increase the fluid volume. Of all the water that passes into the small intestine, 90% is absorbed. This absorption process also causes vitamins and electrolytes to pass into the body at this point in digestion.

From the small intestine, digestion proceeds to the large intestine. As with other portions of the digestive system, movement through the large intestine occurs through peristalsis. However, the peristaltic movement in the large intestine is more sluggish and irregular than in the small intestine. Bacteria inhabit the large intestine and manufacture several vitamins. Although the large intestine has absorptive capabilities, it typically absorbs only water, a few minerals, and the vitamins manufactured by its bacteria.

Feces consist of the materials left after digestion has taken place. Feces are composed of undigested fiber, inorganic material, undigested nutrients, water, and bacteria. Peristalsis carries the feces through the large intestine, through the **rectum**, and finally through the **anus**, where they are eliminated.

In summary, the digestive system turns food into nutrients by a process that begins in the mouth with the breakdown of food into smaller particles. Digestive juices continue to act on food particles in the stomach, but digestion of most types of nutrients occurs in the small intestine. Digestion is completed with the elimination of the undigested residue. The digestive system is plagued by more diseases and disorders than any other body system. Many digestive disorders are not of active concern to health psychology, but several, such as obesity, anorexia nervosa, bulimia, and binge eating, have important behavioral components. In addition, maintaining a stable weight depends on behaviors—eating and activity.

FACTORS IN WEIGHT MAINTENANCE

Stable weight occurs when the calories absorbed from food equal those expended for body metabolism plus physical activity. This balance is not a simple calculation but rather the result of a complex set of actions and interactions. Caloric content varies with foods, with fat having more calories per volume than carbohydrates or proteins. The degree of absorption depends on how rapidly food passes through the digestive system and even the nutrient composition of the foods. Furthermore, metabolic rates can differ from person to person and from time to time. Activity level is another source of variability, with greater activity requiring greater caloric expenditures.

To obtain calories, people (and other animals) eat. Eating and weight balance have regulating components in the nervous system, forming both a short-term and a long-term regulation system. A variety of hormones and neurotransmitters are important for regulating eating and weight, and they function in an interrelated and complex manner (Erlanson-Albertsson, 2005). **Leptin**, a protein hormone discovered in 1994 (Horvath, 2005), is produced by adipose tissue (fat) and acts on receptors in the central nervous system as part of a signaling system involved in the long-term regulation of weight. Low leptin levels signal low fat stores, prompting eating. High levels signal adequate fat stores and satiation. *Insulin* is a second hormone involved in weight maintenance. Produced by the pancreas, this hormone allows body cells to take in glucose for their use. (Deficiency in insulin production or use results in diabetes, which is covered in Chapter 11.) High insulin production leads to the intake of more glucose than cells can use, and the excess is converted into fat in the body. In the brain,

insulin acts on the **hypothalamus**, sending signals of satiation and decreasing appetite (Erlanson-Altertsson, 2005; Horvath, 2005).

The hormone **ghrelin**, a peptide hormone discovered in 1999, also seems to be involved in eating (Cummings & Schwartz, 2003; Erlanson-Albertsson, 2005). This hormone is produced primarily in the stomach, and its level rises before and falls after meals; thus, ghrelin seems to be involved in the short-term regulation of food intake by prompting eating. Ghrelin acts in the hypothalamus to activate *neuropeptide Y*, which secretes *Agouti-related peptide*. This peptide stimulates appetite and decreases metabolism, thus affecting the weight balance equation in two ways. Ghrelin also interacts with the *orexins*, two other peptide hormones that are related to appetite and eating. Melanin-concentrating hormone is yet another brain peptide that is related to increased food intake.

A variety of hormones are related to feelings of satiation and thus tend to decrease or terminate eating. The hormone **cholecystokinin (CCK)**, a peptide hormone produced by the intestines, acts on the brain to produce feelings of satiation. CCK, *glucagon-like peptide 1*, and *peptide Y* are all produced in the intestines but act on the hypothalamus to signal satiation. Thus, the picture of hormone and neurotransmitter action in relation to hunger and eating is very complex, with one system to initiate eating and one to produce satiation and thus decrease eating. Table 14.1 lists each set of hormones and shows where they are produced. Notice that many are produced in the

TABLE 14.1

Hormones Involved in Appetite and Satiation

Hormones That Increase Appetite		Hormones That Increase Satiation	
Hormone	Produced in	Hormone	Produced in
Ghrelin	Stomach	Leptin	Adipose tissue
Neuropeptide Y	Hypothalamus	Insulin	Pancreas
Orexins	Hypothalamus	Cholecystokinin (CCK)	Intestines
Agouti-related peptide	Hypothalamus	Glucagon-like peptide 1	Intestines
Melanin-concentrating hormone (MCH)	Hypothalamus	Peptide YY	Intestines

hypothalamus, and all may act on different nuclei in the hypothalamus to form a complex mechanism for the short-term and long-term regulation of weight (Erlanson-Albertsson, 2005; Zigman & Elmquist, 2003).

To understand the complexities of weight metabolism and weight maintenance, consider an extreme example: an experiment in which participants were systematically starved.

Experimental Starvation

More than 60 years ago, Ancel Keys and his colleagues (Keys, Brozek, Henschel, Mickelsen, & Taylor, 1950) began a study on the physical effects of human starvation. The research took place during World War II; the participants were conscientious objectors who volunteered to be part of the study as an alternative to military service. In most ways these volunteers were quite

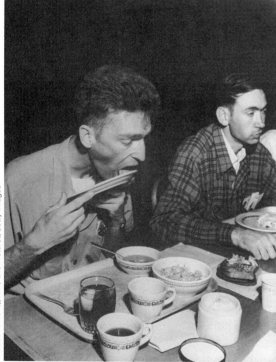

Experimental starvation produced an obsession with food and a variety of negative changes in the behavior of these volunteers.

normal young men; their weights were normal, their IQs were in the normal to bright range, and they were emotionally stable.

For the first three months of the project, the 36 volunteers ate regularly and established their normal caloric requirements. Next, the men were put on half their previous rations, with the goal of reducing their body weight to 75% of previous levels. Although the researchers cut the participants' caloric intake in half, they were careful to give them adequate nutrients so that the men were never in any danger of actually starving.

At first these men lost weight rapidly. They were constantly hungry, but the initial pace of weight loss did not last. To continue losing weight, the men had to consume even fewer calories, which led to considerable suffering. Nevertheless, most stayed with the project through the entire six months, and most met their goal of losing 25% of their body weight.

The behaviors that accompanied the semistarvation were quite surprising to Keys and his colleagues. At the beginning, the men were optimistic and cheerful, but these feelings soon vanished. The men became irritable, aggressive, and began to fight among themselves, behavior that was completely out of character. Although the men continued this bellicose behavior throughout the six months of the starvation phase, they also became apathetic and avoided physical activity as much as they could. They became neglectful of their dormitory, their own physical appearance, and their girlfriends.

The men were, of course, hungry, and they became increasingly obsessed with thoughts of food. Mealtimes became the center of their lives; they tended to eat very slowly and to be very sensitive to the taste of their food. At the beginning of the period of caloric reduction, the researchers saw no need to place physical restrictions on the men to prevent them from cheating on their diets. But about three months into the starvation, the men felt that they would be tempted to cheat if they left the dormitory alone. As a result, they were allowed to go out only in pairs or in larger groups. These dedicated, polite, normal, stable young men had become abnormal and unpleasant under conditions of semistarvation.

Obsession with food and continued negative outlook also characterized the refeeding phase of the project. During refeeding, the plan was for the men to regain the weight they had lost. This phase was to have lasted three months, with food introduced at gradually increasing levels, but the men objected so strongly that the pace of refeeding was accelerated. As a result, the men ate as much and as often as they could, some as many as five large meals a day. By the end of the refeeding period, most men had regained their preexperimental weight; in fact, many were slightly heavier. About half were still preoccupied with food, and for many, their prestarvation optimism and cheerfulness had not completely returned.

Experimental Overeating

A study of experimental starvation does not seem very attractive, but an experiment on overeating might sound appealing to many people. Ethan Allen Sims and his associates (Sims, 1974, 1976; Sims et al., 1973; Sims & Horton, 1968) found a group of people who should have been especially interested and appreciative—prisoners. Inmates at the Vermont State Prison volunteered to gain 20 to 30 pounds as part of an experiment on overeating. Sims's interest was analogous to Keys's—an understanding of the physical and psychological components of overeating. Special living arrangements were made for these prisoners, including plentiful and delicious food. In addition, the experiment included a restriction of physical activity to make weight gain easier.

Did these men gain weight? With an increase in calories and a decrease in physical activity, weight gain was nearly assured. At first they gained fairly easily. But soon the rate of weight gain slowed, and the participants had to eat more and more to continue gaining. As with the men in the starvation study, these men needed about 3,500 calories to maintain their weight at normal levels, but many had to double that amount to continue gaining. Not all the men were able to attain their weight goals, regardless of how much they ate. One man did not reach his goal even though he ate more than 10,000 calories per day.

Were the overeating prisoners as miserable as the starving conscientious objectors? No, but they did find overeating unpleasant. Food became repulsive to them, despite the excellent quality and preparation. They had to force themselves to eat, and many considered dropping out of the study.

When the weight gain phase of the study was over, the prisoners cut down their food intake dramatically and lost weight. Not all lost as quickly as others, and two had some trouble returning to their original weight. An examination of these two men's medical backgrounds revealed some family history of obesity, although the men themselves had never been overweight. These results indicate that normal weight people have trouble increasing their weight substantially and that, even if they do, the increased weight is difficult to maintain.

IN SUMMARY

Weight maintenance depends largely on two factors: the number of calories absorbed through food intake and the number expended through body metabolism and physical activity. Underlying this balance is a complex set of hormones and neurotransmitters that have selective effects on various brain sites, including the hypothalamus. Weight gain occurs when more nutrients are present than are required for maintenance of body metabolism and physical activity. Weight loss occurs when insufficient nutrients are present to furnish the necessary energy for body metabolism and activity. An experiment in starvation showed that loss of too much weight leads to irritability, aggression, apathy, lack of interest in sex, and preoccupation with food. Another experiment in overeating showed that some people find gaining weight almost as difficult as losing it.

OVEREATING AND OBESITY

Overeating is not the sole cause of obesity, but it is an important part of the weight maintenance equation. As the studies on experimental starvation and overeating show, metabolic level changes with food intake as well as with energy output to alter the efficiency of nutrient use by the body. Thus, individual variations in body metabolism allow some people to burn calories faster than others. Two people who eat the same amount may have different weights, but obese people usually eat more than normal weight people (Jeffery & Harnack, 2007; Wing & Polley, 2001).

Although many overweight people say that they eat less than others, these self-reports are not very accurate, and objective measurements usually indicate that obese people eat more. They are especially likely to eat food rich in fat, which has a higher caloric density than carbohydrates or protein. They may eat less food but more calories. Overweight individuals also have a tendency to be less physically active than leaner people, which contributes to overweight. These behaviors contribute to obesity and its related health consequences, but the underlying reasons for obesity and even its definition remain controversial.

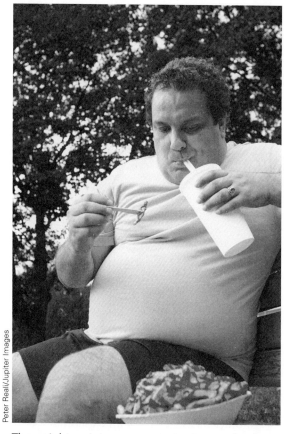

Peter Reali/Jupiter Images

The weight maintenance equation is complex, but overeating is a cause of obesity.

What Is Obesity?

Answers to the question of what obesity is vary by personal and social standards. Should obesity be defined in terms of health? Appearance? Body mass? Percentage of body fat? Weight charts? Total weight? No good definition of obesity would consider only body weight, because some individuals have a small skeletal frame, whereas others are larger, and some people's weight is in muscle, whereas others carry weight in fat. Muscle tissue and bone weigh more than fat, so some people can be heavier yet leaner, as athletes often are.

Traditionally, charts that provide normal weight ranges for various heights and body frame sizes were the standard for determining normal weight and overweight. The charts, published by the Metropolitan Life Insurance Company, are based on statistics from the Society of Actuaries and thus reflect weight ranges with the lowest mortality. Table 14.2 shows both the 1959 and 1983 charts; a comparison shows that being overweight was redefined in an upward direction.

Despite the convenience of weight charts, an accurate measure of percentage of body fat is a better index of obesity than total weight. Determining percentage and distribution of body fat is not as easy as consulting a chart, and several different methods exist to assess body fat (Skybo & Ryan-Wenger, 2003). Many new technologies for imaging the body—computer tomography, ultrasound, magnetic resonance imaging, and PET scanning—can be applied to assessing fat content, but these methods have the drawbacks of being very expensive and relatively inaccessible. Simpler methods include the skinfold technique, which involves measuring the thickness of a pinch of skin, and bioelectrical impedance measurement, which involves sending a harmless level of electrical current through the body to measure levels of fat in various parts of the body. The bioelectric impedance measurement is more accurate than the skinfold technique.

Another method is the **body mass index (BMI)**, defined as body weight in kilograms (kg) divided by height in meters squared (m^2)—that is, BMI = kg/m^2. Although BMI does not consider a person's age, gender, or body build, this measurement began to gain popularity in the early 1990s.

TABLE 14.2

Metropolitan Life Insurance Company's Desirable Weights, 1959 and 1983

Height	Small Frame		Medium Frame		Large Frame	
	1959	1983	1959	1983	1959	1983
Women						
4 ft. 10 in.	92–98 lb.	102–111 lb.	96–107 lb.	109–121 lb.	104–119 lb.	118–131 lb.
4 11	94–101	103–113	98–110	111–123	106–122	120–134
5 0	96–104	104–115	101–113	113–126	109–125	122–137
5 1	99–107	106–118	104–116	115–129	112–128	125–140
5 2	102–110	108–121	107–119	118–132	115–131	128–143
5 3	105–113	111–124	110–122	121–135	118–134	131–147
5 4	108–116	114–127	113–126	124–138	121–138	134–151
5 5	111–119	117–130	116–130	127–141	125–142	137–155
5 6	114–123	120–133	120–135	130–144	129–146	140–159
5 7	118–127	123–136	124–139	133–147	133–150	143–163
5 8	122–131	126–139	128–143	136–150	137–154	146–167
5 9	126–135	129–142	132–147	139–153	141–158	149–170
5 10	130–140	132–145	136–151	142–156	145–163	152–173
5 11	134–144	135–148	140–155	145–159	149–168	155–176
6 0	138–148	138–151	144–159	148–162	153–173	158–179
Men						
5 ft. 2 in.	112–120 lb.	128–134 lb.	118–129 lb.	131–141 lb.	126–141 lb.	138–150 lb.
5 3	115–123	130–136	121–133	133–143	129–144	140–153
5 4	118–126	132–138	124–136	135–145	132–148	142–156
5 5	121–129	134–140	127–139	137–148	125–152	144–160
5 6	124–133	136–142	130–143	139–151	138–156	146–164
5 7	128–137	138–145	134–147	142–154	142–161	149–168
5 8	132–141	140–148	138–152	145–157	147–166	152–172
5 9	136–145	142–151	142–156	148–160	151–170	155–176
5 10	140–150	144–154	146–160	151–163	155–174	158–180
5 11	144–154	146–157	150–165	154–166	159–179	161–184
6 0	148–158	149–160	154–170	157–170	164–184	164–188
6 1	152–162	152–164	158–175	160–174	168–189	168–192
6 2	156–167	155–168	162–180	164–178	173–194	172–197
6 3	160–171	158–172	167–185	167–182	178–199	176–202
6 4	164–175	162–176	172–190	171–187	182–204	181–207

Source: "New Weight Standards for Men and Women," by Metropolitan Life Insurance Company, 1959, *Statistical Bulletin, 40*, p. 1. Copyright © 1959, 1983 by The Metropolitan Life Insurance Company. Adapted by permission.

The National Task Force on the Prevention and Treatment of Obesity (2000) acknowledged that neither the weight charts nor BMI measures body fat but contended that this index can provide a standard for measuring overweight and obesity. This group defined overweight as a BMI of 25 through 29.9 and obesity as a BMI of 30 or more. (A 5'10" man with a BMI of 30 would weigh 207 pounds, and a 5'4" woman with a BMI of 30 would weigh 174.) These numbers are approximately 20% above the weights in the 1983 Metropolitan Life Insurance Company's height–weight charts for people with a medium frame. Table 14.3 shows a sample of BMI levels and their corresponding heights and weights.

Another measure that can be useful in assessing overweight is fat distribution, measured as the ratio of waist to hip size. People who have waists

TABLE 14.3

Body Mass Index Scores and Their Corresponding Heights and Weights

Height in Inches	Body Mass Index (kg/m^2)							
	17.5*	21	23	25	27	30	35	40**
	Weight in Pounds							
60	90	107	118	128	138	153	179	204
61	93	111	122	132	143	158	185	211
62	96	115	126	136	147	164	191	218
63	99	118	130	141	152	169	197	225
64	102	122	134	145	157	174	202	232
65	105	126	138	150	162	180	210	240
66	109	130	142	155	167	186	216	247
67	112	134	146	159	172	191	223	255
68	115	138	151	164	177	197	230	262
69	118	142	155	169	182	203	236	270
70	122	146	160	174	188	207	243	278
71	125	150	165	179	193	215	250	286
72	129	154	169	184	199	221	258	294
73	132	159	174	189	204	227	265	302
74	136	163	179	194	210	233	272	311
75	140	168	184	200	216	240	279	319
76	144	172	189	205	221	246	287	328

*BMI of 17.5 after intentional starvation meets one *DSM-IV* definition of anorexia nervosa.

**BMI of 40 is considered morbid obesity by Bender, Trautner, Spraul, & Berger, 1998.

that approach the size of their hips tend to have fat distributed around their middles, whereas people who have large hips compared to their waists have lower hip-to-waist ratios.

Regardless of the definitions that researchers have used to study obesity, overweight is often defined in terms of social standards and fashion. These definitions usually have little to do with health and are subject to variations by culture and time. Examples are numerous during human history. During times when food supply was uncertain (the most frequent situation throughout history), carrying some supply of fat on the body was a type of insurance and thus often considered attractive (Nelson & Morrison, 2005). Fat could also be considered a mark of prosperity; fat advertised to the world that a person could afford an ample supply of food. Only in very recent history has this standard changed. Before 1920, thinness was considered unattractive, possibly due to its association with diseases or poverty.

Thinness is no longer considered unattractive. In fact, today it is as highly desirable as plumpness was in previous centuries, especially for women. Early studies that examined changes in the body weight of *Playboy* centerfolds and Miss America candidates from 1959 to 1978 (Garner, Garfinkel, Schwartz, & Thompson, 1980), from 1979 to 1988 (Wiseman, Gray, Mosimann, & Ahrens, 1992), and another from 1922 to 1999 (Rubenstein & Caballero, 2000) found that weights for both groups had decreased relative to average weight of the general population. More recent analysis of centerfolds (Seifert, 2005; Sypeck et al., 2006) has confirmed a trend toward thinness over the past 50 years. These ideal bodies are so thin that 99% of centerfolds and 100% of Miss America winners were in the underweight range (Spitzer, Henderson, & Zivian, 1999). This thin ideal for women's bodies has become so widely accepted that even normal weight women often consider themselves too heavy. Surveys of women in the United States (Maynard, Serdula, Galuska, Gillespie, & Mokdad, 2006) and Great Britain (Wardle & Johnson, 2002) revealed that many normal weight women wished to weigh less. Clearly, obesity, like beauty, is in the eye of the beholder, and the ideal body has become thinner over the past 50 years.

Despite the emphasis on thinness, obesity in the United States has become epidemic. From the early 1980s to the late 1990s, adult obesity increased by 50% (NCHS, 2007). Extreme obesity more than doubled during the 1990s. That increase has leveled, but no decline has occurred (Hedley et al., 2004). Researchers have proposed several reasons for the dramatic increase in obesity over the past two decades, including an increase in consumption of fast food and sweetened sodas, growing portion sizes, and a decrease in physical activity. Not only people in the United States (Pereira et al., 2005) but also those in many other countries, including developing nations (Finkelstein, Ruhm, & Kosa, 2005), have begun eating more fast food and viewing more television and videos. Both behaviors are related to a larger body mass index and to weight gain. The consumption of sugar-sweetened sodas is another growing trend that may relate to growing fatter (Bray, 2004; Tam et al., 2006). Large portion size also contributes to

increasing obesity (Young & Nestle, 2002), and people in the United States began to eat more meals in restaurants during this time period (NCHS, 2007). Restaurant portion sizes have grown, and people have been supersized. This trend affects the United States more than European countries (Rozin et al., 2003), but obesity is a growing epidemic around the world (James, 2008).

If obesity is defined as having a BMI of 30 or higher, then 32% of U.S. adults are obese, and an additional 34% are overweight, defined as a BMI of 25.0 to 29.9 (NCHS, 2007). The rates of overweight and obesity are lower in children and adolescents, with 17% overweight, but 31% are at risk. Obese and overweight people are found in both genders, all ethnic groups, all geographic regions, and all educational levels. As Figure 14.2 shows, however, the rates of obesity and overweight vary by gender and ethnic background. The United States shows high rates of overweight and obesity, but other parts of the world have also experienced an increase in obesity, including Canada (Bélanger-Ducharme & Tremblay, 2005), Great Britain (Wardle & Johnson, 2002), Australia (Thorburn, 2005), Latin America (Fraser, 2005), Iran (Rashidi, Mohammadpour-Ahranjani, Vafa, & Karandish, 2005), and many countries in Europe (Berghöfer et al., 2008).

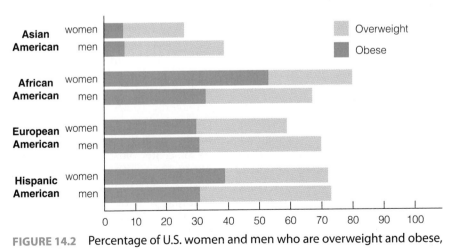

FIGURE 14.2 Percentage of U.S. women and men who are overweight and obese, by ethnic group.

Source: Data from *Statistical Abstract of the United States, 2008*, by U.S. Census Bureau, 2008, Washington, DC: U.S. Government Printing Office, Table 199, p. 132.

Why Are Some People Obese?

Understanding the biology of eating and energy regulation is challenging, but explaining why that regulation fails to work for some people is even more difficult. Several models attempt to explain why some people are obese and others maintain a normal weight. These models, which should be able to explain both the development and the maintenance of obesity, include the setpoint model, genetic explanations, and the positive incentive model.

The Setpoint Model The setpoint model holds that weight is regulated around a **setpoint**, a type of internal thermostat. When fat levels rise above or fall below a certain level, physiological and psychological mechanisms are activated that encourage a return to setpoint. The discovery of leptin is consistent with this view. This hormone is produced by body fat and acts as a signaling system to the hypothalamus in the brain. The findings from the study on experimental starvation and the studies on experimental overeating are also consistent with the concept of a setpoint, which predicts that deviations from normal weight in either direction are achieved only with difficulty. When fat levels fall below setpoint, the body takes action to preserve its fat stores. Part of that action includes slowing the metabolic process to require fewer calories, thus making the body more conservative in its energy expenditures. People on diets have difficulty in continuing to lose weight because their bodies fight against the depletion of fat stores. With conditions of prolonged and serious starvation, this slowed metabolism is expressed behaviorally as listlessness and apathy—both of which were exhibited by Keys's starving volunteers.

Increased hunger is the body's other corrective action when fat supplies fall below setpoint. Again, this mechanism seems to be consistent with the action of leptin and the results of the Keys et al. study on starvation. When fat stores fall, leptin levels decrease, which activates the hypothalamus in ways that result in hunger (Erlanson-Albertsson, 2005; Horvath, 2005). In Keys's study, the men who dieted to 75% of their normal body weight became miserable and hungry, and they stayed that way until they were back to their original weight. During the entire time they were below their normal weight (which would be below setpoint), they were obsessed with food. When they were allowed to eat, they preferred the high-calorie foods that tended to increase their fat stores most rapidly, a situation that is consistent with setpoint theory.

The experiment on overeating also fits with setpoint theory. The prisoners who tried to gain more than their normal weight were fighting their natural setpoint and the increased amount of leptin produced by their added fat cells. This signal should have translated into something like "Stop eating," which seems to have happened— the prisoners found eating unpleasant.

Questions remain concerning the setpoint model, including why the setpoint should vary so much from person to person and why some people have a setpoint that is set at obese. One answer may be that the setpoint is at least partly established through a hereditary component.

Genetic Explanations of Obesity One genetic explanation of obesity looks to prehistory to explain why people have a tendency to put on weight, hypothesizing that humans (and other animals) have evolved a "thrifty" metabolism that tends to store fat (Cummings & Schwartz, 2003). This tendency would be adaptive if food supplies were scarce, as they have been throughout most of history. With the plentiful supply of food available to most people in industrialized societies, this thrifty metabolism results in overweight and obesity. Indeed, some speculation holds that this availability makes obesity almost inevitable (Walker, Walker, & Adam, 2003). However, not all people are obese, and within any environment, some individuals are fatter than others. Some of that variation is attributable to the inheritance of specific genes rather than the general tendency to store fat.

Obesity tends to run in families, which suggests the possibility of a genetic basis. However, eating patterns are also shared in families, so researchers have examined twins and adopted children to disentangle genetic and environmental influences in weight. Evidence from studies of adopted children (Stunkard et al., 1986) and of identical twins reared together or apart (Stunkard, Harris, Pedersen, & McClean, 1990) has suggested a role for heredity

WOULD YOU BELIEVE . . . ?

You May Need a Nap Rather Than a Diet

Would you believe that sleep deprivation is related to obesity? It's not that being awake longer creates more opportunities for eating (which may be true) or that nighttime snacking may lead to obesity (which it may; Coles, Dixon, & O'Brien, 2007). Rather, sleep may be related to weight regulation, and missing sleep may produce problems in this system.

A suggestion of the importance of sleep for weight regulation came from the observation that sleep deprivation has become increasingly common for large numbers of people, and this trend has coincided with the growth in obesity. Researchers began to wonder: Is this relationship a coincidence or is there some underlying connection?

First, researchers attended to the basic question: Does inadequate sleep correlate with overweight? An examination of the sleep habits of a representative sample of the U.S. population (Gangwisch, Malaspina, Boden-Albala, & Heymsfield, 2005) led to the conclusion that individuals who get less than 7 hours of sleep per night are more likely to be overweight or obese than people who sleep more. This relationship also occurs in obese children (Latzer, Tzischinsky, & Roer, 2007). Thus, overweight and sleep deprivation are correlated in both adults and children.

Next, researchers attempted to connect lack of sleep with hormonal mechanisms that might underlie the relationship between sleep deprivation and obesity. Reviews of that research (Knutson & van Cauter, 2008; van Cauter et al., 2007) led to the conclusion that the type of partial sleep deprivation that is so common is also capable of altering the regulation of the hormones involved in appetite and eating in ways that may cause weight gain and insulin resistance. Specifically, sleep deprivation increases ghrelin, which stimulates eating, and decreases leptin, which acts as a satiation signal (Knutson & van Cauter, 2008). These stimulation effects may occur through the action of the orexins, which are involved in both appetite regulation and waking. Missing sleep may increase the risks for obesity and diabetes by altering the brain chemistry that underlies weight regulation. Thus, getting adequate sleep may be more beneficial than keeping you well rested—sleeping may protect against obesity.

in weight. Adopted children's weights were more similar to their biological parents' than to their adoptive parents', and the weights of twins were highly correlated, even when the twins had not been raised together. A study of twins (Schousboe et al., 2004) found a high degree of heritability for BMI and also for fat distribution on the body. Confirmation for a genetic basis for fat distribution came from a study that was part of the Framingham Heart Study (Fox et al., 2004). However, this project also furnished evidence for an environmental component; obesity showed some signs of contagion, spreading throughout networks of friends and family (Christakis & Fowler, 2007).

These studies suggest that weight and fat distribution have strong genetic components, but no authorities claim that most human obesity is determined by a single gene (Cummings & Schwartz, 2003). Indeed, authorities are now focusing on the interaction among genes, behavior, and environment to understand weight regulation and obesity (Levin, 2005; Morrison, 2008). Some combinations of genes may function in faulty ways that dysregulate the setpoint system and produce obesity, but research is also turning toward the contributions of eating and how food choices may act to disrupt body weight regulation, producing obesity (Erlanson-Albertsson, 2005; Mercer & Archer, 2008).

This emphasis is well founded—obesity occurs in a specific environment; a person cannot be obese without an adequate food supply. Thus, the genetic components of obesity may explain some of the variation in weight among people in a given environment. However, the increase in obesity that is occurring around the world has developed too rapidly to be the result of genes, so researchers must look beyond inheritance to attain a complete explanation of obesity. (See Would You Believe . . . ? box for another suggestion of an environmental influence on the development of obesity.)

The Positive Incentive Model The shortcomings of setpoint theory and genetics in explaining all factors related to eating and obesity led to the formulation of the *positive incentive model*. This model holds that the positive reinforcers of eating have important consequences for weight maintenance. This view suggests that people have several types of motivation to eat, including personal pleasure and social context as well as biological factors (Pinel, Assanand, & Lehman, 2000). The personal pleasure factors revolve around the pleasures of eating, including the taste of food and how pleasurable eating is at any given time. The social context of eating includes the cultural background of the person eating as well as the people present, whether or not they are eating, and the type and tastiness of available food. Biological factors include the length of time since eating and blood glucose levels. In addition, some proponents of the positive incentive theory (Pinel et al., 2000) take an evolutionary view, contending that humans have an evolved tendency to eat in the presence of food. Scarcity of food has built animals that survived when they laid on fat, making eating and the selection of food an important evolved ability. Therefore, this model includes biological factors but holds that eating is a process involving self-regulation, with important individual, learned, and cultural components (Epstein, Leddy, Temple, & Faith, 2007; Finlayson, King, & Blundell, 2007).

The setpoint model ignores the factors of taste, learning, and social context in eating, and these factors are unquestionably important (Rozin, 1999; Rozin et al., 2003; Stroebe, 2008). For each person in each instance, the act of choosing something to eat has a long history of personal experience and cultural learning. But a preferred food will not be equally appealing under all circumstances. For example, some foods—such as pickles and ice cream—do not seem to go together (at least for most people), even if both foods are individually tasty.

Social setting is important to eating, which is often a social activity. People tend to eat more in the presence of others, unless they believe that the others are judging them, and then they eat less (Herman, Roth, & Polivy, 2003), suggesting that social norms govern eating situations (Herman & Polivy, 2005). Culture provides an even wider context for eating, and various cultures have restrictions (and requirements) on what, when, and how much to eat. People tend to get hungry on a schedule that corresponds to mealtimes, but people in the United States are much more likely to eat cereal for breakfast than for dinner. In contrast, people in Spain do not eat cold cereal, and the lack of cultural tradition for this type of food made marketing it difficult in that country (Visser, 1999). These cultural and learned factors also affect the caloric value of chosen foods and how much a person eats, and these choices influence body weight. For example, when people choose "comfort foods," they often choose either food that carries personal nostalgic emotions or food that represents a personal indulgence (Locher, Yoels, Maurer, & Van Ells, 2005).

The positive incentive view predicts a variety of body weights, depending on food availability, individual experience with food, cultural encouragement to eat various foods, and the cultural ideal for body weight. Thus, the availability of an abundant food supply is necessary but not sufficient to produce obesity. People must overeat to become obese, and the quantity of food a person eats is related to how palatable the food is. Some tastes, such as sweet, are innately determined through the action of taste buds, and an overabundance of sweet food may be a factor in the dysregulaton of body weight (Erlanson-Albertsson, 2005). In industrialized countries, a huge food industry promotes food products as desirable through massive advertising campaigns, and many of these foods are high in fat and sugar. This situation influences individual food choices that promote population-wide obesity (Brownell & Horgen, 2004). Indeed, even rats eat more when food cues are abundant in the environment (Polivy, Coelho, Hargreaves, Fleming, & Herman, 2007).

Another factor that promotes overeating in industrialized countries is the availability of a variety of foods. Eating a very desirable food leads to a decreased evaluation of how pleasant

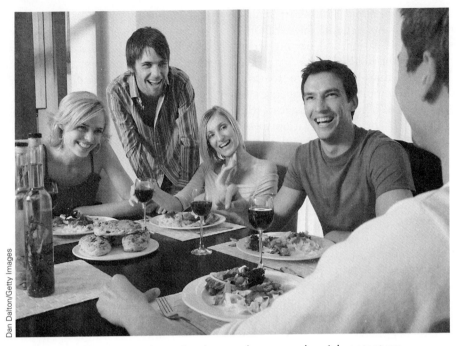

According to the positive incentive theory, pleasure and social context are important factors in eating.

that food is (Hetherington & Rolls, 1996); that is, people become satiated for any particular food. When food supplies are limited in variety (but not in quantity), this factor can lead to lower levels of food consumption, but a new taste can tempt someone who is full to eat more. Indeed, if eating a sufficient amount terminated a meal, dessert would not be so popular (Pinel, 2009).

Variety is important in boosting eating, even in rats. A large body of research (Ackroff et al., 2007; Raynor & Epstein, 2001; Sclafani, 2001) indicates that variety is important in the amount eaten, for rats and for humans. An early study (Sclafani & Springer, 1976) showed that a "supermarket" diet produced weight gains of 269% in laboratory rats. The diet consisted of a changing variety of foods chosen from the supermarket, including chocolate chip cookies, salami, cheese, bananas, marshmallows, chocolate, peanut butter, and sweetened condensed milk. The combination of high fat and high sugar plus the changing variety led to enormous weight gain.

Are humans very different? The availability of a wide variety of tasty food should produce widespread obesity, which is exactly the situation that exists in a number of countries today. This wide variety of foods allows people to always have some foods that furnish a new taste, and people in such situations never become satiated for all available foods.

However, fat may be more important than other ingredients in producing obesity. Not only is fat denser in calories, but some evidence indicates that fat intake is a behavior capable of affecting the biology of weight regulation. One hypothesis (Erlanson-Albertsson, 2005; Tremblay, 2004) holds that ingestion of foods high in fat and sugar disrupts satiation signals and boosts appetite signals in the brain. Thus, eating a diet high in fat and sugar increases appetite rather than leading to satiation. Results from a twin study (Rissanen et al., 2002) support this contention. To control for genetics, this study examined twin pairs in which one twin was obese and the other was normal weight. This procedure assured that the weight difference was due to environmental rather than genetic factors. The results indicated that the obese twins not only ate a diet higher in fat than their leaner twins but also reported memories of preferences for such foods from adolescence and young adulthood.

Thus, the positive incentive theory of eating and weight maintenance takes into account factors that the setpoint model ignores, including individual food preferences, cultural influences on eating, cultural influences on body composition, and the relationship between food availability and obesity. Both models draw on biological factors and inheritance, and many advocates of the setpoint theory acknowledge that the factors highlighted by the positive incentive theory are important to weight regulation and contribute to obesity.

How Unhealthy Is Obesity?

Overweight and obesity are undesirable from a social point of view, but does overweight endanger health? These effects depend partly on the degree of overweight and the distribution of fat on the body. Research has not implicated being slightly overweight as a health risk (McGee, 2005). However, being obese places a person at an elevated risk for several types of health problems and premature death.

A U-shaped relationship has appeared between weight and poor health; that is, the very thinnest and the very heaviest people seem to be at greatest risk for all-cause mortality (Flegal, Graubard, Williamson, & Gail, 2005). Low body weight is not as much of a risk as obesity, and some researchers

(Pinel et al., 2000) have argued that low body weight can be healthier than normal weight. In any case, overweight is more hazardous.

Without any question, obesity is a health risk, but those who are overweight yet not obese may not experience much more risk than those in the normal weight range. For example, studies from the United States (Flegal et al., 2005) and the European Union (Banegas, López-García, Gutiérrez-Fisac, Guallar-Castillón, & Rodríguez-Artalejo, 2003) found little elevation in risk for people who were overweight but substantial risk for those who were obese. A large-scale study from Germany (Bender, Trautner, Spraul, & Berger, 1998) showed no increased mortality risk for men with BMI scores up to 32 and only a very weak relationship for women in this range, but BMI scores over 40 doubled the mortality. A summary of these levels of risk appears in Table 14.4.

Other studies show similar results: Obesity is associated not only with increased mortality but also with increased use of health care (Bertakis & Azari, 2005) and increased chances for developing Type 2 diabetes, gallbladder disease, and high blood pressure (Must et al., 1999). Obesity also raises the risks for migraine headache (Horev, Wirguin, Lantsberg, & Ifergane, 2005); kidney stones (Taylor, Stampfer, & Curhan, 2005); and sleep apnea, respiratory problems, liver disease, osteoarthritis, reproductive problems in women, and colon cancer (National Task Force on the Prevention and Treatment of Obesity, 2000). Mortality risk is lowest for women with BMIs between 22 and 23.4 and for men with BMIs between 23.5 and 24.9 (Calle, Thun, Petrelli, Rodriguez, & Heath, 1999).

TABLE 14.4

Categories of Obesity and Risks for All-Cause Mortality Based on Body Mass Index (BMI)

Degree of Obesity	BMI Range	Risk for Men	Relative Risk	Risk for Women	Relative Risk
Moderate	25 to 32	None	1.0	Very low	1.1
Obese	32 to 36	Low	1.3	Low	1.2
Gross	36 to 40	High	1.9	Low	1.3
Morbid	40>	Very high	3.1	Very high	2.3

Source: Based on Bender et al. (1998).

Both age and ethnicity complicate the interpretation of risk from obesity. For young and middle-aged adults, being obese is a risk for all-cause mortality and especially for death due to cardiovascular disease (McGee, 2005). Indeed, being overweight during childhood and adolescence predicts increased mortality in the years to come (Bjørge, Engeland, Tverdal, & Smith, 2008). After age 65, the relationship no longer exists (Baik et al., 2000), and losing weight after age 50 increases risk (Diehr et al., 1998). For African American men and women, the healthiest BMI levels were around 27, which is in the range considered overweight but not obese.

Another weight-related factor associated with morbidity and mortality is weight distribution. People who accumulate excess weight around their abdomen are at greater risk than people who carry their excess weight on their hips and thighs, and the tendency for this distribution has a genetic component (Fox et al., 2004). A variety of studies have shown that patterns of body weight and the waist-to-hip ratio may be better predictors of all-cause mortality than the body mass index (Folsom et al., 2000). Excess abdominal fat raises the risk for Type 2 diabetes (Hu, 2003) and cardiovascular disease (Pi-Sunyer, 2004).

The dangers of "beer bellies" were noted more than 20 years ago (Hartz, Rupley, & Rimm, 1984), but more recently this pattern of fat distribution has been integrated into a pattern of risk factors called the *metabolic syndrome*, a collection of factors proposed to elevate the risk for cardiovascular disease and diabetes. In addition to excess abdominal fat, components of the metabolic syndrome include elevated blood pressure, insulin resistance, and problems with the levels of two components of cholesterol. A large waistline is the most visible symptom of this syndrome, and research has indicated that abdominal fat is positively related to the metabolic syndrome, but fat on the thighs has a negative relationship (Goodpaster et al., 2005).

In conclusion, obese people have heightened risks of developing certain health problems, especially diabetes, gallstones, and cardiovascular disease. Table 14.5 summarizes studies showing that obesity and fat distributed around the waist both relate to increased mortality rates, especially from heart disease.

IN SUMMARY

Obesity can be defined in terms of health or social standards, and the two are not always the same. The ideal weight for health is reflected in the Metropolitan Insurance Company weight charts or the body mass index (BMI). Social standards, however, have dictated a standard of thinness with a lower body weight than is ideal for health.

Obesity has been explained by the setpoint model, genetic factors, and the positive incentive model. Setpoint theory explains weight regulation in terms of biological control systems that are sensitive to body fat. This model hypothesizes that obesity is a defect in this control mechanism. Such a defect is the primary component of genetic models of obesity, which hypothesize that obesity occurs when a person inherits some configuration of defective genes that affect the neurochemicals that signal hunger or satiation. However, neither of these models takes learned and environmental factors of eating into account, but the positive incentive model does. This view holds that people (and other animals) gain weight when they have ready access to an abundant and varied supply of tasty food.

DIETING

Many people in the United States have some knowledge of the risks of obesity and even know about the risks of an unfavorable waist-to-hip ratio, but media portrayals of idealized thin bodies are even more influential in the motivation to diet (Wiseman, Sunday, & Becker, 2005). Despite the idealization of thinness, obesity in the United States rose sharply during the 1990s and has not decreased since (NCHS, 2007). Acceptance of the ideal body as thin, combined with the growing

TABLE 14.5

The Relationship Between Weight and Disease or Death

Study	Sample	Results
Effects of Obesity		
Flegal et al., 2005	U.S. population	Obesity is a risk for all-cause mortality.
Banegas et al., 2003	Adults from 15 members of the European Union	Obesity is a stronger risk than overweight, but both contribute to mortality.
Bertakis & Azari, 2005	Obese and normal weight adults	Obese adults sought health care more often than normal weight adults.
Must et al., 1999	Overweight and obese adults	Obesity is related to diabetes, gallbladder disease, and hypertension.
Horev et al., 2005	Obese women	Headaches are more common among obese women.
Taylor et al., 2005	Men, older women, younger women	Obesity is a risk for kidney stones.
McGee, 2005	Young and middle-aged adults	Obesity increases risk for all-cause mortality.
Bender et al., 1998	Obese men	No increase in all-cause mortality up to BMI of 32. Morbid obesity carries a threefold risk for men and more than a double risk for women.
Bjørge et al., 2008	Overweight children and adolescents	Overweight during childhood and adolescence raises the risk for later mortality.
Effects of Abdominal Fat		
Hu, 2003	Women	Central fat is related to Type 2 diabetes and all-cause mortality.
Pi-Sunyer, 2004	Review of studies, including cross-cultural	Central fat is related to the development of cardiovascular disease.
Folsom et al., 2000	Middle-aged and older women	Waist/hip ratio is a better predictor than BMI of all-cause mortality.
Goodpaster et al., 2005	Older women and men	Abdominal fat is related to the metabolic syndrome.

prevalence of overweight, produces a situation in which dieting and weight loss are the subjects of a great many people's concern. What are people doing to try to lose weight, and how well do these strategies work?

People are inundated with messages about diets—television, magazine, and newspapers are filled with advertisements for miracle diets that take off pounds almost effortlessly. Those diets may seem too good to be true, and they are. In September 2002, the U.S. Federal Trade Commission issued a report that described how widespread false and misleading diets have become ("Federal Trade Commission," 2002). Despite the customer testimonials and the before-and-after photos, these "miracle" diets do not work. U.S. Surgeon General Richard Carmona said, "There is no such thing as a miracle pill for weight loss. The surest and safest way to weight loss and healthier living is by combining healthful eating and exercising" ("Federal Trade Commission," 2002, p. 8). Despite this prudent advice, many people fail to make wise choices when they want to lose weight. For example, people may concentrate on cutting fat in their diet without attending to the amount of sugar and other sweeteners they consume (Bray, Nielsen, & Popkin, 2004), or they cut carbohydrates yet eat a high-fat diet.

Other unwise decisions abound in dieting, both in terms of the number of people dieting and the methods they use. The trend toward dieting has become more severe in the past few decades. During the mid-1960s, only 10% of overweight adults were dieting (Wyden, 1965), but during subsequent years those percentages steadily increased; in 2007, 60% of high school girls and 30% of high school boys were trying to lose weight (Eaton et al., 2008). Adults, too, are increasingly likely to diet. A survey of adults (Kruger, Galuska, Serdula, & Jones, 2004) showed that almost 38% of women and 24% of men were trying to lose weight. However, many of these adolescent and adult dieters do not have sufficient excess weight to put them at risk for disease or death, and many take unwise approaches to losing weight.

Approaches to Losing Weight

To lose weight or keep from gaining weight, people have several choices. They can (1) reduce portion size, (2) restrict the types of food they eat, (3) increase their level of exercise, (4) rely on drastic medical procedures such as fasting, diet pills, or surgery, or (5) use a combination of these approaches. Regardless of the approach, *all diets that prompt weight loss do so through restriction of calories.*

Restricting Types of Food Maintaining a diet consisting of a variety of foods with smaller portions is a reasonable and healthy strategy. The Weight Watchers program emphasizes eating a healthy variety of foods. This program proved most effective in an evaluation of a variety of dieting strategies (Dansinger et al., 2005), producing the best combination of weight loss and low dropout rate of any of the programs in this study. Other studies have compared a variety of popular dieting programs, including Atkins, Ornish, LEARN, Mediterranean, and Zone diets. These diets vary in terms of the amount of fat and carbohydrates allowed, with diets such as the Atkins and Zone diets restricting carbohydrates, and programs such as the Ornish and LEARN diets focusing on fat restriction.

Several long-term, well-controlled comparison studies have revealed slight differences among these programs in terms of weight loss and

effects on health risks. Despite warnings from nutritionists about the dangers of high-fat, low-carbohydrate diets, overweight people who follow these diets have not experienced unfavorable changes in cholesterol levels or risks for cardiovascular disease (Gardner et al., 2007; Shai et al., 2008). To the contrary, the Atkins diet prompted greater weight loss and more favorable cholesterol changes than the low-fat diets after 12 months (Gardner et al., 2007) and 24 months (Shai et al., 2008). This program also produced a more rapid initial weight loss, a tendency to regain some of the lost weight, and higher dropout rates than other programs. However, low-carbohydrate diets were slightly more successful than other programs in producing long-term weight loss, especially for men (Shai et al., 2008). For women, the Mediterranean diet was more successful. None of the diets produced an impressive weight loss for any group—a loss of an average of 10 to 12 pounds in the most successful group.

Some diets are more extreme, restricting the dieter to a limited group of foods or even a single food. All-fruit diets, egg diets, cabbage soup diet, and even the ice cream diet fall into this category. Of course, such diets are nutritional disasters. They produce weight loss by restricting calories; dieters get tired of the monotony of one food and eat less than they would if they were eating a variety. "All the hard-boiled eggs you want" turns out to be not many!

Taking monotony a step further are the liquid diets, which exist in a variety of forms and under various brand names. Liquid diets have the advantage of being nutritionally more balanced than most restricted food diets. Still, liquid diets and their equivalent meals in the form of puddings or bars have the disadvantage of being monotonous and repetitive, and they tend to be low in fiber. Like all other diets, these work by restricting calorie intake. Although current researchers may disagree on the advantages of low-fat or low-carbohydrate diets, they are likely to agree that diets high in fiber from fruits and vegetables are good choices (Schenker, 2001). However, these diets can be effective. An intensive behavioral program using meal replacements (Anderson, Conley, & Nicholas, 2007) was successful for very overweight people, producing weight losses of 50 to 100 pounds, with better maintenance rates than most diet programs.

In conclusion, all food restriction strategies can be successful in producing weight loss, but many are bad approaches. Many of these diets fail to teach new eating habits that people can maintain over the long term. Thus, people who lose weight on one of these diets—especially one of the more extreme diets—will be likely to regain that weight, and they will have the experience of a period of unhealthy eating, which may have health consequences.

Behavior Modification Programs Although dieting should be seen as a permanent modification in one's eating habits, such change is difficult. The behavior modification approach toward treating obesity begins with the assumption that eating is a behavior that is subject to change. This application of behavioral theory was originated by Richard Stuart (1967), who reported a much higher success rate than that achieved through previous approaches. Most behavior modification programs focus on eating and exercise, helping overweight people to monitor and change their behavior. Clients in these programs often keep eating diaries to focus their awareness on the types of foods they eat and under what circumstances, as well as to provide data the therapist can use to devise a personal plan for changing unhealthy eating habits. The outcome of a recent weight loss trial (Hollis et al., 2008) indicated that dieters who kept a diary lost twice as much weight as those on the same program who did not. In addition, exercise goals are a typical component of behavior modification programs. The most common format for these programs is a group setting with weekly meetings that include instruction in nutrition and in self-monitoring to attain individual goals (Wing & Polley, 2001). Almost all weight control programs include some modification of eating or lifestyle, and these programs may be referred to as behavioral or behavior modification programs (Wadden, Crerand, & Brock, 2005).

Because weight loss is not a behavior, these behavioral programs tend to reinforce good eating habits rather than the number of pounds lost.

In other words, the behaviors, not the consequences, are the targets for reward and change. People who are overweight to moderately obese may be fairly successful in these types of programs. The goal is typically gradual weight loss and maintenance of that loss. The average amount of weight lost is about 20 pounds over six months, but dieters maintain only about 60% of that loss over a year (Wing & Polley, 2001). Thus, even moderate, gradual weight loss may be difficult to maintain.

Exercise The importance of exercise in weight loss has become increasingly apparent (Manson, Skerrett, Greenland, & VanItallie, 2004). Because metabolic rate slows down when food intake decreases, some form of physical activity is necessary to speed up metabolism in dieters. Exercise is known to counteract metabolic slowdown and thus may be an indispensable part of weight reduction programs. In a large-scale survey of dieters ("Federal Trade Commission," 2002), exercising at least three times a week was a strategy shared by 73% of successful dieters. Exercise can also change body composition, adding muscle while dieting decreases fat levels. (The role of exercise is discussed more fully in Chapter 15.)

Drastic Methods of Losing Weight People sometimes take drastic measures to lose weight, and physicians sometimes recommend drastic measures for severely obese patients. Even with medical supervision, some weight reduction programs present risks, sometimes to the point of being life threatening.

One approach that turned out to be more dangerous than initially believed was taking drugs to reduce appetite. In the 1950s and 1960s, diet pills were widely prescribed. These drugs were amphetamines, stimulant drugs that increase the activity of the nervous system, speed up metabolism, and suppress appetite. Unfortunately, the effects are short term, and dependence may become a more serious problem than obesity. Increasing evidence of the dangers of amphetamines led to the development of other diet drugs, but the quest for a safe, effective drug that helps people lose weight has proven difficult. Currently available drugs include sibutramine (Meridia) and orlistat

(Xenical) in the United States and rimonabant (Acomplia) in Europe, all of which offer the possibility of modest weight loss (Rucker, Padawal, Li, Curioni, & Lau, 2007). The developing knowledge of hormones and neurochemicals related to weight regulation offer the promise of more effective drugs, but a growing number of obese people are turning to surgery as a way to manage their weight.

Several types of surgery can affect weight, but most current surgeries either restrict the size of the stomach by gastric banding (placing a band around the stomach) or gastric bypass (routing food around most of the stomach and part of the intestines) (Buchwald et al., 2004). People are candidates for these surgeries if their BMI is 35 or higher and if they have health problems that make weight loss imperative. These procedures are successful in promoting drastic weight loss and in improving diabetes, hypertension, and other risk factors for cardiovascular disease. Like any surgery, these procedures carry some risks, and patients typically must be prepared to monitor their food intake and to take nutritional supplements for the rest of their lives (Tucker, Szomstein, & Rosenthal, 2007). Despite the risks and maintenance requirements, these surgeries are increasingly popular, with an overall 600% increase between 1998 and 2002 (Smoot, Xu, Kuppersmith, Singh, & Hilserath, 2006).

Another surgical approach to weight loss is to remove adipose tissue through a fat-suctioning technique called liposuction. The technique produces a recontouring of the body rather than an overall weight loss (Sattler, 2005). This procedure is not useful in controlling the health complications of obesity; rather, it is a cosmetic procedure to change body shape and has little impact on disease risks associated with obesity (S. Klein et al., 2004). Despite the discomfort and expense of the surgery, liposuction is the most common type of plastic surgery worldwide (Sattler, 2005). Like all surgery, it presents risks such as infection and reactions to anesthesia.

Drastic means of losing weight are poor solutions to obesity for most people. However, they are fairly common. High school girls reported using such drastic strategies for weight loss as fasting (16.4%), taking appetite suppressant drugs (7.5%), and using laxatives or purging (6.4%); a majority (53%) admitted chronic dieting (Eaton et al., 2008). Having a friend who uses these methods increases adolescent girls' risks for doing so (Eisenberg, Neumark-Sztainer, Story, & Perry, 2005), and being overweight raises the percentages of those who have used such methods to 40% for girls and 20% for boys (Neumark-Sztainer et al., 2007). All these drastic means of losing weight can be dangerous. In addition, all are difficult to maintain long enough to produce significant weight loss. Even when dieters succeed with these strategies, they usually regain the weight they have lost because these approaches do not enable them to learn how to make good diet choices for permanent weight loss. Indeed, keeping weight off is a major challenge, regardless of weight loss method.

Maintaining Weight Loss In Chapters 12 and 13, we saw that about two-thirds of the people who initially quit smoking or stop drinking will eventually relapse. For people who succeed in losing weight, maintaining that loss is comparably difficult. A systematic review of commercial weight loss programs (Tsai & Wadden, 2005) indicated that people who managed to lose weight on these programs (not all do) had a high probability of regaining 50% of the weight they lost within one to two years. However, this review evaluated highly selected dieters, including those who were extremely obese and those who sought professional help in losing weight. For those people, weight control is now considered to be a chronic illness, with continued professional assistance needed to maintain weight loss (Kubetin, 2001).

Effective formal weight reduction interventions typically include posttreatment programs to help dieters maintain weight loss. These programs are usually more successful than those that lack a posttreatment phase. For example, researchers compared two follow-up interventions in dieters who had completed a six-month weight loss program (Svetkey et al., 2008). Dieters who received no follow-up were compared to those in an intervention that involved brief personal contact on a monthly basis and another that consisted of an interactive technology-based intervention. The personal follow-up was more effective, but both interventions produced dieters who weighed less than before they started the program. However, some simple changes can be effective. For example, people who lost weight and weighed themselves daily were less likely to regain the lost weight than those who did not step on the scales so often (Wing et al., 2007).

A survey by *Consumer Reports* ("The Truth About Dieting," 2002) supplied information about a wide selection of dieters, both successful and unsuccessful. This survey included more than 32,000 dieters, 25% of whom had lost at least 10% of their starting weight and kept it off for at least a year. This number confirmed that people have problems both with losing weight and with maintaining weight loss, but it also showed that some people are successful.

Most of the dieters in the *Consumer Reports* survey lost weight on their own rather than through a formal weight loss program. Consistent with the systematic review of commercial programs (Tsai & Wadden, 2005), more of the unsuccessful dieters (26%) than successful dieters (14%) tried a program such as Weight Watchers or Jenny Craig. Those who were successful tended to use a variety of approaches, including exercising and increasing physical activity, eating fewer fatty and sweet foods, increasing consumption of fruits and vegetables, and cutting down on portion size. Not surprisingly, those dieters who were successful in maintaining their weight loss rarely used any of the drastic means of losing weight reviewed in the prior section, except for surgery; individuals who undergo surgery to lose weight tend to lose large amounts of weight and maintain some of that weight loss (Douketis, Macie, Thabane, & Williamson, 2005). People who lose weight without surgery and keep it off tend to alter their eating and physical activity, forming new habits that they are able to maintain.

Childhood obesity has increased, even among children as young as preschool age, and has become a topic of widespread concern (Sherry, 2007). Interventions may include strategies for preventing the development of overweight, dietary programs, family interventions, physical activity programs, or some combination of these elements. Programs with a dietary modification component showed some effectiveness in reducing weight among overweight children (Collins, Warren, Neve, McCoy, & Stokes, 2007). A meta-analysis of family-based behavioral interventions (Young, Northern, Lister, Drummond, & O'Brien, 2007) and residential weight loss programs for children (Gately et al., 2005) indicated that both approaches can be effective in changing eating and physical activity habits.

Is Dieting a Good Choice?

Although dieting can produce weight loss, it may not be a good choice for everyone. Dieting has psychological costs, may not be effective in improving health, and may be a signal of body dissatisfaction that is a risk for eating disorders. A group of dieters rated their overall experience as positive (Jeffery, Kelly, Rothman, Sherwood, & Boutelle, 2004), but as the dieting continued, positive feelings decreased. Some dieters exhibit strong reactions, behaving very much like starving people: They are irritable, obsessed with food, finicky about taste, easily distractible, and hungry. These behavioral reactions make dieting foolish for those who are close to the best weight for their health. Losing weight may be a good choice for those who are sufficiently overweight to endanger their health, but many dieters are not. Developing reasonable and healthy eating patterns is a far better choice than dieting. That is, dieting is not the same as eliminating overeating (Herman, van Strien, & Polivy, 2008). The former may not be a good choice, whereas the latter is.

Ironically, weight loss may be a health risk for some people and a health benefit for others. Involuntary weight loss is often associated with disease, so the association between unintentional weight loss and mortality is no surprise. However, several studies (Dyer, Stamler, & Greenland, 2000; Sørensen, Rissanen, Korkeila, & Kaprio, 2005) have explored the mortality risks of weight loss and found an increased risk, even for those who lost weight intentionally. Weight loss is also

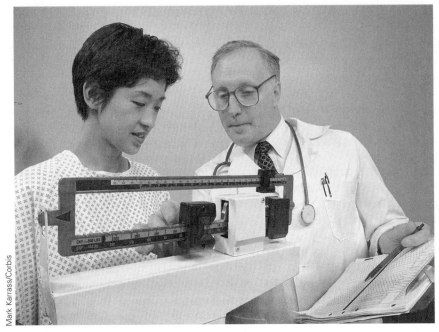

Mark Karrass/Corbis

Dieting is common, even among those who do not need to lose weight for health reasons.

associated with the onset of dementia, including Alzheimer's disease (Grundman, 2005). This increased risk is puzzling because losing weight is beneficial for some conditions. For example, middle-aged and older adults who lost weight and maintained the lower weight improved their cardiovascular risks and risk for hypertension (Moore et al., 2005). Individuals who lost weight through gastric surgery also experienced an improvement of most risk factors for diabetes and cardiovascular disease (Sjöström et al., 2004). Older men decreased their mortality risk if they were substantially overweight and if they intentionally lost weight, but unintentional weight loss increased their risks (Wannamethee, Shaper, & Lennon, 2005). Older women who lost weight decreased their risk for breast cancer (Eliassen, Colditz, Rossner, Willett, & Hankinson, 2006).

Thus, the benefits of weight loss may not apply equally to all people. Even modest weight loss can be important for individuals who are obese and who can maintain the loss. However, the

risks of dieting may be greater than the risks of moderate, stable overweight (Gaesser, 2003).

IN SUMMARY

The near obsession with thinness in our culture has led to a plethora of diets, many of which are neither safe nor permanently effective. Most diets will produce some initial weight loss in response to the restriction of caloric intake, but maintaining the reduced weight levels is a matter of permanent changes in basic eating habits and activity levels. Despite attempts to be thin, people in the United States are now heavier than ever because they have increased the number of calories they consume and lowered their amount of physical activity.

Losing weight is easier than maintaining weight loss, but programs that include posttreatment and frequent follow-up can be successful in helping people maintain a healthy weight. Whether part of a formal program or a personal attempt, eating a variety of healthy foods and maintaining physical activity are more likely than drastic programs to result in long-term weight loss. Like programs for adults, programs for obese children and adolescents face similar challenges and include the same effective components—healthy food choices and physical activity.

Dieting is a good choice for some people but not for others. Obese people and those with a high waist-to-hip ratio should try to lose weight and keep it off. However, most people who diet for cosmetic reasons would be healthier (and happier) if they did not diet, and even people who are slightly overweight may not benefit from dieting.

EATING DISORDERS

The eating disorders that have received the most attention, both in the popular media and in the scientific literature, are anorexia nervosa and bulimia, but binge eating is also an eating disorder diagnosis. The term *anorexia nervosa* literally means lack of appetite due to a nervous or psychological condition; *bulimia* means continuous, morbid hunger. Neither meaning, however, is quite accurate. People with anorexia nervosa have not lost their appetite. Ordinarily, they are perpetually hungry, but they insist that they do not wish to eat. Like Mary-Kate Olsen, these people become preoccupied with losing weight, and their self-induced starvation may result in a life-threatening condition. After failing to mention anorexia for four years, Mary-Kate finally admitted that she was anorexic and said that the disorder had nearly killed her (Barbarich, 2008).

Bulimia has come to mean more than continuous morbid hunger. The chief identifying mark of this eating disorder is repeated bingeing and purging, the purge usually coming after eating huge quantities of food, typically high in calories and loaded with carbohydrates, fat, or both. Eating large quantities of food is critical to the definition of binge eating, but these people who binge do not purge, resulting in overweight and obesity.

These three eating disorders obviously have much in common. Indeed, some authorities regard anorexia and bulimia as two dimensions of the same illness. Others see the three as separate but related disorders (Polivy & Herman, 2002). For example, binge eating is common to all three. In addition, the core components of all three include body dissatisfaction combined with preoccupation with food, weight, and body shape. The basis for body dissatisfaction is easy to understand: Overweight and obesity have become more common, yet the ideal body is thin. This combination has created a discontent that touches everyone in the culture. Children as young as early elementary school age express body dissatisfaction (McCabe & Ricciardelli, 2003; Phares, Steinberg, & Thompson, 2004), and discontent with body shape is so common among women that it is the norm (Rodin, Silberstein, & Striegel-Moore, 1985). However, only a small percentage of people with body dissatisfaction develop eating disorders, indicating that other factors operate to produce these disorders (Tylka, 2004).

Janet Polivy and Peter Herman (2002, 2004) suggested that body dissatisfaction constitutes an essential precursor to the development of eating disorders, but those who develop eating problems must also come to see being thin as a solution to other problems in their lives. People who channel their distress into body concerns and focus on their bodies as a way to change their dissatisfaction have the cognitions that lead to eating disorders (Evans, 2003). Such cognitions include the feeling that being thin will lead to happiness.

Other risks for eating disorders include family and personality correlates such as a great deal of negative family interaction, a history of sexual abuse during childhood, low self-esteem, and high levels of negative mood, anxiety, and depression (Polivy & Herman, 2002). In addition, some genetic or neuroendocrine predisposition may contribute to the development of eating disorders; the neurotransmitter serotonin has been implicated (Kaye, 2008), but research on the hormone leptin revealed no direct involvement with either anorexia or bulimia (Monteleone, DiLieto, Castaldo, & Maj, 2004). A test of factors related to unhealthy weight control strategies (Neumark-Sztainer, Wall, Story, & Perry, 2003) revealed that concern about body weight was the most important factor in eating disorders.

Anorexia Nervosa

This chapter opened with a description of Mary-Kate Olsen, who was hospitalized and treated for anorexia. In this section, we see how her case matches or deviates from a composite model of thousands of cases of anorexia nervosa.

Despite recent publicity on anorexia, neither the disorder nor the term is new. The first two documented cases of intentional self-starvation were reported by Richard Morton in 1689 (Sours, 1980). Morton wrote about an 18-year-old English girl who had died of the effects of anorexia some 25 years earlier and about an 18-year-old boy who had survived. Both had shown a remarkable indifference to starvation, and both had been described as sad and anxious. In London, Sir William Gull (1874) studied several cases of intentional self-starvation during the 1860s. He regarded the condition as a psychological disorder and coined the term *anorexia nervosa* to indicate loss of appetite due to "nervous" causes—that is, psychological factors. From that time until about 1910, Gull's psychopathological conception pervaded the psychological and psychiatric literature. From about 1910 until the late 1930s, some medical authorities tried to link anorexia nervosa with atrophy of the anterior lobe of the pituitary gland, but this medical view soon lost favor.

During the 1940s and 1950s, speculation proliferated concerning the causes and cures of anorexia nervosa. Some psychiatrists hypothesized that the ailment was a denial of femininity and a fear of motherhood. Other theorists suggested that it represented an attempt on the part of the young woman to reestablish unity with her mother. Unfortunately, none of these hypotheses proved fruitful in expanding the scientific understanding of anorexia nervosa. The past four decades have seen a shift away from this sort of speculation and a turn toward the view that anorexia involves a complex of sociocultural, family, and biological factors (Polivy & Herman, 2002). Recent emphasis has been on describing the disorder in terms of behaviors and their physiological effects, demographic correlates, and effective treatment procedures.

What Is Anorexia? Anorexia nervosa is an eating disorder characterized by intentional self-starvation or semistarvation, sometimes to the point of death. People with anorexia are extremely afraid of gaining weight and have a distorted body image, seeing themselves as being too heavy even though they are exceedingly thin. Mary-Kate Olsen expressed such distorted perceptions, wondering why her image in the mirror was so ugly when her twin Ashley was so pretty ("Olsen Treated," 2004). Mary-Kate was not unique in seeing her own body in a distorted way; research using brain imaging (Sachdev, Mondraty, Wen, & Gulliford, 2008) has revealed that women who are anorexic process images of their own bodies differently than they do images of other women's bodies—even when the two bodies are the same weight.

The *Diagnostic and Statistical Manual of Mental Disorders* (4th edition, text revision [*DSM-IV-TR*]) of the American Psychiatric Association (APA, 2000) defines *anorexia nervosa* as intentional weight loss to a point that the person weighs less than 85% of the weight considered normal by the Metropolitan Life Insurance tables or has a body mass index of 17.5 or less, along with a fear of being fat, a distorted body image, and for women, **amenorrhea**, the cessation of menstrual periods for at least three cycles.

The *DSM-IV-TR* (APA, 2000) identifies two subtypes of anorexia: the restricting type and the binge-purge type. Anorexics with the restricting type eat almost nothing, losing weight by dieting, fasting, exercising, or a combination of these strategies. Anorexics with the binge-purge type may eat large quantities of food and use vomiting or laxatives to purge the food they have eaten. Alternatively, these anorexics may eat small amounts of food and purge. Research has confirmed that these two subtypes are distinct (Kaye, 2008). Purging is typical of bulimia, and binge eating occurs in binge eating disorder, but bulimics use purging to maintain a normal body weight. Anorexics purge to lose weight.

Mary-Kate Olsen seems to provide an example of the restricting type of anorexia. Her friends reported that they never saw her eat, and before she received treatment, her parents hired someone to watch her eat to be sure that she swallowed her food ("Inside Mary-Kate's Two Year Ordeal," 2004). She also shares other characteristics typical of many anorexics, who are often young European American women who are outwardly compliant and high achievers. They are preoccupied with food, usually like to cook for others (no reports say that Mary-Kate did), insist that others eat their food, but eat almost nothing themselves. They lose from 15% to 50% of their body weight, yet continue to see themselves as overweight. Like Mary-Kate, they tend to be ambitious, perfectionist, and unhappy with their bodies, and to come from high-achieving families. Mary-Kate is certainly ambitious—she and her sister began appearing in the TV sitcom *Full House* when they were 9 months old and have been involved in entertainment and merchandising ever since. Anorexics are preoccupied with body fat, which usually leads to a strenuous program of exercise—dancing, jogging, doing calisthenics, or playing tennis. Excessively active and energetic behavior continues until their weight loss reaches a level that produces fatigue and weakness, making further activity impossible.

After substantial weight loss has occurred, individual differences tend to disappear, and accounts of individuals with the disorder are remarkably similar. Interestingly, most of the descriptions are also consistent with the sketch of starving conscientious objectors drawn by Keys et al. (1950). Thus, these conditions are probably an effect of starvation and not its cause. As weight loss reaches more than 25% of one's previous normal weight, the person constantly feels chilled, grows a soft, downy covering of body hair, loses scalp hair, loses interest in sex, and develops an unusual preoccupation with food. As starvation nears a perilous level, the anorexic becomes more hostile toward family and friends who try to reverse the weight loss. Mary-Kate Olsen appears not to have reached this level—she remained on good terms with her family and agreed with the family decision to go into treatment.

Many authorities, including Hilde Bruch (1973, 1978, 1982), have regarded anorexia nervosa as a means of gaining control. Bruch, who spent more than 40 years studying eating disorders and the effects of starvation, reported that prior to dieting, anorexics typically are troubled girls who feel incapable of changing their lives. These young women often see their parents as overdemanding and in absolute control of their life, yet they remain too compliant to rebel openly. They try to seize control of their life in the most personal manner possible: by changing the shape of their body. Short of force-feeding, no one can stop these young women from controlling their own body size and shape. This description seems consistent with Mary-Kate Olsen's life. Anorexics take great pleasure and pride in doing something that is difficult and often compare their superior willpower with that of others who are overweight or who shun exercise. Bruch (1978) reported that anorexics enjoy being hungry and eventually regard any food in the stomach as dirty or damaging.

Who Is Anorexia? Although anorexia is associated with Western culture, it appears in non-Western cultures around the world (Keel & Klump, 2003) and cuts across ethnic groups (Franko, Becker, Thomas, & Herzog, 2007). This diagnosis is more common among upper-middle-class and upper-class women of European ancestry in North America and Europe, but this description matches individuals who have better access to health care and thus are more likely to receive a diagnosis. Anorexia has become more common than it was 50 years ago (Keel & Klump, 2003), but anorexia nervosa is still a very rare disorder in the general population. The *DSM-IV-TR* (APA, 2000) estimated the lifetime prevalence of anorexia at 0.5% for women and one-tenth that for men; other analyses (Hudson, Hiripi, Pope, & Kessler, 2007) yield higher (but still low) estimates—0.9% for women and 0.3% for men. However, among some groups the incidence rates are much higher. For example, 26% of young women who had competed in beauty pageants reported that they believed they had or had received a diagnosis of an eating disorder (Thompson & Hammond, 2003). The competitive, weight-conscious atmosphere of professional schools for dance and modeling prompt the development of anorexia, and 6.5% of dance students and 7% of modeling students met the diagnostic criteria for anorexia nervosa (Garner & Garfinkel, 1980). Even young women who study dance are at elevated risk (Anshel, 2004); more elite dancers experience more frequent and severe

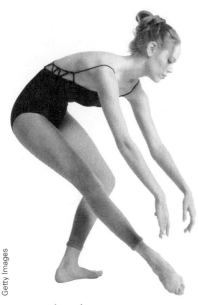

Getty Images

Eating disorders are more common among models, dancers, and athletes whose sports demand thinness.

symptoms of eating disorders (Thomas, Keel, & Heatherton, 2005). Athletes are also at increased risk, especially female athletes who participate in sports that emphasize appearance, thin body type, or low body fat (Torstveit, Rosenvinge, & Sundgot-Borgen, 2008).

Individuals with anorexia often report family difficulties, but it is difficult to determine if the difficulties precede the onset of eating problems or are a result of them (Polivy & Herman, 2002). Family environment is important in several ways. Families with children who have eating disorders tend to include a lot of negative emotion and little emotional support. Family violence—either as an observer or a target—is a risk for eating disorders for both men and women (Bardy, 2008). In addition, a family member with an eating disorder raises the risk for others in the family (Tylka, 2004), but so does having friends with unhealthy weight control practices (Eisenberg et al., 2005) or joining a sorority (Allison & Park, 2004). Thus, disordered eating is affected by social context and not only by family dynamics. In addition, physical or sexual abuse is a more

common experience in the history of those who are anorexic than for individuals who eat normally (Rayworth, 2004).

Over the years, a large majority of those diagnosed as anorexic have been women, and research and treatment have focused on women. Men make up about 10% of all anorexics (APA, 2000). This estimate—that 90% or more of all anorexics are women—has remained constant over a period of years, but it is based mostly on clinical impressions rather than complete population data. A review of eating disorders in men (Woodside, 2002) claimed that community surveys of eating disorders reveal much higher numbers, with men constituting at least 25% of cases. Thus, this eating disorder may be more common among men than the clinical impressions suggest.

Male anorexics are quite similar to female anorexics in terms of social class and family configuration, symptoms, treatment, and prognosis, but they differ in terms of the factors that pushed them toward disordered eating (Ricciardelli, McCabe, Williams, & Thompson, 2007). In addition, some studies have found that sexual orientation is a factor that differs for male and female anorexics, with more male anorexics being gay, but a comparison of symptoms and characteristics (Crisp et al., 2006) revealed many more similarities than differences.

Boys and young men may take drastic measures to achieve their ideal body, just as girls and young women do (Olivardia, Pope, & Phillips, 2000). The ideal body for boys is muscular, and escaping this indoctrination is as difficult as avoiding the thin body ideal is for girls. However, both ideals share the abhorrence of fat. Thus, both women and men have concerns about body shape and size that may appear as disordered eating.

Treatment for Anorexia Treatment for anorexia suffers from an unfortunate dilemma: This disorder has the highest mortality rate of any psychiatric diagnosis, but treatment does not show a high success rate (Guarda, 2008). Between 5% and 10% of all anorexics die from their disorder. Most die of cardiac arrhythmia, but suicide is also a frequent cause of death for those with the bingeing-purging type of anorexia (Foulon et al.,

2007). Despite the very real possibility of death, anorexia nervosa remains one of the most difficult behavior disorders to treat. About 50% of anorexics recover; 30% improve but struggle with eating-related body image problems, obsessive-compulsive disorder, or depression (Berkman, Lohr, & Bulik, 2007); and 20% experience continued eating pathology.

An initial complication for treatment is that most anorexics see nothing wrong with their eating behavior, resent suggestions that they are too thin, and resist any attempt to change their eating. That attitude appears on a number of websites hosted by individuals who are anorexic and promote it as a lifestyle alternative rather than a disorder (Davis, 2008). Readiness for change predicts more successful treatment (McHugh, 2007). Motivating anorexics to seek treatment is thus a major challenge that may be addressed by the application of motivational interviewing (Hogan & McReynolds, 2004). This technique is a directive intervention to change attitudes about problems and make people more willing to work toward change.

As starvation continues, anorexics eventually reach the point of fatigue, exhaustion, and possible physical collapse, and they are forced into treatment. This situation seems undesirable, but the immediate aim of almost any treatment program for anorexia is medical stabilization of any danger from the physical symptoms of starvation (Fairburn & Harrison, 2003; Hay, 2004). Then, anorexics need to work toward restoration of normal weight, healthy eating, and improved body image. Some authorities believe that hospitalization is required, especially for medical stabilization and restoration of weight; others believe that outpatient treatments can be effective; still others focus on drug treatments or a combination of drug and behavioral treatments. Recommendations concerning the methods of achieving these goals are not universally accepted, and systematic reviews have yet to reach firm conclusions concerning what treatments are effective for people with anorexia (Hay, 2004; Bulik, Berkman, Brownley, Sedway, & Lohr, 2007).

Since the mid-1970s, cognitive behavior therapy has become increasingly popular as a treatment for anorexia nervosa, and it has shown some success in changing both cognitive distortions that accompany body image problems and eating behavior (Fairburn & Harrison, 2003). Cognitive behavior therapists attack these irrational beliefs while maintaining a warm and accepting attitude toward patients. Anorexics are taught to discard the absolutist, all-or-nothing thinking pattern expressed in such self-statements as "If I gain one pound, I'll go on to gain a hundred." Addressing cognitive distortions may be more important than previously recognized—a developing body of research indicates that anorexics experience significant cognitive distortions that apply to the processing of food-related words (Nikendei et al., 2008). In addition, people with anorexia are more likely than others to believe that they cannot control their thoughts, and half reported that they used cognitive strategies to make themselves feel worse (Woolrich, Cooper, & Turner, 2008). The cognitive component of cognitive behavioral therapy could address these problems.

Many hospital-based programs consist of individual and group cognitive behavioral therapy plus supervised meals, meal planning, and nutrition education (Williamson, Thaw, & Varnado-Sullivan, 2001). However, cognitive behavioral therapy may be underutilized as a therapy for eating disorders (Fairburn & Harrison, 2003). Despite some evidence for its effectiveness (Bulik et al., 2007), this approach is not among the most frequently used, which may partially explain why anorexia treatment success rates are as low as they are. For example, the treatment facility in which Mary-Kate Olsen received her treatment used a program based on the 12-step approach that originated with Alcoholics Anonymous ("Inside Mary-Kate's Two Year Ordeal," 2004), which is not the most effective therapy available for eating disorders.

For adolescents, parents may or may not be actively involved in cognitive behavioral treatment programs, but one approach emphasizes the role of parents in treatment. Developed at the Maudsley Hospital in London, this approach is family based (Locke, le Grange, Agras, & Dare, 2001). Rather than treating parents as part of the problem, this approach accepts them as an essential part of the solution. Acknowledging that it is relatively easy to get anorexics to gain weight in the hospital, this approach focuses on helping them eat at home by equipping parents with strategies to get their children to eat. This family-centered approach has demonstrated effectiveness with adolescents whose anorexia is a recent development (Bulik et al., 2007; Locke & le Grange, 2005) but is not effective for adults.

Drugs have also been used in the treatment of anorexia. The drug fluoxetine (Prozac) is often a component of treatment. However, a systematic review found insufficient evidence to recommend this treatment for anorexia (Claudino et al., 2006). Another systematic review (Court, Mulder, Hetrick, Purcell, & McGorry, 2008) failed to find evidence that antipsychotic drugs were an effective therapy for anorexia. Thus, the arsenal for treating this difficult disease remains understocked.

Relapse always remains a possibility. Even with intensive therapy that targets irrational eating patterns and distorted body image, some anorexics retain elements of these maladaptive thought processes. Some slip back to self-starvation, some attempt suicide, some become depressed, and some develop other eating disorders (Carter, Blackmore, Sutandar-Pinnock, & Woodside, 2004). Despite her intention to continue treatment, rumors of a relapse for Mary-Kate Olsen appeared in 2005 ("Mary-Kate's Relapse Rumors," 2005) and again in 2007 ("Is Mary-Kate Olsen Anorexic," 2007). Follow-up care is often included in comprehensive programs, and cognitive behavioral therapy seems especially useful to prevent relapses (Pike, Timothy, Vitousek, Wilson, & Bauer, 2003).

Bulimia

Bulimia is often regarded as a companion disorder to anorexia nervosa, and some cases have been identified of individuals who have moved from one diagnosis to the other (Eddy et al., 2007). Unlike anorexics, who rely mostly on strict fasts to lose more and more weight, bulimics engage in binge eating; that is, they consume huge quantities of food in an uncontrolled manner and then purge, either by vomiting or by taking laxatives. The seemingly bizarre practice of binge eating followed by purging is not new. The ancient Romans sometimes indulged in very similar eating rituals.

After they had feasted on great quantities of rich food, these Romans would retire to the vomitorium, empty their stomachs, and then return to eat some more (Friedländer, 1968). Unlike bulimia, this practice may not have been oriented toward weight control. Today, bulimia is defined as an eating disorder and affects millions of people.

What Is Bulimia? As defined by the *Diagnostic and Statistical Manual of Mental Disorders* (*DSM-IV-TR*) of the American Psychiatric Association (APA, 2000), *bulimia nervosa* involves recurrent episodes of binge eating, a sense of lack of control over eating, and inappropriate, drastic measures to compensate for the binge. Some bulimics fast or exercise excessively, but most use self-induced vomiting or laxatives and maintain a relatively normal weight.

One factor that distinguishes bulimia from anorexia is lack of impulse control (Polivy & Herman, 2002), although this characteristic may apply to some people who are bulimic more strongly than to others (T. C. Myers et al., 2006). Bulimics often experience problems related to impulsivity, such as a history of alcohol or drug abuse, sexual promiscuity, suicide attempts, and stealing or shoplifting. This factor may be critical; a person may become bulimic rather than anorexic if she or he cannot resist the impulse to eat, yet feels the body dissatisfaction that is common to both of these disorders.

Childhood experiences with sexual abuse, physical abuse, and posttraumatic stress are additional correlates of bulimia (Rayworth, 2004; Treur, Koperdák, Rózsa, & Füredi, 2005). A survey of a representative sample of bulimic women in the United States (Wonderlich, Wilsnack, Wilsnack, & Harris, 1996) revealed that nearly one-fourth of all female victims of childhood sexual abuse displayed bulimic behaviors later on. These women tend to have more severe symptoms than others (Treur et al., 2005). A relationship also exists between bulimia and depression, but childhood sexual abuse is also related to depression, as are suicide attempts. Body image and eating disorders tend to precede the development of depression in adolescent girls (Kaye, 2008; Stice & Bearman, 2001), which suggests a developmental sequence and may allow the establishment of a chain of causality for the development of bulimia.

Personality factors also differ in bulimics; those who binge and purge fall into different categories (Duncan et al., 2005; Wonderlich et al., 2005). One subgroup of bulimics exhibited more pathology than the other, including more concomitant mental disorders and stronger symptoms of bulimia, whereas another group showed less pathology and less severe symptoms of bulimia. However, depression and anxiety are part of the experience of bulimia.

Who Is Bulimic? In at least one way, the population of bulimics is quite similar to that of anorexics. Both eating disorders occur far more often in women than in men, with about 90% to 95% of those diagnosed in both groups being women (APA, 2000). Whereas anorexia appears primarily among upper-middle-class and upper-class European Americans, bulimia is more democratic, occurring with equal prevalence in various social classes and ethnic groups (Franko et al., 2007).

How prevalent is bulimia? Is its incidence increasing or decreasing? Approximately 1% to 3% of American women and 0.2% of men meet the current diagnostic criteria for bulimia (APA, 2000), making this disorder much more common than anorexia. In a survey of high school students (Eaton et al., 2008), 6.4% of girls and 2.2% of boys said that they had vomited or used laxatives to lose or avoid gaining weight. These percentages reflect a high rate of these behaviors, which suggests a growing prevalence of bulimia. An analysis of the history of this disorder (Keel & Klump, 2003) indicated a substantial increase during the second half of the 20th century. Furthermore, bulimia is restricted to Western cultures and those cultures influenced by Western values, making this eating disorder a culture-bound syndrome.

Is Bulimia Harmful? To many people, bingeing and purging may seem an acceptable means of controlling weight. For others, guilt is a nearly inevitable part of bulimia, and some mental health problems accompany this disorder. However, the question remains: Is bulimia harmful to physical health? Unlike anorexia nervosa, which has a mortality rate of 5% to 10% (Brown, Mehler, & Harris, 2000), bulimia is very seldom fatal. Nevertheless, bulimia has serious detrimental consequences.

The combination of binge eating and purging is harmful in several ways. First, the intake of large quantities of sweets can result in **hypoglycemia**, or a deficiency of sugar in the blood. This may seem paradoxical because the typical binge eater consumes huge amounts of sugar, but the metabolism of sugar prompts insulin release, which drives down blood sugar levels. Low blood sugar results in dizziness, fatigue, depression, and cravings for more sugar, which may prompt another binge. Second, binge eaters seldom eat a balanced diet, and poor nutrition may lead to lethargy and depression. Third, binge eating is expensive. Bulimics can spend more than $100 a day on food, and this expense can lead to other problems, such as financial difficulties or stealing. Also, binge eaters are preoccupied with food in an obsessive way, thinking and planning the next binge. This obsession may leave bulimics with limited time to attend to other activities (Polivy & Herman, 2002).

Purging also leads to several physical problems (McGilley & Pryor, 1998). One of the most common consequences of frequent vomiting is damaged teeth; hydrochloric acid from the stomach erodes the enamel that protects the teeth. Many longtime bulimics need extensive dental work, and dentists are sometimes the first health care professionals to see evidence of bulimia. Hydrochloric acid may also lead to damage in the mouth and esophagus. Bleeding and tearing of the esophagus are not common among bulimics but are very dangerous. Some longtime sufferers report reverse peristalsis, an involuntary regurgitation of food, often after eating quite moderately. Other potential dangers of frequent purging include **anemia**, a reduction in the number of red blood cells; **electrolyte imbalance** caused by the loss of minerals such as sodium, potassium, magnesium, and calcium; and **alkalosis**, an abnormally high level of alkaline in the body tissues resulting from the loss of hydrochloric acid. These conditions may lead to weakness and fatigue. Purging through excessive use of laxatives and diuretics may lead to kidney damage, dehydration, and a spastic colon or the loss of voluntary control over excretory functions. In addition, ingredients in the substances used as laxatives may have toxic properties, adding to the dangers (Steffen, Mitchell, Roerig, & Lancaster, 2007). In summary, bulimia is not a benign eating practice but a serious disorder with a multitude of harmful consequences.

Treatment for Bulimia In one important respect, the treatment of bulimia has a critical advantage over therapy programs for anorexia nervosa—bulimics are more motivated to change their eating behaviors. Unfortunately, this motivation does not guarantee that bulimics will seek therapy.

Cognitive behavior therapy is an effective treatment for bulimia (Butler, Chapman, Forman, & Beck, 2006; Wilson, Fairburn, Agras, Walsh, & Kraemer, 2002). Cognitive behavior therapists work toward changing both distorted cognitions, such as obsessive body concerns, and behaviors, such as bingeing, vomiting, and laxative use. Specific techniques may include keeping a diary on the factors related to bingeing and on feelings after purging, monitoring caloric intake, eating slowly, eating regular meals, and clarifying distorted views of eating and weight control. A review of the effectiveness of cognitive behavioral treatment (Butler et al., 2006) revealed its effectiveness. Applied to bulimia, this treatment is very effective (Compas, Haaga, Keefe, Leitenberg, & Williams, 1998); the average reduction in the frequency of binge eating was 80%, an unusually high percentage of success for any type of therapy.

Interpersonal psychotherapy has also been used successfully in treating bulimics (Wilson et al., 2002). Interpersonal psychotherapy is a nonintrospective, short-term therapy that was originally applied to depression. It focuses on present interpersonal problems and not on eating, taking the approach that eating problems tend to appear in late adolescence when interpersonal issues present major developmental challenges. In this view, eating problems represent maladaptive attempts to cope. The success rate of interpersonal therapy is comparable to that of cognitive behavioral therapy (Wilson et al., 2002), but it does not work as quickly. Some research (Constantino, Arnow,

Blasey, & Agras, 2005) indicates that matching patient characteristics and expectations to therapy intervention improves the success of both cognitive behavioral and interpersonal therapy.

Drugs, especially the antidepressant fluoxetine (Prozac), have been used for some time in the treatment of bulimia with good success (Mitchell & Selders, 2005). Psychotherapy is a better choice for most patients than drugs alone. The combination of drugs and psychotherapy may also be a good choice for some bulimic patients (Trunko, Rockwell, Curry, Runfola, & Kaye, 2007).

Preventing bulimia would be more desirable than treatment, and some programs attempt to change the attitudes that put people at risk. These programs are aimed at young women with the risk factors of low self-esteem, poor body image, high acceptance of the thin body ideal, a strong need for perfection, a history of repeated dieting, and other dysfunctional eating behaviors or attitudes. Some programs are school based, whereas others target young women at high risk. One typical strategy is psychoeducational, which attempts to change the acceptance of the thin body ideal and boost self-esteem. Programs that aim to reduce unhealthy dieting have demonstrated some success (O'Brien & LeBow, 2007). Better success occurred through adding a weight control component oriented toward building healthy eating while controlling weight (Stice, Presnell, Groesz, & Shaw, 2005; Stice, Trost, & Chase, 2003). Thus, programs that address the cognitive component of bulimia and offer a healthy way to manage body concerns may be more successful in averting development of this disorder.

Binge Eating Disorder

Many people eat too much at times, such as parties or holidays, but binge eating disorder is more than an occasional overindulgence. Binge eating consists of the same type of out-of-control eating that is symptomatic of bulimia, but without any form of purging. This category is under consideration for inclusion as a disorder in the *DSM* by the American Psychiatric Association (APA, 2000). To be diagnosed with this disorder, people must exhibit frequent (at least twice a week for at least six months) binge eating episodes with

BECOMING HEALTHIER

1. Develop your eating competence (Stotts et al., 2007) by getting good information about nutrition and using that information in deciding on a healthy diet.

2. Be more concerned with eating a healthy diet than with your weight.

3. Consult a chart that contains height–weight recommendations or body mass index rather than a fashion magazine to determine what is the correct weight for you.

4. Give up dieting, but also give up overeating.

5. Concentrate less on food restriction and more on exercise as a way to change your body shape.

6. Do not skip meals as a way to lose weight, especially breakfast; people who eat breakfast are less likely to be overweight than those who skip breakfast (Purslow et al., 2008).

7. Do not compare your body to those of models and actors or actresses. These images furnish unrealistic and unattainable body images that tend to make people unhappy with their own bodies.

8. Understand that losing weight will not solve all your problems.

9. If you lose weight, know when to stop. Listen to people who tell you that you have lost enough.

10. Do not hide how little you weigh from friends or family by wearing baggy clothing.

11. When you make dietary changes, find ways to keep eating a pleasurable activity. Feelings of deprivation and going without favorite foods can make you too miserable to care about eating correctly.

12. Do not use diet drugs, fast, or go on a very low calorie diet to lose weight, even if you are very obese.

13. Do not vomit as a way to keep from gaining weight.

14. Learn how to see someone who is normal weight or slightly overweight as attractive. Look for such people in the news and in the media.

feelings of a lack of control, and they must experience distress over this behavior.

Who Are Binge Eaters? Eating large quantities of food would seem to be a risk for obesity, and it is (Stice, Presnell, & Spangler, 2002). Many individuals who are obese experience binge eating. An examination of women with eating disorders (Striegel-Moore et al., 2004) revealed that binge eaters had higher BMIs than women with other eating disorders and experienced an even greater degree of body dissatisfaction. Binge eating is common to bulimia and, to a lesser degree, to anorexia; thus, it is not surprising that individuals with any of these eating disorders exhibit similar self-esteem, body dissatisfaction, and weight concerns (Decaluwé & Braet, 2005; Grilo et al., 2008). Alcohol problems are also common to both bulimics and binge eaters (Krahn, Kurth, Gomberg, & Drewnowski, 2005).

As with anorexics, binge eaters are more likely to be female than male, but binge eating is more common among men than anorexia or bulimia is (Hudson et al., 2007). The loss of control that characterizes binge eating occurs among children younger than 12 years old (Tanofsky-Kraff, Marcus, Yanovski, & Yanovski, 2008) and among adolescents (Goldschmidt et al., 2008), representing a major factor in obesity for these age groups. In addition, all ethnic groups are represented, and binge eating occurs in non-Western societies at rates that are similar to those in the United States and Europe (Becker, Burwell, Navara, & Gilman, 2003). Binge eating is also more common than either anorexia or bulimia—the estimated prevalence is at least 2% of the population. As with other eating disorders, most people with symptoms are not diagnosed and thus do not receive treatment.

Like others with eating disorders, people who experience eating binges also tend to have other behavioral or psychiatric problems, which complicates the diagnosis of this disorder (Stunkard & Allison, 2003). Indeed, the presence of personality disorders is one criterion that distinguishes

TABLE 14.6

Comparison of Anorexia, Bulimia, and Binge Eating

	Anorexia	Bulimia	Binge Eating
Body weight	<17.5 BMI	Normal	Overweight
Distorted body image	Yes	Yes	Yes
Percent affected			
Women	0.9%	1–3%	3.5%
Men	0.3%	0.5%	2.0%
Vulnerability			
Gender	Women	Women	Women
Age	Adolescent & young adult	Adolescent & young adult	Adults
Ethnicity	European & European American	All	All
Prominent characteristics	Ambitious, perfectionist, anxiety disorders	Impulsive, sensation-seeking	Personality disorders
Alcohol or drug abuse problems	Not common	Common	Common
Obsessive thoughts	Body fat and control	Food and next binge	Food and next binge
Health risks	5–10% mortality	Hypoglycemia, anemia, electrolyte imbalance	Obesity
Treatment success	50%; relapse is a risk	80%; relapse is a risk	Good success for binges but weight loss is difficult

binge eaters from those who are obese but do not binge (van Hanswijck de Jonge, van Furth, Lacey, & Waller, 2003). Table 14.6 presents a comparison of anorexia, bulimia, and binge eating.

Treatment for Binge Eating Treatments for binge eating face the challenge of changing an established eating pattern plus helping binge eaters lose weight. Cognitive behavioral therapy is effective in helping people control binge eating, but it is not very effective in promoting weight loss (Grilo, Masheb, & Wilson, 2005; Yager, 2008). Nor are obese binge eaters good candidates for weight loss surgery; this drastic intervention does not help in managing binges (Yager, 2008).

Thus, researchers have searched for a component to add to therapy programs. One consideration was antidepressant drugs, such as fluoxetine (Prozac), which has some use in relieving psychiatric problems. However, adding this drug to cognitive behavioral therapy does not boost the effectiveness of the program. Adding

the weight loss drug orlistat, however, proved more effective (Grilo, Masheb, & Salant, 2005), and adding the drug sibutramine may be even more so (Yager, 2008).

Perception of the problem also plays a role in treatment for binge eaters. Some people who experience binges seek treatment for the bingeing behavior, whereas others see their main problem as overweight. Those who focused on their binge eating tended to choose cognitive behavioral therapy; those who saw their problem as weight were more likely to choose a therapy with that goal (Brody, Masheb, & Grilo, 2005). This type of tailoring is an advantage for many therapies and problems.

IN SUMMARY

Some people begin a weight loss program that seemingly gets out of control and turns into an almost total fasting regimen. This eating disorder, called anorexia nervosa, is uncommon but most prevalent among young, high-achieving women who have high body dissatisfaction and believe that being thin will solve their problems. Anorexia is very difficult to treat successfully because people with this disorder continue to see themselves as too fat and thus lack the motivation to change their eating habits. A type of family therapy and cognitive behavioral therapy are more effective than other approaches.

Bulimia is an eating disorder characterized by uncontrolled binge eating, usually accompanied by guilt and followed by vomiting or other purgative methods. In general terms, bulimics are more likely than other people to be depressed and impulsive, which may lead to alcohol and other drug abuse and stealing. In addition, they are more likely to have been victims of childhood family or sexual abuse, to be dissatisfied with their bodies, and to use food as a coping strategy.

Treatment for bulimia has generally been more successful than treatment for anorexia, partly because of bulimics' greater motivation to change. The more successful programs for eating disorders are those that include cognitive behavioral techniques, which seek to change not only eating patterns but also the pathological concerns about weight and eating, and interpersonal therapy, which focuses on relationship issues. Antidepressant drugs have been used with limited success to treat bulimia.

Although not yet officially classified as a disorder in the *DSM*, binge eating presents problems. Those who experience binges are often overweight or obese and share impulse control and other psychological problems common to those with bulimia. Women are more likely to be binge eaters, but more men have this than any other eating disorder. Treatment faces the problems of altering maladaptive eating patterns and body image problems as well as promoting weight loss. Cognitive behavioral therapy is effective with the former, but losing weight is a difficult problem, as we have seen.

ANSWERS

This chapter has addressed six basic questions:

1. How does the digestive system function?

The digestive system turns food into nutrients by breaking down food into particles that can be absorbed. The process of breaking down food begins in the mouth and continues in the stomach, but absorption of most nutrients occurs in the small intestine. A complex signaling system involves hormones produced in the body and brain and received by the hypothalamus and other brain structures to control eating and weight. Hormones such as ghrelin, neuropeptide Y, agouti-related peptide, the orexins, and melanin-concentrating hormone increase appetite and feelings of hunger, whereas leptin, insulin, cholecystokinin (CCK), glucagon-like peptide 1, and peptide YY are involved in satiation.

2. What factors are involved in weight maintenance?

Weight maintenance depends largely on two factors: the number of calories absorbed through food intake and the number expended through body metabolism and physical activity. Experimental starvation has demonstrated that losing weight leads to irritability, aggression, apathy, lack of interest in sex, and preoccupation with food. Initial weight loss may be easy, but the slowing of metabolic rate makes drastic weight loss difficult. Experimental overeating has demonstrated that gaining weight can be almost as difficult and unpleasant as losing it.

3. What is obesity, and how does it affect health?

Obesity can be defined in terms of percent body fat, body mass index (BMI), or social standards, all of which yield different estimates for the prevalence of obesity. Over the past 25 years, obesity has become more common in the United States and other countries, but the ideal body has become thinner. The difficulty of either losing or gaining weight and the discovery of leptin, ghrelin, and the orexins have led many investigators to adopt the notion of a natural setpoint for weight maintenance. Obesity seems to be a deviation from this regulation that has genetic components, but the recent rapid growth of obesity is not compatible with a genetic model. An alternative view holds that positive aspects of eating lead people to overeat when a variety of tasty foods is available, which is the situation in the United States and other industrialized countries.

Obesity is associated with increased mortality, heart disease, Type 2 diabetes, and digestive tract diseases, and the very thinnest and the very heaviest people are at the greatest risk for death. Severe obesity and carrying excess weight around the waist rather than hips are both risks of death from several causes, especially heart disease.

4. Is dieting a good way to lose weight?

A cultural obsession with thinness has led to a plethora of diets, many of which are neither safe nor permanently effective. Changing from overeating to healthier eating patterns and incorporating exercise are wise choices for weight change, whereas liposuction, diet drugs, fasting, and very low calorie diets are not.

5. What is anorexia nervosa, and how can it be treated?

Anorexia nervosa is an eating disorder characterized by self-starvation. This disorder is most prevalent among young, high-achieving women with body image problems but is uncommon, affecting less than 1% of the population. Anorexics are very difficult to treat successfully because they continue to see themselves as too fat and thus lack the motivation to change their eating habits. Cognitive behavioral therapy and a specific type of family therapy are more effective than other approaches.

6. What is bulimia, and how does it differ from binge eating?

Bulimia is an eating disorder characterized by uncontrolled binge eating, usually accompanied by guilt and followed by vomiting or other purgative methods. Bulimia is more common than anorexia, affecting between 1% and 3% of the population. Their motivation to change eating patterns has made bulimics better therapy candidates than anorexics. Treatment for bulimia, especially cognitive behavioral therapy and interpersonal therapy, has generally been successful.

Binge eating is similar to bulimia in terms of binges, but binge eaters do not purge. Thus, they are often overweight or obese, whereas bulimics tend to be normal weight. Binge eating is also more common than bulimia, especially among men. The two disorders are similar in terms of impulsivity, history of family violence, and coexisting personality disorders. Binge eating is more difficult to treat because therapy must address both binge eating and weight problems.

SUGGESTED READINGS

Brownell, K. D., & Horgen, K. B. (2004). *Food fight: The inside story of the food industry, America's obesity crisis, and what we can do about it.* New York: McGraw-Hill. In this controversial book, Kelly Brownell and Katherine Horgen contend that obesity is the result not of a lack of willpower but of a "toxic food environment" created by the food industry.

Bruch, H. (1978). *The golden cage: The enigma of anorexia nervosa.* Cambridge, MA: Harvard University Press. Written by one of the leading authorities on anorexia nervosa, this nontechnical book is a classic in the field of anorexia. Bruch describes anorexia and suggests methods of treating this eating disorder.

Polivy, J., & Herman, C. P. (2004). Sociocultural idealization of thin female body shapes: An introduction to the special issues on body image and eating disorders. *Journal of Social and Clinical Psychology, 23,* 1–6. These prominent researchers provide an interesting perspective on eating and eating disorders that summarizes the findings of articles from a special issue devoted to this topic.

The truth about dieting. (2002, June). *Consumer Reports, 67*(6), 26–31. Although this article in a popular magazine does not contain the latest research on dieting, its review and conclusions remain valid. The article reports on the results of a survey of more than 30,000 dieters—both successful and unsuccessful. From these results, the article presents suggestions about how to change eating patterns for permanent weight loss.

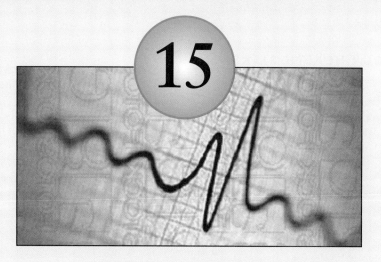

15

EXERCISING

QUESTIONS

This chapter focuses on six basic questions:

1. What are the different types of physical activity?

2. Does physical activity benefit the cardiovascular system?

3. What are some other health benefits of physical activity?

4. Can physical activity be hazardous?

5. How much is enough but not too much?

6. What are some problems in maintaining an exercise program?

CHECK YOUR HEALTH RISKS

Check the items that apply to you.

☐ 1. Whenever the urge to exercise comes over me, I sit down until the urge goes away.

☐ 2. My family history of heart disease means that I am going to have a heart attack whether I exercise or not.

☐ 3. When it comes to exercise, I subscribe to the motto "No pain, no gain."

☐ 4. I have changed jobs in order to have more time to train for competitive athletic events.

☐ 5. I use exercise along with diet as a means of controlling my weight.

☐ 6. People have advised me to start an exercise program, but I just never seem to have the time or energy.

☐ 7. One of the reasons I exercise is that I believe that a person can't be too thin and that exercise will help me continue to lose weight.

☐ 8. I may begin an exercise program when I'm older, but now I'm young and in good shape.

☐ 9. I'm too old and out of shape to begin exercising.

☐ 10. I'd probably have a heart attack if I started to jog or run.

☐ 11. I'd like to exercise, but I can't run, and walking isn't strenuous enough to be good exercise.

☐ 12. I try not to let injuries interfere with my regular exercise routine.

Except for item 5, each of these items represents a health risk from either too little or too much exercise. Count your check marks to evaluate your risks. As you read this chapter, you will learn that some of these items are riskier than others.

REAL-WORLD PROFILE OF JIM FIXX

At age 35, Jim Fixx was 50 pounds overweight, smoked two packs of cigarettes a day, and except for an occasional game of tennis or touch football, generally lived a sedentary life as a magazine editor. But at that point, his life changed dramatically. By his own account, the impetus for this transformation was a pulled leg muscle he incurred while playing tennis. To rehabilitate his leg and avoid another muscle pull, Fixx began a modest exercise program. Painfully he jogged half a mile or so three or four times a week. Gradually he increased both his distance and his speed, and running began to play an increasingly important role in his life.

His exercise routine slowly altered both his physical appearance and his attitude toward his health. He lost weight, stopped smoking, felt physically rejuvenated, and came to believe strongly in the preventive and curative powers of running. Perhaps too much so. On a warm July day in 1984, Jim Fixx died while returning from his afternoon run. The cause of death was listed as sudden **cardiac arrhythmia** due to coronary artery disease.

Because Jim Fixx, like some other runners, died during or immediately after exercising, some controversy arose over the potential hazards of strenuous physical activity. However, Fixx had a family history of heart problems; his father suffered a heart attack at age 35 and died of another one at 43. Fixx, then, outlived his father by 9 years—so perhaps his 17 years of long-distance running provided more benefits than risks. Some people conclude that exercise is hazardous to health. Others, however, argue that Fixx would have died earlier if he had not become a runner.

Although Jim Fixx died more than 20 years ago, his popular books on the joys of running motivated others to begin a running program (Fixx, 1977, 1980). In the years since Fixx's death, most people in the United States have become aware of the health benefits of regular exercise. A substantial portion of the population now believes that regular physical activity plays an important role in people's health.

TYPES OF PHYSICAL ACTIVITY

Although exercise can include hundreds of different kinds of physical activities, physiologically there are only five types of exercise: isometric, isotonic, isokinetic, anaerobic, and aerobic. Each has different goals, different activities, and different advocates. Each can contribute to some aspect of fitness or health, but aerobic exercise produces benefits for cardiorespiratory health.

Isometric exercise is performed by contracting muscles against an immovable object. Although the body does not move in isometric exercise, muscles push hard against each other or against an immovable object and thus produce increases in strength. Pushing hard against a solid wall is an example of isometric exercise. Because joints do not move, it may not be apparent that exercise is occurring, but the contraction of muscles produces gains in strength—but little else. This type of physical activity can improve muscle strength, which can be especially important for older people in preserving independent living.

Isotonic exercise requires the contraction of muscles and the movement of joints. Weight lifting and many forms of calisthenics fit into this category. Programs based on isotonic exercise can improve muscle strength and muscle endurance if the program is sufficiently lengthy. Again, older people can profit from isotonic exercise, but many people in a weight-lifting program are bodybuilders interested in improving the appearance of their body rather than improving health.

In **isokinetic exercise,** exertion is required for lifting, and additional effort is required to return to the starting position. This type of exercise requires specialized equipment that adjusts the amount of resistance according to the amount of force applied. Isokinetic exercise is frequently used to restore muscle strength and muscle endurance in people who have suffered muscle injuries. It is an important adjunct in physical rehabilitation,

helping injured people to regain strength and flexibility with more safety than other types of exercise.

Anaerobic exercises require short, intensive bursts of energy but no increased amount of oxygen use. This form of exercise includes short-distance running, some calisthenics, softball, and other exercises that require intense, short-term energy. Such exercises improve speed and endurance, but they may carry risks for people with coronary heart disease.

Aerobic exercise is any exercise that requires dramatically increased oxygen consumption over an extended period of time. Aerobic exercise includes jogging, walking at a brisk pace, cross-country skiing, dancing, rope skipping, swimming, cycling, and other activities that increase oxygen consumption.

The important characteristics of aerobic exercise are intensity and duration. Exercise must be intense enough to elevate the heart rate into a certain range, which is computed from a formula based on age and the maximum possible heart rate. This type of program requires elevated oxygen use and provides a workout for both the respiratory system, which furnishes the oxygen, and the coronary system, which pumps the blood. Of the various approaches to fitness, aerobic activity is superior to other types of exercise in developing cardiorespiratory health. Although current recommendations call for a person to engage in some aerobic exercise at least three times a week, any is better than none.

Kenneth Cooper (1968, 1982, 1985), one of the early advocates of aerobic exercise, was also one of the first to recommend caution in adopting an aerobic exercise program. First, he recommended a medical examination before beginning a program of aerobic exercise, because potentially dangerous coronary abnormalities can exist without any apparent symptoms. Second, he strongly suggested the use of an exercise electrocardiogram, known as a stress test, to detect any abnormal cardiac activity during exercise. Third, Cooper suggested less strenuous activity than some of his contemporaries. For example, Jim Fixx advocated running long distances 6 or 7 days a week, whereas Cooper maintained that jogging or speed walking 3 miles a day 5 days a week confers an optimum level of cardiovascular fitness. For Cooper, more frequent exercise or greater distance does not confer much additional benefit and may increase the chances of injury. In a later section of this chapter, we examine the question of how much exercise is enough and how much is too much.

REASONS FOR EXERCISING

People exercise for a variety of reasons, some that are consistent with good health and some that are not. Reasons for adhering to a physical activity program include physical fitness, weight control, cardiovascular health, increased longevity, protection against cancer, prevention of osteoporosis, control of diabetes, enhanced self-esteem, and as a buffer against depression, anxiety, and stress. This chapter looks at evidence relating to each of these reasons as well as to the potential hazards of physical activity.

Physical Fitness

Does physical activity help people become physically fit? The effects of exercise on fitness depend both on the duration and intensity of the exercise and on the definition of fitness. To most exercise physiologists, fitness is a complex condition consisting of muscle strength, muscle endurance, flexibility, and cardiorespiratory (aerobic) fitness. Each of the five types of exercise can contribute to these four different aspects of fitness, but no one type fulfills all the requirements.

In addition, fitness can be considered in terms of both organic and dynamic fitness. *Organic fitness* is the capacity for action and movement that is determined by inherent characteristics of the body. These organic factors include genetic endowment, age, and health limitations. *Dynamic fitness* is acquired through various types of physical activity, whereas organic fitness is not. A person can have a good level of organic fitness and yet be "out of shape" and perform poorly. Another person may train and improve dynamic fitness but still be unable to win races because of relatively poor organic fitness. Athletes who want to be champions need to have been very selective about

choosing their biological parents in order to have inherited a high level of organic fitness. Aspiring champions must train in order to gain the dynamic fitness necessary for optimal athletic performance. Michael Phelps, who broke records for swimming in the 2008 Olympics, had an excellent balance of organic and dynamic fitness—he inherited a body suited to swimming, but he needed to work hard to break records. The following discussion is concerned almost exclusively with dynamic fitness and its components, because this type of fitness can be modified through exercise, whereas organic fitness cannot.

Muscle Strength and Endurance Two components of physical fitness are muscle strength and muscle endurance. Muscle strength is a measure of how strongly a muscle can contract. This type of fitness can be achieved through isometric, isotonic, isokinetic, and to a lesser extent, anaerobic exercise. All these types of exercise have the capability to increase muscle strength, because they involve contracting muscles.

Muscle endurance differs from muscle strength in that it requires continued performance. Some strength is necessary for muscle endurance, but the opposite is not true: A muscle may be strong but not have the endurance to continue its performance. Exercises that improve strength require greater exertion for limited repetitions; exercises that improve endurance require less exertion but are performed many times (Knuttgen, 2007). Both muscle strength and muscle endurance improve through similar types of exercises, including isometric, isotonic, and isokinetic.

Flexibility Flexibility is the range-of-motion capacity of a joint. The types of exercises that develop muscle strength and muscle endurance generally do not improve flexibility. Moreover, flexibility is specific to each joint, so that exercises designed to develop flexibility tend to be quite varied. In addition to being a component of fitness, flexibility also decreases the likelihood of injury in other types of physical activity, especially aerobic and anaerobic exercise.

Flexibility is best attained through slow, sustained stretching exercises. Fast, jerky, bouncing movements are not recommended, as they can cause soreness and injury. Flexibility training is typically not as intense as strength and endurance training. Yoga and tai chi provide the types of movements that increase flexibility.

Aerobic Fitness Of all the types of physical activity, aerobic exercise contributes most to cardiorespiratory fitness. When people acquire aerobic fitness, they improve cardiorespiratory health in several ways. First, they increase the amount of oxygen that can be used during strenuous exercise, and second, they increase the amount of blood pumped with each heartbeat. These changes result in a lowering of both resting heart rate and resting blood pressure and increase the efficiency of the cardiovascular system (Cooper, 2001). This type of exercise helps protect both men and women from heart disease and a variety of other diseases (Murphy et al., 2007).

Weight Control

In recent years, obesity has become a worldwide problem, with many people adopting a sedentary lifestyle, spending much of their time watching television, viewing videos, playing computer games, surfing the Internet, and talking on cell phones. This epidemic of obesity suggests that physical activity contributes to weight control and that activity also relates to body composition—that is, the ratio of fat to muscle. Research confirms these two suggestions.

Most experts see obesity as a long-term accumulation of excess body fat (Forbes, 2000; Hansen, Shriver, & Schoeller, 2005). Although the exact formula of dietary fat to amount of physical activity is not fully understood, most exercise physiologists believe that exercise is an important element in the development of obesity. However, the level of exercise needed for cardiovascular health is not necessarily the same as that needed for weight control. For example, a study in Finland (Barengo et al., 2004) found that 15 minutes of walking or cycling to and from work reduced both cardiovascular mortality and all-cause mortality. This and dozens of other studies have found that relatively low levels of physical activity can benefit cardiovascular health. However, the

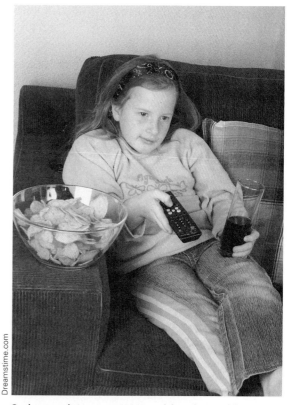

Sedentary leisure activities add to the problem of childhood obesity.

amount of exercise necessary to prompt weight loss is far greater. Some authorities (Jakicic & Otto, 2005) now recommend that obese people need to spend at least 60 minutes a day engaged in moderate to heavy physical activity to bring about initial weight loss and to maintain that loss. Other sources agree (Hill & Wyatt, 2005), suggesting that formerly obese people must spend 60 to 90 minutes performing moderate to intense physical activity to maintain weight loss. Length and intensity of physical activity seem to be required for long-lasting weight control, which seems to require more exercise than the amount needed for cardiovascular health.

A second consideration deals with exercise as a means of sculpting an ideal body shape. Unfortunately, exercise is quite limited as a method of spot reduction. Muscle and fat have little to do with one another, and it is possible to have both in the same part of the body. Both fat and muscle tissue are depleted when people lose weight. If people exercise during weight reduction, they build muscle tissue while losing fat, which may build a more attractive body shape. Spot reduction appears to be the result, because fat tends to be lost from the places where it was most abundant. However, fat distribution is under strong genetic control, and people with large hips or thighs in relation to other body parts will have large hips or thighs after they lose weight. Despite some exercise promoters' claims, a particular callisthenic exercise will not reduce fat in a specific part of the body.

Inactive people who are concerned about weight and who have recently stopped smoking should strongly consider beginning a physical activity program. Steven Blair and Tim Church (2004) claimed that such an exercise program would be at least as effective as dieting in controlling weight and much better than dieting in changing the ratio of fat to muscle tissue. An early study supported this view. Investigators randomly assigned sedentary obese men to one of three groups: dieters, runners, or controls (Wood et al., 1988). The dieters did not exercise, the runners did not diet, and the controls did neither. After a year, people in both the exercise group and the dieting group had lost about the same amount of weight, and both of these groups had lost more than people in the control group. However, some important differences emerged in comparing the dieters and the runners. Although both groups had lost an equal amount of weight, the dieters lost both fat and lean tissue, whereas the runners lost only fat tissue and retained more lean muscle tissue.

Exercise does not produce much weight loss through burning calories; for example, more than 30 minutes of tennis is required to work off the calories in two doughnuts. However, sitting and eating doughnuts is a risk for obesity in two ways—the sitting and the eating. Rather, most of the weight loss associated with exercise comes from elevation of the metabolic rate, the rate at which the body metabolizes calories. The resulting increase in the number of calories burned can produce changes in weight that exceed the number of calories spent in any activity.

IN SUMMARY

All physical activity can be subsumed under one or more of five basic categories: isometric, isotonic, isokinetic, anaerobic, and aerobic. Each of these five exercise types has advantages and disadvantages for improving physical fitness, but only aerobic exercise benefits cardiorespiratory health.

People have a variety of reasons for maintaining an exercise regimen, including physical fitness, aerobic health, and weight control. The various types of exercise can increase dynamic fitness, strengthen muscles, improve endurance, and increase flexibility. Aerobic fitness reduces death not only from cardiovascular disease but also from all causes.

One popular reason for remaining physically active is to control weight and achieve a sculpted body. Physical activity can help people lose weight, but its capacity for spot reduction is very limited. Overweight people can lose weight through moderate physical activity, highly active thin people can maintain lean body mass through proper diet, and people of moderate weight can increase lean body weight without an overall weight gain.

Physical Activity and Cardiovascular Health

During the early years of the 20th century, physicians often advised patients with heart disease to avoid strenuous physical activity, based on the belief that too much physical activity could damage the heart and threaten a person's life. (Figure 9.7 in Chapter 9 paints a dramatic picture of the rise and fall of death rates from cardiovascular disease throughout the 20th century.) During the middle of that century, some cardiologists began to rethink this advice and to recommend aerobic exercise both as an adjunct to standard treatment and as a protection against heart disease. At about the same time, many people (some influenced by Jim Fixx) began running, not only for cardiovascular health, but also for a variety of other reasons. Later in this section, we examine the evidence for the cardiovascular benefits of exercise, but first we look briefly at the history of studies that examined exercise and cardiovascular health.

Early Studies

During the early 1950s, Jerremy Morris and his colleagues (Morris, Heady, Raffle, Roberts, & Parks, 1953) made history with their observation that physical activity was related to cardiovascular disease. This observation took place in England and involved London's famous double-decker buses. Morris and his colleagues discovered that physically active male conductors differed from the sedentary drivers in their incidence of heart disease. This study, of course, did not prove that physical activity decreases the chances of coronary heart disease (CHD), because these two groups of workers may have been selected for jobs on the basis of body type, personality, or some other factor associated with a high or low risk of CHD.

Ten years later, Harold Kahn (1963) investigated the relationship between physical activity and heart disease among postal workers in Washington, D.C. When Kahn compared the death rates among sedentary postal workers versus the more active mail carriers, he found lower CHD death rates among the active men. A more important finding was that the potential benefits from past activity disappeared after a few years. When mail carriers switched to more sedentary clerical jobs, their rates of CHD changed. After more than five years of working as a clerk, former carriers had an incidence of death from CHD equal to that of men who had always been clerks. This finding suggested that exercise should be incorporated into one's lifestyle on a continuing basis.

These studies seemed to indicate that workers who are physically active have a reduced risk of coronary heart disease. However, the studies did not address the problem of self-selection that clouds any conclusion about exercise benefits. Also, after five years, the postal workers were five years older than they were at the beginning of the study, and age is a factor in heart disease. Furthermore, none of the early studies measured the workers' activity levels *off* the job. Most of these

issues have been addressed in more recent studies, including a series of investigations by Ralph Paffenbarger, who was a professor of epidemiology at Stanford University School of Medicine and the Harvard School of Public Health. He investigated the relationship between physical activity and health in two large populations of participants: San Francisco longshoremen and Harvard alumni.

The San Francisco longshoremen study began in 1951 to examine CHD deaths over time (Paffenbarger, Gima, Laughlin, & Black, 1971; Paffenbarger, Laughlin, Gima, & Black, 1970). In general, they found that CHD death rates were much higher for workers with low versus high activity. In these studies, the problem of initial self-selection was not a major factor, because all workers in both the high- and low-activity groups had begun their employment with at least five years of strenuous cargo handling. From these and other studies, Paffenbarger concluded that high-intensity exercise produces a training effect that protects against coronary heart disease.

In the late 1970s, Paffenbarger and his associates (Paffenbarger, Wing, & Hyde, 1978) published a landmark epidemiological study based on extensive medical records of former Harvard University students, their weekly total energy expenditure, and a composite physical activity index that took into account all activity, both on and off the job. Paffenbarger and his colleagues then divided the Harvard alumni into high- and low-activity groups. Of those men whose energy levels could be determined, about 60% expended fewer than 2,000 kcal per week and were thus placed in the low-activity group; the 40% who expended more than 2,000 kcal made up the high-activity group. (Note that 2,000 kcal of energy is approximately that expended in 20 miles of jogging or its equivalent.) The results of this study showed that the least active Harvard alumni had an increased risk of heart attack over their more physically active classmates, with 2,000 kcal per week as the breaking point. In addition, exercise benefited men who smoked, had a history of hypertension, or both. Beyond the 2,000 kcal per week expenditure, increased exercise paid no dividends in

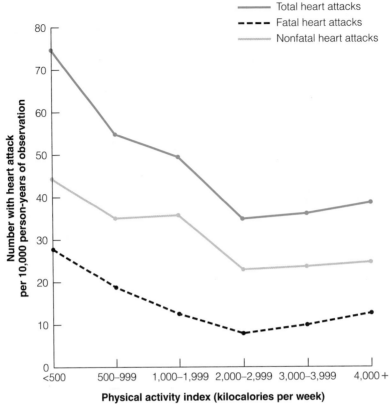

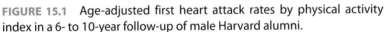

FIGURE 15.1   Age-adjusted first heart attack rates by physical activity index in a 6- to 10-year follow-up of male Harvard alumni.

Source: Adapted from "Physical Activity as an Index of Heart Attack Risk in College Alumni," by R. S. Paffenbarger, Jr., A. L. Wing, and R. T. Hyde, 1978, *American Journal of Epidemiology, 108,* p. 166. Copyright © 1978 by The Johns Hopkins University School of Hygiene and Public Health. Reprinted by permission of Oxford University Press.

terms of reduced risk of fatal or nonfatal heart attacks. Figure 15.1 shows this relationship.

Later Studies

In October 2000, an international panel of scientists met in Toronto to hold a symposium on evidence for a dose–response relationship between physical activity and several measures of health, including cardiovascular disease and all-cause mortality (Bouchard, 2001; Kesaniemi et al., 2001). (Recall that a dose–response relationship is a direct, consistent association between an independent variable, such as physical activity, and a dependent variable, such as heart disease or all-cause mortality.) Panelists at this conference evaluated existing research, giving most weight to randomized, controlled trials. In general, a review of the research found a consistent inverse association between levels of physical activity and cardiovascular disease for both women and men (Kohl, 2001). Even minimal levels of exercise provided some protection against heart disease. Another review from this symposium (Lee & Skerrett, 2001) concluded that a strong dose–response relationship existed between physical activity and premature death; higher levels were proportionately related to lower death rates.

Evidence also shows cardiovascular benefits among people in a variety of nations and different ethnic groups. For example, many Mexican Americans are at risk for obesity, high cholesterol, and other cardiovascular risk factors, which suggests that they can probably profit from a routine exercise program. A study of Mexican Americans in the San Antonio Heart Study (Rainwater et al., 2000) found that changes in physical activity over a five-year period tended to mirror changes in CVD risk factors. The evidence was somewhat stronger for men than for women and for participants who were lean at the beginning of the study than for those who were heavy.

Physical activity appears to offer protection against cardiovascular disease; four decades of studies on this topic have revealed unmistakable patterns (Myers, 2000; Schlicht, Kanning, & Bös, 2007). First, people who are already active receive some gains by increasing their level of activity, but the largest gains occur when people go from a sedentary lifestyle to an active one. Second, walking, especially for older people, confers protection against CVD (Murphy et al. 2007). Third, an inactive lifestyle has been shown to be equal to diabetes, high cholesterol level, smoking, and high blood pressure as a CVD risk factor. Fourth, physically fit men and women in all age groups can reduce their CVD risk through leisure-time activities. Fifth, exercise accumulated several years ago does not provide much current protection against all-cause mortality. Similarly, people who survive a heart attack and who include physical activity as part of their cardiac rehabilitation program decreased their all-cause mortality as well as their risk for a subsequent heart attack. However, those benefits disappear after five years if participants stop exercising. Thus, because previous physical activity loses its benefit after a few years, heart attack survivors should maintain their exercise program.

Exercise also offers protection against stroke. Researchers from the Nurses' Health Study (Hu et al., 2000) found that the most active women, compared with sedentary women, reduced their risk of death from ischemic stroke by about 34% and that a dose–response relationship existed between levels of physical activity and protection from ischemic stroke. Individuals who had a stroke were less physically active than others, including less physical activity in the week preceding their stroke (Krarup et al., 2007). Similarly, a meta-analysis (Wendel-Vos et al., 2004) found

that high levels of occupational and leisure-time physical activity reduce the risk of both ischemic stroke and hemorrhagic stroke.

These and other reports on cardiovascular disease suggest that a lifestyle that includes at least some physical activity can help protect people against premature cardiovascular disease, including stroke. Even small amounts of activity can help, but more is better, at least to a point. (In a later section, we discuss how much is enough without being too much.)

Do Women and Men Benefit Equally?

All the earlier studies on the cardiovascular effects of exercise had one important limitation: They focused exclusively on men. To complete the picture of the health benefits of exercise, later researchers extended their investigations to women. Gender differences in degree of physical activity, leisure-time activity, and job-related activity might suggest differences between men and women in their level of protection against cardiovascular disease and all-cause mortality.

A number of studies looked exclusively at women to see if the benefits of physical activity extend equally to them. For example, a study of postmenopausal women in Iowa (Kushi et al., 1997) found that older women who exercised moderately at least four times a week had much lower rates of all-cause mortality than women who were sedentary. Even moderate physical activity once a week significantly reduced the chances of death from CVD. In this study, vigorous activity also reduced death rates but was not superior to moderate physical activity. A report from the Nurses' Health Study (Rockhill et al., 2001) showed that active middle-aged and older women reduced their risk of death by 20% to 30%. Paffenbarger and his associates (Oguma, Sesso, Paffenbarger, & Lee, 2002) looked at 37 prospective cohort studies and one retrospective study that dealt with the association between all-cause mortality and both physical activity and physical fitness in women. The results generally indicated that women can gain about as much as men from physical activity. Inactive women were much more likely than active women to have died during the study period. An energy expenditure of about 1,000 kilocalories per week is probably adequate to avoid premature death. (See Figure 15.1 for a relationship between level of kilocalories and first heart attack in men.) Evidence is not as strong concerning a dose–response relationship between levels of physical activity and all-cause mortality in women as it is for men.

In summary, both women and men can improve their cardiovascular health and live longer with light to moderate exercise. Physically active people can expect an average increase in longevity of about two years (Blair, Cheng, & Holder, 2001). A cynic might criticize this finding by pointing out that a person would need to jog a total of about two years between the ages of 20 and 80 to increase longevity by two years. Why live another two years if one must spend that time exercising? However, physical activity does not merely extend the life span two years at the end; it adds quality years throughout a person's life span. Remaining physically active not only protects against disability, disease, and death but also contributes to enhanced health in all age groups. Both women and men who are overweight, who smoke, and who have high cholesterol levels can lower their risks of cardiovascular disease by engaging in light to moderate exercise.

Physical Activity and Cholesterol Levels

How does exercise protect against cardiovascular disease? Current evidence (Hausenloy & Yellen, 2008) suggests that exercise increases high-density lipoprotein (HDL, or "good" cholesterol) while decreasing LDL ("bad" cholesterol). The combination of raising HDL and lowering LDL may leave total cholesterol the same, but the ratio of total cholesterol to HDL becomes more favorable, and the risk for heart disease decreases. Thus, physical activity can benefit cardiac patients in two ways: by lowering LDL and by raising HDL (Szapary, Bloedon, & Foster, 2003).

Some investigators (Kramsch, Aspen, Abramowitz, Kreimendahl, & Hood, 1981) have conducted experiments on animals and found that physical activity can have a positive effect on monkeys' cholesterol and atherosclerosis. These investigators fed all monkeys a very high

cholesterol diet, but some of the monkeys had a sedentary lifestyle, whereas others were forced into a physical activity program. Compared with sedentary monkeys, those that were physically active had significantly higher HDL levels, lower LDL levels, less narrowing of arteries, and fewer sudden deaths. Do these findings also apply to humans?

Studies with humans have generally found that moderate levels of exercise, with or without dietary changes, bring about a favorable ratio of total cholesterol to HDL. Reviews of studies from the Toronto symposium (Leon & Sanchez, 2001; Williams, 2001) generally found that moderate exercise, such as walking and gardening, increases HDL and less frequently decreases both LDL and triglycerides. The combination of a low-fat diet and exercise is even more effective (Varady & Jones, 2005). Thus, moderate activity may lead to a more favorable ratio of total cholesterol to HDL, but prolonged strenuous physical activity does not seem to confer additional protection against heart disease; that is, there is inconsistent evidence for a dose–response relationship between varying levels of physical activity and death from heart disease (Leon & Sanchez, 2001).

If adults can improve their lipid numbers through moderate exercise, could children and adolescents also benefit from regular physical activity? The assessment of fitness and cardiovascular risk factors is complicated by obesity; many children and adolescents who are sedentary are also overweight or obese. In such individuals, low fitness is related to high cholesterol levels and other cardiovascular risk factors for children in Europe (Andersen et al., 2008) and the United States (Eisenmann, Welk, Wickel, & Blair, 2007). Programs to improve these risk factors typically include both weight loss and exercise, yielding little research that evaluates only physical activity (Kelley & Kelley, 2007).

In general, physically active children can profit from exercise, but probably not as much as adults (Tolfrey, 2004). However, children as young as 4 can profit from an enhanced exercise program (Sääkslahti et al., 2004). This research looked at 4- to 7-year-old children and found that both girls and boys with highly active play time had low levels of total cholesterol, high levels of HDL cholesterol, and a favorable ratio between total cholesterol and high-density lipoprotein cholesterol. A study of preadolescent and early adolescent children showed results similar to studies with adults; that is, exercise seems to lower LDL while raising HDL and leaving total cholesterol basically unchanged (Tolfrey, Jones, & Campbell, 2000). Regular aerobic exercise may protect against heart disease in both adults and children by increasing HDL and by improving the ratio of total cholesterol to HDL.

IN SUMMARY

For more than 50 years, evidence has accumulated suggesting that physical activity reduces the incidence of coronary heart disease. The early studies had many flaws and tended to include only men. However, later research has confirmed a strong association between a regimen of moderate physical activity and cardiovascular health, including heart disease and stroke. In addition, physical activity can raise HDL, thereby improving the ratio of total cholesterol to high-density lipoprotein. As a result, regular activity may add as much as two years to one's life while decreasing disability, especially in later years.

OTHER HEALTH BENEFITS OF PHYSICAL ACTIVITY

Although most people who exercise do so for physical fitness, weight control, or cardiovascular health, other benefits accrue to those who adopt a physical activity regimen, including protection against some kinds of cancer, prevention of bone density loss, control of diabetes, and improved psychological health.

Protection Against Cancer

Several comprehensive reviews (Miles, 2007; Thune & Furberg, 2001) have evaluated much of the literature on the connection between physical activity and various cancers. Several key findings emerged from these reviews. Of the hundreds of studies evaluated, most focused on cancers of the colon and rectum, breast, endometrium, prostate, and lung. Physical activity offers protection against each of these types of cancer, with the strongest evidence for colorectal and breast cancer. The protective effects for colorectal cancer seem to be stronger for men, and exercise appears to protect postmenopausal more than premenopausal women from breast cancer. Results from a meta-analysis (Tardon et al., 2005) are consistent with the systematic reviews, suggesting that moderate to high levels of physical activity reduce incidence of lung cancer in both women and men, but the relationship is stronger for women.

Research has begun to focus on how physical activity acts to lower cancer risk (Rogers, Colbert, Greiner, Perkins, & Hursting, 2008). Possibilities exist for beneficial effects on both tumor initiation and growth. Furthermore, physical activity affects proinflammatory cytokines, which are involved in the development of both cardiovascular disease (Stewart et al., 2007) and cancer. Thus, research has not only established the protective benefits of physical activity for cancer but also has begun to show how those benefits may occur.

Exercise may also be helpful for people with cancer. One study (Quist et al., 2006) indicated that cancer patients undergoing chemotherapy benefited from physical activity training by increasing strength, aerobic fitness, and weight. A systematic review of studies (Cramp & Daniel, 2008) also indicated that exercise is beneficial to help manage the fatigue that often accompanies cancer treatment. Thus, physical activity is effective in preventing several types of cancer and is helpful in managing some of the distressing side effects of cancer treatment.

Prevention of Bone Density Loss

Exercise has also been recommended as a protection against **osteoporosis**, a disorder characterized by a reduction in bone density due to calcium loss that results in brittle bones. Is this recommendation valid? An early review of research (Harris, Caspersen, DeFriese, & Estes, 1989) concluded that physical activity offers strong protection against osteoporosis in postmenopausal women but is less effective in preventing this disorder in premenopausal women.

Since this review, evidence has accumulated suggesting that physical activity can protect both men and women against loss of bone mineral density, especially those who were active during their youth. Bone minerals accrue during childhood and early adolescence, and activity during those years may be especially important for bone health (Hind & Burrows, 2007). A history of athletic performance offers opportunities for such activity, and an examination of young retired athletes (Nordström et al., 2005) confirmed both the advantages of exercise and the disadvantages of ceasing to be physically active. These former athletes seemed to have lost some bone mineral density (BMD) after they retired from active sports (Nordström et al., 2005) but still retained more BMD and had fewer fractures at age 60 than those who had not been athletes. Similarly, 70-year-old professional football (soccer) players who had retired from active participation at least 10 years earlier retained much of their bone mineral density (Uzunca, Birtane, Durmus-Altun, & Ustun, 2005).

Both men and women can benefit from high-impact exercise such as running and jumping. However, this type of exercise may leave people (especially older individuals) vulnerable to injuries. We discuss these and other injuries later in this chapter, but as the Would You Believe . . . ? box explains, both older and young people benefit from exercise. An experimental study (Vainionpää, Korpelainen, Leppäluoto, & Jämsä, 2005) indicated that young, premenopausal women in the experimental (high-impact) group had significantly higher bone mineral density than young women in the control group. However, an intervention featuring walking (Palombaro, 2005) and another using tai chi (Wayne et al., 2007) did not demonstrate effectiveness as clearly as the program with higher-impact exercise (Zehnacker, & Bemis-Dougherty, 2007).

Control of Diabetes

Because obesity is a factor in Type 2 diabetes and because exercise is an established means of controlling weight, it follows that physical activity may be a useful weapon in the control of diabetes. Systematic reviews of research on this topic have confirmed the benefits of exercise for improvement of insulin resistance (Plasqui & Westerterp, 2007), for prevention of Type 2 diabetes (Jeon, Lokken, Hu, & van Dam, 2007), and for the management of this condition (Kavookjian, Elswick, & Whetsel, 2007). Thus, the benefits of exercise for Type 2 diabetes are well established.

Does physical activity protect Type 1 diabetics? A meta-analysis of behavior change interventions (Conn et al., 2008) indicated that exercise is an important component in managing Type 1 diabetes. Physically active adolescents with Type 1 diabetes exhibit lower cardiovascular risk factors than those who are less active (Herbst, Kordonouri, Schwab, Schmidt, & Holl, 2007). Although these studies reported a modest protective benefit for physical activity, they do not suggest that exercise is a panacea for the control of diabetes. Nevertheless, they do indicate that physical activity can be a useful component in the treatment of insulin-dependent diabetes and can offer some protection against the development of non-insulin-dependent diabetes.

Psychological Benefits of Physical Activity

The gains from regular physical activity appear to extend to psychological benefits, including a defense against depression, a reduction of anxiety, a buffer against stress, and a contributor to high self-esteem. People who exercise list psychological reasons nearly as often as physiological ones when asked about the benefits they receive from exercise. Does the evidence support these claims?

In general, the link between physical activity and psychological functioning is less clearly established than the one between physical activity and physiological health. In addition, any evaluation of the therapeutic effects of exercise on psychological disorders must consider the problems raised by the placebo effect. For this reason, quality research is difficult, and some areas lack adequate research to evaluate the effects (Larun, Nordheim, Ekeland, Hagen, & Heian, 2006). Nevertheless, evidence suggests that a regular exercise regimen can decrease

WOULD YOU BELIEVE . . . ?

It's Never Too Late—or Too Early

Physical activity is a healthy habit, but would you believe that it's never too late in the life span to start exercising? Or too early?

Older adults benefit from being physically active in many ways. Cardiovascular benefits include lower blood pressure, improved symptoms of congestive heat failure, and decreased risk for cardiovascular disease (Karani, McLaughlin, & Cassel, 2001). In addition, physically active older adults have lower risk for diabetes, osteoporosis, osteoarthritis, and depression. All of these benefits result in lowered sickness and death among physically active older adults (Everett, Kinser, & Ramsey, 2007).

Despite these many benefits, 32% of men and 42% of women in the United States over age 75 are sedentary (USCB, 2007). People tend to become less active as they age, and they also reduce their exercising when they experience pain (Nied & Franklin, 2002). For example, arthritis causes knee and hip joint pain that makes older people less willing to exercise. Also, people who have had a stroke may experience balance or weakness problems that make them feel uneasy about even normal levels of activity. Older people are more likely than younger ones to fall, and resulting broken bones may make a permanent change in their mobility and independence.

Although all of these concerns have some foundation, the risks are manageable. Physical activity offers more benefits than risks for older people, even for those over age 85 and for those who are frail. They may need supervision for their exercise, but older adults benefit from physical activity. Exercise such as tai chi even helps quell fears and risks of falling (Sattin, Easley, Wolf, Chen, & Kutner, 2005; Zijlstra et al., 2007). Almost all older people can decrease health risks and gain mobility from exercising.

It's also never too early to begin an active lifestyle. Physical activity furnishes lifetime benefits, and even young children benefit. Very young children may not seem to be at any risk from inactivity, but they are. To maintain their goals of safety and convenience, parents and caregivers often confine infants in strollers, infant seats, or playpens that limit their movement (National Association for Sport and Physical Education, 2002). These experiences not only limit mobility during infancy but may also delay developmental goals such as crawling and walking. Lack of physical activity during toddlerhood can lead to a sedentary childhood. Inactive children may also lag in developing motor skills and join the growing number of overweight and obese children in the United States (Floriani & Kennedy, 2008).

The National Association for Sport and Physical Education (NASPE, 2002) proposed guidelines for physical activity, beginning during infancy. For all children, NASPE emphasized supervision and safety. The recommendations for infants included allowing them to experience settings in which they can move while maintaining safety, and playing a variety of games such as peekaboo and hide-and-seek. NASPE recommended at least 30 minutes a day of structured physical activity for toddlers, and 60 minutes for preschool children. Scott Roberts (2002) went a step further, recommending workouts for children. He argued that the prohibitions against weight lifting and other types of strength training for children have no research basis. On the contrary, Roberts maintained that children experience the same benefits from this type of exercise as do adults, including protection against cardiovascular disease, hypertension, and obesity as well as improved strength, flexibility, and posture.

Would you believe that age—any age—is not an excuse to be inactive? It's never too late to benefit from exercise, and it's never too early to begin an active lifestyle. Remember, physical activity brings lifetime benefits, so it's never to early—or too late—to begin a lifetime exercise program.

depression, reduce anxiety, buffer stress, and raise self-esteem.

Decreased Depression The *Diagnostic and Statistical Manual of Mental Disorders* (4th edition, text revision [*DSM-IV-TR*]) of the American Psychiatric Association (APA, 2000) defines a major depressive episode as "a period of at least 2 weeks during which there is either depressed mood or the loss of interest or pleasure in nearly all activities" (p. 349). During a lifetime, as many as 25% of women and 12% of men may suffer from major depression (APA, 2000). If physical activity can relieve major depression, then millions of people can benefit from a therapy that is easily available to nearly everyone.

People who exercise regularly are generally less depressed than sedentary people (Martinsen, 2005). When groups of exercisers are compared to groups of sedentary people on different measures of depression, highly active people are usually less depressed. One possible explanation is that, rather than improving mood, exercising may be restricted to healthy people. Depressed people may simply be less motivated to exercise.

However, experimental studies have begun to determine the direction of causation. For example, one randomized, controlled trial (Annesi, 2005) divided moderately depressed individuals into an experimental group that performed 10 weeks of moderate physical activity three times a week for 20 to 30 minutes and a control group that did not exercise. Clear differences emerged between the two groups, with those who exercised experiencing much lower levels of depression than participants in the control group. A similar research design (Dunn, Trivedi, Kampert, Clark, & Chambliss, 2005) investigated the possibility of a dose–response relationship between exercise and relief of depression and found evidence for such a relationship.

The evidence is beginning to accumulate for the benefits of exercise for depression (Daley, 2008). Exercise is certainly more effective than no treatment and may be comparable to cognitive therapy (Donaghy, 2007) or antidepressant medication (Daley, 2008). The long-term effects, however, have not been substantiated. Nevertheless, an evaluation of the significance of exercise programs (Rethorst, Wipfli, & Landers, 2007) determined that such programs not only produced statistically significant differences but also clinically significant effects. In summarizing the effects of physical activity on depression, Rod Dishman (2003) emphasized the benefits, saying that people who can maintain an exercise program receive benefits comparable to those of other forms of therapy

for depression. Dishman explained: "I am not proposing that exercise is a replacement for psychotherapy or drug therapy, but these findings about exercise are not trivial and suggest that physical activity may be an important addition or complement to standard treatment for mild depression" (p. 45).

Reduced Anxiety Many people report that they exercise to feel more relaxed and less anxious. Does exercise play a role in anxiety reduction? The answer may depend on the type of anxiety under study. **Trait anxiety** is a general personality characteristic or trait that manifests itself as a more or less constant feeling of dread or uneasiness. **State anxiety** is a temporary, affective condition that stems from a specific situation. Feelings of worry or concern over a final examination or a job interview are examples of state anxiety. This type of anxiety is usually accompanied by physiological changes, such as increased perspiration and rapid heart rate.

Research on the effects of physical activity on state anxiety suffers from many of the same methodological limitations as research on physical activity and depression; that is, only a few of the studies have had an adequate number of participants and have used random assignment to experimental and placebo or control groups (Dunn, Trivedi, & O'Neal, 2001). A meta-analysis of randomized, controlled trials (Wipfli, Rethorst, & Landers, 2008) indicated that exercise is more effective than no treatment and has comparable or superior effects to other forms of therapy. Moreover, exercise need not be aerobic or vigorous to be effective; the evidence for a dose–response relationship is lacking (Dunn et al., 2001; Wipfli et al., 2008).

How does physical activity help reduce anxiety? One hypothesis is that exercise simply provides a change of pace—a chance to relax and forget one's troubles. In support of this change-of-pace hypothesis, exercise demonstrated no stronger therapeutic effect than meditation (Bahrke & Morgan, 1978). Studies have shown that other techniques to reduce anxiety, including biofeedback, transcendental meditation, "timeout" therapy, and even beer drinking in a pub atmosphere, can also be effective (Morgan, 1981). Each of these interventions provides a change of pace, and all have been demonstrated to be associated with reduced levels of state anxiety.

Another hypothesis concerning the effects of physical activity on anxiety involves changes in brain chemistry. Studies with rats (Greenwood et al., 2005) have indicated that exercise changes the transport of the neurotransmitter serotonin, which is related to positive mood. Studies with humans (Broocks et al., 2003) have also suggested that changes occur in the metabolism of this neurotransmitter after exercise. Thus, physical activity may reduce anxiety by providing a change of pace, by altering neurotransmitter activity, or through some combination of the two.

Buffer Against Stress Two questions arise in relation to exercise and stress: (1) Can exercise enhance psychological well-being? (2) Can it protect people against the harmful effects of stress? Research on the first question has generally produced an affirmative answer. For example, some investigators (Ensel & Lin, 2004; Galper, Trivedi, Barlow, Dunn, & Kampert, 2006) found that participants who exercised regularly raised their level of psychological well-being significantly higher than those who did not exercise. A somewhat related study (Atlantis, Chow, Kirby, & Fiatarone Singh, 2004) placed workers from a single worksite into a program that included aerobic exercise, weight training, and behavior modification, or on a waiting list to act as a control group. After 24 weeks, workers in the exercise group demonstrated a significantly higher quality of life and lower stress than those in the control group. Finally, a meta-analysis (Netz, Wu, Becker, & Tenenbaum, 2005) found that physical activity relates to psychological well-being, but longer exercise duration does not always lead to continuing increases in feelings of well-being. Thus, even moderate exercise can boost well-being.

Answers to the second question are more difficult, because a direct causal link between stress and subsequent physical illness has not yet been firmly established (see Chapter 6 on stress and disease). However, several studies suggest that physical activity helps people deal with stress. Fitness appears to act as a buffer for both physical and psychological stress (Ensel & Lin, 2004); individuals who were more fit experienced less distress. Some studies have explored the physiology of this relationship, examining blood pressure and immune system responses. Exercise moderates the increase in blood pressure that accompanies psychological stress (Hamer, Taylor, & Steptoe, 2006). The immune system response of proinflammatory cytokines to exercise stress is moderated in fit individuals (Hamer & Steptoe, 2007). Thus, exercise acts to decrease stress, on both a psychological and a physiological level.

The duration of exercise required to produce positive effects is not extreme; as little as 10 minutes of moderately strenuous exercise is capable of elevating mood (Hansen, Stevens, & Coast, 2001). The results of the studies on stress buffering do not indicate a strong effect for exercise, but physical activity is a strategy that many people use to help them manage stress. Figure 15.2 shows some of the positive effects of exercise.

Increased Self-Esteem We have seen that people who exercise regularly decrease their risk of cardiovascular disease, cancer, and diabetes; improve their cholesterol ratio; have lower levels of depression; decrease anxiety level; and have fewer stress-related illnesses. Exercise may not be the direct cause of enhanced feelings of self-esteem, but it may contribute indirectly through each of these factors. Alternatively, exercise may not raise global self-esteem but may be limited to physical self-esteem (Ryan, 2008). However, participation in an exercise program is related to feeling good about oneself both for children and adolescents (Ekeland, Heian, Hagen, Abbott, & Nordheim, 2004) and for adults (Alfermann & Stoll, 2000).

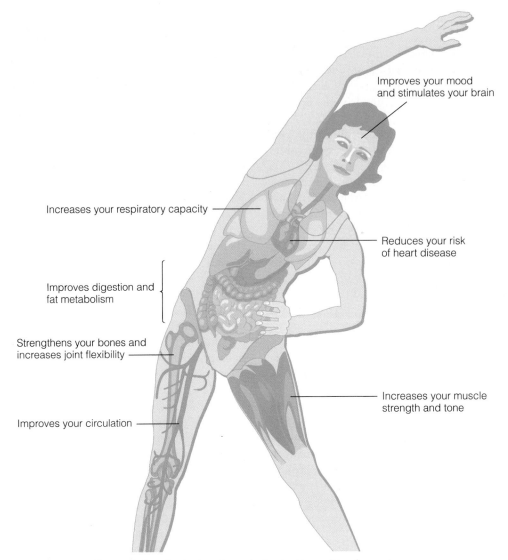

Improves your mood
and stimulates your brain

Increases your respiratory capacity

Reduces your risk
of heart disease

Improves digestion and
fat metabolism

Strengthens your bones and
increases joint flexibility

Increases your muscle
strength and tone

Improves your circulation

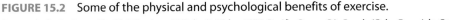

FIGURE 15.2 Some of the physical and psychological benefits of exercise.

Source: An Invitation to Health (7th ed., p. 493), by D. Hales, 1997, Pacific Grove, CA: Brooks/Cole. Copyright © 1997 by Brooks/Cole Publishing Company. Reprinted by permission.

IN SUMMARY

During the past 50 years, research has accumulated to support the hypothesis that physical activity is associated with health and improved psychological functioning. Regular moderate physical activity can reduce the incidence of cardiovascular disease, including heart disease and stroke. Exercise improves both blood pressure and cholesterol profile, showing some ability to raise HDL. Physical activity also shows benefits for decreasing the risk for the development of diabetes and several types of cancer, including colon and breast cancer. Exercise can also promote bone growth in young people and slow the loss of bone minerals in older individuals. Moreover, physical activity shows psychological benefits.

Indeed, exercise may be a useful intervention for depression. Benefits also appear for reducing anxiety, increasing feelings of well-being, and enhancing the ability to perform daily tasks.

An earlier section of this chapter examined several reasons why people exercise. Table 15.1 lists some of these reasons, summarizes research evidence, and cites at least one study pertaining to each reason.

TABLE 15.1

Reasons for Exercising and Research Supporting These Reasons

Reasons for Exercising	Findings	Principal Source(s)
Weight control	Obesity can be reduced through exercise; 60 to 90 minutes a day may be necessary.	Hansen et al., 2005; Hill & Wyatt, 2005; Jakicic & Otto, 2005
Weight control	Exercise is as effective as dieting; sculpting the perfect body won't work.	Blair & Church, 2004; Wood et al., 1988
Heart disease and aerobic fitness	Light to moderate exercise provides sufficient protection.	Barengo et al., 2004; Cooper, 2001; Lee & Skerrett 2001; Paffenbarger et al., 1978
	Dose–response effect.	Bouchard, 2001
	Both women and men need routine exercise.	Kesaniemi et al., 2001; Kohl, 2001
	Both physical fitness and physical activity have a dose–response relationship with aerobic health.	Blair et al., 2001; Lee & Skerrett, 2001
	Walking confers benefits for older people.	Murphy et al., 2007
Stroke	Active women reduce risk of stroke.	Hu et al., 2000
	Inactive people are more likely to have strokes.	Krarup et al., 2007
	Physical activity can reduce two types of stroke.	Wendel-Vos et al., 2004
All-cause mortality	Moderate exercise four times per week reduces deaths.	Kushi et al., 1997
	Nurses' Health Study reviewed 37 prospective cohort studies.	Rockhill et al., 2001; Oguma et al, 2002
Cholesterol level	Exercise increases HDL and decreases LDL.	Hausenloy & Yellen, 2008; Szapary et al., 2003
	Exercise reduces LDL and triglycerides.	Leon & Sanchez, 2001
	Low fitness is related to high cholesterol in children and adolescents.	Andersen et al., 2008; Eisenmann et al., 2007
	Exercise relates to low cholesterol in children.	Sääkslahti et al., 2004; Tolfrey, 2004; Tolfrey et al., 2000
Cancer	Meta-analyses show inverse relationship between exercise and cancer of various sites.	Miles, 2007; Thune & Furberg, 2001
	Exercise reduces risk for lung cancer, with a stronger relationship for women.	Tardon et al., 2005
	Exercise may protect against both tumor initiation and growth.	Rogers et al., 2008
	Physical activity helps people with cancer manage the effects of cancer treatment.	Cramp & Daniel, 2008; Quist et al., 2006

(Continued)

TABLE 15.1 Reasons for Exercising and Research Supporting These Reasons—*Continued*

Reasons for Exercising	Findings	Principal Source(s)
Bone density loss (osteoporosis)	Exercise can protect both men and women against bone loss.	Harris et al., 1989
	Exercise helps build bone mass in children and adolescents	Hind & Burrows, 2007
	Retired male athletes retain much of bone mineral density.	Nordström et al., 2005; Uzunca et al., 2005
	High-impact activity can delay loss of bone minerals in women.	Korpelainin et al., 2005
	Low-impact activities are not as effective as high-impact exercise.	Palombaro, 2007; Wayne et al., 2007; Zehnacker et al., 2007
Diabetes	Exercise improves insulin resistance.	Plasqui & Westerterp, 2007
	Exercise lowers risk for Type 2 diabetes.	Jeon et al., 2007
	Exercise can help in managing Type 2 diabetes.	Kavookjian et al., 2007
	Exercise is an important component in managing Type 1 diabetes.	Conn et al., 2008
	Exercise lowers risk for CVD in individuals with Type 1 diabetes.	Herbst et al., 2007
Decreased depression	Moderate exercise 3 times a week for 20 to 30 minutes reduces depression.	Annesi, 2005
	A dose–response relationship occurs with exercise and depression.	Dunn et al., 2005
	Exercise compares with cognitive therapy and antidepressant medication in effectiveness.	Daley, 2008; Donaghy, 2007
	Benefits of exercise are clinically significant.	Rethorst et al., 2007
Reduced anxiety	Moderate exercise can reduce state anxiety.	Dunn et al., 2001; Wipfli et al., 2008
Buffer against stress	Exercise enhances feelings of well-being.	Ensel & Lin, 2004; Galper et al., 2006
	Weight training reduces stress.	Atlantis et al., 2004
	Exercise increases well-being, but more is not always better.	Netz et al., 2005
	Exercise affects blood pressure and immune system response to stress.	Hamer et al., 2006; Hamer & Steptoe, 2007
Enhance self-esteem	Exercise can enhance self-esteem of children and adolescents.	Ekeland et al., 2004
	Exercise can enhance self-esteem for adults, especially physical self-esteem.	Alfermann & Stoll, 2000; Ryan, 2008

HAZARDS OF PHYSICAL ACTIVITY

Although physical activity can enhance physical functioning, reduce anxiety, stress, and depression, and increase feelings of self-esteem, it also poses hazards to one's physical and psychological health. Some athletes overtrain to the point of staleness and, as a consequence, suffer from negative mood, fatigue, and depression (Tobar, 2005). In addition, some highly active people suffer from exercise-related injuries; others allow exercise to assume an almost addictive importance in their lives. In this section, we look at some of these potential hazards related to physical activity.

Exercise Addiction

Some people become so involved with exercise that they ignore injuries to continue exercising or allow their exercise regimen to interfere with other parts of their lives such as work or family responsibilities. These people are often labeled as having an *exercise addiction*, but their behavior may not match the description of an addiction. In Chapter 13, we saw that addictions produce tolerance, dependence, and withdrawal symptoms.

William Morgan (1979) compared the process of excessive exercising to the development of other addictions. Initially, the tolerance for running is low, and it has many unpleasant side effects. But persistence eases the unpleasant aspects, and the pleasure of meeting goals becomes a powerful reinforcer. Like most social drinkers who have a casual, nonobsessive relationship with alcohol, most exercisers are able to incorporate physical activity into their lives without drastic changes in lifestyle. Other exercisers, however, cannot. Those who continue to increase their exercise must make changes in their lives to accommodate the time required, with consequences for other responsibilities and activities.

A high level of commitment to exercise is not the same as addiction (Terry, Szabo, & Griffiths, 2004). Some people's exercise habits reflect a high degree of commitment, whereas others fit the description of dependence, showing a strong emotional attachment to exercise (Ackard, Brehm, & Steffen, 2002) and exhibiting withdrawal symptoms such as depression and anxiety when prevented from exercising (Hausenblas & Symons Downs, 2002a, 2002b). Committed exercisers tend to have rational reasons for their exercise behavior such as extrinsic rewards, whereas addicted exercisers tend to use exercise as a way to manage negative emotions and problems in their lives (Warner & Griffiths, 2006). Research to establish the physiological basis of exercise addiction (Hamer & Karageorghis, 2007) has progressed, opening the possibility that exercise addiction may be analogous to other types of addiction. This contentions remains controversial, however, and some authorities prefer the term *obligatory exercise* or *exercise dependence* rather than exercise addiction.

Obligatory exercisers share several characteristics with people with eating disorders, especially anorexia. For example, they continue their chosen activity even when they are injured, continuing behavior that is harmful and even self-destructive. They also show a progressive self-absorption, with a great deal of concentration on internal experiences. In addition, many people who are anorexic experience a compulsion to exercise excessively (D. Klein et al., 2004). This observation prompted the proposal that teenage female anorexics and addicted male runners are analogous (Davis & Scott-Robertson, 2000); both show the need for mastery of the body, unusually high expectations of self, tolerance or denial of physical discomfort and pain, and a single-minded commitment to endurance. Other researchers (Ackard et al., 2002) found that obligatory exercisers exhibited body obsession, were more likely to have eating disorders, and showed symptoms of other psychological problems. The motivation for excessive exercise is a critical mediating factor that connects exercise to eating disorders (Cook & Hausenblas, 2008). For these individuals, the connection between exercising and eating disorders is a strong emotional attachment to exercise. These individuals experience injuries yet continue to exercise, neglect their personal relationships, and shortchange their jobs to devote time to exercise. Perhaps this fanaticism can be best expressed in the words of one obligatory runner:

> One day last spring I was having an exceptionally good run. I was running about 10 miles a day at that time and on this particular day I had decided to extend my workout. I was around the 14-mile point and I was preparing to cross a one-lane bridge when all of a sudden a large cement mixer turned the corner and began to cross the bridge. I never thought for a second about stopping and letting the truck pass. I simply continued and said to myself, "Come on you son-of-a-bitch and I'll split you right down the middle—there will be concrete all over the

road!" The driver slammed on the brakes and swerved to the side as I sailed by. That was really scary afterward, but at the time I really felt good. I have felt equally strong and indestructible many times since, but never have taken on a cement truck again. (Morgan, 1979, pp. 63, 67)

Injuries From Physical Activity

Excluding head-to-head challenges with cement trucks, what are the chances of experiencing injuries from exercise? Many people with a regular exercise program accept minor injuries and soreness as an almost inevitable component of their program. However, irregular exercise produces even more injuries and more discomfort, with "weekend athletes" accounting for a disproportional number of injuries.

Musculoskeletal injuries are common, and the greater the frequency and intensity of exercise, the more likely it is that people will injure themselves (Cosca & Navazio, 2007; Lowry et al., 2007). The Surgeon General's report (USDHHS, 1996) found that about half of runners had experienced an injury during the past year. This review also found, as expected, that the injury rate was lower for walkers than for joggers and that previous injury is a risk factor for subsequent injury. Physical activity is the source of 83% of all musculoskeletal injuries, and at least one-fourth of exercisers must interrupt their regimen because of such injuries (Hootman et al., 2002). The decision to decrease exercise in response to injury is a wise one; "working through the pain" is an exercise myth that is associated with further injury.

Besides muscular and skeletal injuries, avid exercisers encounter a number of other health hazards. Heat, cold, dogs, and drivers can all be sources of danger. During exercise, body temperature rises. Both heat and cold present problems, some of which can be dangerous (Roberts, 2007). Fluid intake before, after, and even during exercise can protect against overheating by allowing cooling through sweating. However, conditions of extremely high air temperature, high humidity, and sunlight can combine to raise body temperature and prevent sweat from evaporating from the skin surface. If the body is prevented from cooling itself, dangerous overheating may occur. Managing

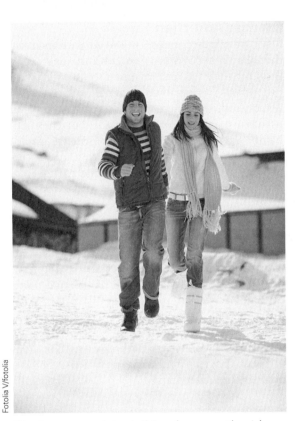

Fotolia V/fotolia

Wearing appropriate clothing decreases the risks of injury during exercise.

the risks for heat stress is a challenge for those who manage sports teams (Cleary, 2007).

Cold temperatures can also be dangerous for outdoor exercising (Roberts, 2007), but proper clothing can provide protection. Layered clothing for the body and gloves, hat, and even a facemask can protect against temperatures of 20°F and below (Pollock, Wilmore, & Fox, 1978). Temperatures below zero, especially when combined with wind, can be dangerous even to people who are not exercising.

Death During Exercise

Many patients who have had a heart attack are put into cardiac rehabilitation programs that include an exercise program, which generally includes close supervision. Although these coronary patients are at elevated risk during exercise, the cardiovascular benefit they receive from exercising ordinarily outweighs the risk (USDHHS, 1996). Nevertheless, individuals who have been diagnosed as having coronary heart disease should undertake exercise only with a physician's permission and under the supervision of specialists in cardiac rehabilitation.

What about people who have no known disease? Heart-related deaths are more likely during exercise, but those people experience a predictable risk. Is it possible for a person who looks and feels well to die unexpectedly during exercise? Yes—but it is also possible to die unexpectedly while watching TV or sleeping. However, exercise increases the risk of such sudden death (Thompson et al., 2007). A 12-year follow-up analysis of male physicians (Albert et al., 2000) showed that sudden death was more than 16 times more likely during or immediately after vigorous physical exertion than during other times. However, the risk was very low for any specific episode of exercise—1 death per 1.5 million episodes of exercise. This study also showed that the benefits of exercise outweighed the risks: Men who exercised regularly were less likely to die during exercise than those who were unaccustomed to exertion. Although the men in this follow-up study (Albert et al., 2000) did not identify themselves as having cardiovascular disease when the study began, either they were affected without their knowledge or developed this disease during the 12 years of the study. Indeed, most sudden deaths during exercise are the result of some type of heart disease, but people may be unaware of their risks.

Under most circumstances, exercise shows benefits for the cardiovascular system, but for those with CVD and for those who have exercised heavily for years of their lives (Raum, Rothenbacher, Ziegler, & Brenner, 2007), this pattern of physical activity is a risk. Even young people may be vulnerable to sudden cardiac death during exercise (Virmani, Burke, & Farb, 2001). In children, adolescents, and young adults, the cause of sudden cardiac death is most often congenital heart abnormalities or arrhythmias (abnormal heartbeat patterns). Among adults, about 60% of sudden cardiac deaths are caused by blood clots that precipitate heart attacks, the typical case of the most frequent cause of death in the United States. Thus, most sudden deaths during exercise are those of individuals who had underlying cardiovascular problems, whether they knew it or not.

Reducing Exercise Injuries

Adequate caution can decrease the probability of injury. For people who have or are at risk for cardiovascular disease, supervised training is a wise precaution, especially when initiating an exercise program. Others, such as people who have been sedentary for a long time, may also benefit from supervision or training. With the guidance of a trainer, people will be less likely to attempt exercise that is inappropriate for their fitness level or to continue to exercise for too long as they start a program. In addition, an exercise professional will teach proper warm-up and stretching routines that are important in preventing injuries (Cooper, 2001).

Regardless of the level of fitness, the use of appropriate equipment decreases injuries. For example, proper running shoes are a necessity for running, jogging, or even exercise walking (Cooper, 2001). The correct type and amount of clothing are also important, either to allow for cooling or to retain heat. In addition to dressing properly for heat or cold, exercisers need to recognize the symptoms of heat stress. These include dizziness, weakness, nausea, muscle cramps, and headache. Each of these symptoms is a signal to stop exercising.

IN SUMMARY

Exercise has hazards as well as benefits. Potential hazards include exercise addiction—that is, a compulsive need to devote long periods of time to strenuous physical activity. Also, exercise may lead to injuries, the majority of which are musculoskeletal and relatively minor. Exercisers should avoid working out in extreme temperatures, and they should know how to avoid dogs, drivers, and darkness.

Death during exercise is a possibility. Those most vulnerable are individuals with cardiovascular disease, who are often older, but young people with heart abnormalities are also at risk. Nevertheless, people who exercise regularly are much less likely than sporadic exercisers to die of a heart attack during intense physical exertion. Exercise-related injuries can be reduced by appropriate preparation such as choosing the appropriate level of exercise, using appropriate equipment, and recognizing signs of trouble and reacting appropriately.

How Much Is Enough but Not Too Much?

During the 1980s, many people, perhaps led by devoted runners/writers such as Jim Fixx, believed that they had to achieve aerobic fitness through vigorous exercise if they wanted to enhance their health. At the same time, health professionals were advising people to structure their exercise program around at least 20 minutes of sustained activity at an intensity level of 50% to 85% of their maximum heart rate 4 or 5 days a week. At the apex of the running epoch, Kenneth Cooper (1985) said that anyone who ran more than 15 miles a week was running for reasons other than health. That statement, which seemed quite moderate at the time, remains valid. If anything, the recommended amount of exercise needed to enhance health may be less than the equivalent of walking 15 miles per week.

How much physical activity is enough but not too much? In recent years, estimates have decreased for the amount of exercise that produces health benefits. In 2007, the American College of Sports Medicine and the American Heart Association revised its recommendations for the amount and type of activity for health benefits (American College of Sports Medicine, 2007). These recommendations clarified earlier recommendations, taking new research into account. According to this official view, a healthy adult under age 65 should participate in 30 minutes of moderately vigorous activity 5 times a week or vigorous activity 20 minutes 3 times a week. In addition, people should engage in 8 to 10 strength training exercises for 12 repetitions at least twice a week. These experts described this level of exercise as adequate to protect against chronic disease, including cardiovascular disease.

The moderately vigorous activity recommendations reflect the evidence that less intense

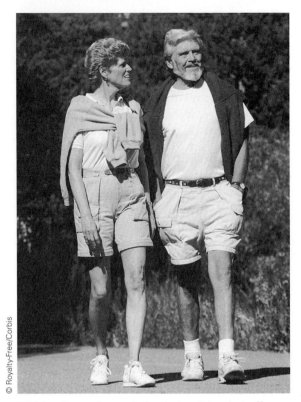

© Royalty-Free/Corbis

Walking is one form of physical activity that offers more advantages than hazards for most people.

exercise produces health benefits and that vigorous exercise is not necessary. For example, a program of walking decreased cardiovascular risk factors in previously sedentary individuals (Murphy et al., 2007). Indeed, moderate exercise may be superior to more intense activity for some cardiovascular risk factors (J. L. Johnson et al., 2007). However, moderately vigorous activity three times a week will not prompt weight loss or maintain weight loss; those goals require more lengthy and more intense exercise (American College of Sports Medicine, 2007). Therefore, how much is enough depends on the health goals.

Adhering to a Physical Activity Program

Adherence to nearly all medical and health regimens is a serious problem (see Chapter 4), and exercise is no exception. Only 48% of adults in

BECOMING HEALTHIER

1. If you don't exercise, make specific plans to start a program of regular physical activity, concentrating on choosing an activity that is convenient and that you feel capable of performing (and even enjoying).

2. If you are overweight and over 40, consult a physician before beginning.

3. Don't start too fast. Once you have determined that you are ready to begin an exercise program, start slowly. The first day you may feel as though you can run a mile. Don't give in to that temptation.

4. Exercising too vigorously on the first day will result in injuries or at least sore muscles. If you are stiff and sore the next day, you overdid it, and you won't feel like exercising.

5. If you are exercising for weight control, don't weigh yourself every day, and try not to become preoccupied with your weight or body shape.

6. If you are in the process of quitting smoking, use exercise as a way to prevent weight gain.

7. Choose and use correct equipment when you exercise.

8. If you jog or cycle in a location unfamiliar to you, check out your surroundings before you begin. Dogs, ditches, and dangerous detours may be in your path.

9. Remember that in order to receive maximum health benefits from your exercise program, you must stick to it. Don't expect quick or dramatic results.

10. To acquire muscle tone as well as aerobic fitness, include a combination of types of exercise such as working out with weights or other isotonic exercise as well as aerobics.

the United States meet the physical activity requirements for health (USBC, 2007); the percentage is similar in the United Kingdom (Adams & White, 2003). For individuals who participate in prescribed exercise regimens, the dropout rates closely parallel the relapse rates reported in smoking and alcohol cessation programs.

Predicting Dropouts

When people consider an exercise program, they weigh the advantages and disadvantages of exercise. For those who move from contemplation to action, the advantages outweigh the disadvantages. To maintain their exercise regimen, the advantages must continue to dominate; otherwise people will relapse into a sedentary lifestyle. Unrealistic expectations about exercise may contribute to feeling discouraged and demoralized. When people's expectations (including unrealistic expectations) about the benefits of exercise are unmet, then they may reassess their reasons for exercising and begin to see more disadvantages than advantages. This reassessment can lead to dropping out (Jones, Harris, Waller, & Coggins, 2005; Polivy & Herman, 2000).

Personal factors contribute to discontinuing exercise, but environmental factors can also present barriers to physical activity. The conviction that exercise is important in promoting health and quality of life is a personal factor, but positive attitudes about exercise are only a first step toward maintaining an activity regimen; changing behavior patterns is much more difficult (Dishman, 2003). Many people cite lack of time and the amount of effort required as barriers to continuing a program of physical activity. In addition, women reported self-consciousness about their physical appearance as a barrier to exercise (King, Touyz, & Charles, 2000).

Maintaining a program of physical activity relates to prior behavior and personal attitudes. Individuals who were physically active when they were young are more likely to maintain an exercise program years later, but even those who were actively involved in exercise or sports may quit at any time (Telama et al., 2005). Those who manage to include exercise in their lives tend to value physical activity and to be motivated to continue by factors within themselves (Haase & Kinnafick, 2007). Self-efficacy also appears as a factor in staying with an exercise program (Millen & Bray, 2008), which is consistent with its role in adherence to various types of behavior change.

Environmental conditions may also present barriers to beginning or to continuing an exercise program. A study that included Hispanic American, African American, Native American, and European American women (King et al., 2000) confirmed the importance of convenience as a factor in exercise maintenance. Women with caregiving duties were particularly at risk for quitting. Finding a convenient time to exercise is a challenge for both women and men. In some high-crime neighborhoods, safety is a concern that may deter participation (Griffin, 2008).

A very common reason for stopping is injury. Of the people who engage in high-intensity physical activity, as many as 50% per year develop injuries serious enough to force them to stop (USDHHS, 1996). As noted earlier, the more frequent and more intense the activity, the greater the chance that an injury will lead to temporary or permanent dropout. Thus, intense, frequent physical activity is one of the best predictors of discontinuing an exercise program.

Increasing Maintenance

Interventions designed to maintain a healthy exercise program are about as effective as other health maintenance programs; that is, these interventions are not much more effective than programs aimed at stopping smoking, eating a healthy diet, or halting alcohol abuse.

Psychologists trained in behavior modification and cognitive behavioral methods have had some success in reducing the dropout rate of exercisers. These programs ordinarily rely on reinforcement for healthy behavior—that is, adhering to exercise programs. Other psychological techniques include writing contracts with the therapist, self-monitoring, instruction, modeling, goal setting, increased self-efficacy, relapse prevention, and a variety of other strategies, most of which we discussed in earlier chapters. Applied to adherence to exercise programs, behavioral programs aimed at increasing social cognition and self-efficacy (Annesi & Unruh, 2007) and offering behavioral support (Annesi, 2007) appeared to be more effective

than other types of interventions. Individually tailoring the regimen to fit the person's stage of behavior change also shows some promise in boosting adherence (Adams & White, 2003), as does making the activity culturally appropriate (Hovell et al., 2008).

An important part of relapse prevention is protection against letting slips lead to full relapse. G. Alan Marlatt and Judith Gordon (1980) called this phenomenon the *abstinence violation effect* (see Chapter 12). When people go five or six days without exercising, they tend to adopt the attitude "I'm out of shape now. It would take too much energy and pain to start over again." As with the smoker or the abuser of alcohol, this exerciser is allowing one lapse to turn into a full-blown relapse. Research with dropouts from an exercise program (Sears & Stanton, 2001) attempted to warn participants that they may be tempted to permanently quit exercising after a period of inactivity but that resuming exercise is a better choice than continued inactivity.

Although behavioral and cognitive behavioral strategies have demonstrated some success, especially when used in combination, maintenance remains a serious problem in most health-related exercise programs. William P. Morgan (2001), one of the leading authorities in this area, has called for a new way of thinking about physical activity. Rather than aiming to boost physical activity to meet some fitness goal for some targeted group of people, Morgan argued that researchers should concentrate on small groups of people and emphasize exercising for a purpose, such as gardening or playing golf, rather than meaningless physical activity. Morgan contended that many people who have tried to meet recommendations for physical activity have dropped out because they viewed the activity as drudgery. Rather than urging people to start physical activity programs, Morgan advocates changing to a more active and enjoyable lifestyle.

IN SUMMARY

In the United States and other industrialized countries, a sedentary lifestyle is more common than a physically active one; about 52% of adults fail to comply with recommendations for regular, vigorous exercise. Maintaining an exercise program may be difficult if the exercise program does not fulfill the person's expectations. In addition, personal and environmental barriers may include time constraints, alternative obligations, and a lack of commitment to physical activity. People are more likely to maintain a convenient and enjoyable exercise program than one that is troublesome and too difficult.

Although avoiding injuries is important, some exercisers quit their program after one uncomfortable experience. Programs designed to improve adherence to physical activity can boost maintenance, and behaviorally oriented components are most effective. Self-efficacy is a factor that boosts adherence to exercise regimens as well as other types of behavior change. However, adherence remains a major problem for exercise, as for other health-related behaviors.

ANSWERS

This chapter has addressed six basic questions:

1. **What are the different types of physical activity?**

   All physical activity can be subsumed under one or more of five basic categories: isometric, isotonic, isokinetic, anaerobic, and aerobic. Each of these five exercise types has advantages and disadvantages for improving physical fitness. Most people who exercise do so for the benefits from one or another of these five types of physical activity, but no one type of exercise promotes all types of fitness.

2. **Does physical activity benefit the cardiovascular system?**

   Most results on the health benefits of exercise have confirmed a positive relationship between regular physical activity and enhanced cardiovascular health, including weight control and a favorable cholesterol ratio. This research suggests that a regimen of moderate, brisk physical activity should be prescribed as one of several components in a program of coronary health.

3. **What are some other health benefits of physical activity?**

   In addition to improving cardiovascular health, regular physical activity may protect against some kinds of cancer, especially colon and breast cancer; help prevent bone density loss, thus lowering one's risk of osteoporosis; prevent and control Type 2 diabetes and help manage Type 1 diabetes; and help people live longer.

   Besides improving physical fitness and health, regular exercise can confer certain psychological benefits. Specifically, research has demonstrated that exercises can decrease depression, reduce anxiety, buffer against the harmful effects of stress, and enhance feelings of self-esteem.

4. **Can physical activity be hazardous?**

   Several hazards accompany both regular and occasional exercise. Some runners appear to be addicted to exercise, becoming obsessed with body image and fearful of being prevented from following their exercise regimen. Injuries are frequent among those who exercise regularly, especially if they train intensively. However, the most serious hazard is sudden death while exercising, which almost always occurs in people with cardiovascular disease. People who exercise regularly are much less likely than occasional exercisers to die of a heart attack during heavy physical exertion.

5. **How much is enough but not too much?**

   During the past 30 years, authorities have decreased their estimation of the amount of physical activity necessary to benefit cardiovascular health. The current pronouncement from the American College of Sports Medicine allowed for two routes to achieve acceptable levels of physical activity. One possibility is moderately vigorous exercise for 30 minutes 5 times per week and the other involves intense exercise for 20 minutes 3 times a week. In addition, individuals should participate in strength training. Although the less intense program of physical activity is not sufficient to promote a high level of fitness, health benefits occur at lower levels of exercise. For cardiovascular health, almost any amount of exercise is better than no exercise.

6. What are some problems in maintaining an exercise program?

More than 50% of adults in the United States are too sedentary for good health. Many of those who begin an exercise program drop out. Personal and environmental factors such as unfulfilled expectations for exercise benefits, injuries, time constraints, alternative obligations, and lack of a safe and convenient place to exercise all contribute to relapsing to a sedentary lifestyle. Psychological interventions have had some limited success in improving compliance with health-related exercise programs.

SUGGESTED READINGS

Burfoot, A. (2005, August). Does running lower your risk of cancer? *Runner's World, 40,* 60–61. In this article, Amby Burfoot looks at some of the research on exercise and cancer and takes issue with Ken Cooper's statement that anyone who exercises more than the equivalent of 15 miles a week is running for something other than health. Burfoot considers the growing evidence that physical activity may protect against cancer as well as help people recover from cancer.

Dishman, R. K. (2003). The impact of behavior on quality of life. *Quality of Life Research,* 12(Suppl. 1), 43–49. This article presents a speech by exercise authority Rod Dishman in which he summarizes the benefits of exercise, the level of activity required for health benefits versus fitness, and the barriers that many people cite as reasons for remaining sedentary.

Plymire, D. C., & Bennett, S. J. (2002). Running, heart disease, and the ironic death of Jim Fixx. *Research Quarterly for Exercise and Sport, 73,* 38–46. Darcy Plymire and Simon Bennett provide an interesting look at factors underlying the death of Jim Fixx and discuss the potentially deadly way of life of some obligatory runners.

Silver, J. K., & Morin, C. (Eds.). (2008). *Understanding fitness: How exercise fuels health and fights disease.* Westport, CT: Praeger Publishers/Greenwood Publishing Group. This book provides an explanation of the biological processes that occur when people exercise, including a review of the many diseases that exercise can help prevent.

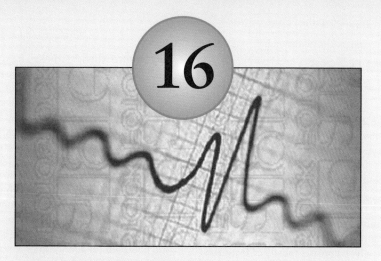

16

FUTURE CHALLENGES

QUESTIONS

This chapter focuses on three basic questions:

1. What role does health psychology play in contributing to the goals of *Healthy People 2010*?

2. What is the outlook for the future of health psychology?

3. How can you use health psychology to cultivate a healthier lifestyle?

REAL-WORLD PROFILE OF DWAYNE AND ROBYN

Dwayne Brown* is a 21-year-old college junior who seldom thinks about his health—either his present or his future health. Dwayne feels good, believes that his present lack of obvious illness is a sign that he is in good health, and assumes that he will always be free of disease and disability.

Dwayne should probably be more concerned because he has a number of habits that have consequences for his health. Probably his riskiest health practice is his diet, which consists mostly of fast-food burgers, with an occasional fried fish sandwich for variety. However, variety is not a high priority for Dwayne, who eats three meals a day, six days a week at the same fast-food restaurant. Breakfast usually consists of a biscuit, scrambled eggs, sausage, and a soft drink (because he doesn't like coffee). For lunch, he has a burger, fries, and another soft drink. Dinner is a repeat of lunch. He also snacks and often chooses ice cream and candy bars. Despite his "junk food" diet, Dwayne is not overweight.

Dwayne holds other attitudes, beliefs, and behaviors that present risks. He seldom exercises or wears seat belts and has few close friends. He believes that his future health is beyond his personal control—that genetics and fate are the underlying determinants of heart disease, cancer, and accidents. Thus, he has thought little about ways of maintaining his health or decreasing his chances of chronic illness or premature death. He does not see a physician regularly. When he feels ill, he takes over-the-counter medication, hoping that he will feel better.

However, Dwayne does some things right. He does not smoke cigarettes or drink alcohol and considers his life as low stress. His abstinence from drinking is based on religious rather than health beliefs, and his avoidance of smoking can be traced to an incident during his adolescence when he smoked a cigarette and became sick. His score on the Social Readjustment Rating Scale (Holmes & Rahe, 1967; see Chapter 5) was as low as anyone's could be, including only one stressful life event—Christmas. Dwayne sees himself as a healthy person.

Robyn Green* is also a 21-year-old college junior, but her attitudes and behaviors concerning health differ a great deal from Dwayne's. Her differences include a basic attitude—that she has the primary responsibility for her health. Consistent with this attitude, Robyn has adopted a lifestyle that she believes will keep her healthy. Like Dwayne, she does not smoke; she took a puff from a cigarette when she was in fourth grade and coughed for a long time, which discouraged her from smoking. Her father was a smoker during her childhood and adolescence, but she and her mother convinced him to stop smoking in their home. Their argument included the dangers of passive smoking, and for that reason, Robyn avoids enclosed places where people are smoking. Unlike Dwayne, Robyn drinks alcohol. Her drinking is moderate, and she does not binge drink. Her parents are also moderate drinkers, and Robyn has grown up in a home in which alcohol is consumed but not abused.

Robyn's diet differs from Dwayne's in dramatic ways. She seldom eats eggs, whole milk products, beef, or pork; she concentrates on eating lots of fruits and vegetables (yet is not vegetarian). She occasionally allows herself a dessert. Robyn is careful about choosing a low-fat diet because she is concerned about cholesterol. Her grandfather died of heart disease at age 63, and she is convinced that his smoking and high-fat, high-cholesterol diet hastened his death. Robyn has also begun an exercise program, which she finds somewhat difficult to maintain with her school schedule. She is enrolled in an aerobic dance class three days a week; she walks 30 minutes a day on those days with no dance class. So far, she has been faithful in maintaining this workout schedule. Robyn sees herself as a healthy person.

* The names have been changed to protect these persons' privacy.

These two students are typical of college students in some ways and extreme in other ways. Dwayne is less knowledgeable and concerned with his health than most college students, whereas Robyn is more so. Examining their perceptions and behaviors gives us a basis for reviewing the health issues and concerns specific to college students, including a way to personalize health psychology. But first, let's look at health care and the challenges facing not only health psychologists but also all health care providers in the United States and around the world.

CHALLENGES FOR HEALTHIER PEOPLE

People in the United States, Canada, and other high-income countries are inundated with health information telling about the dangers of smoking, abusing alcohol, eating improperly, and not exercising regularly. Knowledge does not always translate into action, and people have difficulty in adopting these healthy habits. Still, over the past 35 years U.S. residents have managed to make some healthy changes in their lifestyles, and these changes are reflected in the declining mortality for heart disease, stroke, cancer, homicide, and unintentional injuries (USCB, 2007). However, unhealthy and risky behaviors continue to contribute to an increasing rate of obesity, diabetes, and lower respiratory disease.

Health goals became part of U.S. national policy with the publication of *Healthy People 2000* (USDHHS, 1991), a report that detailed three broad goals, 22 priority areas, and 300 main objectives for improving the health of people in the United States. The broad goals were increasing the span of healthy life, reducing health disparities among Americans, and achieving access to preventive services for all people in the United States.

Healthy People 2010: Understanding and Improving Health (2nd ed., USDHHS, 2000) built on the successes and shortcomings of the previous goals to establish health objectives for the first decade of the 21st century. These objectives include 28 focus areas and 467 specific goals, along with 10 leading indicators, which appear in Table 16.1. These indicators represent areas of major concern that were selected on the basis of the availability of data to measure them and their relation to health. Notice that most of these indicators are major areas of concern to health psychologists. In addition, two overarching goals summarize the focus of this report: to increase quality and years of healthy life and to eliminate health disparities. Those goals are ambitious and have presented many challenges (USDHHS, 2007).

Increasing the Span of Healthy Life

The first goal—to increase the span of healthy life—is a bit different from increasing life expectancy. Rather than striving for longer lives, many

TABLE 16.1

Leading Health Indicators for Healthy People 2010

Physical activity
Overweight and obesity
Tobacco use
Substance abuse
Responsible sexual behavior
Mental health
Injury and violence
Environmental quality
Immunization
Access to health care

people are now trying to increase their number of well-years. A **well-year** is "the equivalent of a year of completely well life, or a year of life free of dysfunction, symptoms, and health-related problems" (Kaplan & Bush, 1982, p. 64). A concept closely related to well-years is **health expectancy,** defined as the number of years a person can anticipate spending free from disability (Robine & Ritchie, 1991). For example, life expectancy in the United States at age 65 is about 16 additional years for men and 19 years for women, but health expectancy is only 8 more years for men and 10 more years for women, leaving both men and women with a discrepancy that represents years of disability (Robine & Ritchie, 1991; Robine, Jagger, Mathers, Crimmins, & Suzman, 2003). The situation in the United Kingdom is similar: Men and women at age 65 can expect to live another 15 and 19 years, respectively, but only 12 (men) and 11 (women) of those years will be free of disability (Jagger et al., 2007). Thus, health expectancy has not grown as rapidly as life expectancy in the United States or the United Kingdom. In the United States, years of life have increased, but years of life without chronic illness have declined (USDHHS, 2007).

U.S. residents are not benefiting from increases in healthy life expectancy as much as residents of many other countries (Mathers et al., 2004). Although people in the United States may expect 69.3 years of healthy life, this figure ranks 29th in the world in terms of disability-free life expectancy. The United States trails most other

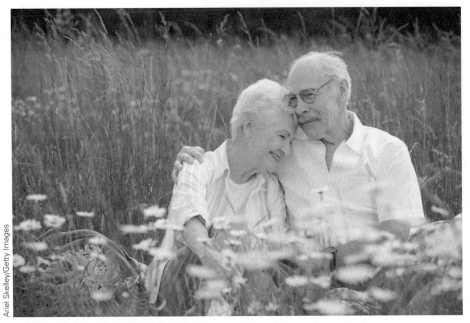

Ariel Skelley/Getty Images

Increasing the span of healthy life is a goal for health psychologists.

industrialized countries because of high rates of smoking-related disease, violence, and AIDS-related health problems. Table 16.2 shows the healthy life expectancy for a selection of countries with both high and low values.

The differences between life expectancy and health expectancy are even larger when comparing the richest and poorest countries, or even the richest and poorest segments of the population within a country (Bossuyt, Gadeyne, Deboosere, & van Oyen, 2004; Mathers et al., 2004; Matthews, Jagger, & Hancock, 2006). Wealthy people not only live longer but also have more years of healthy life.

Health expectancy is influenced by disorders that may differ from those that shorten life. That is, the diseases that kill people are not necessarily the same as those that compromise health. For example, circulatory disorders head both lists, but disorders producing restricted movement and respiratory disorders are responsible for producing lost health expectancy, whereas cancer and accidents are major sources of lost life expectancy. Thus, interventions aimed at increasing life expectancy will not necessarily improve health expectancy and quality of life.

The need to increase the health of older people is important not only to improve their quality of life but also to help manage health care costs. Because of their tendency to have chronic illnesses, older people use health care services more heavily than younger people, with a rate of physician contacts twice as high for those over 75 as for those between ages 18 and 44 (USCB, 2007). In an editorial in the *New England Journal of Medicine*, Andrew Kramer (1995) advocated a change of emphasis in health care for the elderly. Rather than concentrating on acute care delivered in hospitals, Kramer argued for the promotion of primary care and long-term care, strategies that might help improve quality of life for the elderly. Following this suggestion, several types of programs have demonstrated effectiveness in improving quality of life for chronically ill older people (Boult, Kane, & Brown, 2000). These programs include providing care with an interdisciplinary team of health care providers rather than exclusively through physicians, teaching self-management skills so that older people are better able to care for themselves, making group rather than individual physician appointments, and providing in-home services rather than hospital-based

TABLE 16.2

Healthy Life Expectancy for Selected Nations, 2002

Ranking	Country	Healthy Life Expectancy
1	Japan	75.0
2	San Marino	73.4
3	Sweden	73.3
4	Switzerland	73.2
6	Iceland	72.8
8	Australia	72.6
11	Canada	72.0
14	Germany	71.8
24	United Kingdom	70.6
29	USA	69.3
36	Costa Rica	67.2
44	Mexico	65.4
55	China	64.1
71	Colombia	62.0
85	Vietnam	61.3
100	Brazil	59.8
114	Russian Federation	58.4
136	India	53.5
144	Iraq	50.1
163	Haiti	43.8
179	Somalia	36.8
190	Angola	33.4
192	Sierra Leone	28.6

Source: Data from Annex Table 4, *World Health Report 2004,* by World Health Organization. Retrieved January 10, 2006, from www.who.int/whr.

services. Unfortunately, implementation of these innovative programs has been slow and resistance among hospitals and physicians has been high. Without innovative changes, the goal of increasing healthy years of life will not be attained.

Reducing Health Disparities

The United States progressed toward achieving the objectives of *Healthy People 2000*, and set higher goals for *Healthy People 2010*. However, most of those improvements have occurred among higher socioeconomic groups, with college-educated European Americans meeting the *Healthy People 2010* goals more often than members of other educational and ethnic groups

(USDHHS, 2007). Overall, huge discrepancies in health status continue to exist among various socioeconomic and ethnic groups (Agency for Healthcare Quality Research [AHQR], 2004) and between men and women (Govender & Penn-Kekana, 2008; Zoller, 2005).

With *Healthy People 2010* (USDHHS, 2000), the emphasis shifted away from targeting special groups and toward high standards of improved health for everyone. With such a plan, the Department of Health and Human Services hopes to eliminate disparities in infant mortality, cancer screening, cardiovascular disease, diabetes, HIV/AIDS, sedentary lifestyle, obesity, and other health areas that have shown large discrepancies between the general population and at least one ethnic group. However, those goals are proving elusive; no progress toward eliminating disparities occurred between 2000 and 2005 (USDHHS, 2007). Even more discouraging, although much research has explored the types and sources of health disparities, little research has focused on effective ways to reduce these disparities (Davis, Vinci, Okwuosa, Chase, & Huang, 2007).

In the United States, ethnicity is not separable from social, economic, and educational factors that contribute to disease as well as to seeking and receiving health care (Kawachi, Daniels, & Robinson, 2005). Being poor with a low educational level elevates risks for many diseases and provides a poorer prognosis for those who are ill. These disadvantages also apply to children in these socioeconomic groups (Wen, 2007). African Americans, Hispanic Americans, and Native Americans have lower average educational levels and incomes than European Americans and Asian Americans (USDHHS, 2000), and education relates to income. Thus, the factor of ethnicity is difficult to separate from income and education, complicating the interpretation of the underlying reasons for health disparities among people of different ethnic backgrounds.

For example, African Americans, compared with European Americans, have a shorter life expectancy as well as a higher infant mortality rate, more homicide deaths, higher rates of cardiovascular disease, higher cancer mortality, and more tuberculosis and diabetes (USCB, 2007).

They also experience lower health expectancy (USDHHS, 2007). Inadequate medical treatment may be a factor: African Americans receive poorer care than European Americans on about two-thirds of the quality measures of health care (AHQR, 2004). But even when equating for income (De Lew & Weinick, 2000) and access to health care (Schneider, Zaslavsky, & Epstein, 2002), African Americans have poorer outcomes than European Americans. Part of the discrepancy may be due to limited **health literacy**, the ability to read and understand health information to make health-related decisions (Paasche-Orlow, Parker, Gazmararian, Nielsen-Bohlman, & Rudd, 2005; Rudd, 2007).

Inadequate medical treatment for African Americans presents the possibility that discrimination may be a factor (D. R. Brown et al., 2008; Smiles, 2002). For example, African Americans receive less aggressive treatment for symptoms of coronary heart disease and are less likely

to be referred to a cardiologist than European Americans, are less likely to receive kidney dialysis, and are less likely to receive the most effective treatments for HIV infection (Institute of Medicine, 2002). Many physicians believe that race or ethnicity plays no role in the care they provide (Lillie-Blanton, Maddox, Rushing, & Mensah, 2004), but these results and the reports of African Americans (D. R. Brown et al., 2008) indicate otherwise.

Low economic status, lack of access to medical care, and poor health literacy affect Native Americans at least as strongly as African Americans (USDHHS, 2007). Native Americans have a shorter life expectancy, a higher mortality rate, higher infant mortality, and higher rates of infectious illness than European Americans (Hayes-Bautista et al., 2002). Many Native Americans receive health care from the Indian Health Service, but that organization has a history of poor funding as well as mistreatment of Native American patients that has led to mistrust (Keltner, Kelley, & Smith, 2004). In addition, many Native Americans live in rural settings in which health care services are limited. These circumstances contribute to decreased access to health care, which is related to poor health, but Native Americans who live in urban areas also experience poor health and limited access to health care (Castor et al., 2006). Native Americans also exhibit many risky behaviors that influence their health, including high rates of smoking and alcohol abuse, poor diet, and behaviors that increase injuries and deaths from violence. Native Americans, then, are one of the groups poorly served by the current system of health care and health education in the United States.

Many Hispanic Americans also experience low income and educational status. However, Hispanics in the United States include a variety of groups, and their health and longevity tend to vary with income and education. Cuban Americans generally have higher education and economic levels than Mexican Americans or Puerto Ricans, and Cuban Americans are more likely to have access to regular health care and physician visits (LaVeist, Bowie, & Cooley-Quille, 2000). Cubans have better health and Puerto

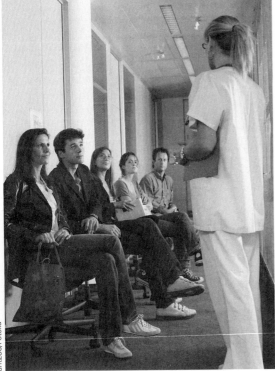

ant236/Fotolia

Many people in the United States face barriers in obtaining medical care.

Ricans tend to have poorer health than other groups of Hispanics in the United States (Borrell, 2005). Puerto Ricans and Mexican Americans have lower life expectancy than other Hispanics in the United States.

Hispanic Americans are much more likely to develop diabetes, obesity, and hypertension than European Americans (USDHHS, 2000). Hispanic American young men are at sharply increased risk of violent death (Hayes-Bautista et al., 2002), which may be the reason for the overall lower life expectancy of Hispanic Americans. In other age groups, Hispanics fare about the same as or better than European Americans on some health and mortality measures. Hispanic Americans have a lower death rate than many other ethnic groups, including European Americans, for heart disease, stroke, and lung cancer (NCHS, 2007). These low death rates seem puzzling, given the high rates of smoking, obesity, and hypertension among Hispanic Americans. The poor health habits of Hispanic Americans, combined with their low disease prevalence, may reflect a transition in which immigrants are in the process of adopting American lifestyles but have not yet had time to develop the chronic diseases typical of the United States (Borrell, 2005).

The trend toward developing diseases typical of the U.S. population applies to all immigrant groups—those who adopt the lifestyle of the United States soon have the patterns of disease and death characteristic of this country. This acculturation is a partial explanation for the lower mortality among Hispanics in the United States—lower rates of smoking and alcohol abuse are related to lower mortality (Abraído-Lanza, Chao, & Flórez, 2005). Especially for Mexican Americans, recent immigrant status seems to be a health advantage, and longer residence means adoption of behaviors that constitute health risks. For example, acculturation (measured in terms of years lived in the United States) was the best predictor of eating habits and obesity among Hispanic women and men in California (Hubert, Snider, & Winkleby, 2005). Similarly, Hispanic and Asian American adolescents who speak English at home (a measure of acculturation) were more likely to smoke than those who did not speak English at home (Unger et al., 2000); they also tended to exercise less and to eat more fast food (Unger et al., 2004). Thus, Hispanic and Asian Americans who have adopted Western habits increase their risks. However, Asian Americans still have more favorable health status and life expectancy than other ethnic groups (NCHS, 2007).

Asian Americans have lower infant mortality, longer life expectancy, fewer lung and breast cancer deaths, and lower cardiovascular death rates than other ethnic groups (NCHS, 2007). Like Hispanic Americans, Asian Americans come from a variety of ethnicities, including Chinese, Korean, Japanese, Vietnamese, and Cambodian. Many Asian cultures share values that promote good health, such as strong social and family ties, but other factors present barriers to good health. For example, Vietnamese and Cambodian cultures show a higher tolerance for family violence than European American culture (Weil & Lee, 2004). Overall, Asian Americans have the longest life expectancy and best health of any ethnic group in the United States.

Low income has an obvious connection to lower standards of health care. After adjusting for poverty, many of the health disadvantages of ethnicity disappear (Krieger, Chen, Waterman, Rehkopf, & Subramanian, 2005). One health care disadvantage related to poverty is lack of insurance, which makes access to health care more difficult in the United States. However, universal access to health care does not completely remove the disparities among socioeconomic groups (Lasser, Himmelstein, & Woolhandler, 2006; Martikainen, Valkonen, & Martelin, 2001). Even in countries that have universal access to health care, health disparities between poor and wealthy people persist, suggesting that factors other than access to health care are involved in maintaining health.

Education and socioeconomic level are two factors that may influence health status—independent of access to health care. Across ethnic groups and in countries around the world, people who have higher education and income also have better health and longevity than those with lower education and income (Crimmins & Saito, 2001; Mackenbach et al., 2008). As the Chapter 1

WOULD YOU BELIEVE . . . ?

Terence Was Right

Would you believe that Terence, the Roman playwright who lived during the second century B.C., was mostly right when he advised moderation in all things? Except for cigarette smoking, most of your health behaviors should follow Terence's counsel.

In Chapter 13, we discussed evidence that moderation in alcohol consumption was healthier for people's hearts than either heavy drinking or complete abstinence. For example, a meta-analysis (Rimm et al., 1999) showed that abstinence, heavy drinking, or binge drinking has no cardiovascular benefits. However, light to moderate drinking (defined as two drinks a day or less) is associated with lower incidence of heart disease deaths.

In Chapter 14, we reviewed research showing a relationship between obesity and health problems. That relationship is U-shaped, indicating that the heaviest people and the thinnest people had a

greater risk for poor health than people who have avoided extremes of weight (Flegal et al., 2005). As body mass index moves substantially in either direction away from moderate levels, mortality rate goes up.

In Chapter 15, we saw that the devoted runners of 20 years ago were not improving their health through excessive physical activity but were running for reasons other than health. Although marathon running may not be harmful to cardiovascular health, it can lead to other types of health problems, including serious injuries (Cosca & Navazio, 2007; Lowry et al., 2007). But if long-distance running can be harmful, a sedentary lifestyle is even more dangerous. The American College of Sports Medicine (2007) recommends that adults accumulate 30 minutes of moderate physical activity a day through such activities as brisk walking, gardening, bicycling, climbing stairs, or

swimming at least 5 days a week as well as participate in some type of strength training. More strenuous exercise is an option but not a requirement for improving or maintaining health.

Moderation also applies to less important health practice such as eating candy. Consuming candy may seem like a guilty pleasure, but if you are not diabetic and you eat moderately, you may live longer than people who do not eat candy. This result appeared in a study that questioned the "puritanical stance toward pleasure" that is conveyed by the popular belief "if it tastes that good, it can't be healthy" (Lee & Paffenbarger, 1998, p. 1683). A longitudinal study of men in the Harvard Health study confirmed that even eating candy in moderation was related to longer life span than refraining or overindulging. As with so many other things in life, moderation appears to be the key. Once again, Terence was right.

Would You Believe . . . ? box detailed, people who attend college have many health advantages. Compared to those with a high school education or less, those who attend college live longer and healthier, with lower rates of infectious and chronic diseases and unintentional injuries (NCHS, 2007). These advantages should not be surprising, considering the low rate of smoking among those who attend or graduate from college compared to people with fewer than 12 years of education; smoking is a leading contributor to ill health and death.

In addition, people with low education and low socioeconomic status are more likely to have risky health habits, such as eating a high-fat diet and leading a sedentary life, than people with higher incomes and more education. Although

improved access to health care and decreased discrimination in health care delivery will probably eliminate some of the health disparities among ethnic groups, changes in health-related behaviors and improved living conditions will also be necessary to achieve the goal of eliminating health disparities in the United States. The Would You Believe . . . ? box discusses the value of healthy habits.

IN SUMMARY

People in the United States and other industrialized countries are becoming more health conscious, and both government policy and individual behavior reflect this concern. *Healthy*

People 2010 built upon the success of *Healthy People 2000* and stated two overarching goals for the U.S. population: (1) to increase the quality and years of healthy life and (2) to eliminate health disparities. The first goal includes increasing the number of well-years or health expectancy—that is, years free of dysfunction, disease symptoms, and health-related problems. The second goal—eliminating disparities in health care—is far from being met, in part because people at the upper socioeconomic level continue to make greater gains in health status than do those at the lower levels. Ethnicity remains a factor in health and health care, not only in the United States but also in other countries. In the United States, African Americans and Native Americans experience great disadvantages compared to Asian Americans and European Americans. Some Hispanics experience health advantages and others disadvantages. The factors of education and income are intertwined with ethnicity, complicating understanding of the source of disparities in health.

OUTLOOK FOR HEALTH PSYCHOLOGY

Since the founding of health psychology more than 30 years ago, the field has blossomed, prompting a plethora of research and clinical applications to a variety of health-related behaviors and outcomes. That progress has touched many areas of health care, but social and economic forces will influence the future of the field.

Progress in Health Psychology

In 1969, William Schofield published an article in the *American Psychologist* that provided a major impetus to health psychology. Analyzing the research publications in psychology that dealt with health, he found that only 19% of the research articles dealt with topics other than the traditional mental health concerns of psychology. This finding brought about a call for a wider scope of psychological services and research. The American Psychological Association (APA) appointed a task force to perform a further analysis, and this task force concluded that health was not a common area of research for psychologists (APA Task Force on Health Research, 1976). However, during the past 30 years, psychology research on health issues has accelerated to the point that it has changed the field of psychology, making health-related issues common topics in psychology journals; health psychologists have also become frequent contributors to journals in medicine and health care.

The current mission statement of the American Psychological Association includes the declaration that psychology is a "means for promoting health, education, and human welfare" (APA, 2005). The inclusion of health in this mission is a validation of the influence of health psychology (Smith & Suls, 2004) and highlights the impact of health psychology on the entire field.

Despite the growth of health psychology and its ability to contribute to health care, the field faces several challenges. One major challenge is acceptance by other health care practitioners, an acceptance that continues to grow. Health psychologists will be challenged by the most serious problem within health care—namely, escalating costs. In an environment of limited resources, psychologists will be forced to justify the costs that their services add to health care (Tovian, 2004). Although the diagnostic and therapeutic techniques used by health psychologists have demonstrated effectiveness, these procedures also have financial costs. Health psychology must meet the challenges of justifying its costs by offering services that meet the needs of individuals and society while fitting within a troubled health care system.

Future Challenges for Health Care

Health care in the United States faces enormous challenges. The two goals of *Healthy People 2010*—to add years of healthy life and to eliminate disparities in providing health care—are proving difficult to achieve. Adding years of healthy life to an aging population is a daunting task. As the population ages, chronic illnesses and chronic pain become more common.

The number of people in the United States 65 years old or older has increased from about 3 million in 1900 to almost 37 million in 2003. In 1900, only 4% of the population was over 65;

in 2006, more than 12% of U.S. citizens had reached that age (USCB, 2007). During this same period, life expectancy increased from 47 years to more than 77 years. By the year 2010, life expectancy is projected to be more than 78 years (see Figure 16.1), with more than 18 million people, or 6.2% of the total population, over age 75.

As the population continues to age during the next few decades, psychology will play an important role in helping older people achieve and maintain healthy and productive lifestyles and adjust to the problems of chronic illness. As we have seen, health psychology has a role in preventing illness, promoting healthy aging, and helping people cope with pain. In old age, lifestyles can still be changed to help prevent illness, but health psychology's alliance with gerontology will more likely produce an emphasis on promoting and maintaining health, managing pain, and formulating health care policy.

The elimination of health disparities based on gender, ethnicity, age, income, educational level, and disability has proven difficult, and increasing diversity will continue to challenge the health care system. The health and life expectancy disadvantage for African Americans exists throughout the life span (Wen, 2007; Whitfield, Weidner, Clark, & Anderson, 2002), and Hispanic Americans and Native Americans also have shorter life and health expectancies than European Americans and Asian Americans. Many of these disparities can be traced back to economic and educational differences among ethnic groups (Lasser et al., 2006; USDHHS, 2007). The health disparity attributable to gender is not so easy to understand. Women receive poorer health care yet have longer life expectancies. This survival advantage was small in 1900, grew to more than 7 years during the 1970s, and has declined to about 5 years (NCHS, 2007). Efforts to trace this

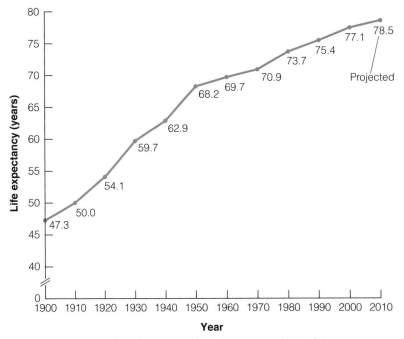

FIGURE 16.1 Actual and projected life expectancy, United States, 1900–2010.

Sources: Data from *Historical Statistics of the United States: Colonial Times to 1970* (p. 55), by U.S. Department of Commerce, Bureau of the Census, 1975, Washington, DC: U.S. Government Printing Office; *Statistical Abstracts of the United States: 2001* (p. 73), by U.S. Bureau of the Census, 2001, Washington, DC: U.S. Government Printing Office.

gender difference to biology have been largely unsuccessful, but health-related behaviors, social support, and coping strategies favor women (Whitfield et al., 2002).

Woven throughout these issues is escalating costs—the primary challenge facing health care in the United States. The health care system is in turmoil over the rising cost of medical care. Insurance costs continue to increase, and a growing number of people have no insurance and cannot afford to pay for care (NCHS, 2007). The changes in patterns of death and disability that occurred during the 20th century also have an impact on the cost of health care because the system of providing care has not accommodated to those changes. Both changing needs for health care and health care costs will influence the future of health psychology.

Controlling Health Care Costs The richest nation in the world is having trouble paying its health care bills. Health care costs in the United States have escalated at a higher rate than inflation and other costs of living (Bodenheimer, 2005a; Mongan, Ferris, & Lee, 2008), leaving many people unable to afford health care and others in the position of fearing that they will not be able to do so in the future.

A number of factors have contributed to the high costs. Many of those factors can be traced to the system that provides care and the economic forces within that system (Bodenheimer, 2005b, 2005c; Mongan et al., 2008). The problems stem from a combination of proliferation of expensive technology, a large proportion of physicians who are specialists, inefficient administration, inappropriate treatments, and a profit-oriented system that resists controls.

Figure 16.2 shows where health care dollars go. Hospitals receive 31% and physicians 21% of the dollars spent (USCB, 2007). Health care costs could be lower if the number of hospital beds matched the demand for beds, but hospitals have overbuilt, resulting in the need to fill these hospital beds and a high cost for doing so. Indeed, areas of the country with more hospital beds have higher rates of hospitalization than areas with fewer beds (Fisher et al., 2003). Some national policy to control hospital overbuilding could help control this situation.

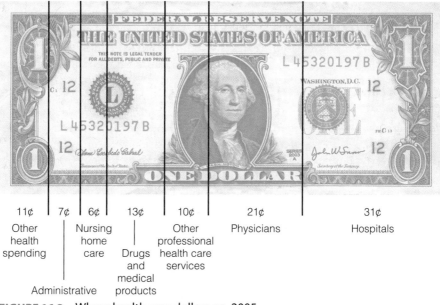

11¢	7¢	6¢	13¢	10¢	21¢	31¢
Other health spending		Nursing home care		Other professional health care services	Physicians	Hospitals
			Drugs and medical products			
	Administrative					

FIGURE 16.2   Where health care dollars go, 2005.

Source: Health, United States, 2007, 2007, by National Center for Health Statistics, Table 124.

Although physicians receive less of the health care dollar than hospitals, their fees contribute significantly to the high cost of health care (Bodenheimer, 2005c). Managed care curtailed physicians' fees during the late 1980s and early 1990s, but the backlash against managed care loosened these restrictions, and physicians' fees began to increase again in the late 1990s. The number of specialists adds to the cost of medical care, and the scarcity of primary care/family practitioners (and the lack of incentive for going into primary care) also plays a role (Sepulveda, Bodenheimer, & Grundy, 2008). Ironically, more physicians created competition, but rather than decreasing costs, this situation has contributed to higher costs (Weitz, 2007).

Administrative costs contribute substantially to high health care costs in the United States (Bodenheimer, 2005a; Mongan et al., 2008). The complex system of insurance, private physicians, private and public hospitals, and government-supported medical programs such as Medicare has produced different procedures, forms, payment plans, expenses allowed, maximum payments, and deductibles involved in payment for medical services. Thus, payment is a complex matter of filling out and filing forms, not only by patients but also by health care providers. In addition to the costs of inefficiency, this over-complicated system adds to people's frustration in dealing with the health care system and creates possibilities for errors and fraud.

Health care reform has been recognized as an urgent priority for the United States, but many conflicting interests have prevented widespread changes (Bodenheimer, 2005c; Mongan et al., 2008). During the 1980s, health maintenance organizations (HMOs) proliferated as a way to control costs (Weitz, 2007). Originally, HMOs were nonprofit organizations oriented toward preventive care, but corporations entered the HMO market and profit became a motive. The growth of HMOs and the restriction of care received through these organizations contributed to slowing the health care cost escalation. A backlash against the restrictions on care imposed by HMOs produced patients' rights movements, which have edged the system back toward high spending.

Examining other countries that face similar health problems and their solutions can give direction about ways to provide health care in the United States. Other industrialized countries such as Canada, Japan, Australia, the countries of western Europe, and Scandinavia share certain factors with the United States—aging populations with high rates of cardiovascular disease, cancer, and other chronic diseases—that pose similar challenges for their health care systems (Bodenheimer, 2005b). Many of these countries do a better job of providing health care to a larger percentage of their residents at lower cost than does the U.S. system. Their longer life expectancies and health expectancies are testimony to the effectiveness of their systems.

Germany, Canada, and Great Britain have all faced the problems of escalating health care costs, and these nations have also struggled to contain rising costs (Weitz, 2007). The history of health care costs in these countries and the United States appears in Figure 16.3. These countries have managed to contain health care expenditures by controlling at least some of the factors that account for the rise in medical costs in the United States: Canada has a single payer system, which minimizes administrative costs; Great Britain limits access to high-technology medicine; Germany imposes some limits on payments to physicians and limits hospitals' purchases of high-technology equipment.

All of the strategies for cost containment have drawbacks. For example, people have quicker access to medical procedures such as MRIs, mammograms, and knee replacement surgery in the United States than in Canada, but these procedures are significantly more expensive in the United States (Bodenheimer, 2005b). Time delays for some services may pose risks, but in other cases, patients in the United States are over-treated, and limiting access could actually boost health and life expectancy (Emanuel & Fuchs, 2008; Research and Policy Committee, 2002). Canadians' longer life expectancy suggests that the delays they experience do not pose major threats (Lasser et al., 2006).

By devising systems in which all people have access to health care, Germany, Canada, and

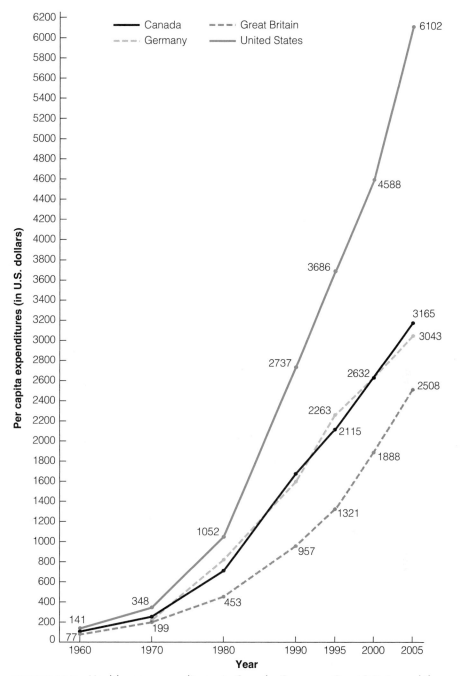

FIGURE 16.3   Health care expenditures in Canada, Germany, Great Britain, and the United States, 1960–2004.

Source: Health, United States, 2007, 2007, by National Center for Health Statistics, Hyattsville, MD: U.S. Government Printing Office, Table 120.

Great Britain have diminished competitive profit making, which remains a central feature of the U.S. system (Mahar, 2006). These three countries have different systems for paying for health care, and all have experienced cost problems, but each has universal coverage, whereas a growing percentage of people in the United States have limited access to health care.

Limiting access to care may decrease costs but also results in poorer health, and good care is the purpose of the system (Mongan et al., 2008). Finding ways to avoid hospitalization and use of emergency rooms can help to contain costs (Bodenheimer & Fernandez, 2005). Avoiding medical errors is another way to lower health care costs: Mistakes tend to increase hospitalization and move less serious disease to more serious illness.

About 70% of the cost of health care is spent on 10% of the population, whereas healthy people (about 50% of the population) account for about 3% of health care expenditures (Bodenheimer & Fernandez, 2005). These statistics highlight the importance of maintaining and promoting health as a way to contain health care costs. Thus, health psychologists can have a role in reducing health care costs because unhealthy behaviors are related to the chronic diseases that generate the majority of expenses, such as cardiovascular disease, cancer, diabetes, and chronic lower respiratory disease. People with a healthy lifestyle are much less likely to develop these diseases. Those with good health habits have lifetime medical costs about half those for people with poor health habits. However, people who live longer have years to accrue medical costs, so even good health can be costly in the long run (van Baal et al., 2008). Promotion of good health habits is an important way to decrease the need for medical services in the short run.

Reducing the demand for medical services is another approach to controlling health care costs (Fries, 1998), which may be a good strategy to move people toward self-care. The availability of a wide range of medical technology has led to the widespread belief that modern medicine can cure any disease, and this belief has fostered an over-reliance on medicine to heal rather than a reliance on good health habits to avoid disease and self-management for people with chronic conditions. Building feelings of personal efficacy for health can help reduce the demand for medical services, and this approach has potential benefits for health in U.S. society. For example, encouraging individuals with chronic health problems to join self-help groups may reduce their need for intensive medical care (Humphreys & Moos, 2007). Additional research in this area may reveal that this approach can be a good strategy for containing health care costs.

Controlling health care costs will require substantial changes in the U.S. health care system. Insurance companies, hospitals, and physicians will all be affected and have all fought against changes (Mongan et al., 2008). As the examination of health care systems in other countries showed, no system can provide a good quality of medical care for low costs, but many countries do a better job than the United States. The health care systems of all industrialized countries are faced with the problem of providing care to an aging population whose health concerns stem predominantly from chronic illnesses.

Adapting to Changing Health Care Needs In 1900, infectious diseases were the major health concern, but that situation changed during the 20th century. By the beginning of the 21st century, chronic illnesses were the leading cause of death and disability in the United States and other industrialized countries. The health care system, however, remains oriented toward providing acute care for sick people rather than providing services that will prevent, ameliorate, or manage chronic conditions. That is, the health care system has not responded to meet the needs created by changed patterns of disease that occurred during the 20th century (Bodenheimer, 2005c). Thus, people need services that may not be available and may receive (and pay for) services that do not best suit their health needs. Controlling chronic illness can occur through two routes: management to control these disabling conditions and prevention to avoid them.

Management of chronic illness is a current need that will become more important in the future. Cardiovascular disease, cancer, chronic lower respiratory disease, and diabetes account for more than 70% of deaths in the United States (Bodenheimer & Fernandez, 2005). However, health care for these and other chronic illnesses is plagued by undertreatment, overtreatment, and mistreatment. For example, overtreatment was detected for 30% of individuals attending a primary care clinic, who were diagnosed with asthma and prescribed inhaled corticosteroids despite a lack of evidence for symptoms of asthma (Lucas, Smeenk, Smeele, & van Schayck, 2008). Undertreatment appeared in an analysis of management of hypertension in patients who had experienced a stroke (Elkins, 2006), 20% to 30% of whom did not receive treatment for diagnosed hypertension. Such treatment has been identified as a way to control this major risk for future strokes. Mistreatment occurs when health care providers make medical errors, which occurs with alarming frequency (HealthGrades, 2004). Creating a system that will provide more effective management of chronic illnesses will demand a shift from hospital- and physician-based care to a team approach that includes access to medical care and patient education to improve monitoring and self-care.

Self-care is also a priority for prevention, which is a strategy that can reduce the need for medical services. However, primary prevention offers more savings than secondary prevention. *Primary prevention* consists of immunizations and programs that encourage lifestyle changes; this type of prevention is usually a good bargain. Immunizations have some potential for harm but remain good choices unless the risk from side effects of the immunization is comparable to the risk of catching the disease. Programs that encourage people to quit smoking, eat properly, exercise, and moderate their drinking generally have low cost and little potential to do harm (Clark, 2008). In addition, some of these behaviors, such as smoking and inactivity, are risks for many health problems, and efforts oriented toward changing these behaviors can pay off by decreasing risks for several disorders. For example, a study of people who led a life that included the recommended exercise, body mass index, eating habits, and no history of smoking (Fraser & Shavlik, 2001) showed a significant life extension that led to the conclusion that healthy lifestyle can add 10 years of life. Thus, primary prevention efforts pose few risks and offer many potential benefits.

Most prevention efforts are aimed at young and middle-aged adults who feel the need to change their behavior for health reasons, but a broadened emphasis may be more productive. A review of health behaviors in older people (Siegler, Bastian, Steffens, Bosworth, & Costa, 2002) concluded that not only lifelong health habits but also healthy behavior begun after age 65 can add healthy years to life. Efforts to build health-promoting behaviors in adolescents would be even more advantageous, but this group has been even more neglected in terms of lifestyle interventions (Williams, Holmbeck, & Greenley, 2002). Most of the health research and interventions for adolescents have centered on injury prevention and smoking deterrence, but adolescents build a foundation for a lifetime of health-related behaviors. Thus, primary prevention efforts tailored for people throughout the life span have the potential to improve health and life expectancy.

Secondary prevention consists of screening people at risk for developing a disease in order to find potential problems in their early and more treatable stages. However, such efforts can be costly because the number of people at risk may be much larger than the number who will develop the disease. Based on the economic considerations of cost–benefit analysis—that is, how much money is spent and how much is saved—secondary prevention may cost more than it saves.

However, neither hospitals nor physicians are ideally suited to provide prevention services. Hospitals are oriented toward acute care, and physicians' time is very expensive to be devoted to health education. Providing health education and even immunizations is more cost efficient when handled by public health agencies, health educators, and health psychologists than by hospitals and physicians. Making these changes in the health care system would provide better care as well as offer the potential for controlling health care costs.

Will Health Psychology Continue to Grow?

What do the problems in the U.S. health care system mean for health psychology? Those problems have an impact on people in clinical health psychology and behavioral medicine; these practitioners must work within that troubled system and demonstrate that the services they provide have value (Tovian, 2004). However, health psychologists are also working to reform the system. Their commitment to the biopsychosocial model has helped to promote this model as a more comprehensive view of health and to end the false dichotomy between mental and physical health (Suls & Rothman, 2004). Clinical health psychologists have firmly established their expertise as consultants, but health psychologists may become even more prominent as health care providers. Kaiser Permanente of northern California designated psychologists as primary health care providers in its health maintenance facilities more than a decade ago (Bruns, 1998), and programs are currently in place for training health psychologists to be primary providers (McDaniel & le Roux, 2007). These psychologists typically become behavioral health or behavioral medicine specialists and serve as part of teams that implement an integrated care approach to health care services. According to a message to graduate students in psychology, primary care psychology is one of the "hot" areas for postgraduate training (Packard, 2007).

Health psychology research has contributed to the field of health by developing a knowledge base that continues to expand. The vision of the 1976 American Psychological Association Task Force on Health Research has been fulfilled: Psychologists have taken a leading role in creating a scientific understanding of the behavioral factors in disease development and prevention. This approach was new to health care because the biomedical model dominated medicine at the time. The biomedical model is being questioned, even among physicians, as health care researchers and practitioners from all backgrounds come to realize that psychological and social factors also contribute to health and disease (Suls & Rothman, 2004). Within psychology, the view that psychology is a health profession is rising (Tovian, 2004).

The problems in the health care system present major challenges for the future of health psychology. The short history of health psychology shows that the field has developed rapidly and made substantial contributions to research and practice in health care. The rapid gains of the 1980s slowed in the 1990s, but health psychology continued to grow steadily. The 21st century has already seen continued growth for health psychology.

IN SUMMARY

Health psychology has made significant contributions to health care research and practice, but health psychology must meet a number of challenges to continue to grow. Several of these challenges are tied to the troubled health care system in the United States. Health care costs have risen in the United States more rapidly than in other industrialized countries, many of which manage to provide health care to a wider segment of their population and with a better outcome in terms of life expectancy and health expectancy. The United States needs to reform its inefficient health care system so that a larger segment of the population can receive quality health care services.

The future of health care will demand better management of chronic illnesses and a greater emphasis on prevention. The aging population will increase the need for management of chronic conditions that are more common among older people. Prevention may be the key both to better health and to controlling health care costs. Health psychology has a role to play in both the management and prevention of chronic illness, as reflected in the growth of the field of primary care psychology.

MAKING HEALTH PSYCHOLOGY PERSONAL

At the beginning of this chapter, we met Dwayne Brown and Robyn Green, two college students with varying attitudes toward health and differing health-related behaviors. You may see similarities and differences between Dwayne's and Robyn's behavior and your own. By contrasting their behavior with that of typical college students and analyzing their actions and attitudes, you may be able to understand your risks and form a plan to adopt health behaviors that will lead you to a healthier and longer life.

Understanding Your Risks

Both Dwayne and Robyn expressed an attitude that is widespread among young people—the perception of good health. More than 90% of college students expressed similar opinions, rating their health as *good*, *very good*, or *excellent* (American College Health Association [ACHA], 2006). That perception is consistent with statistics on morbidity and mortality (USCB, 2007); young adults have a lower incidence of disease and death than older adults (but higher than children between ages 5 and 14, who have the lowest mortality rate). The perception of good health may be beneficial, but that view may also create hazards by leading young adults (like Dwayne) to believe that they are invulnerable and that their good health will continue, regardless

of their behavior. That view is dangerously incorrect and may even increase the risks for the leading cause of death to this age group—unintentional injury (accidents). Indeed, both unintentional injury and intentional violence are leading causes of injury and death for people before age 45.

Injury and Violence As the leading killers of young people, injuries and violence are responsible for more lost years of life than any other source. For example, each cancer-related death accounts for an average of 18 lost years of life, but each death due to unintentional injury subtracts an average of 34 years from life expectancy (USCB, 2007). Most deaths among college students are the result of behaviors that contribute to either unintentional or intentional injuries.

Automobile crashes are by far the leading cause of fatal injuries among adolescents and young adults. For young people 15 to 24, about three-fourths of fatalities from unintentional injuries are due to motor vehicle crashes (USCB,

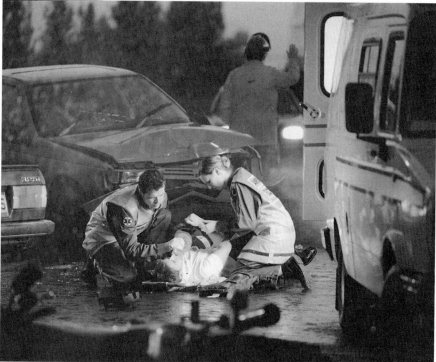

Automobile crashes are the leading cause of fatal injuries for adolescents and young adults in the United States.

Getty Images

2007). Alcohol has been identified as contributing to nearly half these motor vehicle deaths (Hingson, Heeren, Winter, & Wechsler, 2005), and this problem is not restricted to the United States. In countries around the world, driving after drinking is a common practice for college students, and countries with higher rates of this practice also have higher rates of traffic fatalities (Steptoe et al., 2004). Unfortunately, college students are more likely than their nonstudent peers to drive after drinking (Hingson et al., 2005). College students are also more likely than their peers to use cell phones while driving, which is another behavior that sharply increases the risk of a crash (Cramer, Mayer, & Ryan, 2007).

Failure to use seat belts also contributes to the injury and death rate for automobile crashes; unrestrained drivers are 5 times more likely to be injured than those using restraints (Bustamante, Zhang, O'Connell, Rodriguez, & Borroto-Ponce, 2007). A substantial difference appears for male and female college students for these risks, and Dwayne and Robyn are typical in this respect—college men are less likely to use seat belts than college women (Henson, Carey, Carey, & Maisto, 2006), but women are more likely to use their cell phones while driving (Cramer et al., 2007).

College students are also victims (and perpetrators) of intentional violence, including assaults, robberies, rapes, and murders, but at a lower rate than nonstudents of comparable age (Carr, 2007). That is, college campuses are safer than life outside the campus. Crime rates in general have decreased in the United States, and that trend has also appeared on college campuses; only about one-fourth of campus injuries are the result of intentional violence. However, many campus crimes go unreported, and people fail to report sexual and partner violence more often than they report these acts of violence.

A survey of college students (ACHA, 2006) indicated that 2% of college women and 0.8% of college men had been raped within the past school year. This percentage is small but represents thousands of people per year. In addition, the percentage is cumulative; by the end of college life, the chance of a college woman's experiencing a rape or attempted rape is more than 20% (Carr, 2007). Unwanted sexual touching and threats

are much more common. Sexual victimization is related to a variety of health risks for women, including smoking, drug use, thoughts of suicide, and eating disorders (Gidycz, Orchowski, King, & Rich, 2008). Thus, sexual violence can initiate a cascade of health problems.

Dating violence is also a common experience during college, although emotionally abusive relationships are much more common (13% within the past year) than physically abusive ones (2% within the past year) (Carr, 2007). Women who are involved in physically abusive relationships are at increased risk for sexual violence and for victimization by a stalker, a form of victimization that is more common among college students than other groups. However, both women and men are perpetrators as well as victims of dating violence. A large, international study of dating violence (Straus, 2008) revealed that women are almost as likely as men to initiate dating violence. Couples in which one partner is more dominant than the other are at increased risk for violent behavior.

Suicide and suicide attempts are other forms of intentional violence that occur among college students. About 11% of college women and 9% of college men reported that they had seriously

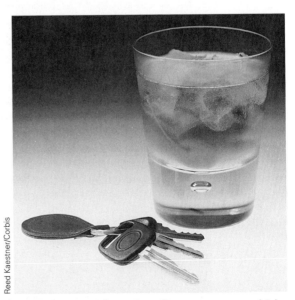

Reed Kaestner/Corbis

Alcohol is a significant contributor to motor vehicle crashes, and college students are more likely than others to binge drink.

considered suicide within the past school year (ACHA, 2006); 1.5% had attempted suicide within that time span. Feelings of hopelessness and depression, involvement in an abusive relationship, and being lesbian, gay, or bisexual increased the risk for suicidal thoughts and suicide attempts (Carr, 2007). As Joetta Carr (2007) commented, "Some campus violence is a reflection of society's sexism, racism, and homophobia" (p. 311). Drinking, drug use, and mental health problems magnify the risks for all types of campus violence. However, college campuses are safer environments than most places, and students are safer on campus than in most communities.

Lifestyle Choices In addition to the hazards from intentional and unintentional violence as leading causes of death and injury, young adulthood is also a time during which individuals adopt health-related behaviors that will have an impact on their health for decades. These health behaviors contribute to the risks for the leading causes of death during middle age and later. Dwayne and Robin exhibit both risky and protective health behaviors, the most important of which is their status as nonsmokers. That choice is typical of college students; a lower percentage of college students smoke than of those who have not attended college (Wetter et al., 2005). Indeed, education is currently the best predictor of smoking status. The choice to refrain from smoking is a major factor in the statistic that individuals with a college education live longer and experience better health than others.

Dwayne's abstention from alcohol and Robyn's social drinking are patterns that appear among college students, but many students choose less wisely and engage in binge drinking. That choice represents the most dangerous pattern of drinking among young people. Continued heavy drinking can bring many health problems, and almost 8% of college students reported that drinking had interfered with their academic performance (ACHA, 2006). Even occasional binge drinking is risky because of its association with injury and violence. Almost half of those between ages 18 to 24 engage in this practice (NCHS, 2007), and college students are more likely than others to do so.

College students often fail to eat a healthy diet. When students begin college, they often enter a new living situation in which they make dietary choices rather than eating at home. A study of college students in Greece (Papadaki, Hondros, Scott, & Kapsokefalou, 2007) indicated that living arrangement was a critical factor in diet. Those students who moved away from home tended to change their diet to less healthy choices that included more sugar, alcohol, and fast food and fewer of the food choices for the healthy Mediterranean diet typical of that country. Those who continued to live at home made few changes. Like Dwayne, few college students in the United States meet the guidelines for fruit and vegetable consumption (Adams & Colner, 2008). Like Robyn, those who do tend to adhere to other healthy behaviors, including using seat belts, engaging in physical activity, and sleeping well, along with decreased chances of smoking and driving after drinking.

College students are less likely than the general population to be overweight and more likely to engage in physical exercise, but significant percentages of students fall short of those health goals. One study of eating, weight, and physical activity among college students (Burke, Lofgren, Morrell, & Reilly, 2007) indicated that 33% of male and 22% of female college students were overweight; 11% and 7% were obese. A third of the women and 23% of the men accumulated less than 30 minutes of physical activity per day. As would be expected, these students showed elevated cholesterol and blood pressure, laying the foundations for cardiovascular disease. Neither Dwayne nor Robyn is overweight, but Dwayne's diet and lack of exercise puts him at greater risk for high cholesterol and high blood pressure than Robyn, who recalls her grandfather's experience with heart disease and does not want to repeat it.

College students also encounter stress, and Robyn's rating of her stress is more typical than Dwayne's rating, which was very low. Most college students report many more sources of stress. Indeed, a survey of college students (ACHA, 2006) revealed that stress appeared as the most frequently named reason for academic problems. Stress management strategies and problem-solving skills proved more important than perceived stress in terms of physical symptoms of stress among college students (Largo-Wight, Peterson, & Chen, 2005). These results suggest that stress is a major challenge for college students, but developing problem-focused strategies to manage stress is important. Indeed, college students can lead healthy lives during their college years by cultivating a healthy lifestyle, and these habits provide the basis for a longer life as well as a healthier one.

Cultivating a Healthy Lifestyle

Health psychologists and other health researchers have created a massive amount of information about health and health-related behaviors. Although it may seem that a lot of information would help people make wise choices concerning their health, such is not the case. Electronic media, including television and the Internet, inundate people with health information. The media carry stories daily about current research findings, but people may be confused by what they perceive as an overwhelming amount of information, which even seems contradictory at times (Kickbusch, 2008). Evaluating all the information and translating it into personal terms is a substantial task, which requires *health literacy*—the ability to read and understand health information to make health decisions. This ability is related, of course, to literacy in general but goes further to include an understanding and evaluation of scientific information related to health (White, Chen, & Atchison, 2008; Zaarcadoolas, Pleasant, & Greer, 2005).

Increase Your Health Literacy Despite their educational level, college students do not necessarily have a high degree of health literacy. They actively seek health information but tend to consult friends and family rather than more authoritative sources (Baxter, Egbert, & Ho, 2008). To increase your health literacy, begin to evaluate health claims critically, considering the source of the claim. Expertise matters, so listen to the experts. Health research has produced a large body of evidence that allows health researchers to make recommendations. The massive research findings from health psychology represent an authoritative source, with recommendations on

smoking, drinking alcohol, eating a healthy diet, exercising, decreasing the risk of unintentional injury, and managing stress.

Adopt Good Health Behaviors—Now One way to summarize the recommendations from health research is to work toward integrating the findings from the Alameda County study into your life. Recall that this study identified five behaviors that led to better health and lower mortality (Belloc, 1973; Berkman & Breslow, 1983). These behaviors were (1) refraining from smoking cigarettes, (2) engaging in regular physical exercise, (3) drinking alcohol in moderation or not at all, (4) maintaining a healthy weight, and (5) sleeping 7 to 8 hours per night.

Of these habits, avoiding tobacco is probably the most important health behavior you can adopt. The damage from tobacco takes years to become apparent, but smoking cigarettes and being exposed to tobacco smoke are hazardous. The evidence is also overwhelming concerning the benefits of adopting an active lifestyle. For individuals of any age, physical activity can boost health and prevent disease and disability. These two health habits are more important for long-term health benefits than for immediate ones, but nonsmokers who exercise regularly experience short-term health advantages as well as longer life expectancies.

Moderating alcohol intake is also an important health behavior. The evidence concerning levels of drinking is clear: Light drinkers are healthier than those who drink more, and probably than those who do not drink. However, these findings apply to older adults more strongly than to younger ones. Drinking presents many risks to college students, who are more likely to binge drink than any other age group. Thus, good advice for college students is to work toward moderating drinking and avoiding the hazards of mixing alcohol and motor vehicles. Also, alcohol increases the risk of all types of violence, which is the leading cause of death for young adults. Avoiding heavy or binge drinking is the wise choice for college students.

Maintaining a healthy weight is important, but so are food choices. The foundation for cardiovascular disease begins during adolescence and young adulthood, and food choices are important. A high-fat diet is a component in this process. Even if you are able to maintain close to an ideal weight while eating a high-fat diet (as Dwayne was), this choice is a bad one. Evidence is strong that diet with lots of fruits and vegetables provides many health benefits. Choosing such a diet while balancing work, school, and personal demands is not an easy task but will lead to short-term benefits through weight maintenance and long-term advantages through decreasing the risks for cardiovascular disease, diabetes, and cancer.

The fifth recommendation from the Alameda County study may be the most difficult for college students to follow: Get 7 to 8 hours of sleep a night. Later research has confirmed the relationship: People who sleep more than 8 or less than 6 hours per night experienced higher death rates (Patel et al., 2004). Setting a priority on sleep may be difficult but will also pay off immediately in terms of energy, concentration, and perhaps even improved immune function (Motivala & Irwin, 2007).

A final recommendation from the Alameda County study emphasized the importance of social support (Camacho & Wiley, 1983; Wiley & Camacho, 1980). People with a social network are healthier than those with few social contacts. College students have many opportunities to form a social network of friends, which they may add to their families as sources of social support. Remember that social support provides one type of coping strategy, but it is wise to cultivate a range of such strategies, including problem-focused as well as emotion-focused strategies, and use them appropriately.

The combination of these health behaviors will extend your life and improve your health, not only in the future but during your college years.

IN SUMMARY

Improving the health of college students requires understanding the risks specific to this group and finding ways to diminish those risks, including changes in their health-related behaviors. Injuries from intentional and unintentional violence are major health threats to young adults, including college students. Vehicle crashes are the most common threat, but injuries and deaths occur as a result of assault, rape, partner violence, suicide, and homicide. Alcohol is a factor in all of those types of violence.

Health habits adopted during young adulthood lay the foundation for health or disease in later years. To make healthy choices, individuals need to develop their health literacy so that they can evaluate the health information that that they receive from others and from the media. A good guideline for cultivating a healthy lifestyle comes from the Alameda County study, which found that people are healthier and live longer if they (1) refrain from smoking cigarettes, (2) engage in physical activity regularly, (3) drink alcohol in moderation or not at all, (4) maintain a healthy weight, and (5) sleep 7 to 8 hours per night. In addition, developing a social support network enhances health.

ANSWERS

This chapter has addressed three basic questions:

1. What role does health psychology play in contributing to the goals of _Healthy People 2010_?

Health psychology is one of several disciplines that have a role in helping the nation achieve the goals and objectives of _Healthy People 2010_. The two broad goals of this document are (1) increasing the span of healthy life and (2) eliminating health disparities among various ethnic groups. Health psychologists emphasize adding healthy years of life, not merely more years. They cooperate with other health professionals in understanding and reducing health discrepancies among different ethnic groups, but this goal has proven difficult to accomplish.

2. What is the outlook for the future of health psychology?

Health psychology faces challenges in the 21st century. Finding ways to control health care costs is a major goal for all health care providers. Health psychologists can contribute to that goal through their expertise in understanding and treating the chronic diseases that have become the leading causes of death in industrialized countries. Even more important, health psychologists have advocated for prevention, which has the potential to decrease the need for health care. Prevention through behavior change can help in controlling health care costs. To be included in future health care, health psychologists must continue to add to both the research and practice components of the field: Build a research base, and develop more effective strategies for behavior change.

3. How can you use health psychology to cultivate a healthier lifestyle?

The habits that you adopt during young adulthood form a foundation for your health-related behavior throughout middle and older adulthood, so the choices you make now are important for your future health. Health psychology offers suggestions concerning how to cultivate healthy choices in terms of smoking, drinking and drug use, diet, exercise, and stress management. Increasing your health literacy and relying on research rather than information from the media or from friends provides a strategy for making good health choices.

SUGGESTED READINGS

Kickbusch, I. (2008). Health literacy: An essential skill for the twenty-first century. *Health Education, 108*, 101–104. This article examines the challenges to developing health literacy and emphasizes the importance of doing so in light of the ever-increasing complexity of health research.

Mongan, J. J., Ferris, T. G., & Lee, T. H. (2008). Options for slowing the growth of health care costs. *New England Journal of Medicine, 358*, 1509–1514. This recent article examines some possibilities for controlling health care costs without a drastic overhaul of the U.S. health care system.

Whitfield, K. E., Weidner, G., Clark, R., & Anderson, N. B. (2002). Sociodemographic diversity in behavioral medicine. *Journal of Consulting and Clinical Psychology, 70*, 463–481. Keith Whitfield and his colleagues provide a comprehensive review of ethnic, gender, and economic factors that affect health and life expectancy, analyzing the risks and protective factors associated with each demographic group.

GLOSSARY

A-beta fibers Large sensory fibers involved in rapidly transmitting sensation and possibly in inhibiting the transmission of pain. (Chapter 7)

A-delta fibers Small sensory fibers that are involved in the experience of "fast" pain. (Chapter 7)

absolute risk A person's chances of developing a disease or disorder independent of any risk that other people may have for that disease or disorder. (Chapter 2)

acetylcholine One of the major neurotransmitters of the autonomic nervous system. (Chapter 5)

acquired immune deficiency syndrome (AIDS) An immune deficiency caused by viral infection and resulting in vulnerability to a wide range of bacterial, viral, and malignant diseases. (Chapter 6)

acrolein A yellowish or colorless, pungent liquid produced as a by-product of tobacco smoke; one of the aldehydes. (Chapter 12)

acupressure The application of pressure rather than needles to the points used in acupuncture. (Chapter 8)

acupuncture An ancient Chinese form of analgesia that consists of inserting needles into specific points on the skin and continuously stimulating the needles. (Chapter 8)

acute pain Short-term pain that results from tissue damage or other trauma. (Chapter 7)

addiction Dependence on a drug such that stopping its use results in withdrawal symptoms. (Chapter 13)

adherence A patient's ability and willingness to follow recommended health practices. (Chapter 4)

adrenal cortex The outer layer of the adrenal glands; secretes glucocorticoids. (Chapter 5)

adrenal glands Endocrine glands, located on top of each kidney, that secrete hormones and affect metabolism. (Chapter 5)

adrenal medulla The inner layer of the adrenal glands; secretes epinephrine and norepinephrine. (Chapter 5)

adrenocortical response The response of the adrenal cortex, prompted by ACTH, that results in the release of glucocorticoids including cortisol. (Chapter 5)

adrenocorticotropic hormone (ACTH) A hormone produced by the anterior portion of the pituitary gland that acts on the adrenal gland and is involved in the stress response. (Chapter 5)

adrenomedullary response The response of the adrenal medulla, prompted by sympathetic nervous system activation, that results in the release of epinephrine. (Chapter 5)

aerobic exercise Exercise that requires an increased amount of oxygen consumption over an extended period of time. (Chapter 15)

afferent neurons Sensory neurons that relay information from the sense organs toward the brain. (Chapter 7)

agoraphobia An anxiety state characterized by fear about or avoidance of places or situations from which escape might be difficult. (Chapter 6)

alarm reaction The first stage of the general adaptation syndrome (GAS), in which the body's defenses are mobilized against a stressor. (Chapter 5)

alcohol dehydrogenase A liver enzyme that metabolizes alcohol into aldehyde. (Chapter 13)

aldehyde dehydrogenase An enzyme that converts aldehyde to acetic acid. (Chapter 13)

aldehydes A class of organic compounds obtained from alcohol by oxidation and also found in cigarette smoke; they cause mutations and are related to the development of cancer. (Chapter 12)

alkalosis An abnormally high level of alkaline in the body. (Chapter 14)

allergy An immune system response characterized by an abnormal reaction to a foreign substance. (Chapter 6)

allostasis The concept that different circumstances require different levels of physiological activation. (Chapter 5)

alternative medicine A group of diverse medical and health care systems, practices, and products that are not currently considered part of conventional medicine and are used as alternatives to conventional treatment. (Chapter 8)

amenorrhea Cessation of the menses. (Chapter 14)

amphetamines One type of stimulant drug. (Chapter 13)

anabolic steroids Steroid drugs that increase muscle bulk and decrease body fat but also have toxic effects. (Chapter 13)

anaerobic exercise Exercise that requires short, intensive bursts of energy but does not require an increased amount of oxygen use. (Chapter 15)

analgesic drugs Drugs that decrease the perception of pain. (Chapter 7)

anemia A low level of red blood cells, leading to generalized weakness and lack of vitality. (Chapter 14)

anesthesia Loss of sensations of temperature, touch, or pain. (Chapter 13)

angina pectoris A disorder involving a restricted blood supply to the myocardium, which results in chest pain and restricted breathing. (Chapter 9)

anorexia nervosa An eating disorder characterized by intentional starvation, distorted body image, excessive amounts of energy, and an intense fear of gaining weight. (Chapter 14)

antibodies Protein substances produced in response to a specific invader or antigen, marking it for destruction and thus creating immunity to that invader. (Chapter 6)

antigens Substances that provoke the immune system to produce antibodies. (Chapter 6)

anus Opening through which feces are eliminated. (Chapter 14)

arteries Vessels carrying blood away from the heart. (Chapter 9)

arterioles Small branches of an artery. (Chapter 9)

arteriosclerosis A condition marked by loss of elasticity and hardening of arteries. (Chapter 9)

asthma A chronic disease that causes constriction of the bronchial tubes, preventing air from passing freely and causing wheezing and difficulty breathing during attacks. (Chapters 6, 11)

atheromatous plaques Deposits of cholesterol and other lipids, connective tissue, and muscle tissue. (Chapter 9)

atherosclerosis The formation of plaque within the arteries. (Chapter 9)

autoimmune diseases Disorders that occur as a result of the immune system's failure to differentiate between body cells and foreign cells, resulting in the body's attack and destruction of its own cells. (Chapter 6)

autonomic nervous system (ANS) The part of the peripheral nervous system that primarily serves internal organs. (Chapter 5)

aversion therapy A type of behavioral therapy, based on classical conditioning techniques, that uses some aversive stimulus to countercondition the patient's response. (Chapter 13)

Ayurveda A system of medicine that originated in India more than 2,000 years ago; it emphasizes the attainment of health through balance and connection with all things in the universe. (Chapter 8)

B-cell A variety of lymphocyte that attacks invading microorganisms. (Chapter 6)

barbiturates Synthetic sedative drugs used medically to induce sleep. (Chapter 13)

behavior modification Shaping behavior by manipulating reinforcement in order to obtain a desired behavior. (Chapter 7)

behavioral medicine An interdisciplinary field concerned with developing and integrating behavioral and biomedical sciences. (Chapter 1)

benign Limited in cell growth to a single tumor. (Chapter 10)

beta-carotene A form of vitamin A found in abundance in vegetables such as carrots and sweet potatoes. (Chapter 10)

bile salts Salts produced in the liver and stored in the gall bladder that aid in digestion of fats. (Chapter 14)

biofeedback The process of providing feedback information about the status of a biological system to that system. (Chapter 8)

biomedical model A perspective that considers disease to result from exposure to a specific disease-causing organism. (Chapter 1)

biopsychosocial model The approach to health that includes biological, psychological, and social influences. (Chapter 1)

body mass index (BMI) An estimate of obesity determined by body weight and height. (Chapter 14)

bronchitis Any inflammation of the bronchi. (Chapter 12)

bulimia An eating disorder characterized by periodic bingeing and purging, the latter usually taking the form of self-induced vomiting or laxative abuse. (Chapter 14)

C fibers Small-diameter nerve fibers that provide information concerning slow, diffuse, lingering pain. (Chapter 7)

cancer A group of diseases characterized by the presence of new cells that grow and spread beyond control. (Chapter 10)

capillaries Very small vessels that connect arteries and veins. (Chapter 9)

carcinogenic Cancer-inducing. (Chapter 10)

carcinoma Cancer of the epithelial tissues. (Chapter 10)

cardiac arrhythmia Irregularity in the heartbeat rhythm. (Chapter 15)

cardiac rehabilitation A complex of approaches designed to restore heart patients to cardiovascular health. (Chapter 9)

cardiologist A medical doctor who specializes in the diagnosis and treatment of heart disease. (Chapter 9)

cardiovascular disease (CVD) Disorders of the circulatory system, including coronary artery disease and stroke. (Chapter 9)

cardiovascular reactivity (CVR) An increase in blood pressure and heart rate as a reaction to frustration or harassment. (Chapter 9)

cardiovascular system The system of the body that includes the heart, arteries, and veins. (Chapter 9)

case–control study A retrospective epidemiological study in which people affected by a given disease (cases) are compared to others not affected (controls). (Chapter 2)

catecholamines A class of chemicals containing epinephrine and norepinephrine. (Chapter 5)

catharsis The spoken or written expression of strong negative emotion, which may result in improvement in physiological or psychological health. (Chapter 5)

central control trigger A nerve impulse that descends from the brain and influences the perception of pain (Chapter 7)

central nervous system (CNS) All the neurons within the brain and spinal cord. (Chapter 5)

cholecystokinin (CCK) A peptide hormone released by the intestines that may be involved in feelings of satiation after eating. (Chapter 14)

chronic pain Pain that endures beyond the time of normal healing; frequently experienced in the absence of detectable tissue damage. (Chapter 7)

chronic recurrent pain Alternating episodes of intense pain and no pain. (Chapter 7) cilia Tiny, hairlike structures lining parts of the respiratory system. (Chapter 12)

cirrhosis A liver disease resulting in the production of non-functional scar tissue. (Chapter 13)

clinical trial A research design that tests the effects of medical treatment. Many clinical trials are randomized, controlled trials that allow researchers to determine whether a new treatment is or is not effective. (Chapter 2)

cluster headache A type of severe headache that occurs in daily clusters for 4 to 16 weeks. Symptoms are similar to migraine, but duration is much briefer. (Chapter 7)

cocaine A stimulant drug extracted from the coca plant. (Chapter 13)

cognitive behavioral therapy (CBT) A type of therapy that aims to develop beliefs, attitudes, thoughts, and skills to make positive changes in behavior. (Chapter 5)

cognitive therapy A type of therapy that aims to change attitudes and beliefs, assuming that behavior change will follow. (Chapter 7)

complementary medicine A group of diverse medical and health care systems, practices, and products that are not currently considered part of conventional medicine and are used in addition to conventional techniques. (Chapter 8)

coping Strategies that individuals use to manage the distressing problems and emotions in their lives. (Chapter 5)

coronary artery disease (CAD) A disorder of the myocardium arising from atherosclerosis and/or arteriosclerosis. (Chapter 9)

coronary heart disease (CHD) Any damage to the myocardium resulting from insufficient blood supply. (Chapter 9)

correlation coefficient Any positive or negative relationship between two variables. Correlational evidence cannot prove causation, but only that two variables vary together. (Chapter 2)

correlational studies Studies designed to yield information concerning the degree of relationship between two variables. (Chapter 2)

cortisol A type of glucocorticoid that provides a natural defense against inflammation and regulates carbohydrate metabolism. (Chapter 5)

cross-sectional study A type of research design in which subjects of different ages are studied at one point in time. (Chapter 2)

crowding A person's perception of discomfort in a high-density environment. (Chapter 5)

cytokines Chemical messengers secreted by cells in the immune system, forming a communication link between the nervous and immune systems. (Chapter 6)

daily hassles Everyday events that people experience as harmful, threatening, or annoying. (Chapter 5)

delirium tremens A condition induced by alcohol withdrawal and characterized by excessive trembling, sweating, anxiety, and hallucinations. (Chapter 13)

delta alcoholism A drinking pattern characterized by an inability to abstain from alcohol. (Chapter 13)

dependence A condition in which a drug becomes incorporated into the functioning of the body's cells so that it is needed for "normal" functioning. (Chapters 7, 13)

diabetes mellitus A disorder caused by insulin deficiency. (Chapters 6, 11)

diaphragm The partition separating the cavity of the chest from that of the abdomen. (Chapter 12)

diastolic pressure A measure of blood pressure between contractions of the heart. (Chapter 9)

diathesis–stress model A theory of stress that suggests that some individuals are vulnerable to stress-related illnesses because they are genetically predisposed to those illnesses. (Chapter 6)

disulfiram A drug that causes an aversive reaction when taken with alcohol; used to treat alcoholism; Antabuse. (Chapter 13)

dopamine A neurotransmitter that is especially important in mediating the reward associated with taking psychoactive drugs. (Chapter 13)

dorsal horns The part of the spinal cord away from the stomach that receives sensory input and that may play an important role in the perception of pain. (Chapter 7)

dose–response relationship A direct, consistent relationship between an independent variable, such as a behavior, and a dependent variable, such as an illness. For example, the greater the number of cigarettes one smokes, the greater the likelihood of lung cancer. (Chapter 2)

double-blind design An experimental design in which neither the subjects nor those who dispense the treatment condition have knowledge of who receives the treatment and who receives the placebo. (Chapter 2)

eating disorder Any serious and habitual disturbance in eating behavior that produces unhealthy consequences. (Chapter 14)

efferent neurons Motor neurons that convey impulses away from the brain. (Chapter 7)

electrolyte imbalance A condition caused by loss of body minerals. (Chapter 14)

electromyograph (EMG) biofeedback Feedback that reflects activity of the skeletal muscles. (Chapter 8)

emotion-focused coping Coping strategies oriented toward managing the emotions that accompany the perception of stress. (Chapter 5)

emotional disclosure A therapeutic technique whereby people express their strong emotions by talking or writing about the events that precipitated them. (Chapter 5)

emphysema A chronic lung disease in which scar tissue and mucus obstruct the respiratory passages. (Chapter 12)

endocrine system The system of the body consisting of ductless glands. (Chapter 5)

endorphins Naturally occurring neurochemicals whose effects resemble those of the opiates. (Chapter 7)

environmental tobacco smoke (ETS) The smoke of spouses, parents, or coworkers to which nonsmokers are exposed; passive smoking. (Chapter 12)

epidemiology A branch of medicine that investigates the various factors that contribute either to positive health or to the frequency and distribution of a disease or disorder. (Chapter 2)

epinephrine A chemical manufactured by the adrenal medulla that accounts for much of the hormone production of the adrenal glands; sometimes called adrenaline. (Chapter 5)

esophagus The tube leading from the pharynx to the stomach. (Chapter 14)

essential hypertension Elevations of blood pressure that have no known cause. (Chapter 9)

ethanol The variety of alcohol used in beverages. (Chapter 13)

ex post facto design A scientific study in which the values of the independent variable are not manipulated, but selected by the experimenter after the groups have naturally divided themselves. (Chapter 2)

exhaustion stage The final stage of the general adaptation syndrome (GAS), in which the body's ability to resist a stressor has been depleted. (Chapter 5)

feces Any materials left over after digestion. (Chapter 14)

fetal alcohol syndrome (FAS) A pattern of physical and psychological symptoms found in infants whose mothers drank heavily during pregnancy. (Chapter 13)

fibromyalgia A chronic pain condition characterized by tender points throughout the body; this condition produces symptoms of fatigue, headache, cognitive difficulties, anxiety, and sleep disturbances. (Chapter 7)

formaldehyde A colorless, pungent gas found in cigarette smoke; it causes irritation of the respiratory system and has been found to be carcinogenic; one of the aldehydes. (Chapter 12)

gall bladder A sac on the liver in which bile is stored. (Chapter 14)

gamma alcoholism A drinking pattern characterized by loss of control. (Chapter 13)

gastric juices Stomach secretions that aid in digestion. (Chapter 14)

gate control theory A theory of pain holding that structures in the spinal cord act as a gate for sensory input that is interpreted as pain. (Chapter 7)

general adaptation syndrome (GAS) The body's generalized attempt to defend itself against stress; consists of alarm reaction, resistance, and exhaustion. (Chapter 5)

ghrelin A peptide hormone produced primarily in the stomach, the level of which rises before and falls after meals. (Chapter 14)

glucagon A hormone secreted by the pancreas that stimulates the release of glucose, thus elevating blood sugar level. (Chapter 11)

granulocyte A type of lymphocyte that acts rapidly to kill invading organisms. (Chapter 6)

health expectancy The period of life that a person spends free from disability. (Chapter 16)

health literacy The ability to read and understand health information to make health decisions. (Chapter 16)

health psychology A field of psychology that contributes to both behavioral medicine and behavioral health; the scientific study of behaviors that relate to health enhancement, disease prevention, and rehabilitation. (Chapter 1)

high-density lipoprotein (HDL) A form of lipoprotein that confers some protection against coronary artery disease. (Chapter 9)

hormones Chemical substances released into the blood and having effects on other parts of the body. (Chapter 5)

human immunodeficiency virus (HIV) A virus that attacks the human immune system, depleting the body's ability to fight infection; the infection that causes AIDS. (Chapter 11)

humoral immunity Immunity created through the process of exposure to antigens and production of antibodies in the bloodstream. (Chapter 6)

hydrocyanic acid A poisonous acid produced by treating a cyanide with an acid; one of the products of cigarette smoke. (Chapter 12)

hypertension Abnormally high blood pressure, with either a systolic reading in excess of 160 or a diastolic reading in excess of 105. (Chapter 9)

hypoglycemia Deficiency of sugar in the blood. (Chapter 14)

hypothalamus A small structure beneath the thalamus, involved in the control of eating, drinking, and emotional behavior. (Chapter 14)

illness behavior Those activities undertaken by people who feel ill and who wish to discover their state of health, as well as suitable remedies. Illness behavior precedes formal diagnosis. (Chapter 3)

immune surveillance theory A theoretical model suggesting that cancer is the result of an immune system dysfunction. (Chapter 6)

immunity A response to foreign microorganisms that occurs with repeated exposure and results in resistance to a disease. (Chapter 6)

incidence A measure of the frequency of new cases of a disease or disorder during a specified period of time. (Chapter 2)

induction The process of being placed into a hypnotic state. (Chapter 8)

inflammation A general immune system response that works to restore damaged tissue. (Chapter 6)

insulin A hormone that enhances glucose intake to the cells. (Chapter 11)

integrative medicine The approach to treatment that attempts to integrate techniques from both conventional and alternative medicine. (Chapter 8)

interneurons Neurons that connect sensory neurons to motor neurons; association neurons. (Chapter 7)

ischemia Restriction of blood flow to tissue or organs; often used with reference to the heart. (Chapter 9)

islet cells The part of the pancreas that produces glucagon and insulin. (Chapter 11)

isokinetic exercise Exercise requiring exertion for lifting and additional effort for returning weight to the starting position. (Chapter 15) isometric exercise Exercise performed by contracting muscles against an immovable object. (Chapter 15)

isotonic exercise Exercise that requires the contraction of muscles and the movement of joints, as in weight lifting. (Chapter 15)

Kaposi's sarcoma A malignancy characterized by multiple soft, dark blue or purple nodules on the skin, with hemorrhages. (Chapter 10)

laminae Layers of cell bodies. (Chapter 7)

leptin A protein hormone produced by fat cells in the body that is related to eating and weight control. (Chapter 14)

leukemia Cancer originating in blood or blood-producing cells. (Chapter 10)

life events Major events in a person's life that require change or adaptation. (Chapter 5)

lipoproteins Substances in the blood consisting of lipid and protein. (Chapter 9)

liver The largest gland in the body; it aids digestion by producing bile, regulates organic components of the blood, and acts as a detoxifier of blood. (Chapter 14)

longitudinal study A type of research design in which one group of subjects is studied over a period of time. (Chapter 2)

low-density lipoprotein (LDL) A form of lipoprotein found to be positively related to coronary artery disease. (Chapter 9)

lymph Tissue fluid that has entered a lymphatic vessel. (Chapter 6)

lymph nodes Small nodules of lymphatic tissue spaced throughout the lymphatic system that help clean lymph of debris. (Chapter 6)

lymphatic system System that transports lymph through the body. (Chapter 6)

lymphocytes White blood cells found in lymph that are involved in the immune function. (Chapter 6)

lymphoma Cancer of the lymphoid tissues, including lymph nodes. (Chapter 10)

macrophage A type of lymphocyte that attacks invading organisms. (Chapter 6)

malignant Having the ability not only to grow but also to spread to other parts of the body. (Chapter 10)

medulla The structure of the hindbrain just above the spinal cord. (Chapter 7)

meta-analysis A statistical technique for combining results of several studies when these studies have similar definitions of variables. (Chapter 2)

metastasize To undergo metastasis, the spread of malignancy from one part of the body to another by way of the blood or lymph systems. (Chapter 10)

migraine headache Recurrent headache pain originally believed to be caused by constriction and dilation of the vascular arteries but now accepted as involving neurons in the brain stem. (Chapter 7)

model A set of related principles or hypotheses constructed to explain significant relationships among concepts or observations. (Chapter 2)

motivational interviewing A therapeutic approach that originated within substance abuse treatment that attempts to change a client's motivation and prepares the client to enact changes in behavior. (Chapter 4)

mucociliary escalator The mechanism by which debris is moved toward the pharynx. (Chapter 12)

myelin A fatty substance that acts as insulation for neurons. (Chapter 7)

myocardial infarction Heart attack. (Chapter 9)

myocardium The heart muscle. (Chapter 9)

natural killer (NK) cell A type of lymphocyte that attacks invading organisms. (Chapter 6)

naturopathy A medical system that arose in Europe during the 19th century that holds that nature contains the power to heal and the human body has the ability to maintain and to return to a state of health. (Chapter 8)

negative reinforcement Removing an unpleasant or negatively valued stimulus from a situation, thereby strengthening the behavior that precedes this removal. (Chapter 4)

neoplastic Characterized by new, abnormal growth of cells. (Chapter 10)

neuroendocrine system Those endocrine glands that are controlled by and interact with the nervous system. (Chapter 5)

neurons Nerve cells. (Chapter 5)

neurotransmitters Chemicals that are released by neurons and that affect the activity of other neurons. (Chapter 5)

nitric oxide A colorless gas prepared by the action of nitric acid on copper and also produced in cigarette smoke; it affects oxygen metabolism and may be dangerous. (Chapter 12)

nocebo effect Adverse effect of a placebo. (Chapter 2)

nociceptors Sensory receptors in the skin and organs that are capable of responding to various types of stimulation that may cause tissue damage. (Chapter 7)

non-Hodgkin's lymphoma A malignancy characterized by rapidly growing tumors that are spread through the circulatory or lymphatic systems. (Chapter 10)

norepinephrine One of two major neurotransmitters of the autonomic nervous system. (Chapter 5)

oncologist A physician who specializes in the treatment of cancer. (Chapter 10)

opiates Drugs derived from the opium poppy, including codeine, morphine, and heroin. (Chapter 13)

optimistic bias The belief that other people, but not oneself, will develop a disease, have an accident, or experience other negative events. (Chapters 3, 4, 9, 12)

osteoarthritis Progressive inflammation of the joints. (Chapter 7)

osteoporosis A disease characterized by a reduction in bone density, brittleness of bones, and a loss of calcium from the bones. (Chapter 15)

pancreas An endocrine gland, located below the stomach, that produces digestive juices and hormones. (Chapter 11)

pancreatic juices Acid-reducing enzymes secreted by the pancreas into the small intestine. (Chapter 14)

parasympathetic nervous system A division of the autonomic nervous system that promotes relaxation and functions under normal, nonstressful conditions. (Chapter 5)

passive smoking The exposure of nonsmokers to the smoke of spouses, parents, or coworkers; environmental tobacco smoke. (Chapter 12)

pathogen Any disease-causing organism. (Chapter 1)

pepsin An enzyme, produced by gastric mucosa, that initiates digestive activity. (Chapter 14)

periaqueductal gray An area of the midbrain that, when stimulated, decreases pain. (Chapter 7)

peripheral nervous system (PNS) The nerves that lie outside the brain and spinal cord. (Chapter 5)

peristalsis Contractions that propel food through the digestive tract. (Chapter 14)

personal control Confidence that people have in their ability to control the events that shape their lives. (Chapter 5)

phagocytosis The process of engulfing and killing foreign particles. (Chapter 6)

phantom limb pain The experience of chronic pain in an absent body part. (Chapter 7)

pharynx Part of the digestive tract between the mouth and the esophagus. (Chapter 14)

pituitary gland An endocrine gland that lies within the brain and whose secretions regulate many other glands. (Chapter 5)

placebo An inactive substance or condition that has the appearance of an active treatment and that may cause improvement or change because of people's belief in the placebo's efficacy. (Chapter 2)

plasma cells Cells, derived from B-cells, that secrete antibodies. (Chapter 6)

population density A physical condition in which a large population occupies a limited space. (Chapter 5)

positive reinforcement Adding a positively valued stimulus to a situation, thereby strengthening the behavior it follows. (Chapter 4)

positive reinforcer Any positively valued stimulus that, when added to a situation, strengthens the behavior it follows. (Chapter 7)

posttraumatic stress disorder (PTSD) An anxiety disorder caused by experience with an extremely traumatic event and characterized by recurrent and intrusive reexperiencing of the event. (Chapters 5, 6)

prechronic pain Pain that endures beyond the acute phase but has not yet become chronic. (Chapter 7)

prevalence The proportion of a population that has a disease or disorder at a specific point in time. (Chapter 2)

primary afferents Sensory neurons that convey impulses from the skin to the spinal cord. (Chapter 7)

primary appraisal One's initial appraisal of a potentially stressful event (Lazarus and Folkman). (Chapter 5)

proactive coping A coping strategy that involves anticipating a problem and taking steps to avoid it. (Chapter 5)

problem-focused coping Coping strategies aimed at changing the source of the stress. (Chapter 5)

prospective studies Longitudinal studies that begin with a disease-free group of subjects and follow the occurrence of disease in that population or sample. (Chapter 2)

prudent diet A dietary pattern high in fruits, vegetables, whole grains, low-fat dairy products, fish, and poultry and low in red meat and refined grains. (Chapter 10)

psychoneuroimmunology (PNI) A multidisciplinary field that focuses on the interactions among behavior, the nervous system, the endocrine system, and the immune system. (Chapter 6)

punishment The presentation of an aversive stimulus or the removal of a positive one. Punishment sometimes, but not always, weakens a response. (Chapter 4)

Raynaud's disease A vasoconstrictive disorder characterized by inadequate circulation in the extremities, especially the fingers or toes, resulting in pain. (Chapter 8)

reappraisal One's nearly constant reevaluation of stressful events (Lazarus and Folkman). (Chapter 5)

reciprocal determinism Bandura's model that includes environment, behavior, and person as mutually interacting factors. (Chapter 4)

rectum The end of the digestive tract leading to the anus. (Chapter 14)

relative risk The risk a person has for a particular disease compared with the risk of other people who do not have that person's condition or lifestyle. (Chapter 2)

reliability The extent to which a test or other measuring instrument yields consistent results. (Chapter 2)

resistance stage The second stage of the general adaptation syndrome (GAS), in which the body adapts to a stressor. (Chapter 5)

retrospective studies Longitudinal studies that look back at the history of a population or sample. (Chapter 2)

rheumatoid arthritis An autoimmune disorder characterized by a dull ache within or around a joint. (Chapters 6, 7)

risk factor Any characteristic or condition that occurs with greater frequency in people with a disease than it does in people free from that disease. (Chapter 2)

salivary glands Glands that furnish moisture that helps in tasting and digesting food. (Chapter 14)

sarcoma Cancer of the connective tissues. (Chapter 10)

secondary appraisal One's perceived ability to control or cope with harm, threat, or challenge (Lazarus and Folkman). (Chapter 5)

secondary hypertension Elevations in blood pressure that are triggered by other diseases. (Chapter 9)

sedatives Drugs that induce relaxation and sometimes intoxication by lowering the activity of the brain, the neurons, the muscles, the heart, and even by slowing the metabolic rate. (Chapter 13)

selenium A trace element found in grain products and in meat from grain-fed animals. (Chapter 10)

self-efficacy The belief that one is capable of performing the behaviors that will produce desired outcomes in any particular situation. (Chapters 3, 4)

self-selection A condition of an experimental investigation in which subjects are allowed, in some manner, to determine their own placement in either the experimental or the control group. (Chapter 2)

setpoint A hypothetical ratio of fat to lean tissue at which a person's weight will tend to stabilize. (Chapter 14)

sick role behavior Those activities undertaken by people who have been diagnosed as sick that are directed at getting well. (Chapter 3)

single-blind design A design in which the participants do not know if they are receiving the active or inactive treatment, but the providers are not blind to treatment conditions. (Chapter 2)

social contacts Number and kinds of people with whom one associates; members of one's social network. (Chapter 5)

social isolation The absence of specific role relationships. (Chapter 5)

social network The number and kinds of people with whom one associates; social contacts. (Chapter 5)

social support Both tangible and intangible support a person receives from other people. (Chapters 4, 5)

somatic nervous system The part of the PNS that serves the skin and voluntary muscles. (Chapter 5)

somatosensory cortex The part of the brain that receives and processes sensory input from the body. (Chapter 7)

somatosensory system The part of the nervous system that carries sensory information from the body to the brain. (Chapter 7)

spleen A large organ near the stomach that serves as a repository for lymphocytes and red blood cells. (Chapter 6)

spontaneous remission Disappearance of problem behavior or illness without treatment. (Chapter 13)

state anxiety A temporary condition of dread or uneasiness stemming from a specific situation. (Chapter 15)

stroke Damage to the brain resulting from lack of oxygen; typically the result of cardiovascular disease. (Chapter 9)

subject variable A variable chosen (rather than manipulated) by a researcher to provide levels of comparison for groups of subjects. (Chapter 2)

substantia gelatinosa Two layers of the dorsal horns of the spinal cord. (Chapter 7)

sympathetic nervous system A division of the autonomic nervous system that mobilizes the body's resources in emergency, stressful, and emotional situations. (Chapter 5)

synaptic cleft The space between neurons. (Chapter 5)

syndrome A cluster of symptoms that characterize a particular condition. (Chapter 7)

synergistic effect The combined effect of two or more variables that exceeds the sum of their individual effects. (Chapter 10)

systolic pressure A measure of blood pressure generated by the heart's contraction. (Chapter 9)

T-cells The cells of the immune system that produce immunity. (Chapter 6)

tension headache Pain produced by sustained muscle contractions in the neck, shoulders, scalp, and face, as well as by activity in the central nervous system. (Chapter 7)

thalamus Structure in the forebrain that acts as a relay center for incoming sensory information and outgoing motor information. (Chapter 7)

theory A set of related assumptions from which testable hypotheses can be drawn. (Chapter 2)

thermal biofeedback Feedback concerning changes in skin temperature. (Chapter 8)

thermister A temperature-sensitive resistor used in thermal biofeedback. (Chapter 8)

thymosin A hormone produced by the thymus. (Chapter 6)

thymus An organ located near the heart that secretes thymosin and thus processes and activates T-cells. (Chapter 6)

tolerance The need for increasing levels of a drug in order to produce a constant level of effect. (Chapters 7, 13)

tonsils Masses of lymphatic tissue located in the pharynx. (Chapter 6)

trait anxiety A personality characteristic that manifests itself as a more or less constant feeling of dread or uneasiness. (Chapter 15)

tranquilizers A type of sedative drug that reduces anxiety. (Chapter 13)

transcutaneous electrical nerve stimulation (TENS) Treatment for pain involving electrical stimulation of neurons from the surface of the skin. (Chapter 7)

triglycerides A group of molecules consisting of glycerol and three fatty acids; one of the components of serum lipids that has been implicated in the formation of atherosclerotic plaque. (Chapter 9)

urban press The many environmental stressors that affect city living, including noise, crowding, crime, and pollution. (Chapter 5)

vaccination A method of inducing immunity in which a weakened form of a virus or bacterium is introduced into the body. (Chapter 6)

validity Accuracy; the extent to which a test or other measuring instrument measures what it is supposed to measure. (Chapter 2)

veins Vessels that carry blood to the heart. (Chapter 9)

venules The smallest veins. (Chapter 9)

well-year The equivalent of a year of complete wellness. (Chapter 16)

withdrawal Adverse physiological reactions exhibited when a drug-dependent person stops using that drug; the withdrawal symptoms are typically unpleasant and opposite to the drug's effects. (Chapter 13)

REFERENCES

Abbott, R. B., Hui, K.-K., Hays, R. D., Li, M.-D., & Pan, T. (2007). A randomized controlled trial of tai chi for tension headaches. *Evidence Based Complementary and Alternative Medicine, 4*, 107–113.

Abel, E. L. (2004). Paternal contribution to fetal alcohol syndrome. *Addiction Biology, 9*, 127–133.

Abi-Saleh, B., Iskandar, S. B., Elgharib, N., & Cohen, M. V. (2008). C-reactive protein: The harbinger of cardiovascular diseases. *Southern Medical Journal, 101*, 525–533.

Abnet, C. C. (2007). Carcinogenic food contaminants. *Cancer Investigation, 25*, 189–196.

Abraído-Lanza, A. F., Chao, M. T., & Flórez, K. R. (2005). Do healthy behaviors decline with greater acculturation? Implications for the Latino mortality paradox. *Social Science and Medicine, 61*, 1243–1255.

Ackard, D. M., Brehm, B. J., & Steffen, J. J. (2002). Exercise and eating disorders in college-aged women: Profiling excessive exercisers. *Eating Disorders, 10*, 31–47.

Ackroff, L., Bonacchi, K., Magee, M., Yijn, Y.-M., Graves, J. V., & Sclafani, A. (2007). Obesity by choice revisited: Effects of food availability, flavor variety and nutrient composition on energy intake. *Physiology and Behavior, 92*, 468–478.

Acme Celebs. (2002). *Drew Barrymore*. Retrieved March 29, 2005, from http://www.acmecelebs.com/drew_barrymore/biography.htm

Adams, B., Aranda, M. P., Kemp, B., & Takagi, K. (2002). Ethnic and gender differences in distress among Anglo American, African American, Japanese American, and Mexican American spousal caregivers of persons with dementia. *Journal of Clinical Geropsychology, 8*, 279–301.

Adams, J., & White, M. (2003). Are activity promotion interventions based on the transtheoretical model effective? A critical review. *British Journal of Sports Medicine, 37*, 106–114.

Adams, R. E., & Boscarino, J. A. (2005). Stress and well-being in the aftermath of the World Trade Center attack: The continuing effects of a communitywide disaster. *Journal of Community Psychology, 33*, 175–190.

Adams, T. B., & Colner, W. (2008). The association of multiple risk factors with fruit and vegetable intake among a nationwide sample of college students. *Journal of American College Health, 56*, 455–461.

Adamson, J., Ben-Shlomo, Y., Chaturvedi, N., & Donovan, J. (2003). Ethnicity, socio-economic position and gender: Do they affect reported health-care seeking behavior? *Social Science and Medicine, 47*, 895–904.

Ader, R., & Cohen, N. (1975). Behaviorally conditioned immunosuppression. *Psychosomatic Medicine, 37*, 333–340.

Agency for Healthcare Quality Research (AHQR). (2004). *2004 National healthcare disparities report*. AHRQ Publication No. 05-0014. Rockville, MD: U.S. Department of Health and Human Services.

Ahrens, M. (2004). Smoking and fire. *American Journal of Public Health, 94*, 1075–1076.

Ai, A. L., Peterson, C., Tice, T. N., Bolling, S. F., & Koenig, H. G. (2004). Faith-based and secular pathways to hope and optimism subconstructs in middle-aged and older cardiac patients. *Journal of Health Psychology, 9*, 435–452.

Ajzen, I. (1985). From intentions to actions: A theory of planned behavior. In J. Kuhland & J. Beckman (Eds.), *Action-control: From cognitions to behavior* (pp. 11–39). Heidelberg, Germany: Springer.

Ajzen, I. (1988). *Attitudes, personality, and behavior*. Chicago: Dorsey Press.

Ajzen, I. (1991). The theory of planned behavior. *Organizational Behavior and Human Decision Processes, 50*, 179–211.

Ajzen, I., & Fishbein, M. (1980). *Understanding attitudes and predicting social behavior*. Englewood Cliffs, NJ: Prentice-Hall.

Ajzen, I., & Fishbein, M. (2004). Questions raised by a reasoned action approach: Comment on Ogden (2003). *Health Psychology, 23*, 431–434.

Alaejos, M. S., González, V., & Afonso, A. M. (2008). Exposure to heterocyclic aromatic amines from the consumption of cooked red meat and its effect on human cancer risk: A review. *Food Additives and Contaminants, 25*, 2–24.

Albert, C. M., Mittleman, M. A., Chae, C. U., Lee, I.-M., Hennekens, C. H., & Manson, J. E. (2000). Triggering of sudden death from cardiac causes by vigorous exertion. *New England Journal of Medicine, 343*, 1355–1361.

Aldana, S. G., Greenlaw, R., Salberg, A., Merrill, R. M., Hager, R., & Jorgensen, R. B. (2007). The effects of an intensive lifestyle modification program on carotid artery intima-media thickness: A randomized trial. *American Journal of Health Promotion, 21*, 510–516.

Aldridge, A. A., & Roesch, S. C. (2007). Coping and adjustment in children and cancer: A meta-analytic study. *Journal of Behavioral Medicine, 30*, 115–129.

Alexander, F. (1950). *Psychosomatic medicine*. New York: Norton.

Alfermann, D., & Stoll, O. (2000). Effects of physical exercise on self-concept and well-being. *International Journal of Sport Psychology, 31*, 47–65.

Allen, K. (2003). Are pets a healthy pleasure? The influence of pets on blood pressure. *Current Directions in Psychological Science, 12*, 236–239.

Allison, K. C., & Park, C. L. (2004). A prospective study of disordered eating among sorority and nonsorority women. *International Journal of Eating Disorders, 35*, 354–358.

Alper, J. (1993). Ulcers as infectious diseases. *Science, 260*, 159–160.

Alzheimer's Organization. (2004). *Text of President Reagan's letter announcing his own Alzheimer's diagnosis, November 5, 1994.* Retrieved July 1, 2005, from http://www.alz.org/Media/newsreleases/ronaldreagan/ reaganletter.asp

Amabile, N., Susini, G., Pettenati-Soubayroux, I., Bonello, L., Gil, J.-M., Arques, S., et al. (2008). Severity of periodontal disease correlates to inflammatory systemic status and independently predicts the presence and angiographic extent of stable coronary artery disease. *Journal of Internal Medicine, 263*, 644–652.

Amato, P. R., & Hohmann-Marriott, B. (2007). A comparison of high- and low-distress marriages that end in divorce. *Journal of Marriage and Family, 69*, 621–638.

American Cancer Society. (2007). *Macrobiotic diet.* Retrieved May 5, 2008, from http://www.cancer.org/docroot/ETO/content/ETO_5_3X_Macrobiotic_Diet.asp

American Cancer Society. (2008). *Cancer facts and figures 2008.* Atlanta: American Cancer Society.

American College Health Association (ACHA). (2006). American College Health Association National College Health Assessment (ACHA-NCHA) spring 2005 reference group data report. *Journal of American College Health, 55*, 5–16.

American College of Sports Medicine. (2007). *Guidelines for healthy adults under age 65.* Retrieved August 16, 2008, from http://www.acsm.org/AM/Template.cfm?Section=Home_Page&TEMPLATE=/CM/HTMLDisplay.cfm&CONTENTID=7764

American Lung Association. (2007). *Trends in asthma morbidity and mortality.* Retrieved August 3, 2008, from http://www.lungusa.org/site/c.dvLUK9O0E/b.33347/

American Psychiatric Association (APA). (2000). *Diagnostic and statistical manual of mental disorders* (4th ed., text revision). Washington, DC: Author.

American Psychological Association (APA). (2002). Ethical principles of psychologists and code of conduct. *American Psychologist, 57*, 1060–1073.

American Psychological Association (APA). (2005). Bylaws of the American Psychological Association, Article I, 1. Retrieved August 5, 2005, from http://www.apa.org/governance/bylaws/art1.html

American Psychological Association (APA) Task Force on Health Research. (1976). Contributions of psychology to health research: Patterns, problems, and potentials. *American Psychologist, 31*, 263–274.

Andel, R., Crowe, M., Pedersen, N. L., Mortimer, J., Crimmins, E., Johansson, B., et al. (2005). Complexity of work and risk of Alzheimer's disease: A population-based study of Swedish twins. *Journal of Gerontology Series B: Psychological Sciences and Social Sciences, 60B*(5), 251–258.

Andersen, L. B., Sardinha, L. B., Froberg, K., Riddoch, C. J., Page, A. S., & Anderssen, S. A. (2008). Fitness, fatness and clustering of cardiovascular risk factors in children from Denmark, Estonia and Portugal: The European Youth Heart Study. *International Journal of Pediatric Obesity, 3*(Suppl. 1), 58–66.

Anderson J. L., Horne, B. D., Jones, H. U., Reyna, S. P., Carlquist, J. F., Bair, T. L., et al. (2004). Which features of the metabolic syndrome predict the prevalence and clinical outcomes of angiographic coronary artery disease? *Cardiology, 101*, 185–193.

Anderson, J. W., Conley, S. B., & Nicholas, A. S. (2007). One hundred pound weight losses with an intensive behavioral program: Changes in risk factors in 118 patients with long-term follow-up. *American Journal of Clinical Nutrition, 86*, 301–307.

Anderson, K. O., Syrjala, K. L., & Cleeland, C. S. (2001). How to assess cancer pain. In D. C. Turk & R. Melzack (Eds.), *Handbook of pain assessment* (2nd ed., pp. 579–600). New York: Guilford Press.

Anderson, P. (2006). Global use of alcohol, drugs and tobacco. *Drug and Alcohol Review, 25*, 489–502.

Andersson, K., Melander, A., Svensson, C., Lind, O., & Nilsson, J. L. G. (2005). Repeat prescriptions: Refill adherence in relation to patient and prescriber characteristics, reimbursement level and type of medication. *European Journal of Public Health, 15*, 621–626.

Andrasik, F. (2001). Assessment of patients with headache. In D. C. Turk & R. Melzack (Eds.), *Handbook of pain assessment* (2nd ed., pp. 454–474). New York: Guilford Press.

Andrasik, F. (2003). Behavioral treatment approaches to chronic headache. *Neurological Science, 24*, S80–S85.

Andrasik, F. (2006). Psychophysiological disorders: Headache as a case in point. In F. Andrasik (Ed.), *Comprehensive handbook of personality and psychopathology: Vol. 2. Adult psychopathology* (pp. 409–422). Hoboken, NJ: Wiley.

Aneshensel, C. S., Botticello, A. L., & Yamamoto–Mitani, N. (2004). When caregiving ends: The course of depressive symptoms after bereavement. *Journal of Health and Social Behavior, 45*, 422–440.

Anisman, H., Merali, Z., Poulter, M. O., & Hayley, S. (2005). Cytokines as a precipitant of depressive illness: Animal and human studies. *Current Pharmaceutical Design, 11*, 963–972.

Annesi, J. J. (2005). Changes in depressed mood associated with 10 weeks of moderate cardiovascular exercise in formerly sedentary adults. *Psychological Reports, 96*, 855–862.

Annesi, J. J. (2007). Effects of a computer feedback treatment and behavioral support protocol on drop out from a newly initiated exercise program. *Perceptual and Motor Skills, 105*, 55–66.

Annesi, J. J., & Unruh, J. L. (2007). Effects of the Coach Approach® intervention on drop-out rates among adults initiating exercise programs at nine YMCAs over three years. *Perceptual and Motor Skills, 104,* 459–466.

Anshel, M. H. (2004). Sources of disordered eating patterns between ballet dancers and non-dancers. *Journal of Sport Behavior, 27,* 115–133.

Antall, G. F., & Kresevic, D. (2004). The use of guided imagery to manage pain in an elderly orthopaedic population. *Orthopaedic Nursing, 23,* 335–340.

Antoni, M. H., Ironson, G., & Scheiderman, N. (2007). *Cognitive-behavioral stress management workbook.* New York: Oxford University Press.

Antoni, M. H., & Lutgendorf, S. (2007). Psychosocial factors in disease progression in cancer. *Current Directions in Psychological Science, 16,* 42–46.

Apkarian, A. V., Bushnell, M. C., Treede, R.-D., & Zubieta, J.-K. (2005). Human brain mechanisms of pain perception and regulation in health and disease. *European Journal of Pain, 9,* 463–484.

Arbisi, P. A., & Butcher, J. N. (2004). Relationship between personality and health symptoms: Use of the MMIP-2 in medical assessments. *International Journal of Clinical and Health Psychology, 4,* 571–595.

Arbisi, P. A., & Seime, R. J. (2006). Use of the MMPI-2 in medical settings. In J. N. Butcher (Ed.), *MMPI-2: A practitioner's guide* (pp. 273–299). Washington, DC: American Psychological Association.

Arias, A. J., Steinberg, K., Banga, A., & Trestman, R. L. (2006). Systematic review of the efficacy of meditation techniques as treatments for medical illness. *Journal of Alternative and Complementary Medicine, 12,* 817–832.

Armeli, S., Tennen, H., Todd, M., Carney, A., Mohr, C., Affleck, G., et al. (2003). A daily process examination of the stress-response dampening effects of alcohol consumption. *Psychology of Addictive Behaviors, 17,* 266–276.

Armitage, C. J., & Conner, M. (2000). Social cognition models and health behaviour: A structured review. *Psychology & Health, 15,* 173–189.

Armitage, C. J., & Conner, M. (2001). Efficacy of the theory of planned behaviour: A meta-analytic review. *British Journal of Social Psychology, 40,* 471–499.

Armitage, C. J., Sheeran, P., Conner, M., & Arden, M. A. (2004). Stages of change or changes of stage? Predicting transitions in transtheoretical model stages in relation to healthy food choice. *Journal of Consulting and Clinical Psychology, 72,* 491–499.

Armor, D. J., Polich, J. M., & Stambul, H. B. (1976). *Alcoholism and treatment.* Santa Monica, CA: Rand.

Armour, B. S., Woollery, T., Malarcher, A., Pechacek, T. F., & Husten, C. (2005). Annual smoking-attributable mortality, years of potential life lost, and productivity losses—United States, 1997–2001. *Mortality and Morbidity Weekly Reports, 54*(25), 625–628.

Arnold, R., Ranchor, A. V., Sanderman, R., Kempen, G. I. J. M., Ormel, J., & Suurmeijer, T. P. B. M. (2004). The relative contribution of domains of quality of life to overall quality of life for different chronic diseases. *Quality of Life Research, 13,* 883–896.

Arntz, A., & Claassens, L. (2004). The meaning of pain influences its experienced intensity. *Pain, 109,* 20–25.

Aro, A. R., De Koning, H. J., Schreck, M., Henriksson, M., Anttila, A., & Pukkala, E. (2005). Psychological risk factors of incidence of breast cancer: A prospective cohort study in Finland. *Psychological Medicine, 35,* 1515–1521.

Arora, N. K., Rutten, L. J. F., Gustafson, D. H., Moser, R., & Hawkins, R. P. (2007). Perceived helpfulness and impact of social support provided by family, friends, and health care providers to women newly diagnosed with breast cancer. *Psycho-Oncology, 16,* 474–486.

Artham, S. M., Lavie, C. J., Milani, R. V. (2008). Cardiac rehabilitation programs markedly improve high-risk profiles in coronary patients with high psychological distress. *Southern Medical Journal, 101,* 262–267.

Arthur, C. M., Katkin, E. S., & Mezzacappa, E. S. (2004). Cardiovascular reactivity to mental arithmetic and cold pressor in African Americans, Caribbean Americans, and White Americans. *Annals of Behavioral Medicine, 27,* 31–37.

Ashley, M. J., Rehm, J., Bondy, S., Single, E., & Rankin, J. (2000). Beyond ischemic heart disease: Are there other health benefits from drinking alcohol? *Contemporary Drug Problems, 27,* 735–778.

Ashton, W., Nanchahal, K., & Wood, D. (2001). Body mass index and metabolic risk factors for coronary heart disease in women. *European Health Journal, 22,* 46–55.

Askay, S. W., Patterson, D. R., Jensen, M. P., & Sharar, S. R. (2007). A randomized controlled trial of hypnosis for burn wound care. *Rehabilitation Psychology, 52,* 247–253.

Aspden, P., Wolcott, J., Bootman, J. L., & Cronenwett, L. R. (Eds.). (2007). *Preventing medication errors: Quality chasm series.* Washington, DC: National Academies Press.

Aspinwall, L. G., & Taylor, S. E. (1997). A stitch in time: Self-regulation and proactive coping. *Psychological Bulletin, 121,* 417–436.

Associated Press. (2004). Clinton leaves hospital after surgery. *Associated Press Heart Health.* Retrieved June 16, 2005, from http://www.msnbc.msn.com/id/5906976/

Asthma Action America. (2004). *Children and asthma in America.* Retrieved July 7, 2005, from http://www.asthmainamerica.com/frequency.html

Astin, J. A. (1998). Why patients use alternative medicine. *Journal of the American Medical Association, 279,* 1548–1553,

Astin, J. A. (2004). Mind-body therapies for the management of pain. *Clinical Journal of Pain, 20,* 27–32.

Atlantis, E., Chow, C.-M., Kirby, A., & Fiatarone Singh, M. (2004). An effective exercise-based intervention for improving mental health and quality of life measures: A randomized controlled trial. *Preventive Medicine, 39,* 424–434.

Averbuch, M., & Katzper, M. (2000). A search for sex differences in response to analgesia. *Archives of Internal Medicine, 160,* 3424–3428.

Awad, G. H., Sagrestano, L. M., Kittleson, M. J., & Sarvela, P. D. (2004). Development of a measure of barriers to HIV testing among individuals at high risk. *AIDS Education and Prevention, 16*, 115–125.

Back, S. E., Gentilin, S., & Brady, K. T. (2007). Cognitive-behavioral stress management for individuals with substance use disorders: A pilot study. *Journal of Nervous and Mental Disease, 195*, 662–668.

Baer, H. A. (2008). The growing legitimation of complementary medicine in Australia: Successes and dilemmas. *Australian Journal of Medical Herbalism, 20*, 5–11.

Bahrke, M. S., & Morgan, W. P. (1978). Anxiety reduction following exercise and meditation. *Cognitive Therapy and Research, 2*, 323–334.

Baik, I., Ascherio, A., Rimm, E. B., Giovannucci, E., Spiegelman, D., Stampfer, M. J., et al. (2000). Adiposity and mortality in men. *American Journal of Epidemiology, 152*, 264–271.

Bailey, B. N., Delaney-Black, V., Covington, C. Y., Ager, J., Janisse, J., Hannigan, J. H., et al. (2004). Prenatal exposure to binge drinking and cognitive and behavioral outcomes at age 7 years. *American Journal of Obstetrics and Gynecology, 191*, 1037–1042.

Bailis, D. S., Segall, A., Mahon, M. J., Chipperfield, J. G., & Dunn, E. M. (2001). Perceived control in relation to socioeconomic and behavioral resources for health. *Social Science and Medicine, 52*, 1661–1676.

Baker, F., Ainsworth, S. R., Dye, J. T., Crammer, C., Thun, M. J., Hoffmann, D., et al. (2000). Health risks associated with cigar smoking. *Journal of the American Medical Association, 284*, 735–740.

Baker, S. G., Lichtenstein, P., Kaprio, J., & Holm, N. (2005). Genetic susceptibility to prostate, breast, and colorectal cancer among Nordic twins. *Biometrics, 61*, 55–63.

Bala, M., Strzeszynski, L., & Cahill, K. (2008). Mass media interventions for smoking cessation in adults. *Cochrane Database of Systematic Reviews*, Cochrane AN: CD004704.

Baliki, M. N., Geha, P. Y., Apkarian, A. V., & Chialvo, D. R. (2008). Beyond feeling: Chronic pain hurts the brain, disrupting the default-mode network dynamics. *Journal of Neuroscience, 28*, 1398–1403.

Balkrishnan, R., & Jayawant, S. S. (2007). Medication adherence research in populations: Measurement issues and other challenges. *Clinical Therapeutics, 29*, 1180–1183.

Ball, D. (2008). Addiction science and its genetics. *Addiction, 103*, 360–367.

Banaji, M. R., & Steele, C. M. (1989). The social cognition of alcohol use. *Social Cognition, 7*, 137–151.

Bandura, A. (1986). *Social foundations of thought and action: A social cognitive theory.* Englewood Cliffs, NJ: Prentice-Hall.

Bandura, A. (1997). *Self-efficacy: The exercise of control.* New York: Freeman.

Bandura, A. (2001). Social cognitive theory: An agentic perspective. *Annual Review of Psychology, 52*, 1–26.

Banegas, J. R., López-García, E., Gutiérrez-Fisac, J. L., Guallar-Castillón, P., & Rodríguez-Artalejo, F. (2003). A simple estimate of mortality attributable to excess weight in the European Union. *European Journal of Clinical Nutrition, 57*, 201–208.

Bánóczy, J., & Squier, C. (2004). Smoking and disease. *European Journal of Dental Education, 8*, 7–10.

Barbarich, D. (2008, February 4). Mary-Kate Olsen "Anorexia nearly killed me." Retrieved July 21, 2008, from http://www.entertainmentwise.com/news/40362/marykate-olsen-anorexia-nearly-killed-me

Barber, J. (1996). A brief introduction to hypnotic analgesia. In J. Barber (Ed.), *Hypnosis and suggestion in the treatment of pain: A clinical guide.* New York: Norton.

Barber, T. X. (1984). Hypnosis, deep relaxation, and active relaxation: Data, theory, and clinical applications. In R. L. Woolfolk & P. M. Lehrer (Eds.), *Principles and practice of stress management.* New York: Guilford Press.

Barber, T. X. (2000). A deeper understanding of hypnosis: Its secrets, its nature, its essence. *American Journal of Clinical Hypnosis, 42,* 208–272.

Bardia, A., Tleyjeh, I. M., Cerhan, J. R., Sood, A. K., Limburg, P. J. Erwin, P., J., et al. (2008). Efficacy of antioxidant supplementation in reducing primary cancer incidence and mortality: Systematic review and meta-analysis. *Mayo Clinic Proceedings, 83*, 23–34.

Bardy, S. S. (2008). Lifetime family violence exposure is associated with current symptoms of eating disorders among both young men and women. *Journal of Traumatic Stress, 21*, 347–351.

Barengo, N. C., Hu, G., Lakka, T. A., Pekkarinen, H., Nissinen, A., & Tuomilehto, J. (2004). Low physical activity as predictor for total and cardiovascular disease mortality in middle-aged men and women in Finland. *European Heart Journal, 25*, 2204–2211.

Barlow, J. H., & Ellard, D. R. (2004). Psycho-educational interventions for children with chronic disease, parents and siblings: An overview of the research evidence base. *Child: Care, Health and Development, 30*, 637–645.

Barnes, P. J. (2008). Immunology of asthma and chronic obstructive pulmonary disease. *Nature Reviews Immunology, 8*, 183–192.

Barnes, P. M., Powell-Griner, E., McFann, K., & Nahin, R. L. (2004). Complementary and alternative medicine use among adults: United States, 2002. *Advance Data from Vital and Health Statistics,* No. 343. Hyattsville, MD: National Center for Health Statistics.

Barnett, R. C., & Hyde, J. S. (2001). Women, men, work, and family: An expansionist theory. *American Psychologist, 56*, 781–796.

Barron, F., Hunter, A., Mayo, R., & Willoughby, D. (2004). Acculturation and adherence: Issues for health care providers working with clients of Mexican origin. *Journal of Transcultural Nursing, 15*, 331–337.

Barth, J., Critchley, J., & Bengel, J. (2008). Psychosocial interventions for smoking cessation in patients with coronary heart disease. *Cochrane Database of Sytematic Reviews*, AN: CD006886.

Barton-Donovan, K., & Blanchard, E. B. (2005). Psychosocial aspects of chronic daily headache. *Journal of Headache and Pain, 6,* 30–39.

Baseman, J. G., & Koutsky, L. A. (2005). The epidemiology of human papillomavirus infections. *Journal of Clinical Virology, 32,* 16–24.

Bassman, L. E., & Uellendahl, G. (2003). Complementary/alternative medicine: Ethical, professional, and practical challenges for psychologists. *Professional Psychology: Research and Practice, 34,* 264–270.

Batty, G. D., Shipley, M. J., Mortensen, L. H., Boyle, S. H., Barefoot, J., Grønbæk, M., et al. (2008). IQ in late adolescence/early adulthood, risk factors in middle age and later all-cause mortality in men: The Vietnam Experience Study. *Journal of Epidemiology and Community Health, 62,* 522–531.

Baum, A., Perry, N. W., Jr., & Tarbell, S. (2004). The development of psychology as a health science. In R. G. Frank, A. Baum, & J. L. Wallander (Eds.), *Handbook of clinical health psychology* (Vol. 3, pp. 9–28). Washington, DC: American Psychological Association.

Baumann, M. H., Xiaoying, W., & Rothman, R. B. (2007). 3,4- Methylenedioxymethamphetamine (MDMA) neurotoxicity in rats: A reappraisal of past and present findings. *Psychopharmacology, 189,* 407–424.

Baumann, P., Schild, C., Hume, R. F., & Sokol, R. J. (2006). Alcohol abuse—A persistent preventable risk for congenital anomalies. *International Journal of Gynecology and Obstetrics, 95,* 66–72.

Baxter, L., Egbert, N., & Ho, E. (2008). Everyday health communication experiences of college students. *Journal of American College Health, 56,* 427–436.

Beadnell, B., Baker, S. A., Gillmore, M. R., Morrison, D. M., Huang, B., & Stielstra, S. (2008). The theory of reasoned action and the role of external factors on heterosexual men's monogamy and condom use. *Journal of Applied Social Psychology, 38,* 97–134.

Beaglehole, R., Bonita, R., & Kjellström, T. (1993). *Basic epidemiology.* Geneva: World Health Organization.

Beck, A. T. (1976). *Cognitive therapy and the emotional disorders.* New York: International Universities Press.

Beck, A. T., Ward, C. H., Mendelson, M., Mock, J., & Erbaugh, J. (1961). An inventory for measuring depression. *Archives of General Psychiatry, 4,* 561–571.

Becker, A. E., Burwell, R. A., Navara, K., & Gilman, S. E. (2003). Binge eating and binge eating disorder in a small-scale, indigenous society: The view from Fiji. *International Journal of Eating Disorders, 34,* 423–431.

Becker, M. H. (1979). Understanding patient compliance: The contributions of attitudes and other psychosocial factors. In S. J. Cohen (Ed.), *New directions in patient compliance* (pp. 1–31). Lexington, MA: Lexington Books.

Becker, M. H., & Rosenstock, I. M. (1984). Compliance with medical advice. In A. Steptoe & A. Mathews (Eds.), *Health care and human behavior.* London: Academic Press.

Bédard, M., Kuzik, R., Chambers, L., Molloy, D. W., Dubois, S., & Lever, J. A. (2005). Understanding burden differences between men and women caregivers: The contribution of care-recipient problem behaviors. *International Psychogeriatrics, 17,* 99–118.

Beecher, H. K. (1946). Pain of men wounded in battle. *Annals of Surgery, 123,* 96–105.

Beecher, H. K. (1955). The powerful placebo. *Journal of the American Medical Association, 149,* 1602–1607.

Beecher, H. K. (1956). Relationship of significance of wound to pain experience. *Journal of the American Medical Association, 161,* 1609–1613.

Beecher, H. K. (1957). The measurement of pain. *Pharmacological Review, 9,* 59–209.

Beilin, L., & Huang, R.-C. (2008). Childhood obesity, hypertension, the metabolic syndrome and adult cardiovascular disease. *Clinical and Experimental Pharmacology and Physiology, 35,* 409–411.

Bélanger-Ducharme, F., & Tremblay, A. (2005). Prevalence of obesity in Canada. *Obesity Reviews, 6,* 183–186.

Belar, C. D. (1997). Clinical health psychology: A specialty for the 21st century. *Health Psychology, 16,* 411–416.

Belar, C. D. (2008). Clinical health psychology: A health care specialty in professional psychology. *Professional Psychology: Research and Practice, 39,* 229–233.

Belar, C. D., Brown, R. A., Hersch, L. E., Hornyak, L. M., Rozensky, R. H., Sheridan, E. P., et al. (2001). Self-assessment in clinical health psychology: A model for ethical expansion of practice. *Professional Psychology: Research and Practice, 32,* 135–141.

Bell, R. A., Kravitz, R. L., Thom, D., Krupat, E., & Azari, R. (2001). Unsaid but not forgotten: Physician-patient relationship. *Archives of Internal Medicine, 161,* 1977–1983.

Bell, R. A., Kravitz, R. L., Thom, D., Krupat, E., & Azari, R. (2002). Unmet expectations for care and the patient-physician relationship. *Journal of General Internal Medicine, 17,* 817–824.

Belloc, N. (1973). Relationship of health practices and mortality. *Preventive Medicine, 2,* 67–81.

Benaim, C., Froger, J., Cazottes, C., Gueben, D., Porte, M., Desnuelle, C., et al. (2007). Use of the Faces Pain Scale by left and right hemispheric stroke patients. *Pain, 128,* 52–58.

Bendapudi, N. M., Berry, L. L., Frey, K. A., Parish, J. T., & Rayburn, W. L. (2006). Patients' perspectives on ideal physician behaviors. *Mayo Clinic Proceedings, 81,* 338–344.

Bender, R., Trautner, C., Spraul, M., & Berger, M. (1998). Assessment of excess mortality in obesity. *American Journal of Epidemiology, 147,* 42–48.

Benedetti, F. (2006). Placebo analgesia. *Neurological Sciences, 27*(Suppl. 2), S100–S102.

Bennett, G. G., Merritt, M. M., Sollers, J. J., III, Edwards, C. L., Whitfield, K. E., Brandon, D. T., et al. (2004). Stress, coping, and health outcomes among African-Americans: A review of the John Henryism hypothesis. *Psychology and Health, 19,* 369–383.

Benyamini, Y., Leventhal, E. A., & Leventhal, H. (1997). Attributions and health. In A. Baum, S. Newman, J. Weinman, R. West, & C. McManus (Eds.), *Cambridge* handbook of psychology, health and medicine (pp. 72–77). Cambridge, UK: Cambridge University Press.

Benyamini, Y., Leventhal, E. A., & Leventhal, H. (2000). Gender differences in processing information for making self-assessments of health. *Psychosomatic Medicine, 62,* 354–364.

Berghöfer, A., Pischon, T., Reinhold, T., Apovian, C. M., Sharma, A. M., & Willich, S. N. (2008). Obesity prevalence from a European perspective: A systematic review. *BMC Public Health, 8,* 200–209.

Berkman, L. F., & Breslow, L. (1983). *Health and ways of living: The Alameda County Study.* New York: Oxford University Press.

Berkman, L. F., & Syme, S. L. (1979). Social networks, host resistance, and mortality: A nine-year follow-up study of Alameda County residents. *American Journal of Epidemiology, 109,* 186–204.

Berkman, N. D., Lohr, K. N., & Bulik, C. M. (2007). Outcomes of eating disorders: A systematic review of the literature. *International Journal of Eating Disorders, 40,* 293–309.

Berman, J. D., & Straus, S. E. (2004). Implementing a research agenda for complementary and alternative medicine. *Annual Review of Medicine, 55,* 239–254.

Berne, R. M., & Levy, M. N. (2000). *Principles of physiology* (3rd ed.). St. Louis: Mosby.

Bernstein, L., Henderson, B. E., Hanisch, R., Sullivan-Halley, J., & Ross, R. K. (1994). Physical exercise and reduced risk of breast cancer in young women. *Journal of the National Cancer Institute, 86,* 1403–1408.

Bertakis, K. D., & Azari, R. (2005). Obesity and the use of health care services. *Obesity Research, 13,* 372–379.

Bertram, L., & Tanzi, R. E. (2005). The genetic epidemiology of neurodegenerative disease. *Journal of Clinical Investigation, 115,* 1449–1457.

Bhatt, S. P., Luqman-Arafath, T. K., & Guleria, R. (2007). Non-pharmacological management of hypertension. *Indian Journal of Medical Sciences, 61,* 616–624.

Bhogal, S., Zemek, R., & Ducharme, F. M. (2006). Written action plans for asthma in children. *Cochrane Database of Systematic Reviews,* Cochrane AN: CD005306.

Bickel-Swenson, D. (2007). End-of-life training in U.S. medical schools: A systematic literature review. *Journal of Palliative Medicine, 10,* 229–235.

Biener, L., & Siegel, M. (2000). Tobacco marketing and adolescent smoking: More support for a causal inference. *American Journal of Public Health, 90,* 407–411.

Bigal, M. E., & Lipton, R. B. (2008). Concepts and mechanisms of migraine chronification. *Headache, 48,* 7–15.

Bigatti, S., & Cronan, T. A. (2002). A comparison of pain measures used with patients with fibromyalgia. *Journal of Nursing Measurement, 10,* 5–14.

Bipolar-Lives.com. (2007–2008). *Drew Barrymore and bipolar disorder.* Bipolar-Lives.com. Retrieved July 13, 2008, from http://www.bipolar-lives.com/drew-barrymore-and-bipolar-disorder.html

Bird, S. T., Harvey, S. M., Beckman, L. J., & Johnson, C. H. (2000). Getting your partner to use condoms: Interviews with men and women at risk of HIV/STDs. *Journal of Sex Research, 38,* 233–240.

Biron, C., Brun, J., Ivers, H., & Cooper, C. L. (2006). At work but ill: Psychosocial work environment and well-being determinants of presenteeism propensity. *Journal of Public Mental Health, 5,* 26–37.

Birtane, M., Uzunca, K., Tastekin, N., & Tuna, H. (2007). The evaluation of quality of life in fibromyalgia syndrome: A comparison with rheumatoid arthritis by using SF-36 Health Survey. *Clinical Rheumatology, 26,* 679–684.

Bisson, J., & Andrew, M. (2007). Psychological treatment of post-traumatic stress disorder (PTSD). *Cochrane Database of Systematic Reviews,* Cochrane AN: CD003388.

Bjørge, T., Engeland, A., Tverdal, A., & Smith, G. D. (2008). Body mass index in adolescence in relation to cause-specific mortality: A follow-up to 230,000 Norwegian adolescents. *American Journal of Epidemiology, 168,* 30–37.

Black, E., Holst, C., Astrup, A., Toubro, S., Echwald, S., Pedersent, O., et al. (2005). Long-term influences of body-weight changes, independent of the attained weight, on risk of impaired glucose tolerance and Type 2 diabetes. *Diabetic Medicine, 22,* 1100–1205.

Black, P. H. (2003). The inflammatory response is an integral part of the stress response: Implications for atherosclerosis, insulin resistance, Type II diabetes and metabolic syndrome X. *Brain, Behavior and Immunity, 17,* 350–364.

Blackmore, E. R., Stansfeld, S. A., Weller, I., Munce, S., Zagorski, B. M., & Stewart, D. E. (2007). Major depressive episodes and work stress: Results from a national population survey. *American Journal of Public Health, 97,* 2088–2093.

Blair, S. N., Cheng, Y., & Holder, J. S. (2001). Is physical activity or physical fitness more important in defining health benefits? *Medicine and Science in Sports & Exercise, 33,* S379–S399.

Blair, S. N., & Church, T. (2004). The fitness, obesity, and health equation: Is physical activity the common denominator? *Journal of the American Medical Association, 292,* 1232–1234.

Blalock, J. E., & Smith, E. M. (2007). Conceptual development of the immune system as a sixth sense. *Brain, Behavior and Immunity, 21,* 23–33.

Blalock, S. J. (2007). Predictors of calcium intake patterns: A longitudinal analysis. *Health Psychology, 26,* 251–258.

Blanchard, E. B., & Andrasik, F. (1985). *Management of chronic headaches: A psychological approach.* New York: Pergamon Press.

Blanchard, E. B., Appelbaum, K. A., Radniz, C. L., Morrill, B., Michultka, D., Kirsch, C., et al. (1990). A controlled evaluation of thermal biofeedback and thermal biofeedback combined with cognitive therapy in the treatment of vascular headache. *Journal of Consulting and Clinical Psychology, 58,* 216–224.

Blanchard, J., & Lurie, N. (2004). R-E-S-P-E-C-T: Patient reports of disrespect in health care setting and its impact on care. *Journal of Family Practice, 53,* 721–730.

Blascovich, J., Spencer, S. J., Quinn, D., & Steele, C. (2001). African Americans and high blood pressure: The role of stereotype threat. *Psychological Science, 12,* 225–229.

Bleil, M. E., Gianaros, P. J., Jennings, J. R., Flory, J. D., & Manuck, S. B. (2008). Trait negative affect: Toward an integrated model of understanding psychological risk for impairment in cardiac autonomic function. *Psychosomatic Medicine, 70,* 328–337.

Bloomfield, K., Stockwell, T., Gmel, G., & Rehn, N. (2003). *International comparison of alcohol consumption.* National Institute of Alcoholism and Alcohol Abuse. Retrieved April 12, 2005, from http://www.niaaa.nih.gov/ publications/arh27–1/95–109.htm

Bloor, M. (2005). Observations of shipboard illness behavior: Work discipline and the sick role in a residential work setting. *Qualitative Health Research, 15,* 766–777.

Blows, S., Ivers, R. Q., Connor, J., Ameratunga, S., Woodward, M., & Norton, R. (2005). Marijuana use and car crash injury. *Addiction, 100,* 604–611.

Blumenthal, J. A., Babyak, M. A., Carney, R. M., Huber, M., Saab, P. G., Burg, M. M., et al. (2004). Exercise, depression, and mortality after myocardial infarction in the ENRICHD trial. *Medicine and Science in Sports and Exercise, 36,* 746–755.

Bode, C., & Bode, J. C. (1997). Alcohol absorption, metabolism, and production in the gastrointestinal tract. *Alcohol Health & Research World, 21,* 82–83.

Bodenheimer, T. (2005a). High and rising health care costs: Part 1. Seeking an explanation. *Archives of Internal Medicine, 142,* 847–854.

Bodenheimer, T. (2005b). High and rising health care costs: Part 2. Technologic innovation. *Archives of Internal Medicine, 142,* 932–937.

Bodenheimer, T. (2005c). High and rising health care costs: Part 3. The role of health care providers. *Archives of Internal Medicine, 142,* 996–1002.

Bodenheimer, T., & Fernandez, A. (2005). High and rising health care costs: Part 4. Can costs be controlled while preserving quality? *Archives of Internal Medicine, 143,* 26–31.

Bödvarsdóttir, I., & Elklit, A. (2004). Psychological reactions in Icelandic earthquake survivors. *Scandinavian Journal of Psychology, 45,* 3–13.

Boffetta, P. (2004). Epidemiology of environmental and occupational cancer. *Oncogene, 23,* 6392–6403.

Boffetta, P., Aagnes, B., Weiderpass, E., & Andersen, A. (2005). Smokeless tobacco use and risk of cancer of the pancreas and other organs. *International Journal of Cancer, 114,* 992–995.

Bogart, L. M., & Delahanty, D. L. (2004). Psychosocial models. In T. J. Boll, R. G. Frank, A. Baum, & J. L. Wallander (Eds.), *Handbook of clinical health psychology: Vol. 3. Models and perspectives in health psychology* (pp. 201–248). Washington, DC: American Psychological Association.

Boice, J. D. Jr., Bigbee, W. L., Mumma, M. T., & Blot, W. J. (2003). Cancer mortality in counties near two former nuclear materials processing facilities in Pennsylvania, 1950–1995. *Health Physics, 85,* 691–700.

Bolger, N., Zuckerman, A., & Kessler, R. C. (2000). Invisible support and adjustment to stress. *Journal of Personality and Social Psychology, 79,* 953–961.

Bolognesi, M., Nigg, C. R., Massarini, M., & Lippke, S. (2006). Reducing obesity indicators through brief physical activity counseling (PACE) in Italian primary care settings. *Annals of Behavioral Medicine, 31,* 179–185.

Bonanno, G. A. (2004). Loss, trauma, and human resilience. *American Psychologist, 59,* 20–28.

Bonica, J. J. (1990). Definitions and taxonomy of pain. In J. J. Bonica (Ed.), *The management of pain* (2nd ed., pp. 18–27). Malvern, PA: Lea & Febiger.

Bonilla, K. (2007, June 29). Diabetes, pregnancy and Halle Berry. MyDiabetesCentral.com. Retrieved June 29, 2008, from http://www.healthcentral.com/diabetes/c/5868/13828/halle-berry/

Borrell, L. N. (2005). Racial identity among Hispanics: Implications for health and well-being. *American Journal of Public Health, 95,* 379–381.

Bos, V., Kunst, A. E., Garssen, J., & Mackenbach, J. P. (2005). Socioeconomic inequalities in mortality within ethnic groups in the Netherlands, 1995–2000. *Journal of Epidemiology and Community Health, 59,* 329–335.

Bosch-Capblanch, S., Abba, K., Prictor, M., & Garner, P. (2007). Contracts between patients and healthcare practitioners for improving patients' adherence to treatment, prevention and health promotion activities. *Cochrane Database of Systematic Reviews*, Cochrane AN: CD004808.

Bossuyt, N., Gadeyne, S., Deboosere, P., & van Oyen, H. (2004). Socio-economic inequities in health expectancy in Belgium. *Public Health, 118,* 3–10.

Bottonari, K. A., Roberts, J. W., Ciesla, J. A., & Hewitt, R. G. (2005). Life stress and adherence to antiretroviral therapy among HIV-positive individuals: A preliminary investigation. *AIDS Patient Care and STDs, 19,* 719–727.

Bottos, S., & Dewey, D. (2004). Perfectionists' appraisal of daily hassles and chronic headache. *Headache, 44,* 772–779.

Botvin, G. J., & Griffin, K. W. (2004). Life Skills Training: Empirical findings and future directions. *Journal of Primary Prevention, 25,* 211–232.

Bouchard, C. (2001). Physical activity and health: Introduction to the dose-response. *Medicine and Science in Sports and Exercise, 33,* S347–S350.

Boult, C., Kane, R. L., & Brown, R. (2000). Managed care of chronically ill older people: The US experience. *British Medical Journal, 321,* 1011–1014.

Bowers, S. L., Bilbo, S. D., Dhabhar, F. S., & Nelson, R. J. (2008). Stressor-specific alterations in corticosterone and immune responses in mice. *Brain, Behavior, and Immunity, 22,* 105–113.

Boyd, D. B. (2007). Integrative oncology: The last ten years—A personal retrospective. *Alternative Therapies in Health and Medicine, 13,* 56–64.

Boyle, S. H., Williams, R. B., Mark, D. B., Brummett, B. H., Siegler, I. C., Helms, M. J., et al. (2004). Hostility as a predictor of survival in patients with coronary artery disease. *Psychosomatic Medicine, 66,* 629–632.

Brace, M. J., Smith, M. S., McCauley, E., & Sherry, D. D. (2000). Family reinforcement of illness behavior: A comparison of adolescents with chronic fatigue syndrome, juvenile arthritis, and healthy controls. *Journal of Developmental and Behavioral Pediatrics, 21,* 332–339.

Brantley, P. J., Bodenlos, J., Cowles, M., Whitehead, D., Ancona, M., & Jones, G. (2007). Development and validation of the Weekly Stress Inventory—Short Form. *Journal of Psychopathology and Behavioral Assessment, 29,* 54–59.

Brantley, P. J., Jones, G. N., Boudreaux, E., & Gatz, S. L. (1997). The Weekly Stress Inventory. In C. P. Zalaaquett (Ed.), *Evaluating stress: A book of resources* (pp. 405–420). Lanham, MD: Scarecrow Press.

Bray, G. A. (2004). The epidemic of obesity and changes in food intake: The fluoride hypothesis. *Physiology and Behavior, 82,* 115–121.

Bray, G. A., Nielsen, S. J., & Popkin, B. M. (2004). Consumption of high-fructose corn syrup in beverages may play a role in the epidemic of obesity. *American Journal of Clinical Nutrition, 79,* 537–543.

Brecher, E. M. (1972). *Licit and illicit drugs.* Boston: Little, Brown.

Breibart, W., & Payne, D. (2001). Psychiatric aspects of pain management in patients with advanced cancer. In H. Chochinov & W. Breibart (Eds.), *Handbook of psychiatry in palliative medicine* (pp. 131–199). New York: Oxford University Press.

Breuer, J., & Freud, S. (1955). *Studies on hysteria.* In J. Strachey (Ed. and Trans.), *The standard edition of the complete psychological works of Sigmund Freud* (Vol. 2). London: Hogarth Press. (Original work published 1895)

Bricker, J. B., Petersen, A. V., Andersen, M. R., Rajan, K. B., Leroux, B. G., & Sarason, I. G. (2006). Childhood friends who smoke: Do they influence adolescents to make smoking transitions? *Addictive Behaviors, 31,* 889–900.

Briones, T. L. (2007). Psychoneuroimmunology and related mechanisms in understanding health disparities in vulnerable populations. *Annual Review of Nursing Research, 25,* 219–256.

Britt, E., Blampied, N. M., & Hudson, S. M. (2003). Motivational interviewing: A review. *Australian Psychologist, 38,* 193–201.

Brock, T. P., & Smith, S. R. (2007). Using digital videos displayed on personal digital assistants (PDAs) to enhance patient education in clinical settings. *International Journal of Medical Informatics, 76,* 829–835.

Broderick, J. E., Junghaenel, D. U., & Turk, D. C. (2004). Stability of patient adaptation classifications on the multidimensional pain inventory. *Pain, 109,* 94–102.

Brody, M. L., Masheb, R. M., & Grilo, C. M. (2005). Treatment preferences of patients with binge eating disorder. *International Journal of Eating Disorders, 37,* 352–356.

Broocks, A., Meyer, T., Opitz, M., Bartmann, U., Hillmer-Vogel, U., George, A., et al. (2003). 5–HT-1A responsivity in patients with panic disorder before and after treatment with aerobic exercise, clomipramine or placebo. *European Neuropsychopharmacology, 13,* 153–164.

Brooks, V. L., Haywood, J. R., & Johnson, A. K. (2005). Translation of salt retention to central activation of the sympathetic nervous system in hypertension. *Clinical and Experimental Pharmacology and Physiology, 32,* 426–432.

Brown, B. (1970). Recognition of aspects of consciousness through association with EEG alpha activity represented by a light signal. *Psychophysics, 6,* 442–446.

Brown, D. R., Hernández, A., Saint-Jean, G., Evans, S., Tafari, I., Brewster, L. G., et al. (2008). A participatory action research pilot study on urban health disparities using rapid assessment response and evaluation. *American Journal of Public Health, 98,* 28–38.

Brown, J. M., Mehler, P. S., & Harris, R. H. (2000). Medical complications occurring in adolescents with anorexia nervosa. *Western Journal of Medicine, 172,* 189–193.

Brown, R. A., Palm, K. M., Strong, D. R., Lejuez, C. W., Christopher, W., Zvolensky, M. J., et al. (2008). Distress tolerance treatment for early-lapse smokers: Rationale, program description, and preliminary findings. *Behavior Modification, 32,* 302–332.

Brownell, K. D., & Horgen, K. B. (2004). *Food fight: The inside story of the food industry, America's obesity crisis, and what we can do about it.* New York: McGraw-Hill.

Bruch, H. (1973). *Eating disorders. Obesity, anorexia nervosa and the person within.* New York: Basic Books.

Bruch, H. (1978). *The golden cage: The enigma of anorexia nervosa.* Cambridge, MA: Harvard University Press.

Bruch, H. (1982). Anorexia nervosa: Therapy and theory. *American Journal of Psychiatry, 139,* 1531–1538.

Brumback, T., Cao, D., & King, A. (2007). Effects of alcohol on psychomotor performance and perceived impairment in heavy binge social drinkers. *Drug and Alcohol Dependence, 91,* 10–17.

Brummett, B. H., Barefoot, J. C., Siegler, I. C., Clapp-Channing, N. E., Lytle, B. L., Bosworth, H. B., et al. (2001). Characteristics of socially isolated patients with coronary artery disease who are at elevated risk for mortality. *Psychosomatic Medicine, 63,* 267–272.

Brunner, E. J., Mosdøl, A., Witte, D. R., Martikainen, P., Stafford, M., Shipley, M. J., et al. (2008). Dietary patterns and 15-y risks of major coronary events, diabetes, and mortality. *American Journal of Clinical Nutrition, 87,* 1414–1421.

Bruns, D. (1998). Psychologists as primary care providers: A paradigm shift. *Health Psychologist, 20*(4), 19.

Buchwald, H., Avidor, Y., Braunwald, E., Jensen, M. D., Pories, W., Fahrbach, K., et al. (2004). Bariatric surgery: A systematic review and meta-analysis. *Journal of the American Medical Association, 292,* 1724–1737.

Buddie, A. M. (2004). Alternatives to twelve-step programs. *Journal of Forensic Psychology Practice, 4,* 61–70.

Budney, A. J. (2006). Are specific dependence criteria necessary for different substances: How can research on cannabis inform this issue? *Addiction, 101*(Suppl.), 125–133.

Buffington, A. L. H., Hanlon, C. A., & McKeown, M. J. (2005). Acute and persistent pain modulation of attention-related anterior cingulate fMRI activations. *Pain, 113*, 172–184.

Bulik, C. M., Berkman, N. D., Brownley, K. A., Sedway, J. A., & Lohr, K. N. (2007). Anorexia nervosa treatment: A systematic review of randomized controlled trials. *International Journal of Eating Disorders, 40*, 310–320.

Burckhardt, C. S., & Jones, K. D. (2003a). Adult measures of pain: Short-Form McGill Pain Questionnaire (SF-MPQ). *Arthritis & Rheumatism: Arthritis Care & Research, 49*(Suppl.), S98–S99.

Burckhardt, C. S., & Jones, K. D. (2003b). Adult measures of pain: Short-Visual Analog Scale (VAS). *Arthritis & Rheumatism: Arthritis Care & Research, 49*(Suppl.), S100–S101.

Burke, A., & Upchurch, D. M. (2006). Patterns of acupuncture use: Highlights from the National Health Interview Survey. *American Acupuncturist, 37*, 30–31.

Burke, A., Upchurch, D. M., Dye, C., & Chyu, L. (2006). Acupuncture use in the United States: Findings from the National Health Interview Survey. *Journal of Alternative and Complementary Medicine, 12*, 639–648.

Burke, J. D., Lofgren, I. E., Morrell, J. S., & Reilly, R. A. (2007). Health indicators, body mass index and food selection practices in college age students. *FASEB Journal, 21*, A1063.

Burling, T. A., Burling, A. S., Latini, D. (2001). A controlled smoking cessation trial for substance-dependent inpatients. *Journal of Consulting and Clinical Psychology, 69*, 295–304.

Burns, J. W., Kubilus, A., Bruehl, S., & Harden, R. N. (2001). A fourth empirically derived cluster of chronic pain patients based on the Multidimensional Pain Inventory Evidence for repression within the dysfunctional group. *Journal of Counsulting and Clinical Psychology, 69*, 663–673.

Bussey-Smith, K. L., & Rossen, R. D. (2007). A systematic review of randomized control trials evaluating the effectiveness of interactive computerized asthma patient education programs. *Annals of Allergy, Asthma and Immunology, 98*, 507–516.

Bustamante, M. X., Zhang, G., O'Connell, E., Rodriguez, D., & Borroto-Ponce, R. (2007). Motor vehicle crashes and injury among high school and college aged drivers. Miami–Dade County, FL 20005. *Annals of Epidemiology, 17*, 742.

Butler, A. C., Chapman, J. E., Forman, E. M., & Beck, A. T. (2006). The empirical status of cognitive-behavioral therapy: A review of meta-analyses. *Clinical Psychology Review, 26*, 17–31.

Cagle, C. S. (2004). 3 themes described how self care management was learned and experienced by patients with chronic illness. *Evidence-Based Nursing, 7*(3), 94.

Cahill, S. P., & Foa, E. B. (2007). PTSD: Treatment efficacy and future directions. *Psychiatric Times, 24*, 32–34.

Cai, J., Pajak, A., Li, Y., Shestov, D., Davis, C. E., Rywik, S., et al. (2004). Total cholesterol and mortality in China, Poland, Russia, and the US. *Annals of Epidemiology, 14*, 399–408.

Calhoun, J. B. (1956). A comparative study of the social behavior of two inbred strains of house mice. *Ecological Monogram, 26*, 81.

Calhoun, J. B. (1962, February). Population density and social pathology. *Scientific American, 206*, 139–148.

Calipel, S., Lucaspolomeni, M.-M., Wodey, E., & Ecoffey, C. (2005). Premedication in children: Hypnosis versus midazolam. *Pediatric Anesthesia, 15*, 275–281.

Calle, E. E., Thun, M. J., Petrelli, J. M., Rodriguez, C., & Heath, C. W., Jr. (1999). Body-mass index and mortality in a prospective cohort of U.S. adults. *New England Journal of Medicine, 341*, 1097–1105.

Callister, L. C. (2003). Cultural influences on pain perceptions and behavior. *Home Health Care Management & Practice, 15*, 207–211.

Camacho, T. C., & Wiley, J. A. (1983). Health practices, social networks, and change in physical health. In L. F. Berkman & L. Breslow (Eds.), *Health and ways of living: The Alameda County Study.* New York: Oxford University Press.

Camelley, K. B., Wortman, C. B., Bolger, N., & Burke, C. T. (2006). The time course of brief reactions to spousal loss: Evidence from a national probability sample. *Journal of Personality and Social Psychology, 91*, 476–492.

Cameron, L. D., Booth, R. J., Schlatter, M., Ziginskas, D., & Harman, J. E. (2007). Changes in emotion regulation and psychological adjustment following use of a group psychosocial support program for women recently diagnosed with breast cancer. *Psycho-Oncology, 16*, 171–180.

Cameron, L. D., Leventhal, E. A., & Leventhal, H. (1995). Seeking medical care in response to symptoms and life stress. *Psychosomatic Medicine, 57*, 37–47.

Cameron, L. D., Petrie, K. J., Ellis, C., Buick, D., & Weinman, J. A. (2005). Symptom experiences, symptom attributions, and causal attributions in patients following first-time myocardial infarction. *International Journal of Behavioral Medicine, 12*, 30–38.

Camí, J., & Farré, M. (2003). Drug addiction. *New England Journal of Medicine, 349*, 975–986.

Campbell, J. K., Canene-Adams, K., Lindshield, B. L., Boileau, T. W.-M., Clinton, S. K., & Erdman, J. W., Jr. (2004). Tomato phytochemicals and prostate cancer risk. *Journal of Nutrition, 134*, 3486S–3402S.

Cancian, F. M., & Oliker, S. J. (2000). *Caring and gender.* Thousand Oaks, CA: Pine Forge Press.

Cannon, W. (1932). *The wisdom of the body.* New York: Norton.

Carmen, B., Angeles, M., Ana, M., & María, A. J. (2004). Efficacy and safety of naltrexone and acamprosate in the treatment of alcohol dependence: A systematic review. *Addiction, 99*, 811–828.

Carmody, J., & Baer, R. A. (2008). Relationships between mindfulness practice and level of mindfulness, medical and psychological symptoms and well-being in a mindfulness-based stress reduction program. *Journal of Behavioral Medicine, 31*, 23–33.

Carpenter, M. J., Hughes J. R., & Solomon, U. (2005). Smoking reduction with nicotine replacement and motivational advice reduced smoking in people unmotivated to quit. *Evidence-Based Medicine, 10*, 18.

Carr, D. (2003). A "good death" for whom? Quality of spouse's death and psychological distress among older widowed persons. *Journal of Health and Social Behavior, 44*, 215–232.

Carr, J. L. (2007). Campus violence white paper. *Journal of American College Health, 55*, 304–319.

Carter, J. C., Blackmore, E., Sutandar-Pinnock, K., & Woodside, D. B. (2004). Relapse in anorexia nervosa: A survival analysis. *Psychological Medicine, 34*, 671–679.

Carver, C. S., Smith, R. G., Antoni, M. H., Petronis, V. M., Weiss, S., & Derhagopian, R. P. (2005). Optimistic personality and psychosocial well-being during treatment predict psychosocial well-being among long-term survivors of breast cancer. *Health Psychology, 24*, 508–516.

Caspi, A., Harrington, H., Moffitt, T.E., Milne, B.J., & Poulton, R. (2006). Socially isolated children 20 years later. *Archives of Pediatric Adolescent Medicine, 160*, 805–811.

Caspi, A., Sugden, K., Moffitt, T. E., Taylor, A., Craig, I. W., Harrington, H., et al. (2003). Influence of life stress on depression: Moderation by a polymorphism in the 5-HTT gene. *Science, 301*, 386–389.

Castor, M. L., Smyser, M. S., Taualii, M. M., Park, A. N., Lawson, S. A., & Forquera, R. A. (2006). A nationwide population-based study identifying health disparities between American Indians/Alaska Natives and the general populations living in select urban counties. *American Journal of Public Health, 96*, 1478–1484.

Castro, C. M. Wilson, C., Wang, F., & Schillinger, D. (2007). Babel babble: Physicians' use of unclarified medical jargon with patients. *American Journal of Health Behavior, 31*, S85–S95.

Celebrity central: Lindsay Lohan. (2008). *People.* Retrieved March 6, 2008, from http://www.people.com/people/lindsay_lohan/0,,,00.html

Celentano, D. D., Valleroy. L. A., Sifakis, F., Mackellar, D. A., Hylton, J., Thiede, H., et al. (2006). Associations between substance use and sexual risk among very young men who have sex with men. *Sexually Transmitted Diseases, 33*, 265–271.

Centers for Disease Control and Prevention (CDC). (1992). 1993 revised classification system for HIV infection and expanded surveillance case definition for AIDS among adolescents and adults. *Morbidity and Mortality Weekly Report, 41*, No. RR-17.

Centers for Disease Control and Prevention (CDC). (1993). Cigarette smoking—Attributable mortality and years of potential life lost—United States, 1990. *Morbidity and Mortality Weekly Report, 42*, 645–649.

Centers for Disease Control and Prevention (CDC). (1994). Reasons for tobacco use and symptoms of nicotine withdrawal among adolescent and young adult tobacco users—United States, 1993. *Morbidity and Mortality Weekly Report, 43*, 745–750.

Centers for Disease Control and Prevention (CDC). (2008). *HIV/AIDS surveillance report, 2006* (Vol. 18). Atlanta, GA: U.S. Department of Health and Human Services, Centers for Disease Control and Prevention. Retrieved August 3, 2008, from http://www.cdc.gov/hiv/topics/surveillance/resources/reports/

Central Intelligence Agency (CIA). (2008). *World factbook, 2008*. Washington, DC: Author.

Cha, E. S., Doswell, W. M., Kim, K. H., Charron-Prochownik, D., & Patrick, T. E. (2007). Evaluating the Theory of Planned Behavior to explain intention to engage in premarital sex amongst Korean college students: A questionnaire survey. *International Journal of Nursing Studies, 44*, 1147–1157.

Chakrabarty, S., & Zoorob, R. (2007). Fibromyalgia. *American Family Physician, 76*, 247–254.

Champion, V., Skinner, C. S., Hui, S., Monahan, P., Julian, B., Daggy, J., et al. (2007). The effect of telephone versus print tailoring for mammography adherence. *Patient Education and Counseling, 65*, 416–423.

Chandrashekara, S. Jayashree, K., Veeranna, H. B., Vadiraj, H. S., Ramesh, M. N., Shobha, A., et al. (2007). Effects of anxiety on TNF-a levels during psychological stress. *Journal of Psychosomatic Research, 63*, 65–69.

Chang, L., Ernst, T., Speck. O., Patel, H., DeSilva, M., Leonido-Yee, M., et al. (2002). Perfusion MRI and computerized cognitive test abnormalities in abstinent methamphetamine users. *Psychiatry Research: Neuroimaging Section, 114*, 65–79.

Chapman, C. R., Nakamura, Y., & Flores, L. Y. (1999). Chronic pain and consciousness: A constructivist perspective. In R. J. Gatchel & D. C. Turk (Eds.), *Psychosocial factors in pain: Critical perspectives* (pp. 35–55). New York: Guilford Press.

Charlee, C., Goldsmith, L. J., Chambers, L, & Haynes, R. B. (1996). Provider-patient communication among elderly and nonelderly patients in Canadian hospitals: A national survey. *Health Communication, 8*, 281–302.

Chassin, L., Presson, C. C., Rose, J., & Sherman, S. J. (2007). What is addiction? Age-related differences in the meaning of addiction. *Drug and Alcohol Dependence, 87*, 30–38.

Chei, C. L., Iso, H., Yamagishi, K., Inoue, M., & Tsugane, S. (2008). Body mass index and weight change since 20 years of age and risk of coronary heart disease among Japanese: The Japan Public Health Center–Based Study. *International Journal of Obesity, 32*, 144–151.

Chen, E., & Miller, G. E. (2007). Stress and inflammation in exacerbations of asthma. *Brain, Behavior and Immunity, 21*, 993–999.

Chen, H. (2005). Prevalence and economic implications of chronic pain in the United States. *P&T: Journal for Formulary Management, 30*(Special Suppl.), 15–23.

Chen, H. Y., Shi, Y., Ng, C. S., Chan, S. M., Yung, K. K., Lam, Z., et al. (2007). Auricular acupuncture treatment for insomnia: A systematic review. *Journal of Alternative and Complementary Medicine, 13,* 669–676.

Chen, J. Y., Fox, S. A., Cantrell, C. H., Stockdale, S. E., Kagawa-Singer, M. (2007). Health disparities and prevention: Racial/ethnic barriers to flu vaccinations. *Journal of Community Health, 32,* 5–20.

Cheng, B. M. T., Lauder, I. J., Chu-Pak. L., & Kumana, C. R. (2004). Meta-analysis of large randomized controlled trials to evaluate the impact of statins on cardiovascular outcomes. *British Journal of Clinical Pharmacology, 57,* 640–651.

Cheng, T. Y. L., & Boey, K. W. (2002). The effectiveness of a cardiac rehabilitation program on self-efficacy and exercise. *Clinical Nursing Research, 11,* 10–19.

Cherkin, D. C., Sherman, K. J., Deyo, R. A., & Shekelle, P. G. (2003). A review of the evidence for the effectiveness, safety, and cost of acupuncture, massage therapy, and spinal manipulation for back pain. *Annals of Internal Medicine, 138,* 898–907.

Chia, L. R., Schlenk, E. A., & Dunbar-Jacob, J. (2006). Effect of personal and cultural beliefs on medication adherence in the elderly. *Drugs and Aging, 23,* 191–202.

Chida, T., Hamer, M., & Steptoe, A. (2008). A bidirectional relationship between psychosocial factors and atopic disorders: A systematic review and meta-analysis. *Psychosomatic Medicine, 70,* 102–116.

Chinn, S., Jarvis, D., Melotti, R., Luczynska, C., Ackermann-Liebrich, U., Antó, J. M., et al. (2005). Smoking cessation, lung function, and weight gain: A follow-up study. *Lancet, 365,* 1629–1635.

Chitamun, S., & Finchilescu, G. (2003). Predicting the intention of South African female students to engage in premarital sexual relationship: An application of the theory of reasoned action. *South African Journal of Psychology, 33,* 154–161.

Chou, F., Holzemer, W. L., Portillo, C. J., & Slaughter, R. (2004). Self-care strategies and sources of information for HIV/AIDS symptom management. *Nursing Research, 53,* 332–339.

Chou, R., Qaseem, A., Snow, V., Casey, D., Cross, J. T., Jr., Shekelle, P., & Owens, D. K. (2007). Diagnosis and treatment of low back pain: A joint clinical practice guideline from the American College of Physicians and the American Pain Society. *Annals of Internal Medicine, 147,* 478–491, W118–W120.

Christakis, N. A., & Fowler, J. H. (2007). The spread of obesity in a large social network over 32 years. *New England Journal of Medicine, 357,* 370–379.

Christenfeld, N., Glynn, L. M., Phillips, D. P., & Shrira, I. (1999). Exposure to New York City as a risk factor for heart attack mortality. *Psychosomatic Medicine, 61,* 740–743.

Chumbler, N. R., Grimm, J. W., Cody, M., & Beck, C. (2003). Gender, kinship and caregiver burden: The case of community-dwelling memory impaired seniors. *International Journal of Geriatric Psychiatry, 18,* 722–732.

Chung, M. L., Moser, D. K., Lennie, T. A., Worrall-Carter, L., Bentley, B., Trupp, R., et al. (2006). Gender differences in adherence to the sodium-restricted diet in patients with heart failure. *Journal of Cardiac Failure, 12,* 628–634.

Cibulka, N. J. (2006). HIV infection. *American Journal of Nursing, 106,* 59.

Ciesla, J. A., & Roberts, J. E. (2007). Rumination, negative cognition, and their interactive effects on depressed mood. *Emotion, 7,* 555–565.

Cintron, A., & Morrison, R. S. (2006). Pain and ethnicity in the United States: A systematic review. *Journal of Palliative Medicine, 9,* 1454–1473.

Clark, A. D. (2008). The new frontier of wellness. *Benefits Quarterly, 24,* 23–28.

Clark, A. M., Whelan, H. K., Barbour, R., & MacIntyre, P. D. (2005). A realist study of the mechanisms of cardiac rehabilitation. *Journal of Advanced Nursing, 52,* 362–371.

Clark, L., Jones, K., & Pennington, K. (2004). Pain assessment practices with nursing home residents. *Western Journal of Nursing Research, 26,* 733–750.

Clark, M. M., Decker, P. A., Offord, K. P., Patten, C. A., Vickers, K. S., Croghan, I. T., et al. (2004). Weight concerns among male smokers. *Addictive Behaviors, 29,* 1637–1641.

Clark, P. A. (2006). The need for new guidelines for AIDS testing and counseling: An ethical analysis. *Internet Journal of Infectious Diseases, 5*(2), 8.

Clark, R. (2003). Self-reported racism and social support predict blood pressure reactivity in Blacks. *Annals of Behavioral Medicine, 25,* 127–136.

Clark-Grill, M. (2007). Questionable gate-keeping: Scientific evidence for complementary and alternative medicines (CAM): Response to Malcolm Parker. *Journal of Bioethical Inquiry, 4,* 21–28.

Claudino, A. M., Hay, P., Lima, M. S., Bacaltchuk, J., Schmidt, U., & Treasure, J. (2006). Antidepressants for anorexia nervosa. *Cochrane Database of Systematic Reviews,* Cochrane AN: CD004365.

Claxton, A. J., Cramer, J., & Pierce, C. (2001). A systematic review of the association between dose regimens and medication compliance. *Clinical Therapeutics, 23,* 1296–1310.

Cleary, M. (2007). Predisposing risk factors on susceptibility to exertional heat illness: Clinical decision-making considerations. *Journal of Sport Rehabilitation, 16,* 204–214.

Cleland, J. A., Palmer, J. A., & Venzke, J.W. (2005). Ethnic differences in pain perception. *Physical Therapy Reviews, 10,* 113–122.

Clinton: Angiogram "probably saved my life." (2004, September 23). *CNNAccess.* Retrieved June 16, 2005, from http://www.cnn.com/2004/HEALTH/09/03/clinton.lkl/index.html

Clinton, W. J. (2005, Sept. 25). I was a heart attack waiting to happen. *Parade Magazine.*

Codd, R. T., III, & Cohen, B. N. (2003). Predicting college student intention to seek help for alcohol abuse. *Journal of Social and Clinical Psychology, 22,* 168–191.

Coe, C. L., & Laudenslager, M. L. (2007). Psychosocial influences on immunity, including effects on immune maturation and senescence. *Brain, Behavior and Immunity, 21,* 1000–1008.

Coffman, J. M., Cabana, M. D., Halpin, H. A., & Yelin, E. H. (2008). Effects of asthma education on children's use of acute care services: A meta-analysis. *Pediatrics, 121,* 575–586.

Cohen, S. (2005). Keynote presentation at the eighth International Congress of Behavioral Medicine. *International Journal of Behavioral Medicine, 12*(3), 123–131.

Cohen, S., Doyle, W. J., Turner, R., Alper, C. M., & Skoner, D. P. (2003). Sociability and susceptibility to the common cold. *Psychological Science, 14,* 389–395.

Cohen, S., Frank, E., Doyle, W. J., Skoner, D. P., Rabin, B. S., & Gwaltney, J. M., Jr. (1998). Types of stressors that increase susceptibility to the common cold in healthy adults. *Health Psychology, 17,* 214–223.

Cohen, S., Kamarck, T., & Mermelstein, R. (1983). A global measure of perceived stress. *Journal of Health and Social Behavior, 24,* 385–396.

Cohen, S., Tyrrell, D. A. J., & Smith, A. P. (1991). Psychological stress and susceptibility to the common cold. *New England Journal of Medicine, 325,* 606–612.

Cohen, S., Tyrrell, D. A. J., & Smith, A. P. (1993). Negative life events, perceived stress, negative affect, and susceptibility to the common cold. *Journal of Personality and Social Psychology, 64,* 131–140.

Cohn, L., Elias, J. A., & Chupp, G. L. (2004). Asthma: Mechanisms of disease persistence and progression. *Annual Review of Immunology, 22,* 789–818.

Colby, S. M., Monti, P. M., Tevyaw, T. O., Barnett, N. P., Spirito, A., Rohsenow, D. J., et al. (2005). Brief motivational intervention for adolescent smokers in medical settings. *Addictive Behaviors, 30,* 865–874.

Colditz, G. A., Willett, W. C., Hunter, D. J., Stampfer, M. J., Manson, J. E., Hennekens, C. H., et al. (1993). Family history, age, and risk of breast cancer. *Journal of the American Medical Association, 270,* 338–343.

Cole, S. W., Naliboff, B. D., Kemeny, M. E., Griswold, M. P., Fahey, J. L., & Zack, J. A. (2001). Impaired response to HAART in HIV-infected individuals with high autonomic nervous system activity. *Proceedings of the National Academy of Sciences of the United States of America, 98,* 12695–12700.

Coles, S. L., Dixon, J. B., & O'Brien, P. E. (2007). Night eating syndrome and nocturnal snacking: Association with obesity, binge eating and psychological distress. *International Journal of Obesity, 31,* 1722–1730.

Collins, C. E., Warren, J. M., Neve, M., McCoy, P., & Stokes, B. (2007). Review of interventions in the management of overweight and obese children which include a dietary component. *International Journal of Evidence-Based Healthcare, 5,* 2–53.

Collins, M. A. (2008). Protective mechanisms against neuroinflammatory proteins induced by preconditioning braincultures with moderate ethanol concentrations. *Neurotoxicity Research, 13,* 130.

Collins, R. L., Orlando, M., & Klein, D. J. (2005). Isolating the nexus of substance use, violence and sexual risk for HIV infection among young adults in the United States. *AIDS and Behavior, 9,* 73–87.

Committee on the Use of Complementary and Alternative Medicine by the American Public, Institute of Medicine. (2005). *Complementary and alternative medicine in the United States.* Washington, DC: National Academic Press.

Compas, B. E., Haaga, D. A., Keefe, F. J., Leitenberg, H., & Williams, D. A. (1998). Sampling of empirically supported psychological treatments from health psychology: Smoking, chronic pain, cancer, and bulimia nervosa. *Journal of Consulting and Clinical Psychology, 66,* 89–112.

Concato, J., Shah, N., & Horwitz, R. I. (2000). Randomized, controlled trials, observational studies, and the hierarchy of research. *New England Journal of Medicine, 342,* 1887–1892.

Conger, J. (1956). Reinforcement theory and the dynamics of alcoholism. *Quarterly Journal of Studies on Alcohol, 17,* 296–305.

Conn, V. S., Hafdahl, A. R., LeMaster, J. W., Ruppar, T. M., Cochran, J. E., & Nielsen, P. J. (2008). Meta-analysis of health behavior change interventions in Type 1 diabetes. *American Journal of Health Behavior, 32,* 315–392.

Connor, T. (2004). Methylenedioxymethamphetamine (MDMA, "Ecstasy"): A stressor on the immune system. *Journal of Immunology, 111,* 357–367.

Consedine, N. S., Magai, C., & Chin, S. (2004). Hostility and anxiety differentially predict cardiovascular disease in men and women. *Sex Roles, 50,* 63–77.

Constantino, M. J., Arnow, B. A., Blasey, C., & Agras, W. S. (2005). The association between patient characteristics and the therapeutic alliance in cognitive-behavioral and interpersonal therapy for bulimia nervosa. *Journal of Consulting and Clinical Psychology, 73,* 203–211.

Cook, A. J., Roberts, D. A., Henderson, M. D., Van Winkle, L. C., Chastain, D. C., & Hamill-Ruth, R. J. (2004). Electronic pain questionnaires: A randomized, crossover comparison with paper questionnaires for chronic pain assessment. *Pain, 110,* 310–317.

Cook, B. J., & Hausenblas, H. A. (2008). The role of exercise dependence for the relationship between exercise behavior and eating pathology: Mediator or moderator? *Journal of Health Psychology, 13,* 495–502.

Cooper, B. (2001, March). Long may you run. *Runner's World, 36*(3), 64–67.

Cooper, K. H. (1968). *Aerobics.* New York: Evans.

Cooper, K. H. (1982). *The aerobics program for total well-being.* New York: Evans.

Cooper, K. H. (1985). *Running without fear: How to reduce the risks of heart attack and sudden death during aerobic exercise.* New York: Evans.

Corasaniti, M. T., Amantea, D., Russo, R., & Bagetta, G. (2006). The crucial role of plasticity in pain and cell death. *Cell Death and Differentiation, 13*, 534–536.

Corrao, G., Bagnardi, V., Zambon, A., & La Vecchia, C. (2004). A meta-analysis of alcohol consumption and the risk of 15 diseases. *Preventive Medicine, 38*, 613–619.

Cosca, D. D., & Navazio, F. (2007). Common problems in endurance athletes. *American Family Physician, 76*, 237–244.

Costantini, L. (2006). Compliance, adherence, and self-management: Is a paradigm shift possible for chronic kidney disease clients? *CANNT Journal, 16*, 22–26.

Cottington, E. M., & House, J. S. (1987). Occupational stress and health: A multivariate relationship. In A. Baum & J. E. Singer (Eds.), *Handbook of psychology and health: Vol. 5. Stress* (pp. 41–62). Hillsdale, NJ: Erlbaum.

Couper, J. W. (2007). The effects of prostate cancer on intimate relationships. *Journal of Men's Health and Gender, 4*, 226–232.

Court, A., Mulder, C., Hetrick, S. E., Purcell, R., & McGorry, P. D. (2008). What is the scientific evidence for the use of antipsychotic medical in anorexia nervosa? *Eating Disorders: The Journal of Treatment and Prevention, 16*, 217–223.

Courtney, A. U., McCarter, D. F., & Pollart, S. M. (2005). Childhood asthma: Treatment update. *American Family Physician, 71*, 1959–1968.

Cousins, N. (1979). *Anatomy of an illness as perceived by the patient: Reflections on healing and regeneration.* New York: Norton.

Coussons-Read, M. E., Okun, M. L., & Nettles, C. D. (2007). Psychosocial stress increases inflammatory markers and alters cytokine production across pregnancy. *Brain, Behavior and Immunity, 21*, 343–350.

Covington, E. C. (2000). The biological basis of pain. *International Review of Psychiatry, 12*, 128–147.

Coyne, J. C., Stefanek, M., & Palmer, S. C. (2007). Psychotherapy and survival in cancer: The conflict between hope and evidence. *Psychological Bulletin, 133*, 367–394.

Craig, A. D. (2003). Pain mechanisms: Labeled lines versus convergence in central processing. *Annual Review of Neuroscience, 26*, 1–30.

Cramer, J. A. (2004). A systematic review of adherence with medications for diabetes. *Diabetes Care, 27*, 1218–1224.

Cramer, S., Mayer, J., & Ryan, S. (2007). College students use cell phones while driving more frequently than found in government study. *Journal of American College Health, 56*, 181–184.

Cramp, F., & Daniel, J. (2008). Exercise for the management of cancer-related fatigue in adults. *Cochrane Database of Systematic Reviews*, Cochrane AN: CD006145.

Crandall, C. S., Preisler, J. J., & Aussprung, J. (1992). Measuring life event stress in the lives of college students: The Undergraduate Stress Questionnaire (USQ). *Journal of Behavioral Medicine, 15*, 627–662.

Crepaz, N., Passin, W. F., Herbst, J. H., Rama, S. M., Malow, R. M., Purcell, D. W. et al. (2008). Meta-analysis of cognitive-behavioral interventions on HIV-positive persons' mental health and immune functioning. *Health Psychology, 27*, 4–14.

Crimmins, E. M., Ki Kim, J., Alley, D. E., Karlamangla, A., & Seeman, T. (2007). Hispanic paradox in biological risk profiles. *American Journal of Public Health, 97*, 1305–1310.

Crimmins, E. M., & Saito, Y. (2001). Trends in healthy life expectancy in the United States, 1970–1990: Gender, racial, and educational differences. *Social Science and Medicine, 52*, 1629–1642.

Crisp, A., Gowers, S., Joughin, N., McClelland, L., Rooney, B., Nielsen, S., et al. (2006). Anorexia nervosa in males: Similarities and differences to anorexia nervosa in females. *European Eating Disorders Review, 14*(3), 163–167.

Critchley, J. A., & Capewell, S. (2003). Mortality risk reduction associated with smoking cessation in patients with coronary heart disease: A systematic review. *Journal of the American Medical Association, 290*, 86–97.

Crowell, T. L., & Emmers-Sommer, T. M. (2001). "If I knew then what I know now": Seropositive individuals' perceptions of partner trust, safety and risk prior to HIV infection. *Commnication Studies, 52*, 302–323.

Cruess, D. G., Petitto, J. M., Leserman, J., Douglas, S. D., Gettes, D. R., Ten Have, T. R., et al. (2003). Depression and HIV infection: Impact on immune function and disease progression. *CNS Spectrums, 8*, 52–58.

Cummings, D. E., & Schwartz, M. W. (2003). Genetics and pathophysiology of human obesity. *Annual Review of Medicine, 54*, 453–471.

Cunningham, J. A., Blomqvist, J., Koski-Jännes, A., & Cordingley, J. (2005). Maturing out of drinking problems: Perceptions of natural history as a function of severity. *Addiction Research & Theory, 13*, 79–84.

Cutrona, C. E., Russell, D. W., Brown, A., Clark, L. A., Hessling, R. M., & Gardner, K. A. (2005). Neighborhood context, personality, and stressful life events as predictors of depression among African American women. *Journal of Abnormal Psychology, 114*, 3–15.

Cutting Edge Information. (2004). *Pharmaceutical patient compliance and disease management.* Retrieved July 18, 2004, from http://www.pharmadiseasemanagement.com/metrics.htm

Czerniecki, J. M., & Ehde, D. M. (2003). Chronic pain after lower extremity amputation. *Critical Reviews in Physical and Rehabilitation Medicine, 15*, 309–332.

Dagenais, S., Caro, J., & Haldeman, S. (2008). A systematic review of low back pain cost of illness studies in the United States and internationally. *Spine Journal, 8*, 8–20.

Daley, A. (2008). Exercise and depression: A review of reviews. *Journal of Clinical Psychology in Medical Settings, 15*, 140–147.

Damjanovic, A. K., Yang, Y., Glaser, R., Kiecolt-Glaser, J. K., Huy, N., Laskowski, B., et al. (2007). Accelerated telomere erosion is associated with a declining immune function of caregivers of Alzheimer's disease patients. *Journal of Immunology, 179*, 4249–4254.

Damschroder, L. J., Zikmund-Fisher, B. J., & Ubel, P. A. (2005). The impact of considering adaptation in health state valuation. *Social Science and Medicine, 61,* 267–277.

Danaei, G., Vander Hoorn, S., Lopez, A. D., Murray, C. J. L., & Ezzati, M. (2005). Causes of cancer in the world: Comparative risk assessment of nine behavioural and environmental risk factors. *Lancet, 366,* 1784–1793.

Daniels, M. C., Goldberg, J., Jacobsen, C., & Welty, T. K. (2006). Is psychological distress a risk factor for the incidence of diabetes among American Indians? The Strong Heart Study. *Journal of Applied Gerontology, 25*(Suppl.), 60S–72S.

Danner, D. D., Snowdon, D. A., & Friesen, W. V. (2001). Positive emotions in early life and longevity: Findings from the nun study. *Journal of Personality and Social Psychology, 80,* 804–813.

Dansinger, M. L., Gleason, J. A., Griffith, J. L., Selker, H. P., & Schaefer, E. J. (2005). Comparison of the Atkins, Ornish, Weight Watchers, and Zone diets for weight loss and heart disease risk reduction: A randomized trial. *Journal of the American Medical Association, 293,* 43–53.

Dantzer, R., O'Connor, J. C., Freund, G. C., Johnson, R. W., & Kelley, K. W. (2008). From inflammation to sickness and depression: When the immune system subjugates the brain. *Nature Reviews Neuroscience, 9,* 46–57.

D'Arcy, Y. (2005). Conquering pain: Have you tried these new techniques? *Nursing, 35*(3), 36–42.

Darke, S., Kaye, S., & Duflou, J. (2006). Comparative cardiac pathology among deaths due to cocaine toxicity, opioid toxicity and non-drug-related causes. *Addiction, 101,* 1771–1777.

Datta, S. D., Koutsky, L. A., Ratelle, S., Unger, E. R., Shlay, J., McClain, T., et al. (2008). Human papillomavirus infection and cervical cytology in women screened for cervical cancer in the United States, 2003–2005. *Annals of Internal Medicine, 148,* 493–501.

David, D. H., & Lyons-Ruth, K. (2005). Differential attachment responses of male and female infants to frightening maternal behavior: Tend or befriend versus fight or flight? *Infant Mental Health Journal, 26,* 1–18.

Davidson, K., MacGregor, M. W., Stuhr, J., Dixon, K., & MacLean, D. (2000). Constructive anger verbal behavior predicts blood pressure in a population-based sample. *Health Psychology, 19,* 55–64.

Davidson, R. J., Kabat-Zinn, J., Schumacher, J., Rosenkranz, M., Muller, D., Santorelli, S. F., et al. (2003). Alterations in brain and immune function produced by mindfulness meditation. *Psychosomatic Medicine, 65,* 564–570.

Davies, D. L. (1962). Normal drinking in recovered alcohol addicts. *Quarterly Journal of Studies on Alcohol, 24,* 321–332.

Davis, A. M., Vinci, L. M., Okwuosa, T. M., Chase, A. R., & Huang, E. S. (2007). Cardiovascular health disparities. *Medical Care Research and Review, 64*(Suppl.), 29S–100S.

Davis, C., & Scott-Robertson, L. (2000). A psychological comparison of females with anorexia nervosa and competitive male bodybuilders: Body shape ideals in the extreme. *Eating Behaviors, 1,* 33–46.

Davis, J. (2008). Pro-anorexia sites—A patient's perspective. *Child and Adolescent Mental Health, 13,* 97.

Davis, K. C., Hendershot, C. S., George, W. H., Norris, J., & Heiman, J. R. (2007). Alcohol's effects on sexual decisiom making: An integration of alcohol myopia and individual differences. *Journal of Studies on Alcohol and Drugs, 68,* 843–851.

Davis, K. D. (2000). Studies of pain using functional magnetic resonance imaging. In K. L. Casey & M. C. Bushnell (Eds.), *Pain imaging: Progress in pain research and management* (pp. 195–210). Seattle, WA: IASP Press.

Davis, M. C., Zautra, A. J., Younger, J., Motivala, S. J., Attrep, J., & Irwin, M. R. (2008). Chronic stress and regulation of cellular markers of inflammation in rheumatoid arthritis: Implications for fatigue. *Brain, Behavior and Immunity, 22,* 24–32.

Dawson, D. A., Grant, B. F., Stinson, F. S., Chou, P. S., Huang, B., & Ruan, W. J. (2005). Recovery from DSM-IV alcohol dependence: United States, 2001–2002. *Addiction, 100,* 281–292.

De Andrés, J., & Van Buyten, J.-P. (2006). Neural modulation by stimulation. *Pain Practice, 6,* 39–45.

De Benedittis, G. (2003). Understanding the multidimensional mechanisms of hypnotic analgesia. *Contemporary Hypnosis, 20,* 59–80.

Decaluwé, V., & Braet, C. (2005). The cognitive behavioural model for eating disorders: A direct evaluation in children and adolescents with obesity. *Eating Behaviors, 6,* 211–220.

De Civita, M., & Dobkin, P. L. (2005). Pediatric adherence: Conceptual and methodological considerations. *Children's Health Care, 34,* 19–34.

Dehle, C., Larsen, D., & Landers, J. E. (2001). Social support in marriage. *American Journal of Family Therapy, 29,* 307–324.

de la Fuente-Fernández, R., Schulzer, M., & Stoessl, A. J. (2004). Placebo mechanisms and reward circuitry: Clues from Parkinson's disease. *Biological Psychiatry, 56,* 67–71.

de Leeuw, R., Schmidt, J. E., & Carlson, C. R. (2005). Traumatic stressors and post-traumatic stress disorder symptoms in headache patients. *Headache, 45,* 1365–1374.

DeLeo, J. A. (2006). Basic science of pain. *Journal of Bone and Joint Surgery, 88*(Suppl. 2), 58–62.

De Lew, N., & Weinick, R. M. (2000). An overview: Eliminating racial, ethnic, and SES disparities in health care. *Health Care Financing Review, 21*(4), 1–7.

Delnevo, C. D., Hrywna, A., Abatemarco, D. J., & Lewis, M. J. (2003). Relationships between cigarette smoking and weight control in young women. *Family and Community Health, 26,* 140–146.

DeLongis, A., Folkman, S., & Lazarus, R. S. (1988). The impact of daily stress on health and mood: Psychological and social resources as mediators. *Journal of Personality and Social Psychology, 54,* 486–495.

Delvaux, T., & Nostlinger, C. (2007). Reproductive choice for women and men living with HIV: Contraception, abortion and fertility. *Reproductive Health Matters, 15*(Suppl.), 46–66.

De Marzo, A. M., Platz, E. A., Sutcliffe, S., Xu, J., Grönberg, H., Drake, C. G., et al. (2007). Inflammation in prostate carginogenesis. *Nature Reviews Cancer, 7,* 256–269.

Dembroski, T. M., MacDougall, J. M., Williams, R. B., Haney, T. L., & Blumenthal, J. A. (1985). Components of Type A, hostility, and anger-in: Relationship to angio-graphic findings. *Psychosomatic Medicine, 47,* 219–233.

Deniz, O., Aygül, R., Koçak, N., Orhan, A., & Kaya, M. D. (2004). Precipitating factors of migraine attacks in patients with migraine with and without aura. *Pain Clinic, 16,* 451–456.

Derogatis, L. R. (1977). *Manual for the Symptom Checklist-90, Revised.* Baltimore: Johns Hopkins University School of Medicine.

DeSimone, J. (2007). Fraternity membership and binge drinking. *Journal of Health Economics, 26,* 950–967.

DeVoe, J. E., Baez, A., Angier, H., Krois, L., Edlund, C., & Carney, P. A. (2007). Insurance + access ≠ health care: Typology of barriers to health care access for low-income families. *Annals of Family Medicine, 5,* 511–518.

DeVries, A. C., Glasper, E. R., & Detillion, C. E. (2003). Social modulation of stress responses. *Physiology and Behavior, 79,* 399–407.

Dewaraja, R., & Kawamura, N. (2006). Trauma intensity and posttraumatic stress: Implications of the tsunami experience in Sri Lanka for the management of future disasters. *International Congress Series, 1287,* 69–73.

Dhond, R. P., Kettner, N., & Napadow, V. (2007). Neuroimaging acupuncture effects in the human brain. *Journal of Alternative and Complementary Medicine, 13,* 603–616.

Dickerson, S. S., & Kemeny, M. E. (2004). Acute stressors and cortisol responses: A theoretical integration and synthesis of laboratory research. *Psychological Bulletin, 130,* 355–391.

Diehr, P., Bild, D. E., Harris, T. B., Duxbury, A., Siscovick, D., & Rossi, M. (1998). Body mass index and mortality in nonsmoking older adults: The Cardiovascular Health Study. *American Journal of Public Health, 88,* 623–629.

DiIorio, C., McCarty, F., Resnicow, K., Holstad, M. M., Soet, J., Yeager, K., et al. (2008). Using motivational inter-viewing to promote adherence to antiretroviral medica-tions: A randomized controlled study. *AIDS Care, 20,* 273–283.

Dillard, J., with Hirchman, L. A. (2002). *The chronic pain solution.* New York: Bantam.

DiMatteo, M. R. (2004a). Social support and patient adher-ence to medical treatment: A meta-analysis. *Health Psychology, 23,* 207–218.

DiMatteo, M. R. (2004b). Variations in patients' adherence to medical recommendations: A quantitative review of 50 years of research. *Medical Care, 42,* 200–209.

DiMatteo, M. R., & DiNicola, D. D. (1982). *Achieving patient compliance: The psychology of the medical practitioner's role.* New York: Pergamon Press.

DiMatteo, M. R., Giordani, P. J., Lepper, H. S., & Croghan, T. W. (2002). Patient adherence and medical treatment outcomes: A meta-analysis. *Medical Care, 40,* 794–811.

DiMatteo, M. R., Haskard, K. B., & Williams, S. L. (2007). Health beliefs, disease severity, and patients adherence: A meta-analysis. *Medical Care, 45,* 521–528.

DiMatteo, M. R., Lepper, H. S., & Croghan, T. W. (2000). Meta-analysis of the effects of anxiety and depression on patient adherence. *Archives of Internal Medicine, 160,* 2101–2107.

Dingwall, G. (2005). *Alcohol and crime.* Cullompton, UK: Willan Publishing.

DiNicola, D. D., & DiMatteo, M. R. (1984). Practitioners, patients, and compliance with medical regimens: A social psychological perspective. In A. Baum, S. E. Taylor, & J. E. Singer (Eds.), *Handbook of psychology and health: Vol. 4. Social psychological aspects of health* (pp. 55–84). Hillsdale, NJ: Erlbaum.

di Sarsina, R. (2007). The social demand for a medicine fo-cused on the person: The contribution of CAM to health-care and health genesis. *Evidence-Based Complementary and Alternative Medicine, 4*(Suppl. 1), 45–51.

Dishman, R. K. (2003). The impact of behavior on quality of life. *Quality of Life Research, 12*(Suppl. 1), 43–49.

Distefan, J. M., Pierce, J. P., & Gilpin, E. A. (2004). Do favorite movie stars influence adolescent smoking initia-tion? *American Journal of Public Health, 94,* 239–244.

Dittmann, M. (2005). Publicizing diabetes' behavioral im-pact. *Monitor on Psychology, 36*(7), 35–36.

Dobbins, M., DeCorby, K., Manske, S., & Goldblatt, E. (2008). Effective practices for school-based tobacco use prevention. *Preventive Medicine, 46,* 289–297.

Dobson, R. (2005). High cholesterol may increase risk of testicular cancer. *British Medical Journal, 330,* 1042.

Doevendans, P. A., Van der Smagt, J., Loh, P., De Jonge, N., & Touw, D. J. (2003). Prognostic implications of genetics in cardiovascular disease. *Current Pharmacogenomics, 1,* 217–228.

Doll, R., & Hill, A. B. (1956). Lung cancer and other causes of death in relation to smoking: A second report on the mortality of British doctors. *British Medical Journal, 2,* 1071–1081.

Donaghy, M. E. (2007). Exercise can seriously improve your mental health: Fact or fiction? *Advanced in Physiology, 9*(2), 76–88.

Donohue, K. F., Curtin, J. J., Patrick, C. J., & Lang, A. R. (2007). Intoxication level and emotional response. *Emotion, 7,* 103–112.

Dorenlot, P., Harboun, M., Bige, V., Henrard, J.-C., & Ankri, J. (2005). Major depression as a risk factor for early institutionalization of dementia patients living in the community. *International Journal of Geriatric Psychiatry, 20,* 471–478.

Dorr, N., Brosschot, J. F., Sollers, J. J., & Thayer, J. F. (2007). Damned if you do, damned if you don't: The differential effect of expression and inhibition of anger on cardiovascular recovery in Black and White males. *International Journal of Psychophysiology, 66,* 125–134.

Dougall, A. L., & Baum, A. (2001). Stress, health, and illness. In A. Baum, T. A. Revenson, & J. E. Singer (Eds.), *Handbook of health psychology* (pp. 321–337). Mahwah, NJ: Erlbaum.

Douketis, J. D., Macie, C., Thabane, L., & Williamson, D. F. (2005). Systematic review of long-term weight loss studies in obese adults: Clinical significance and applicability to clinical practice. *International Journal of Obesity, 29,* 1153–1167.

Dresler, C. M., Leon, M. E., Straif, K., Baan, R., & Secretan, B. (2006). Reversal of risk upon quitting smoking. *Lancet, 368,* 348–349.

Droomers, M., Schrijvers, C. T. M., & Mackenbach, J. P. (2002). Why do lower educated people continue smoking? Explanations from the longitudinal GLOBE study. *Health Psychology, 21,* 263–272.

Du, X. L., Meyer, T. E., & Franzini, L. (2007). Meta-analysis of racial disparities in survival in association with socioeconomic status among men and women with color cancer. *Cancer, 109,* 2161–2170.

Dunbar, H. F. (1943). *Psychosomatic diagnosis.* New York: Hoeber.

Duncan, A. E., Neuman, R. J., Kramer, J., Kuperman, S., Hesselbrock, V., Reich, T., & Bucholz, K. K. (2005). Are there subgroups of bulimia nervosa based comorbid psychiatric disorders? *International Journal of Eating Disorders, 37,* 19–25.

Dunn, A. L., Trivedi, M. H., Kampert, J. B., Clark, C. G., & Chambliss, H. O. (2005). Exercise treatment for depression: Efficacy and dose response. *American Journal of Preventive Medicine, 28,* 1–8.

Dunn, A. L., Trivedi, M. H., & O'Neal, H. A. (2001). Physical activity dose-response effects on outcomes of depression and anxiety. *Medicine and Science in Sports and Exercise, 33,* S587–S597.

Durkheim, E. (1967). *The elementary forms of religious life* (Joseph Ward Swain, Trans.). New York: Free Press. (Original work published 1912)

Dusseldrop, E., van Elderen, T., Maes, S., Meulman, J., & Kraaj, V. (1999). A meta-analysis of psychoeducational programs for coronary heart disease patients. *Health Psychology, 18,* 506–519.

Dutra, L., Stathopoulou, G., Basden, S. L., Leyro, T. M., Powers, M. B., & Otto, M. W. (2008). A meta-analytic review of psychosocial interventions for substance use disorders. *American Journal of Psychiatry, 165,* 179–187.

Dyer, A. R., Elliott, P., Stamler, J., Chan, Q., Ueshima, H., & Zhou, B. F. (2003). Dietary intake in male and female smokers, ex-smokers, and never smokers: The INTERMAP Study. *Journal of Human Hypertension, 17,* 641–654.

Dyer, A. R., Stamler, J., & Greenland, P. (2000). Associations of weight change and weight variability with cardiovascular and all-cause mortality in the Chicago Western

Electric Company Study. *American Journal of Epidemiology, 152,* 324–333.

Eaker, E. D., Sullivan, L. M., Kelly-Hayes, M., D'Agostino, R. B, Sr., & Benjamin, E. J. (2007). Marital status, marital strain, and risk of coronary heart disease or total mortality: The Framingham Offspring Study. *Psychosomatic Medicine, 69,* 509–513.

Eaton, D. K., Kann, L., Kinchen, S., Shanklin, S., Ross, J., Hawkins, J., et al. (2008). Youth risk behavior surveillance—United States, 2007. *Morbidity and Mortality Weekly Report, 57*(SS-4), 1–130.

Ebrecht, M., Hextall, J., Kirtley, L.-G., Taylor, A., Dyson, M., & Weinman, J. (2004). Perceived stress and cortisol levels predict speed of wound healing in healthy male adults. *Psychoneuroendocrinology, 29,* 798–809.

Eckhardt, C. I., & Crane, C. (2008). Effects of alcohol intoxication and aggressivity on aggressive verbalizations during anger arousal. *Aggressive Behavior, 34,* 428–436.

Eddy, K. T., Dorer, D. J., Franko, D. L., Tahilani, K., Thompson-Brenner, H., & Herzog, D. B. (2007). Should bulimia nervosa be subtyped by history of anorexia nervosa? A longitudinal validation. *International Journal of Eating Disorders, 40*(Suppl.), S67–S71.

Edwards, A. G. K., Hailey, S., & Maxwell, M. (2004). Psychological interventions for women with metastatic breast cancer. *Cochrane Database of Systematic Reviews,* Cochrane AN: CD004253.

Edwards, C. L., Fillingim, R. B., & Keefe, F. (2001). Race, ethnicity and pain. *Pain, 94,* 133–137.

Edwards, G. (1977). The alcohol dependence syndrome: Usefulness of an idea. In G. Edwards & M. Grant (Eds.), *Alcoholism: New knowledge and new responses.* London: Croom Helm.

Edwards, G. (2000). *Alcohol: The world's favorite drug.* New York: Thomas Dunne Books.

Edwards, G., & Gross, M. M. (1976). Alcohol dependence: Provisional description of a clinical syndrome. *British Medical Journal, 1,* 1058–1061.

Edwards, G., Gross, M. M., Keller, M., Moser, J., & Room, R. (1977). *Alcohol-related disabilities* (WHO Offset Pub. No. 32). Geneva: World Health Organization.

Edwards, L. M., & Romero, A. J. (2008). Coping with discrimination among Mexican descent adolescents. *Hispanic Journal of Behavioral Sciences, 30,* 24–39.

Ee, C. C., Manheimer, E., Pirotta, M. V., & White, A. R. (2008). Acupuncture for pelvic and back pain in pregnancy: A systematic review. *American Journal of Obstetrics and Gynecology, 198,* 254–259.

Eggert, J., Theobald, H., & Engfeldt, P. (2004). Effects of alcohol consumption on female fertility during an 18-year period. *Fertility and Sterility, 81,* 379–383.

Ehrlich, G. E. (2003). Low back pain. *Bulletin of the World Health Organization, 81,* 671–676.

Eisenberg, M. E., Neumark-Sztainer, D., Story, M., & Perry, C. (2005). The role of social norms and friends' influences on unhealthy weight-control behaviors among adolescent girls. *Social Science and Medicine, 60,* 1165–1173.

Eisenberger, N. I., Gable, S. L., & Lieberman, M. D. (2007). Functional magnetic resonance imaging responses relate to differences in real-world social experience. *Emotion, 7*, 745–754.

Eisenberger, N. I., Jarcho, J. M., Lieberman, M. D., & Naliboff, B. D. (2006). An experimental study of shared sensitivity to physical pain and social rejection. *Pain, 126*, 132–138.

Eisenberger, N. I., & Lieberman, M. D. (2004). Why rejection hurts: A common neural alarm system for physical and social pain. *Trends in Cognitive Sciences, 8*, 294–300.

Eisenberger, N. I., Lieberman, M. D., & Williams, K. D. (2003). Does rejection hurt? An fMRI study of social exclusion. *Science, 302*, 290–292.

Eisenmann, J. C., Welk, G. J., Wickel, E. E., & Blair, S. N. (2007). Combined influence of cardiorespiratory fitness and body mass index on cardiovascular disease risk factors among 8–18 year old youth: The Aerobics Center Longitudinal Study. *International Journal of Pediatric Obesity, 2*(2), 66–72.

Ekeland, E., Heian, F., Hagen, K. B., Abbott, J., & Nordheim, L. (2004). Exercise to improve self-esteem in children and young people. *Cochrane Database of Systematic Reviews*, Cochrane AN: CD003683.

Ekelund, U., Brage, S., Franks, P. W., Hennings, S., Emms, S., & Wareham, N. J. (2005). Physical activity energy expenditure predicts progression toward the metabolic syndrome independently of aerobic fitness in middle-aged healthy Caucasians. *Diabetes Care, 28*, 1195–1200.

Eliassen, A. H., Colditz, G. A., Rosner, B., Willett, W. C., & Hankinson, S. E. (2006). Adult weight change and risk of postmenopausal breast cancer. *Journal of the American Medical Association, 296*, 193–201.

Elkins, J. S. (2006). Management of blood pressure in patients with cerebrovascular disease. *Johns Hopkins Advanced Studies in Medicine, 6*(8), 363–369, 349–350.

Eller, N. H., Netterstrøm, B., & Hansen, Å. M. (2006). Psychosocial factors at home and at work and levels of salivary cortisol. *Biological Psychology, 73*, 280–287.

Elliott, J. O., Seals, B. F., & Jacobson, M. P. (2007). Use of the precaution adoption process model to examine predictors of osteoprotective behavior in epilepsy. *Seizure, 16*, 424–437.

Elliott, R. A. (2006). Poor adherence to anti-inflammatory medication in asthma: Reasons, challenges, and strategies for improved disease management. *Disease Management and Health Outcomes, 14*, 223–233.

Ellis, A. (1962). *Reason and emotion in psychotherapy.* New York: Stuart.

Ellis, D. A., Podolski, C.-L., Frey, M., Naar-King, S., Wang, B., & Moltz, K. (2007). The role of parental monitoring in adolescent health outcomes: Impact on regimen adherence in youth with Type 1 diabetes. *Journal of Pediatric Psychology 32*, 907–917.

Ellis, L. (2004). Thief of time. *InteliHealth.* Retrieved July 1, 2005, from http://www.intelihealth.com/IH/ihtIH/WSIHW000/8303/24299.html

Emanuel, E. J., & Fuchs, V. R. (2008). The perfect storm of overutilization. *Journal of the American Medical Association, 299*, 2789–2791.

Emanuel, L., Bennett, K., & Richardson, V. E. (2007). The dying role. *Journal of Palliative Medicine, 10*, 159–168.

Endresen, G. K. M. (2007). Fibromyalgia: A rheumatologic diagnosis? *Rheumatology International, 27*, 999–1004.

Eng, P. M., Fitzmaurice, G., Kubzansky, L. D., Rimm, E. B., & Kawachi, I. (2003). Anger expression and risk of stroke and coronary heart disease among male health professionals. *Psychosomatic Medicine, 65*, 100–110.

Engler, M. B., & Engler, M. M. (2006). The emerging role of flavonoid-rich cocoa and chocolate in cardiovascular health and disease. *Nutrition Reviews, 64*, 109–118.

Ensel, W. M., & Lin, N. (2004). Physical fitness and the stress process. *Journal of Community Psychology, 32*, 81–101.

Epstein, L. H., Leddy, J. J, Temple, J. L., & Faith, M. S. (2007). Food reinforcement and eating: A multilevel analysis. *Psychological Bulletin, 133*, 884–906.

Erblich, J., Lerman, C., Self, D. W., Diaz, G. A., & Bovbjerg, D. H. (2005). Effects of dopamine D2 receptor (DRD2) and transporter (SLC6A3) polymorphisms on smoking cue-induced cigarette craving among African-American smokers. *Molecular Psychiatry, 10*, 407–414.

Erlanson-Albertsson, C. (2005). How palatable food disrupts appetite regulation. *Basic and Clinical Pharmacology and Toxicology, 97*, 61–73.

Ernst, E., Pittler, M. H., Wider, B., & Boddy, K. (2007a). Massage therapy: Is its evidence base getting stronger? *Complementary Health Practice Review, 12*, 179–183.

Ernst, E., Pittler, M. H., Wider, B., & Boddy, K. (2007b). Mind–body therapies: Are the trial data getting stronger? *Alternative Therapies in Health and Medicine, 13*(5), 62–64.

Ernster, V. L., Grady, D., Müke, R., Black, D., Selby, J., & Kerlikowske, K. (1995). Facial wrinkling in men and women by smoking status. *American Journal of Public Health, 85*, 78–82.

Ertekin-Taner, N. (2007). Genetics of Alzheimer's disease: A centennial review. *Neurologic Clinics, 25*, 611–667.

Escamilla, G., Cradock, A. L., & Kawachi, I. (2000). Women and smoking in Hollywood movies: A content analysis. *American Journal of Public Health, 90*, 412–414.

European Vertebral Osteoporosis Study Group. (2004). Variation in back pain between countries: The example of Britain and Germany. *Spine, 29*, 1017–1021.

Evans, G. W., & Stecker, R. (2004). Motivational consequences of environmental stress. *Journal of Environmental Psychology, 24*, 143–165.

Evans, M. A., Shaw, A. R. G., Sharp, D. J., Thompson, E. A., Falk, S., Turton, P., et al. (2007). Men with cancer: Is their use of complementary and alternative medicine a response to needs unmet by conventional care? *European Journal of Cancer Care, 16*, 517–525.

Evans, P. C. (2003). "If only I were thin like her, maybe I could be happy like her": The self-implications of associating a thin female ideal with life success. *Psychology of Women Quarterly, 27,* 209–214.

Everett, M. D., Kinser, A. M., & Ramsey, M. W. (2007). Training for old age: Production functions for the aerobic exercise inputs. *Medicine and Science in Sports and Exercise, 39,* 2226–2233.

Everson, S. A., Lynch, J. W., Kaplan, G. A., Lakka, T. A., Sivenius, J., & Salonen, J. T. (2001). Stress-induced blood pressure reactivity and incident stroke in middle-aged men. *Stroke, 32,* 1263–1270.

Exubera lung cancer warning could be death knell for inhaled insulin. (2008, April 10). *NewsInferno.* Retrieved June 28, 2008, from http://www.newsinferno.com/archives/2881

Ezekiel, J. E., & Miller, F. G. (2001). The ethics of placebo-controlled trials: A middle ground. *New England Journal of Medicine, 345,* 915–920.

Ezzati, M., & Lopez, A. D. (2004). Regional, disease specific patterns of smoking-attributable mortality in 2000. *Tobacco Control, 13,* 388–395.

Ezzo, J., Streitberger, K., & Schneider, A. (2006). Cochrane systematic reviews examine p6 acupuncture-point stimulation for nausea and vomiting. *Journal of Complementary and Alternative Medicine, 12,* 489–495.

Faden, R. R. (1987). Ethical issues in government sponsored public health campaigns. *Health Education Quarterly, 14,* 27–37.

Fairburn, C. G., & Harrison, P. J. (2003). Eating disorders. *Lancet, 361,* 407–416.

Fairhurst, M., Wiech, K., Dunckley, P., & Tracey, I. (2007). Anticipatory brainstem activity predicts neural processing of pain in humans. *Pain, 128,* 101–110.

Fang, C. V., & Myers, H. F. (2001). The effects of racial stressors and hostility on cardiovascular reactivity in African American and Caucasian men. *Health Psychology, 20,* 64–70.

Farber, N., & Olney, J. W. (2003). Drugs of abuse that cause developing neurons to commit suicide. *Developmental Brain Research, 147,* 37–45.

Farley, J. J., Rodrigue, J. R., Sandrik, L. L., Tepper, V. J., Marhefka, S. L., & Sleasman, J. W. (2004). Clinical assessment of medication adherence among HIV-infected children: Examination of the Treatment Interview Protocol (TIP). *AIDS Care, 16,* 323–337.

Farrell, S. P., Hains, A. A., Davies, W. H., Smith, P., & Parton, E. (2004). The impact of cognitive distortions, stress, and adherence on metabolic control in youths with Type 1 diabetes. *Journal of Adolescent Health, 34,* 461–467.

Fauvel, J. P. (2001). Perceived job stress but not individual cardiovascular reactivity to stress is related to higher blood pressure at work [Abstract]. *Journal of the American Medical Association, 286,* 1814.

Favier, I., Haan, J., & Ferrari, M. D. (2005). Chronic cluster headache: A review. *Journal of Headache and Pain, 6,* 3–9.

Federal Trade Commission weighs in on losing weight. (2002). *FDA Consumer, 36,* 8.

Feinglass, J., Lee, C., Rogers, M., Temple, L. M., Nelson, C., & Chang, R. W. (2007). Complementary and alternative medicine use for arthritis pain in 2 Chicago community areas. *Clinical Journal of Pain, 23,* 744–749.

Feist, J., & Feist, G. J. (2006). *Theories of personality* (6th ed.). Boston: McGraw-Hill.

Feldman, P. J., Cohen, S., Gwaltney, J. M., Jr., Doyle, W. J., & Skoner, D. P. (1999). The impact of personality on the reporting of unfounded symptoms and illness. *Journal of Personality and Social Psychology, 77,* 370–378.

Feldt, K. (2007). Pain measurement: Present concern and future directions. *Pain Medicine, 8,* 541–543.

Female Celebrity Smoking List. (2008). *Gwyneth Paltrow.* Retrieved June 12, 2008, from http://smokingsides.com/asfs/P/Paltrow.html

Ferguson, J., Bauld, L., Chesterman, J., & Judge, K. (2005). The English smoking treatment services: One-year outcomes. *Addiction, 100*(Suppl. 2), 59–69.

Fernandez, E., & Sheffield, J. (1996). Relative contributions of life events versus daily hassles to the frequency and intensity of headaches. *Headache, 36,* 595–602.

Fernandez, R., Griffiths, R., Everett, B., Davidson, P., Salamonson, Y., & Andrew, S. (2007). Effectiveness of brief structures interventions on risk factor modification for patients with coronary heart disease: A systematic review. *International Journal of Evidence-Based Healthcare, 5,* 370–405.

Ferri, M., Amato, L., & Davoli, M. (2006). Alcoholics Anonymous and other 12-step programmes for alcohol dependence. *Cochrane Database of Systematic Reviews,* Cochrane AN: CD005032.

Fichtenberg, C. M., & Glantz, S. A. (2002). Effect of smoke-free workplaces on smoking behaviour: *Systematic Review, 325,* 188–195.

Field, T. M. (1998). Massage therapy effects. *American Psychologist, 53,* 1270–1281.

Fifield, J., Mcquillan, J., Armeli, S., Tennen, H., Reisine, S., & Affleck, G. (2004). Chronic strain, daily work stress and pain among workers with rheumatoid arthritis: Does job stress make a bad day worse? *Work and Stress, 18,* 275–291.

Fillmore, K. M., Stockwell, T., Chikritzhs, T., Bostrom, A., & Kerr, W. (2007). Moderate alcohol use and reduced mortality risk: Systematic error in prospective studies and new hypotheses. *Annals of Epidemiology, 17*(Suppl.), S16–S23.

Filozof, C., Fernández Pinilla, M. C., & Fernández-Cruz, A. (2004). Smoking cessation and weight gain. *Obesity Reviews, 5,* 95–103.

Finkelstein, E. A., Ruhm, C. J., & Kosa, K. M. (2005). Economic causes and consequences of obesity. *Annual Review of Public Health, 26,* 239–257.

Finlayson, G., King, N., & Blundell, J. E. (2007). Liking vs. wanting food: Importance for human appetite control and weight regulation. *Neuroscience and Biobehavioral Reviews, 31,* 987–1002.

Finley, J. W., Davis, C. D., & Feng, Y. (2000). Selenium from high selenium broccoli protects rats from colon cancer. *Journal of Nutrition, 130,* 2384–2389.

Finniss, D. G., & Benedetti, F. (2005). The neural matrix of pain processing and placebo analgesia: Implications for clinical practice. *Headache Currents, 2*(6), 132–138.

Fiore, M. C., Bailey, W. C., Cohen, S. J., Dorfman, S. F., Goldstein, M. G., Gritz, E. R., et al. (1996). *Smoking cessation: Clinical practice guideline no. 18.* AHCPR Publication No. 69-0692. Rockville, MD: U.S. Department of Health and Human Services, Public Health Service, Agency for Health Care Policy and Research.

Firenzuoli, F., & Gori, L. (2007). Herbal medicine today: Clinical and research issues. *Evidence Based Complementary and Alternative Medicine, 4*(Suppl. 1), 37–40.

Fishbein, M., & Ajzen, I. (1975). *Belief, attitude, intention, and behavior: An introduction to theory and research.* Reading, MA: Addison-Wesley.

Fisher, E. S., Wennberg, D. E., Stukel, T. A., Gottlieb, D. J., Lucas, F. L., & Pinder, E. L. (2003). The implications of regional variations in Medicare spending: Part 1. The content, quality, and accessibility of care. *Archives of Internal Medicine, 138,* 273–287.

Fitzpatrick, A. L., Kuller, L. H., Ives, D. G., Lopez, O. L., Jagust, W., Breitner, J. C. S., et al. (2004). Incidence and prevalence of dementia in the Cardiovascular Health Study. *Journal of the American Geriatrics Society, 52,* 195–204.

Fixx, J. F. (1977). *The complete book of running.* New York: Random House.

Fixx, J. F. (1980). *Jim Fixx's second book of running.* New York: Random House.

Flegal, K. M., Graubard, B. I., Williamson, D. F., & Gail, M. H. (2005). Excess deaths associated with underweight, overweight, and obesity. *Journal of the American Medical Association, 293,* 1861–1867.

Fleshner, M., & Laudenslager, M. L. (2004). Psychoneuroimmunology: Then and now. *Behavioral and Cognitive Neuroscience Reviews, 3,* 114–130.

Flor, H. (2001). Psychophysiological assessment of the patient with chronic pain. In D. C. Turk & R. Melzack (Eds.), *Handbook of pain assessment* (2nd ed., pp. 70–96). New York: Guilford Press.

Flor, H., Nikolajsen, L. & Staehelin Jensen, T. (2006). Phantom limb pain: A case of maladaptive CNS plasticity? *Nature Reviews Neuroscience, 7,* 873–881.

Flores, G. (2006). Language barriers to health care in the United States. *New England Journal of Medicine, 355,* 229–231.

Floriani, V., & Kennedy, C. (2008). Promotion of physical activity in children. *Current Opinion in Pediatrics, 20,* 90–95.

Folkman, S., & Lazarus, R. S. (1980). An analysis of coping in a middle-aged community sample. *Journal of Health and Social Behavior, 21,* 219–239.

Folkman, S., & Moskowitz, J. T. (2000). Positive affect and the other side of coping. *American Psychologist, 55,* 647–654.

Folkman, S., & Moskowitz, J. T. (2004). Coping: Pitfalls and promise. *Annual Review of Psychology, 55,* 745–774.

Folk-Williams, S. (2002). AIDS girl: An interview with Alora Gale. *The Body: An AIDS and HIV Information Resource.* Retrieved January 27, 2005, from http://www.thebody.com/features/women/profiles_agale.html

Folsom, A. R., Kushi, L. H., Anderson, K. E., Mink, P. J., Olson, J. E., Hong, C.-P., et al. (2000). Associations of general and abdominal obesity with multiple health outcomes in older women. *Archives of Internal Medicine, 160,* 2117–2128.

Foltz, V., St. Pierre, Y., Rozenberg, S., Rossingnol, M., Bourgeois, P., Joseph, L., et al. (2005). Use of complementary and alternative therapies by patients with self-reported chronic back pain: A nationwide survey in Canada. *Joint Bone Spine, 72,* 571–577.

Foran, H., & O'Leary, K. (2008). Problem drinking, jealousy, and anger control: Variables predicting physical aggression against a partner. *Journal of Family Violence, 23,* 141–148.

Forbes, G. B. (2000). Body fat content influences the body composition response to nutrition and exercise. *Annals of the New York Academic of Sciences, 904,* 359–368.

Forcier, K., Stroud, L. R., Papandonatos, G. D., Hitsman, B., Reiches, M., Krishnamoorthy, J., et al. (2006). Links between physical fitness and cardiovascular reactivity and recovery to psychological stressors: A meta-analysis. *Health Psychology, 25,* 723–739.

Ford, E. S., Ajani, U. A., Croft, J. B., Critchley, J. A., Labarthe, D. R., Kottke, T. E., et al. (2007). Explaining the decrease in U. S. deaths from coronary disease, 1980–2000. *New England Journal of Medicine, 356,* 2388–2398.

Fordyce, W. E. (1974). Pain viewed as learned behavior. In J. J. Bonica (Ed.), *Advances in neurology* (Vol. 4). New York: Raven Press.

Fordyce, W. E. (1976). *Behavioral methods for chronic pain and illness.* St. Louis: Mosby.

Forlenza, J. J., & Baum, A. (2004). Psychoneuroimmunology. In R. G. Frank, A. Baum, & J. L. Wallander (Eds.), *Handbook of clinical health psychology* (Vol. 3, pp. 81–114). Washington, DC: American Psychological Association.

Foulon, C., Guelfi, J. d., Kipman, A., Adès, J., Romo, L., Houdeyer, K., et al. (2007). Switching to the bingeing/purging subtype of anorexia nervosa is frequently associated with suicidal attempts. *European Psychiatry, 22,* 513–519.

Fournier, M., de Ridder, D., & Bensing, J. (2002). Optimism and adaptation to chronic disease: The role of optimism in relation to self-care options for Type 1 diabetes mellitus, rheumatoid arthritis and multiple sclerosis. *British Journal of Health Psychology, 7,* 409–432.

Fox, C. S., Heard-Costa, N. L., Wilson, P. W. F., Levy, D., D'Agostino, R. B., Sr., & Atwood, L. D. (2004). Genome-wide linkage to chromosome 6 for waist circumference in the Framingham Heart Study. *Diabetes, 53,* 1399–1402.

Franko, D. L., Becker, A. E., Thomas, J. J., & Herzog, D. B. (2007). Cross-ethnic differences in eating disorder symptoms and related distress. *International Journal of Eating Disorders, 40,* 156–164.

Franz, I. D. (1913). On psychology and medical education. *Science, 38,* 555–566.

Fraser, B. (2005). Latin America's urbanisation is boosting obesity. *Lancet, 365,* 1995–1996.

Fraser, G. E., & Shavlik, D. J. (2001). Ten years of life: Is it a matter of choice? *Archives of Internal Medicine, 161,* 1645–1652.

Frattaroli, J., Weidner, G., Merritt-Worden, T. A., Frenda, S., & Ornish, D. (2008). Angina pectoris and atherosclerotic risk factors in the Multisite Cardiac Lifestyle Intervention Program. *American Journal of Cardiology, 101,* 911–918.

Freedman, D. S., Khan, L. K., Dietz, W. H., Srinivasan, S. R., & Berenson, G. S. (2001). Relationship of childhood obesity to coronary heart disease risk factors in adulthood: The Bogalusa Heart Study. *Pediatrics, 108,* 712–718.

Freedman, L. S., Kipnis, V., Schatzkin, A., & Potischman, N. (2008). Methods of epidemiology: Evaluating the fat-breast cancer hypothesis—Comparing dietary instruments and other developments. *Cancer Journals, 14*(2), 69–74.

Friedländer, L. (1968). *Roman life and manners under the early empire.* New York: Barnes & Noble.

Friedman, M., & Rosenman, R. H. (1974). *Type A behavior and your heart.* New York: Knopf.

Fries, J. F. (1998). Reducing the need and demand for medical services. *Psychosomatic Medicine, 60,* 140–142.

Frisina, P. G., Borod, J. C., & Lepore, S. J. (2004). A meta-analysis of the effects of written emotional disclosure on the health outcomes of clinical populations. *Journal of Nervous and Mental Disease, 192,* 629–634.

Fritz, G. K. (2000). The evolution of psychosomatic medicine. *Brown University Child and Adolescent Behavior Letter, 16*(4), 8.

Frone, M. R. (2008). Are work strssors related to employee substance use? The importance of temporal context assessment of alcohol and illicit drug use. *Journal of Applied Psychology, 93,* 199–206.

Froom, P., Kristal-Boneh, E., Melamed, S., Gofer, D., Benbassat, J., & Ribak, J. (1999). Smoking cessation and body mass index of occupationally active men: The Israeli CORDIS Study. *American Journal of Public Health, 89,* 718–722.

Fuertes, J. N., Mislowack, A., Bennett, J., Paul, L., Gilbert. T. C., Fontan, G., et al. (2007). The physician-patient working alliance. *Patient Education and Counseling, 66,* 29–36.

Fujino, Y., Tamakoshi, A., Iso, H., Inaba, Y., Kubo, T., Ide, R., et al. (2005). A nationwide cohort study of educational background and major causes of death among the elderly population in Japan. *Preventive Medicine, 40,* 444–451.

Fulkerson, J. A., & French, S. A. (2003). Cigarette smoking for weight loss or control among adolescents: Gender and racial/ethnic differences. *Journal of Adolescent Health, 32,* 306–313.

Fumal, A., & Schoenen, J. (2008). Tension-type headache: Current research and clinical management. *Lancet Neurology, 7,* 70–83.

Fung, T. T., Chiuve, S. E., McCullough, M. L., Rexrode, K. M., Logroscino, G., & Hu, F. B. (2008). Adherence to a DASH-style diet and risk of coronary heart disease and stroke in women. *Archives of Internal Medicine, 168,* 713–720.

Furnham, A. (2007). Are modern health worries, personality and attitudes to science associated with the use of complementary and alternative medicine? *British Journal of Health Psychology, 12,* 229–243.

Gaab, J., Blättler, N., Menzi, T., Pabst, B., Stoyer, S., & Ehlert, U. (2003). Randomized controlled evaluation of the effects of cognitive-behavioral stress management on cortisol responses to acute stress in healthy subjects. *Psychoneuroendocrinology, 28,* 767–779.

Gaab, J., Sonderegger, L., Scherrer, S., & Ehlert, U. (2007). Psychoneuroendocrine effects of cognitive-behavioral stress management in a naturalistic setting—A randomized controlled trial. *Psychoneuroendocrinology, 31,* 428–438.

Gabriel, R., Ferrando, L., Cortón, E. S., Mingote, C., García-Camba, E., Liria, A. F., et al. (2007). Psychopathological consequences after a terrorist attack: An epidemiological study among victims, the general population, and police officers. *European Psychiatry, 22,* 339–346.

Gadde, K. M., Yonish, G. M., Foust, M. S., & Allison, D. B. (2006). Atomoxetine for weight reduction in obese women: A preliminary randomised controlled trial. *International Journal of Obesity, 30,* 1138–1142.

Gaesser, G. A. (2003). Weight, weight loss, and health: A closer look at the evidence. *Healthy Weight Journal, 17,* 8–11.

Gagliese, L., Weizblit, N., Ellis, W., & Chan, V. W. S. (2005). The measurement of postoperative pain: A comparison of intensity scales in younger and older surgical patients. *Pain, 117,* 412–420.

Galdas, P. M., Cheater, F., & Marshall, P. (2005). Men and health help-seeking behavior: Literature review. *Journal of Advanced Nursing, 49,* 616–623.

Galea, S., Ahern, J., Resnick, H., Kilpatrick, D., Bucuvalas, M., Gold, J., et al. (2002). Psychological sequelae of the September 11 terrorist attacks in New York City. *New England Journal of Medicine, 346,* 982–987.

Gallagher, B. (2003). Tai chi chuan and qigong. *Topics in Geriatric Rehabilitation, 19,* 172–182.

Gallagher-Thompson, D., & Coon, D. W. (2007). Evidence-based psychological treatments for distress in family caregivers of older adults. *Psychology and Aging, 22,* 37–51.

Galland, L. (2006). Patient-centered care: Antecedents, triggers, and mediators. *Alternative Therapies, 12,* 62–70.

Gallegos-Macias, A. R., Macias, S. R., Kaufman, E., Skipper, B., & Kalishman, N. (2003). Relationship between glycemic control, ethnicity and socioeconomic status in Hispanic and white non-Hispanic youths with Type 1 diabetes mellitus. *Pediatric Diabetes, 4,* 19–23.

Galper, D. I., Trivedi, M. H., Barlow, C. E., Dunn, A. L., & Kampert, J. B. (2006). Inverse association between physical inactivity and mental health in men and women.

Medicine and Science in Sports and Exercise, 38, 173–178.

Galton, F. (1879). Psychometric experiments. *Brain, 2,* 149–162.

Galton, F. (1883). *Inquiries into human faculty and its development.* London: Macmillan.

Gambrill, S. (2008, April). Magic Johnson—Celebrity spokesperson for minority patient recruitment? *Clinical-TrialsToday.* Retrieved June 30, 2008, from http://www.clinicaltrialstoday.com/2008/04/magic-johnsonce.html

Gan, T. J., Gordon, D. B., Bolge, S. C., & Allen, J. G. (2007). Patient-controlled analgesia: Patient and nurse satisfaction with intravenous delivery systems and expected satisfaction with transdermal delivery systems. *Current Medical Research and Opinion, 23,* 2507–2516.

Gangwisch, J. E., Malaspina, D., Boden-Albala, B., & Heymsfield, S. B. (2005). Inadequate sleep as a risk factor for obesity: Analyses of the NHANES I. *Sleep, 28,* 1289–1296.

Gans, J. A., & McPhillips, T. (2003). Medication compliance-adherence-persistence. *Medication Compliance-Adherence-Persistence (CAP) Digest, 1,* 1–32.

Garavello, W., Negri, E., Talamini, R., Levi, F., Zambon, P., Dal Maso, L., et al. (2005). Family history of cancer, its combination with smoking and drinking, and risk of squamous cell carcinoma of the esophagus. *Cancer Epidemiology, Biomarkers, and Prevention, 14,* 1390–1393.

Garber, M. C. (2004). The concordance of self-report with other measures of medication adherence: A summary of the literature. *Medical Care, 42,* 649–652.

García, J., Simón, M. A., Durán, M., Canceller, J., & Aneiros, F. J. (2006). Differential efficacy of a cognitive-behavioral intervention versus pharmacological treatment in the management of fibromyalgic syndrome. *Psychology, Health and Medicine, 11,* 498–506.

Gardner, C. D., Kiazand, A., Alhassan, S., Kim, S., Stafford, R. S., Balise, R. R., et al. (2007). Comparison of the Atkins, Zone, Ornish, and LEARN diets for change in weight and related risk factors among overweight premenopausal women: The A to Z weight loss study: A randomized trial. *Journal of the American Medical Association, 297,* 969–977.

Garner, D. M., & Garfinkel, P. E. (1980). Social-cultural factors in the development of anorexia nervosa. *Psychological Medicine, 10,* 647–656.

Garner, D. M., Garfinkel, P. E., Schwartz, D., & Thompson, M. (1980). Cultural expectations of thinness in women. *Psychological Reports, 47,* 483–491.

Garofalo, R., Herrick, A., Mustanski, B. S., & Donenberg, G. R. (2007). Tip of the iceberg: Young men who have sex with men, the Internet, and HIV risk. *American Journal of Public Health, 97,* 1113–1117.

Garssen, B. (2004). Psychological factors and cancer development. Evidence after 30 years of research. *Clinical Psychology Review, 24,* 115–338.

Gatchel, R. J. (2005). The biopsychosocial approach to pain assessment and management. In R. J. Gatchel (Ed.), *Clinical essentials of pain management* (pp. 23–46). Washington, DC: American Psychological Association.

Gatchel, R. J., & Epker, J. (1999). Psychosocial predictors of chronic pain and response to treatment. In R. J. Gatchel & D. C. Turk (Eds.), *Psychosocial factors in pain: Critical perspectives* (pp. 412–434). New York: Guilford Press.

Gately, P. J., Cooke, C. B., Barth, J. H., Bewick, B. M., Radley, D., & Hill, A. J. (2005). Children's residential weight-loss program can work: A prospective cohort study of short-term outcomes for overweight and obese children. *Pediatrics, 116,* 73–77.

Geary, D. C., & Flinn, M. V. (2002). Sex differences in behavioral and hormonal response to social threat: Commentary on Taylor et al. (2000). *Psychological Review, 109,* 745–750.

Geisser, M. E., Ranavaya, M., Haig, A. J., Roth, R. S., Zucker, R., Ambroz, C., et al. (2005). A meta-analytic review of surface electromyography among persons with low back pain and normal, healthy controls. *Journal of Pain, 6,* 711–726.

Gelhaar, T., Seiffge-Krenke, I., Borge, A., Cicognani, E., Cunha, M., Loncaric, D., et al. (2007). Adolescent coping with everyday stressors: A seven-nation study of youth from central, eastern, southern, and northern Europe. *European Journal of Developmental Psychology, 4,* 129–156.

Gellad, W. F., Haas, J. S., & Safran, D. G. (2007). Race/ethnicity and nonadherence to prescription medications among seniors: Results of a national study. *Journal of General Internal Medicine, 22,* 1572–1578.

Gellaitry, G., Cooper, V., Davis, C., Fisher, M., Date, H. L., & Horne, R. (2005). Patients' perception of information about HAART: Impact on treatment decisions. *AIDS Care, 17,* 367–376.

George, S., Rogers, R. D., & Duka, T. K. (2005). The acute effect of alcohol on decision making in social drinkers. *Psychopharmacology, 182,* 160–169.

George, W. H., & Stoner, S. A. (2000). Understanding acute alcohol effects on sexual behavior. *Annual Review of Sex Research, 11,* 92–122.

Georges, J., Jansen, S., Jackson, J., Meyrieux, A., Sadowsk, A., & Selmes, M. (2008). Alzheimer's disease in real life—The dementia carer's survey. *International Journal of Geriatric Psychiatry, 23,* 546–553.

Gershon, J., Zimand, E., Pickering, M., Rothbaum, B. O., & Hodges, L. (2004). A pilot and feasibility study of virtual reality as a distraction for children with cancer. *Journal of the American Academy of Child and Adolescent Psychiatry, 43,* 1243–1249.

Gidycz, C. A., Orchowski, L. M., King, C. R., & Rich, C. L. (2008). Sexual victimization and health-risk behaviors: A prospective analysis of college women. *Journal of Interpersonal Violence, 23,* 744–763.

Gielen, A. C., McKenzie, L. B., McDonald, E. M., Shields, W. C., Wang, M.-C., Cheng, Y.-J., et al. (2007). Using a computer kiosk to promote child safety: Results of a randomized, controlled trial in an urban pediatric emergency department. *Pediatrics, 120,* 330–339.

Gilbar, O. (1989). Who refuses chemotherapy: A profile. *Psychological Reports, 64,* 1291–1297.

Gilbert, M. T. P., Rambaut, A., Wlasiuk, G., Spira, T. J., Pitchenik, A. E., & Worobey, M. (2007). The emergence of HIV/AIDS in the Americas and beyond. *Proceedings of the National Academy of Sciences of the United States of America, 104,* 18566–18570.

Gildea, K. M., Schneider, T. R., & Shebilske, W. L. (2007). Appraisals and training performance on a complex laboratory task. *Human Factors, 49,* 745–758.

Gillibrand, R., & Stevenson, J. (2006). The extended health belief model applied to the experience of diabetes in young people. *British Journal of Health Psychology, 11,* 155–169.

Gillies, C. L., Abrams, K. R., Lambert, P. C., Cooper, N. J., Sutton, A. J., Hsu, R. T. (2007). Pharmacological and lifestyle interventions to prevent or delay Type 2 diabetes in people with impaired glucose tolerance: Systematic review and meta-analysis. *British Medical Journal, 334,* 299–302.

Gilpin, E. A., White, M. M., Messer, K., & Pierce, J. P. (2007). Receptivity to tobacco advertising and promotions among young adolescents as a predictor of established smoking in young adulthood. *American Journal of Public Health, 97,* 1489–1495.

Giovannucci, E. (1999). Tomatoes, tomato-based products, lycopene, and cancer: Review of the epidemiologic literature. *Journal of the National Cancer Institute, 91,* 317–331.

Giskes, K., Kunst, A. E., Benach, J., Borrell, C., Costa, C., Dahl, E., et al. (2005). Trends in smoking behaviour between 1985 and 2000 in nine European countries by education. *Journal of Epidemiology and Community Health, 59,* 395–401.

Glaser, R. (2005). Stress-associated immune dysregulation and its importance for human health: A personal history of psychoneuroimmunology. *Brain, Behavior and Immunity, 19,* 3–11.

Glasgow, R. E., & Anderson, R. M. (1999). In diabetes care, moving from compliance to adherence is not enough. *Diabetes Care, 22,* 2090–2091.

Glueckauf, R. L., Ketterson, T. U., Loomis, J. S., & Dages, P. (2004). Online support and education for dementia caregivers: Overview, utilization, and initial program evaluation. *Telemedicine Journal and e-Health, 10*(2), np.

Gmel, G., & Rehm, J. (2003). Harmful alcohol use. *Alcohol Research & Health, 27,* 52–62.

Godfrey, J. R. (2004). Toward optimal health: The experts discuss therapeutic humor. *Journal of Women's Health, 13,* 474–479.

Goffaux, P., Redmond, W. J., Rainville, P., & Marchand, S. (2007). Descending analgesia: When the spine echoes what the brain expects. *Pain, 130,* 137–143.

Gold, D. R., & Wright, R. (2005). Population disparities in asthma. *Annual Review of Public Health, 26,* 89–113.

Goldman, R. (2007, November 6). Halle Berry says she cured herself of Type 1 diabetes, but doctors say that's impossible. *ABC News On Call.* Retrieved June 28, 2008, from http://abcnews.go.com/Health/DiabetesResource/Story?id=3822870&page=1

Goldring, M. B., & Goldring, S. R. (2007). Osteoarthritis. *Journal of Cellular Physiology, 213,* 626–634.

Goldschmidt, A. B., Jones, M., Manwaring, J. L., Luce, K. H., Osborne, M. I., Cunning, D., et al. (2008). The clinical significance of loss of control over eating in overweight adolescents. *International Journal of Eating Disorders, 41,* 153–158.

Goldsmith, C. (2004). Fetal alcohol syndrome: A preventable tragedy. *Access, 18*(5), 34–38.

Goldstein, A. (1976). Opioid peptides (endorphins) in pituitary and brain. *Science, 193,* 1081–1086.

Goldston, K., & Baillie, A. J. (2008). Depression and coronary heart disease: A review of the epidemiological evidence, explanatory mechanisms and management approaches. *Clinical Psychology Review, 28,* 289–307.

Gonder-Frederick, L. A., Cox, D. J., & Ritterband, L. M. (2002). Diabetes and behavioral medicine: The second decade. *Journal of Consulting and Clinical Psychology, 70,* 611–625.

Gonzalez, J. S., Penedo, F. J., Antoni, M. H., Durán, R. E., Fernandez, M. I., McPherson-Baker, S., et al. (2004). Social support, positive states of mind, and HIV treatment adherence in men and women living with HIV/AIDS. *Health Psychology, 23,* 413–418.

Gonzalez, R., Nolen-Hoeksema, S., & Treynor, W. (2003). Rumination reconsidered: A psychometric analysis. *Cognitive Therapy and Research, 27,* 247–259.

Goodpaster, B. H., Krishnaswami, S., Harris, T. B., Katsiaras, A., Kritchevsky, S. B., Simonsick, E. M., et al. (2005). Obesity, regional body fat distribution, and the metabolic syndrome in older men and women. *Archives of Internal Medicine, 165,* 777–783.

Goodwin, D. G. (1976). *Is alcoholism hereditary?* New York: Oxford University Press.

Goodwin, R. D., & Friedman, H. S. (2006). Health status and the five-factor personality traits in a nationally representative sample. *Journal of Health Psychology, 11,* 643–654.

Gorin, A. A., & Stone, A. A. (2001). Recall biases and cognitive errors in retrospective self-reports: A call for momentary assessments. In A. Baum, T. A. Revenson, & J. E. Singer (Eds.), *Handbook of health psychology* (pp. 405–413). Mahwah, NJ: Erlbaum.

Gossop, M., Stewart, D., & Marsden, J. (2008). Attendance at Narcotics Anonymous and Alcoholics Anonymous meetings, frequency of attendance and substance use outcomes after residential treatment for drug dependence: A 5-year follow-up study. *Addiciton, 103,* 119–125.

Gottfredson, L. S., & Deary, I. J. (2004). Intelligence predicts health and longevity, but why? *Current Directions in Psychological Science, 13,* 1–4.

Gouzoulis-Mayfrank, E., & Daumann, J. (2006). The confounding problem of polydrug use in recreational ecstacy/MDMA users: A brief overview. *Journal of Psychopharmacology, 20,* 188–193.

Govender, V., & Penn-Kekana, L. (2008). Gender biases and discrimination: A review of health care interpersonal interactions. *Global Public Health, 3*(Suppl. 1), 90–103.

Grafton, K. V., Foster, N. E., & Wright, C. C. (2005). Test-retest reliability of the Short-Form McGill Pain Questionnaire: Assessment of intraclass correlation coefficients and limits of agreement in patients with osteoarthritis. *Clinical Journal of Pain, 21*, 73–82.

Graham, J. E., Christian, L. M., & Kiecolt-Glaser, J. K. (2006). Marriage, health, and immune function. In S. R. H. Beach, M. Z. Wamboldt, N. J. Kaslow, R. E. Heyman, M. B. First, et al. (Eds.), *Relational processes and DSM-V: Neuroscience, assessment, prevention, and treatment* (pp. 61–76). Washington, DC: American Psychiatric Association.

Graig, E. (1993). Stress as a consequence of the urban physical environment. In L. Goldberger & S. Breznitz (Eds.), *Handbook of stress: Theoretical and clinical aspects* (2nd ed., pp. 316–332). New York: Free Press.

Grant, B. F., Hasin, D. S., Chou, S. P., Stinson, F. S., & Dawson, D. A. (2004). Nicotine dependence and psychiatric disorders in the United States. *Archives of General Psychiatry, 61*, 1107–1115.

Greenwood, B. N., Foley, T. E., Day, H. E. W., Burhans, D., Brooks, L., Campeau, S., et al. (2005). Wheel running alters serotonin (5-HT) transporter, 5-HT_{1A}, 5-HT_{1B}, and alpha_{1b}-adrenergic receptor mRNA in the rat raphe nuclei. *Biological Psychiatry, 57*, 559–568.

Griffin, S. F. (2008). Physical activity influences in a disadvantaged African American community and the communities' proposed solutions. *Health Promotion Practice, 9*, 180–190.

Griffing, S., Lewis, C. S., Chu, M., Sage, R. E., Madry, L., & Primm, B. J. (2006). Exposure to interpersonal violence as a predictor of PTSD symptomatology in domestic violence survivors. *Journal of Interpersonal Violence, 21*, 936–954.

Griggs, C., & Jensen, J. (2006). Effectiveness of acupuncture for migraine: Critical literature review. *Journal of Advanced Nursing, 54*, 491–501.

Grilo, C. M., Hrabosky, J, I., White, M. A., Allison, K. C., Stunkard, A. J., & Masheb, R. M. (2008). Overvaluation of shape and weight in binge eating disorder and overweight controls: Refinement of a diagnostic construct. *Journal of Abnormal Psychology, 117*, 414–419.

Grilo, C. M., Masheb, R. M., & Salant, S. L. (2005). Cognitive behavioral therapy guided self-help and orlistat for the treatment of binge eating disorder: A randomized, double-blind, placebo-controlled trial. *Biological Psychiatry, 57*, 1193–1201.

Grilo, C. M., Masheb, R. M., & Wilson, G. T. (2005). Efficacy of cognitive behavioral therapy and fluoxetine for the treatment of binge eating disorder: A randomized double-blind placebo-controlled comparison. *Biological Psychiatry, 57*, 301–309.

Grossman, P., Niemann, L., Schmidt, S., & Walach, H. (2004). Mindfulness-based stress reduction and health benefits: A meta-analysis. *Journal of Psychosomatic Research, 57*, 35–43.

Grover, S. A., Gray-Donald, K., Joseph, L., Abrahamowicz, M., & Coupal, L. (1994). Life expectancy following dietary modification or smoking cessation. *Archives of Internal Medicine, 154*, 1697–1704.

Grundman, M. (2005). Weight loss in the elderly may be a sign of impending dementia. *Archives of Neurology, 62*, 20–22.

Grundy, S. M. (2007). Cardiovascular and metabolic risk factors: How can we improve outcomes in the high-risk patient? *American Journal of Medicine, 120*(Suppl. 1), S3–S8.

Grundy, S. M., Cleeman, J. I., Bairey Merz, C. N., Brewer, B., Jr., Clark, L. T., Hunninghake, D. B., et al. (2004). Implications of recent clinical trials for the National Cholesterol Education Program Adult Treatment Panel III guidelines. *Circulation, 110*, 227–239.

Grzywacz, J. G., Almeida, D. M., Neupert, S. D., & Ettner, S. L. (2004). Socioeconomic status and health: A micro-level analysis of exposure and vulnerability to daily stressors. *Journal of Health and Social Behavior, 45*, 1–16.

Guarda, A. S. (2008). Treatment of anorexia nervosa: Insights and obstacles. *Physiology and Behavior, 94*, 113–120.

Guck, T. P., Kavan, M. G., Elsasser, G. N., & Barone, E. J. (2001). Assessment and treatment of depression following myocardial infarction. *American Family Physician, 64*, 641–656.

Guevara, J. P., Wolf, F. M., Grum, C. M., & Clark, N. M. (2003). Effects of educational interventions for self management of asthma in children and adolescents: Systematic review and meta-analysis. *British Medical Journal, 326*, 1308–1309.

Guidot, D. M., & Roman, J. (2002). Chronic ethanol ingestion increases susceptibility to acute lung injury. *Chest, 122*(Suppl.), 309S–314S.

Guillot, J., Kilpatrick, M., Hebert, E., & Hollander, D. (2004). Applying the transtheoretical model to exercise adherence in clinical settings. *American Journal of Health Studies, 19*, 1–10.

Gull, W. W. (1874). Anorexia nervosa (apepsia hysterica, anorexia hysterica). *Transactions of the Clinical Society of London, 7*, 22–28. [Reprinted in R. M. Kaufman & M. Heiman (Eds.), *Evolution of psychosomatic concepts: Anorexia nervosa, a paradigm.* New York: International University Press, 1964.]

Gump, B. B., Matthews, K. A., Scheier, M. F., Schulz, R., Bridges, M. W., & Magovern, G. J. (2001). Illness representations according to age and effects on health behaviors following coronary artery bypass graft surgery. *Journal of the American Geriatrics Society, 49*, 284–289.

Gunnar, M., & Quevedo, K. (2007). The neurobiology of stress and development. *Annual Review of Psychology, 58*, 145–173.

Guo, Q., Johnson, C. A., Unger, J. B., Lee, L., Xie, B., Chou, C.-P., et al. (2007). Utility of the theory of reasoned and theory of planned behavior for predicting Chinese adolescent smoking. *Addictive Behaviors, 32*, 1066–1081.

Guo, X., Zhou, B., Nishimura, T., Teramukai, S., & Fukushima, M. (2008). Clinical effect of qigong practice on essential hypertension: A meta-analysis of randomized controlled trials. *Journal of Alternative and Complementary Medicine, 14*, 27–37.

Gustafson, E. M., Meadows-Oliver, M., & Banasiak, N. C. (2008). Asthma in childhood. In T. P. Gullotta & G. M. Blau (Eds.), *Handbook of childhood behavioral issues: Evidence-based approaches to prevention and treatment* (pp. 167–186). New York: Routledge/Taylor & Francis.

Gustavsson, P., Jakobsson, R., Nyberg, F., Pershagen, G., Järup, L., & Schéele, P. (2000). Occupational exposure and lung cancer risk: A population-based case-referent study in Sweden. *American Journal of Epidemiology, 152*, 32–40.

Ha, M., Mabuchi, K., Sigurdson, A. J., Freedman, D. M., Linet, M. S., Doody, M. M. (2007). Smoking cigarettes before first childbirth and risk of breast cancer. *American Journal of Epidemiology, 166*, 55–61.

Haak, T., & Scott, B. (2008). The effect of qigong on fibromyaliga (FMS): A controlled randomized study. *Disability and Rehabilitation, 30*, 625–633.

Haan, M. N., & Wallace, R. (2004). Can dementia be prevented? Brain aging in a population-base. *Annual Review of Public Health, 25*, 1–24.

Haase, A. M., & Kinnafick, F. E. (2007). What factors drive regular exercise behavior?: Exploring the concept and maintenance of habitual exercise. *Journal of Sport and Exercise Psychology, 29*(Suppl.), S165.

Hagedoorn, M., Kujer, R. G., Buuk, B. P., DeJong, G. M., Wobbes, T., & Sanderman, R. (2000). Marital satisfaction in patients with cancer: Does support from intimate partners benefit those who need it the most? *Health Psychology, 19*, 274–282.

Hagger, M. S, Chatzisarantis, N. L., & Biddle, S. J. H. (2002). A meta-analytic review of the theories of reasoned action and planned behavior in physical activity: Predictive validity and the contribution of additional variables. *Journal of Sport and Exercise Psychology, 24*, 3–28.

Haimanot, R. T. (2002). Burden of headache in Africa. *Journal of Headache & Pain, 4*, 47–54.

Hale, C. J., Hannum, J. W., & Espelage, D. L. (2005). Social support and physical health: The importance of belonging. *Journal of American College Health, 53*, 276–284.

Hale, S., Grogan, S., & Willott, S. (2007). Patterns of self-referral in men with symptoms of prostate disease. *British Journal of Health Psychology, 12*, 403–419.

Hall, C. B., Verghese, J., Sliwinski, M., Chen, Z., Katz, M., Derby, C., et al. (2005). Dementia incidence may increase more slowly after age 90: Results from the Bronx Aging Study. *Neurology, 65*, 882–886.

Hall, M. A., & Schneider, C. E. (2008). Patients as consumers: Courts, contracts, and the new medical marketplace. *Michigan Law Review, 106*, 643–689.

Hamer, M., & Karageorghis, C. (2007). Psychobiological mechanisms of exercise dependence. *Sports Medicine, 37*, 477–485.

Hamer, M., & Steptoe, A. (2007). Association between physical fitness, parasympathetic control, and proinflammatory responses to mental stress. *Psychsomatic Medicine, 69*, 660–666.

Hamer, M., Taylor, A., & Steptoe, A. (2006). The effect of acute aerobic exercise on stress related blood pressure responses: A systematic review and meta-analysis. *Biological Psychology, 71*, 183–190.

Hammond, D. (2005). Smoking behaviour among young adults: Beyond youth prevention. *Tobacco Control, 14*, 181–185.

Han, A., Judd, M. G., Robinson, V. A., Taixiang, W., Tugwell, P., & Wells, G. (2004). Tai chi for treating rheumatoid arthritis. *Cochrane Database of Systematic Reviews*, Cochrane AN: CD004849.

Hanewinkel, R., & Sargent, J. D. (2007). Exposure to smoking in popular contemporary movies and youth smoking in Germany. *American Journal of Preventive Medicine, 32*, 466–473.

Hanley, M. A., Jensen, M. P., Smith, D. G., Ehde, D. M., Edwards, W. T., & Robinson, L. R. (2007). Preamputation pain and acute pain predict chronic pain after lower extremity amputation. *Journal of Pain, 8*, 102–109.

Hansen, C. J., Stevens, L. C., & Coast, J. R. (2001). Exercise duration and mood state: How much is enough to feel better? *Health Psychology, 20*, 267–275.

Hansen, K., Shriver, T., & Schoeller, D. (2005). The effects of exercise on the storage and oxidation of dietary fat. *Sports Medicine, 35*, 363–373.

Hansen, P. E., Floderus, B., Frederiksen, K., & Johansen, C. B. (2005). Personality traits, health behavior, and risk for cancer: A prospective study of a Swedish twin cohort. *Cancer, 103*, 1082–1091.

Hanson-Turton, T., Ryan, S., Miller, K., Counts, M., & Nash, D. B. (2007). Convenient care clinics: The future of accessible health care. *Disease Management, 10*(2), 61–73.

Hanvik, L. J. (1951). MMPI profiles in patients with low back pain. *Journal of Consulting and Clinical Psychology, 15*, 350–353.

Harandi, A. A., Esfandani, A., & Shakibaei, F. (2004). The effect of hypnotherapy of procedural pain and state anxiety related to physiotherapy in women hospitalized in a burn unit. *Contemporary Hypnosis, 21*, 28–34.

Harburg, E., Julius, M., Kaciroti, N., Gleiberman, L., & Schork, M. A. (2003). Expressive/suppressive anger-coping responses, gender, and types of mortality: A 17–year follow-up (Tecumseh, Michigan, 1971–1988). *Psychosomatic Medicine, 65*, 588–597.

Harder, B. (2004). Asthma counterattack. *Science News, 166*, 344–345.

Harper, C., & Matsumoto, I. (2005). Ethanol and brain damage. *Current Opinion in Pharmacology, 5*, 73–78.

Harrington, A. (2008). *The cure within: A history of mind-body medicine.* New York: Norton.

Harrington, J., Noble, L. M., & Newman, S. P. (2004). Improving patients' communication with doctors: A systematic review of intervention studies. *Patient Education and Counseling, 52*, 7–16.

Harris, M. I. (2001). Racial and ethnic differences in health care access and health outcomes for adults with Type 2 diabetes. *Diabetes Care, 24*, 454–459.

Harris, S. S., Caspersen, C. J., DeFriese, G. H., & Estes, H. (1989). Physical activity counseling for healthy adults as a primary preventive intervention in the clinical setting: Report for the US Preventive Services Task Force. *Journal of the American Medical Association, 261*, 3590–3598.

Harrison, B. J., Olver, J. S., Norman, T. R., & Nathan, P. J. (2002). Effects of serotonin and catecholamine depletion on interleukin-6 activation and mood in human volunteers. *Human Psychopharmacology: Clinical and Experimental, 17*, 293–297.

Hartz, A., Kent, S., James, P., Xu, Y., Kelly, M., & Daly, J. (2006). Factors that influence improvement for patients with poorly controlled Type 2 diabetes. *Diabetes Research and Clinical Practice, 74*, 227–232.

Hartz, A. J., Rupley, D. C., & Rimm, A. A. (1984). The association of girth measurements with disease in 32,856 women. *American Journal of Epidemiology, 119*, 71–80.

Hasin, D. S., Keyes, K. M., Hatzenbuehler, M. L., Aharonovich, E. A., & Alderson, D. (2007). Alcohol consumption and posttraumatic stress after exposure to terrorism: Effects of proximity, loss, and psychiatric history. *American Journal of Public Health, 97*, 2268–2275.

Hasson, D., Arnetz, B., Jelveus, L., & Edelstam, B. (2004). A randomized clinical trial of the treatment effects of massage compared to relaxation tape recordings on diffuse long-term pain. *Psychotherapy and Psychosomatics, 73*, 17–24.

Hatfield, J., & Job, R. F. S. (2001). Optimism bias about environmental degradation: The role of the range of impact of precautions. *Journal of Environmental Psychology, 21*, 17–30.

Hausenblas, H. A., Carron, A. V., & Mack, D. E. (1997). Application of the theories of reasoned action and planned behavior to exercise behavior: A meta-analysis. *Journal of Sport and Exercise Psychology, 19*, 36–51.

Hausenblas, H. A., & Symons Downs, D. (2002a). Exercise dependence: A systematic review. *Psychology of Sport and Exercise, 3*, 89–123.

Hausenblas, H. A., & Symons Downs, D. (2002b). Relationship among sex, imagery, and exercise dependence symptoms. *Psychology of Addictive Behaviors, 16*, 169–172.

Hausenloy, D. J., & Yellon, D. M. (2008). Targeting residual cardiovascular risk: Raising high-density lipoprotein cholesterol levels. *Heart, 94*, 706–714.

Hawkley, L. C., & Cacioppo, J. T. (2003). Loneliness and pathways to disease. *Brain, Behavior and Immunity, 17*, 98–105.

Hawkley, L. C., & Cacioppo, J. T. (2007). Aging and loneliness: Downhill quickly? *Current Directions in Psychological Science, 16*, 187–191.

Hay, P. (2004). Australian and New Zealand clinical practice guidelines for the treatment of anorexia nervosa. *Australian and New Zealand Journal of Psychiatry, 38*, 659–670.

Hayes, S., Bulow, C., Clarke, R., Vega, E., Vega-Perez, E., Ellison, L., et al. (2000). Incidence of low back pain in women who are pregnant. *Physical Therapy, 80*, 34.

Hayes-Bautista, D. E., Hsu, P., Hayes-Bautista, M., Iniguez, D., Chamberlin, C. L., Rico, C., et al. (2002). An anomaly within the Latino epidemiological paradox: The Latino adolescent male mortality peak. *Archives of Pediatrics and Adolescent Medicine, 156*, 480–484.

Haynes, R. B. (1976). Strategies for improving compliance: A methodologic analysis and review. In D. L. Sackett & R. B. Haynes (Eds.), *Compliance with therapeutic regimens* (pp. 69–82). Baltimore: Johns Hopkins University Press.

Haynes, R. B. (1979). Introduction. In R. B. Haynes, D. W. Taylor, & D. L. Sackett (Eds.), *Compliance in health care* (pp. 1–7). Baltimore: Johns Hopkins University Press.

Haynes, R. B. (2001). Improving patient adherence: State of the art, with a special focus on medication taking for cardiovascular disorders. In L. E. Burke & I. S. Ockene (Eds.), *Compliance in healthcare and research* (pp. 3–21). Armonk, NY: Futura.

Haynes, R. B., McDonald, H. P., & Garg, A. X. (2002). Helping patients follow prescribed treatment: Clinical applications. *Journal of the American Medical Association, 288*, 2880–2883.

He, D. (2005). An introduction to Chinese medical qi gong. *New England Journal of Traditional Chinese Medicine, 4*, 42–44.

He, J., Vupputuri. S., Allen, K., Prerost, M. R., Hughes, J., & Whelton, P. K. (1999). Passive smoking and the risk of coronary heart disease: A meta-analysis of epidemiologic studies. *New England Journal of Medicine, 340*, 920–926.

HealthGrades. (2004). *HealthGrades quality study: Patient safety in American hospitals*. Retrieved February 25, 2008, from http://www.healthgrades.com

HealthGrades. (2006). *Third annual patient safety in American hospitals study*. Retrieved February 25, 2008, from http://www.healthgrades.com

Hearn, W. L., Flynn, D. D., Hime, G. W., Rose, S., Cofino, J. C., Mantero-Atienza, E., et al. (1991). Cocaethylene: A unique cocaine metabolite displays high affinity for the dopamine transporter. *Journal of Neurochemistry, 56*, 698–701.

Heather, N. (2006). Controlled drinking, harm reduction and their roles in the response to alcohol-related problems. *Addiction Research and Theory, 14*, 7–18.

Hedley, A. A., Ogden, C. L., Johnson, C. L., Carroll, M. D., Curtin, L. R., & Flegal, K. M. (2004). Prevalence of overweight and obesity among US children, adolescents, and adults, 1999–2002. *Journal of the American Medical Association, 291*, 2847–2850.

Heijmans, M., Rijken, M., Foets, M., de Ridder, D., Schreurs, K., & Bensing, J. (2004). The stress of being chronically ill: From disease-specific to task-specific aspects. *Journal of Behavioral Medicine, 27,* 255–271.

Heimer, R. (2008). Community coverage and HIV prevention: Assessing metrics for estimating HIV incidence through syringe exchange. *International Journal of Drug Policy, 19*(Suppl. 1), S65–S73.

Heinrich, K. M., Lee, R. E., Regan, G. R., Reese-Smith, J. Y., Howard, H. H., Haddock, C. K. et al. (2008). How does the built environment relate to body mass index and obesity prevalence among public housing residents? *American Journal of Health Promotion, 22,* 187–194.

Helgeson, V. S. (2003). Cognitive adaptation, psychological adjustment, and disease progression among angioplasty patients: 4 years later. *Health Psychology, 22,* 30–38.

Helgeson, V. S., Cohen, S., Schulz, R., & Yasko, J. (2000). Group support interventions for women with breast cancer: Who benefits from what? *Health Psychology, 19,* 107–114.

Helgeson, V. S., Reynolds, K. A., Tomich, P. L. (2006). A meta-analytic review of benefit finding and growth. *Journal of Consulting and Clinical Psychology, 74,* 797–816.

Helgeson, V. S., Snyder, P., & Seltman, H. (2004). Psychological and physical adjustment of breast cancer over 4 years: Identifying distinct trajectories of change. *Health Psychology, 23,* 3–15.

Hembree, E. A., & Foa, E. B. (2003). Interventions for trauma-related emotional disturbances in adult victims of crime. *Journal of Traumatic Stress, 16,* 187–199.

Hemminki, K., Försti, A., & Bermejo, J. L. (2006). Gene-environment interactions in cancer. *Annals of the New York Academy of Science, 1076,* 137–148.

Henderson, L. A., Gandevia, S. C., & Macefield, V. G. (2008). Gender differences in brain activity evoked by muscle and cutaneous pain: A retrospective study of singe-trial fMRI data. *NeuroImage, 39,* 1867–1876.

Hendriks, H. F. J. (2007). Moderate alcohol consumption and insulin sensitivity: Observations and possible mechanisms. *Annals of Epidemiology, 17*(Suppl.), S40–S42.

Heneghan, C. J., Glasziou, P., & Perera, R. (2007). Reminder packaging for improving adherence to self-administered long-term medications. *Cochrane Database of Systematic Reviews,* Cochrane AN: CD005025.

Henke-Gendo, C., & Schulz, T. F. (2004). Transmission and disease association of Kaposi's sarcoma–associated herpes virus: Recent developments. *Current Opinion in Infectious Diseases, 17,* 53–57.

Henley, S. J., Thun, M. J., Chao, A., & Calle, E. E. (2004). Association between exclusive pipe smoking and mortality from cancer and other diseases. *Journal of the National Cancer Institute, 96,* 853–861.

Henson, J. M., Carey, M. P., Carey, K. B., & Maisto, S. A. (2006). Associations among health behaviors and time perspective in young adults: Model testing with boot-strapping replication. *Journal of Behavioral Medicine, 29,* 127–137.

Hepler, R. S., & Frank, I. M. (1971). Marijuana smoking and intraocular pressure. *Journal of the American Medical Association, 217,* 1392.

Herbst, A., Kordonouri, O., Schwab, K. O., Schmidt, F., & Holl, R. W. (2007). Impact of physical activity on cardiovascular risk factors in children with Type 1 diabetes. *Diabetes Care, 30,* 2098–2100.

Herman, C. P., & Polivy, J. (2005). Normative influences on food intake. *Physiology and Beahvior, 86,* 762–772.

Herman, C. P., Roth, D. A., & Polivy, J. (2003). Effects of the presence of others on food intake: A normative interpretation. *Psychological Bulletin, 129,* 873–886.

Herman, C. P., van Strien, T., & Polivy, J. (2008). Undereating or eliminating overeating? *American Psychologist, 63,* 202–203.

Hernán, M. A., Jick, S. S., Logroscino, G., Olek, M. J., Ascherio, A., & Jick, H. (2005). Cigarette smoking and the progression of multiple sclerosis. *Brain, 128*(Pt. 6), 1461–1465.

Heron, M. (2007). Deaths: Leading causes for 2004. *National Vital Statistics Reports, 56*(5). Retrieved January 27, 2008, from http://www.cdc.gov/nchs/data/nvsr/nvsr56/nvsr56_05.pdf

Herrmann, S., McKinnon, E., John, M., Hyland, N., Martinez, O. P., Cain, A., et al. (2008). Evidence-based, multifactorial approach to addressing non-adherence to antiretroviral therapy and improving standards of care. *Internal Medicine Journal, 38,* 8–15.

Hetherington, M. M., & Rolls, B. J. (1996). Sensory-specific satiety: Theoretical frameworks and central characteristics. In E. D. Capaldi (Ed.), *Why we eat what we eat: The psychology of eating* (pp. 267–290). Washington, DC: American Psychological Association.

Hilgard, E. R. (1978). Hypnosis and pain. In R. A. Sternbach (Ed.), *The psychology of pain.* New York: Raven Press.

Hilgard, E. R., & Hilgard, J. R. (1994). *Hypnosis in the relief of pain* (Rev. ed.). Los Altos, CA: Kaufmann.

Hill, J. O., & Wyatt, H. R. (2005). Role of physical activity in preventing and treating obesity. *Journal of Applied Physiology, 99,* 765–770.

Hind, K., & Burrows, M. (2007). Weight-bearing exercise and bone mineral accrual in children and adolescents: A review of controlled trials. *Bone, 40,* 14–27.

Hingson, R., Heeren, T., Winter, M., & Wechsler, H. (2005). Magnitude of alcohol-related mortality and morbidity among U.S. college students ages 18–24: Changes from 1998 to 2001. *Annual Review of Public Health, 26,* 259–279.

Hochbaum, G. (1958). *Public participation in medical screening programs* (DHEW Publication No. 572, Public Health Service). Washington, DC: U.S. Government Printing Office.

Hoey, L. M., Ieropoli, S. C., White, V. M., & Jefford, M. (2008). Systematic review of peer-support programs for people with cancer. *Patient Education and Counseling, 70,* 315–337.

Hoeymans, N., van Lindert, H., & Westert, G. P. (2005). The health status of the Dutch population as assessed by the EQ-6D. *Quality of Life Research, 14,* 655–643.

Hoffman, B. M., Papas, R. K., Chatkoff, D. K., & Kerns, R. D. (2007). Meta-analysis of psychological interventions for chronic low back pain. *Health Psychology, 26,* 1–9.

Hogan, B. E., & Linden, W. (2004). Anger responses styles and blood pressure: At least don't ruminate about it! *Annals of Behavioral Medicine, 27,* 38–49.

Hogan, E. M., & McReynolds, C. J. (2004). An overview of anorexia nervosa, bulimia nervosa, and binge eating disorders: Implications for rehabilitation professionals. *Journal of Applied Rehabilitation Counseling, 35*(4), 26–34.

Hogan, N. S., & Schmidt, L. A. (2002). Testing the grief to personal growth model using structural equation modeling. *Death Studies, 26,* 615–634.

Holden, C. (2003, September 8). Party drug paper pulled. *Science Now,* 1–2.

Holick, M. F. (2004). Sunlight and vitamin D for bone health and prevention of autoimmune disease, cancers, and cardiovascular disease. *American Journal of Clinical Nutrition, 80*(Suppl. 6), S1678–S1688.

Hollis, J. F., Gullion, C. M., Stevens, V. J., Brantley, P. J., Appel, L. J., Ard, J. D., et al. (2008). Weight loss during the intensive intervention phase of the weight-loss maintenance trial. *American Journal of Preventive Medicine, 35,* 118–126.

Holmes, T. H., & Rahe, R. H. (1967). The Social Readjustment Rating Scale. *Journal of Psychosomatic Research, 11,* 213–218.

Holsti, L., & Grunau, R. E. (2007). Initial validation of the Behavioral Indicators of Infant Pain (BIIP). *Pain, 132,* 264–272.

Holt-Lunstad, J., Birmingham, W., & Jones, B. Q. (2008). Is there something unique about marriage? The relative impact of marital status, relationship quality, and network social support on ambulatory blood pressure and mental health. *Annals of Behavioral Medicine, 35,* 239–244.

Holtzman, D., Bland, S. D., Lansky, A., & Mack, K. A. (2001). HIV-related behaviors and perceptions among adults in 25 states: 1997 Behavioral Risk Factor Surveillance System. *American Journal of Public Health, 91,* 1882–1888.

Hong, S., Mills, P. J., Loredo, J. S., Adler, K. A., & Dimsdale, J. E. (2005). The association between interleukin-6, sleep, and demographic characteristics. *Brain, Behavior and Immunity, 19,* 165–172.

Hootman, J. M., Macera, C. A., Ainsworth, B. E., Addy, C. L., Martin, M., & Blair, S. N. (2002). Epidemiology of musculoskeletal injuries among sedentary and physically active adults. *Medicine and Science in Sports and Exercise, 34,* 838–844.

Horev, A., Wirguin, I., Lantsberg, L., & Ifergane, G. (2005). A high incidence of migraine with aura among morbidly obese women. *Headache, 45,* 936–938.

Horvath, T. L. (2005). The hardship of obesity: A soft-wired hypothalamus. *Nature Neuroscience, 8,* 561–565.

Hovell, M. F., Mulvihill, M. M., Buono, M. J., Liles, S., Schade, D. H., Washington, T. A., et al. (2008). Culturally tailored aerobic exercise intervention for low-income Latinas. *American Journal of Health Behavior, 22,* 155–163.

Hoving, C., Reubsaet, A., & de Vries, H. (2007). Predictors of smoking stage transitions for adolescent boys and girls. *Preventive Medicine, 44,* 485–489.

Howe, G. W., Levy, M. L., & Caplan, R. D. (2004). Job loss and depressive symptoms in couples: Common stressors, stress transmission, or relationship disruption? *Journal of Family Psychology, 18,* 639–650.

Hróbjartsson, A., & Gøtzsche, P. C. (2001). An analysis of clinical trials comparing placebo with no treatment. *New England Journal of Medicine, 344,* 1594–1602.

Hróbjartsson, A., & Gøtzsche, P. C. (2004). Is the placebo powerless? Update of a systematic review with 52 new randomized trials comparing placebo with no treatment. *Journal of Internal Medicine, 256,* 91–100.

Hsiao, A.-F., Ryan, G. W., Hays, R. D. Coulter, I. D., Andersen, R. M., & Wenger, N. S. (2006). Variations in provider conceptions of integrative medicine. *Social Science and Medicine, 62,* 2973–2987.

Hsiao, A.-F., Wong, M. D., Goldstein, M. S., Becerra, L. S., Cheng, E. M., & Wenger, N. S. (2006). Complementary and alternative medicine use among Asian-American subgroups: Prevalence, predictors, and lack of relationship to acculturation and access to conventional health care. *Journal of Alternative and Complementary Medicine, 12,* 1003–1010.

Hu, F. B. (2003). Overweight and obesity in women: Health risks and consequences. *Journal of Women's Health, 12,* 163–172.

Hu, F. B., Stampfer, M. J., Colditz, G. A., Ascherio, A., Rexrode, K. M., Willett, W. C., et al. (2000). Physical activity and risk of stroke in women. *Journal of the American Medical Association, 283,* 7961–7967.

Huang, J.-Q., Sridhar, S., & Hunt, R. H. (2002). Role of *Helicobacter pylori* infection and non-steroidal anti-inflammatory drugs in peptic-ulcer disease: A meta-analysis. *Lancet, 359,* 14–21.

Hubert, H. B., Snider, J., & Winkleby, M. A. (2005). Health status, health behaviors, and acculturation factors associated with overweight and obesity in Latinos from a community and agricultural labor camp survey. *Preventive Medicine, 40,* 642–651.

Hudson, J. I., Hiripi, E., Pope, H. G., Jr., & Kessler, R. C. (2007). The prevalence and correlates of eating disorders in the National Comorbidity Survey replication. *Biological Psychiatry, 61,* 348–358.

Huebner, D. M., & Davis, M. C. (2007). Perceived antigay discrimination and physical health outcomes. *Health Psychology, 26,* 627–634.

Hufford, D. J. (2003). Evaluating complementary and alternative medicine: The limits of science and of scientists. *Journal of Law, Medicine and Ethics, 31,* 198–212.

Hughes, B. M. (2007). Social support in ordinary life and laboratory measures of cardiovascular reactivity:

Gender differences in habituation-sensitization. *Annals of Behavioral Medicine, 34,* 166–176.

Hughes, J. (1975). Isolation of an endogenous compound from the brain with pharmacological properties similar to morphine. *Brain Research, 88,* 295–308.

Hughes, J. (2003). Motivating and helping smokers to stop smoking. *Journal of General Internal Medicine, 18,* 1053–1057.

Hughes, J., Gulliver, S. B., Fenwick, J. W., Valliere, W. A., Cruser, K., Pepper, S., et al. (1992). Smoking cessation among self-quitters. *Health Psychology, 11,* 331–334.

Hughes, J., Stead, L., & Lancaster, T. (2004). Antidepressants for smoking cessation. *Cochrane Database of Systematic Reviews,* Cochrane AN: CD000031; PMID: 15494986.

Huisman, M., Kunst, A. E., Bopp, M., Borgan, J.-K., Borrell, C., Costa, G., et al. (2005). Educational inequalities in cause-specific mortality in middle-aged and older men and women in eight western European populations. *Lancet, 365,* 493–500.

Humphreys, K., & Moos, R. H. (2007). Encouraging post-treatment self-help group involvement to reduce demand for continuing care services: Two-year clinical and utilization outcomes. *Alcoholism: Clinical and Experimental Research, 31,* 64–68.

Hunt, G., & Evans, K. (2003). Dancing and drugs: A cross-national perspective. *Contemporary Drug Problems, 30,* 779–814.

Hunt, W. A., Barnett, L. W., & Branch, L. G. (1971). Relapse rates in addiction programs. *Journal of Clinical Psychology, 27,* 455–456.

Huq, F. (2007). Molecular modeling analysis of the metabolism of cocaine. *Journal of Pharmacology and Toxicology, 2,* 114–130.

Hutchinson, A. B., Branson, B. M., Kim, A., & Farnham, P. G. (2006). A meta-analysis of the effectiveness of alternative HIV counseling and testing methods to increase knowledge of HIV status. *AIDS, 20,* 1597–1604.

Huth, M. M., Broome, M. E., & Good, M. (2004). Imagery reduces children's post-operative pain, *Pain, 110,* 439–448.

Huxley, R., Ansary-Moghaddam, A., de González, A. B., Barzi, F., & Woodward, M. (2005). Type-II diabetes and pancreatic cancer: A meta-analysis of 36 studies. *British Journal of Cancer, 92,* 2076–2083.

Huxley, R. R., & Neil, H. A. W. (2003). The relation between dietary flavonol intake and coronary heart disease mortality: A meta-analysis of prospective cohort studies. *Journal of Clinical Nutrition, 57,* 904–908.

Iagnocco, A., Perella, C., Naredo, E., Meenagh, G., Ceccarelli, F., Tripodo, E., et al. (2008). Etanercept in the treatment of rheumatoid arthritis: Clinical follow-up over one year by ultrasonography. *Clinical Rheumatology, 27,* 491–496.

Iannotti, R. J., Schneider, S., Nansel, T. R., Haynie, D. L., Plotnick, L. P., Clark, L. M., et al. (2006). Self-efficacy, outcome expectations, and diabetes self-management in adolescents with Type 1 diabetes. *Journal of Developmental and Behavioral Pediatrics, 27,* 98–105.

Ickovics, J. R., Milan, S., Boland, R., Schoenbaum, E., Schuman, P., Vlahov, D. (2006). Psychological resources protect health: 5-year survival and immune function among HIV-infected women from four US cities. *AIDS, 20,* 1851–1860.

Iglesias, S. L., Azzara, S., Squillace, M., Jeifetz, M., Lores Arnais, M. R., Desimone, M. F., et al. (2005). A study on the effectiveness of a stress management programme for college students. *Pharmacy Education, 5,* 27–31.

Iihara, N., Tsukamoto, T., Morita, S., Miyoshi, C., Takabatake, C., & Kurosaki, Y. (2004). Beliefs of chronically ill Japanese patients that lead to intentional non-adherence to medication. *Journal of Clinical Pharmacy and Therapeutics, 29,* 417–424.

Ijadunola, K. T., Abiona, T. C., Odu, O. O., & Ijadunola, M. Y. (2007). College students in Nigeria underestimate their risk of contacting HIV/AIDS infection. *European Journal of Contraception and Reproductive Health Care, 12,* 131–137.

Ilies, R., Schwind, K. M., Wagner, D. T., Johnson, M. D., DeRue, D. S., & Ilgen, D. R. (2007). When can employees have a family life? The effects of daily workload and affect on work-family conflict and social behaviors at home. *Journal of Applied Psychology, 92,* 1368–1379.

Ingraham, B. A., Bragdon, B., & Nohe, A. (2008). Molecular basis for the potential of vitamin D to prevent cancer. *Current Medical Research and Opinion, 24,* 139–149.

Innes, K. E., & Vincent, H. K. (2007). The influence of yoga-based programs on risk profiles in adults with Type 2 diabetes mellitus: A systematic review. *Evidence Based Complementary and Alternative Medicine, 4,* 469–486.

Inside Mary-Kate's two year ordeal. (2004). *US Weekly.* Retrieved December 15, 2008, from http://www.forum.juicyduff.com/archive/index.php/t-4812.html

Institute of Medicine. (2002). *Unequal treatment: Confronting racial and ethnic disparities in health care.* Washington, DC: Author.

International Association for the Study of Pain (IASP), Subcommittee on Taxonomy. (1979). Pain terms: A list with definitions and notes on usage. *Pain, 6,* 249–252.

In'tVeld, B. A., Ruitenberg, A., Hofman, A., Launer, L. J., van Duijn, C. M., Stijnen, T., et al. (2001). Nonsteroidal anti-inflammatory drugs and the risk of Alzheimer's disease. *New England Journal of Medicine, 345,* 1515–1521.

Iribarren, C., Darbinian, J. A., Lo, J. C., Fireman, B. H., & Go, A. S. (2006). Value of the sagittal abdominal diameter in coronary heart disease risk assessment: Cohort study in a large, multiethnic population. *American Journal of Epidemiology, 164,* 1150–1159.

Ironson, G., Weiss, S., Lydston, D., Ishii, M., Jones, D., Asthana, D., et al. (2005). The impact of improved self-efficacy on HIV viral load and distress in culturally diverse women living with AIDS: The SMART/EST women's project. *AIDS Care, 17,* 222–236.

Irwin, M. R. (2008). Human psychoneuroimmunology: 20 years of discovery. *Brain, Behavior and Immunity, 22,* 129–139.

Irwin, M. R., Pike, J. L., Cole, J. C., & Oxman, M. N. (2003). Effects of a behavioral intervention, tai chi chih, on varicella-zoster virus specific immunity and health functioning in older adults. *Psychosomatic Medicine, 65,* 824–830.

Is Mary-Kate Olsen anorexic again at 80 lbs? (2007). *Star.* Retrieved July 21, 2008, from http://ifitandhealthy.com/is-mary-kate-olsen-anorexic-again-at-80-lbs/

Islam, T., Gauderman, W. J., Berhane, K., McConnell, R., Avol, E., Peters, J. M., et al. (2007). Relationship between air pollution, lung function and asthma in adolescents. *Thorax, 62,* 957–963.

Iso, H., Rexrode, K. M., Stampfer, M. J., Manson, J. E., Colditz. G. A., Speizer, F. E., et al. (2001). Intake of fish and omega-3 fatty acids and risk of stroke in women. *Journal of the American Medical Association, 285,* 304–312.

Ito, T., Takenaka, K., Tomita, T., & Agari, I. (2006). Comparison of ruminative responses with negative rumination as a vulnerability factor for depression. *Psychological Reports, 99,* 763–772.

Ivanovski, B., & Malhi, G. S. (2007). The psychological and neurophysiological concomitants of mindfulness forms of meditation. *Acta Neuropsychiatrica, 19*(2), 76–91.

Jackson, G. (2004). Treatment of erectile dysfunction in patients with cardiovascular disease: Guide to drug selection. *Drugs, 64,* 1533–1545.

Jackson, K. M., Sher, K. J., Gotham, H. J., & Wood, P. K. (2001). Transitioning into and out of large-effect drinking in young adulthood. *Journal of Abnormal Psychology, 110,* 378–391.

Jackson, L., Leclerc, J., Erskine, Y., & Linden, W. (2005). Getting the most out of cardiac rehabilitation: A review of referral and adherence predictors. *Heart, 91,* 10–14.

Jacobs, G. D. (2001). Clinical applications of the relaxation response and mind-body interventions. *Journal of Alternative and Complementary Medicine, 7*(Suppl. 1), 93–101.

Jacobson, E. (1938). *Progressive relaxation: A physiological and clinical investigation of muscle states and their significance in psychology and medical practice* (2nd ed.). Chicago: University of Chicago Press.

Jager, R. D., Mieler, W. F., & Miller, J. W. (2008). Age-related macular degeneration. *New England Journal of Medicine, 358,* 2606–2617.

Jagger, C., Matthews, R., Matthews, F., Robinson, T., Robine, J.-M., & Brayne, C. (2007). The burden of diseases on disability-free life expectancy in later life. *Journals of Gerontology Series A: Biological Sciences and Medical Sciences, 62A,* 408–414.

Jakicic, J. M., & Otto, A. D. (2005). Physical activity considerations for the treatment and prevention of obesity. *American Journal of Clinical Nutrition, 82*(Suppl. 1), 226S–229S.

James, W. P. T. (2008). The epidemiology of obesity: The size of the problem. *Journal of Internal Medicine, 263,* 336–352.

Janssen, R. S., Onorato, I. M., Valdiserri, R. O., Durham, T. M., Nichols, W. P., Seiler, E. M., et al. (2003). Advancing HIV prevention: New strategies for a changing epidemic— United States, 2003. *Morbidity and Mortality Weekly Report, 52,* 329–332.

Janssen, S. A. (2002). Negative affect and sensitization to pain. *Scandinavian Journal of Psychology, 43,* 131–137.

Jay, S. M., Elliott, C. H., Woody, P. D., & Siegel, S. (1991). An investigation of cognitive-behavior therapy combined with oral valium for children undergoing painful medical procedures. *Health Psychology, 10,* 317–322.

Jeffery, R. W., & Harnack, L. J. (2007). Evidence implicating eating as a primary driver for the obesity epidemic. *Diabetes, 56,* 2673–2676.

Jeffery, R. W., Kelly, K. M., Rothman, A. J., Sherwood, N. E., & Boutelle, K. N. (2004). The weight loss experience: A descriptive analysis. *Annals of Behavioral Medicine, 27,* 100–106.

Jellinek, E. M. (1960). *The disease concept of alcoholism.* New Haven, CT: College and University Press.

Jemal, D. V. M., Siegel, R., Ward, E., Hao, Y., Xu, J., Murray, T., et al. (2008). Cancer statistics, 2008. *CA: Cancer Journal for Clinicians, 58,* 71–96.

Jenkins, C. D. (1998). Cardiovascular disease. In E. A. Blechman & K. D. Brownell (Eds.), *Behavioral medicine and women: A comprehensive handbook* (pp. 604–614). New York: Guilford Press.

Jenks, R. A., & Higgs, S. (2007). Associations between dieting and smoking-related behaviors in young women. *Drug and Alcohol Dependence, 88,* 291–299.

Jensen, M. P., & Karoly, P. (2001). Self-report scales and procedures for assessing pain in adults. In D. C. Turk & R. Melzack (Eds.), *Handbook of pain assessment* (2nd ed., pp. 15–34). New York: Guilford Press.

Jeon, C. Y., Lokken, R. P., Hu, F. B., & van Dam, R. M. (2007). Physical activity of moderate intensity and risk of Type 2 diabetes: A systematic review. *Diabetes Care, 30,* 744–752.

Jeon, S. Y., & Lee, S. G. (2007). The effect of changes in attitude and subjective norm on treatment compliance in hypertension patients. *Journal of Applied Biobehavioral Research, 11,* 265–287.

Jha, A. P., Krompinger, J., & Baime, M. J. (2007). Mindfulness training modifies subsystems of attention. *Cognitive, Affective and Behavioral Neuroscience, 7,* 109–119.

John, E. M., Savitz, D. A., & Sandler, D. P. (1991). Prenatal exposure to parents' smoking and childhood cancer. *American Journal of Epidemiology, 133,* 123–132.

John, U., Hanke, M., Rumpf, H.-J., & Thyrian, J. R. (2005). Smoking status, cigarettes per day, and their relationship in national adult general population sample. *International Journal of Obesity, 29,* 1289–1294.

John, U., Meyer, C., Rumpf, H.-J., Hapke, U., & Schumann, A. (2006). Predictors of increased body mass index following cessation of smoking. *American Journal of Addictions, 15,* 192–197.

Johnson, A., Sandford, J., & Tyndall, J. (2007). Written and verbal information versus verbal information only for patients being discharged from acute hospital settings to home. *Cochrane Database of Systematic Reviews*, Cochrane AN: CD003716.

Johnson, J. L., Slentz, C. A., Houmard, J. A., Samsa, G. P., Duscha, B. D., Aiken, L. B., et al. (2007). Exercise training amount and intensity effects on metabolic syndrome (from Studies of a Targeted Risk Reduction Intervention through Defined Exercise). *American Journal of Cardiology, 100*, 1759–1766.

Johnson, L. W., & Weinstock, R. S. (2006). The metabolic syndrome: Concepts and controversy. *Mayo Clinic Proceedings, 81*, 1615–1621.

Johnson, M. I. (2006). The clinical effectiveness of acupuncture for pain relief—You can be certain of uncertainty. *Acupuncture in Medicine, 24*, 71–79.

Johnson, R. A., & Gerstein, D. R. (1998). Initiation of use of alcohol, cigarettes, marijuana, cocaine, and other substances in US birth cohorts since 1919. *American Journal of Public Health, 88*, 27–33.

Johnson, S. S., Driskell, M.-M., Johnson, J. L., Dyment, S. J., Prochaska, J. O., Prochaska, J. M., et al. (2006). Transtheoretical model intervention for adherence to lipid-lowering drugs. *Disease Management, 9*, 102–114.

Johnston, L. D., O'Malley, P. M., Bachman, J. G., & Schulenberg, J. E. (2007*). Monitoring the Future: National survey results on drug use, 1975–2006: Vol. 2. College students and adults ages 19–45* (NIH Publication No. 07-6206). Bethesda, MD: National Institute on Drug Abuse.

Johnston, L. D., O'Malley, P. M., Bachman, J. G., & Schulenberg, J. E. (2008). *Monitoring the Future national results on adolescent drug use: Overview of key findings, 2007* (NIH Publication No. 08-6418). Bethesda, MD: National Institute on Drug Abuse.

Jolliffe, C. D., & Nicholas, M. K. (2004). Verbally reinforcing pain reports: An experimental test of the operant model of chronic pain. *Pain, 107*, 167–175.

Jolly, K., Taylor, R. S., Lip, G. Y. H., & Stevens, A. (2006). Home-based cardiac rehabilitation compared with centre-based rehabilitation and usual care: A systematic review and meta-analysis. *International Journal of Cardiology, 111*, 343–351.

Jonas, W. B., Kaptchuk, T. J., & Linde, K. (2003). A critical overview of homeopathy. *Annals of Internal Medicine, 138*, 393–400.

Jones, D. W., Chambless, L. E., Folsom, A. R., Heiss, G., Hutchinson, R. G., Sharrett, A. R., et al. (2002). Risk factors for coronary heart disease in African Americans: The Atherosclerosis Risk in Communities Study, 1987–1997. *Archives of Internal Medicine, 162*, 2565–2571.

Jones, F., Harris, P., Waller, H., & Coggins, A. (2005). Adherence to an exercise prescription scheme: The role of expectations, self-efficacy, stage of change and psychological well-being. *British Journal of Health Psychology, 10*, 359–378.

Joranson, D. E., Ryan, K. M., Gilson, A. M., & Dahl, J. L. (2000). Trends in medical use and abuse of opioid analgesics. *Journal of the American Medical Association, 283*, 1710–1714.

Jorgensen, R. S., & Kolodziej, M. E. (2007). Suppressed anger, evaluative threat, and cardiovascular reactivity: A tripartite profile approach. *International Journal of Psychophysiology, 66*, 102–108.

Juliano, L. M., & Griffiths, R. R. (2004). A critical review of caffeine withdrawal: Empirical validation of symptoms and signs, incidence, severity, and associated features. *Psychopharmacology, 176*, 1–29.

Julien, R. M. (2008). *A primer of drug action* (11th ed.). New York: Worth.

Kabat-Zinn, J. (1993). Mindfulness meditation: Health benefits of an ancient Buddhist practice. In D. Goleman & J. Gurin (Eds.), *Mind/body medicine: How to use your mind for better health* (pp. 259–275). Yonkers, NY: Consumer Reports Books.

Kahende, J. W., Woollery, T. A., Lee, C.-W. (2007). Assessing medical expenditures on 4 smoking-related diseases, 1996–2001. *American Journal of Health Behavior, 31*, 602–611.

Kahn, H. A. (1963). The relationship of reported coronary heart disease mortality to physical activity of work. *American Journal of Public Health, 53*, 1058–1067.

Kaholokula, J. K., Saito, E., Mau, M. K., Latimer, R., & Seto, T. B. (2008). Pacific Islanders' perspectives on heart failure management. *Patient Education and Counseling, 70*, 281–291.

Kalant, H. (2004). Adverse effects of cannabis on health: An update of the literature since 1996. *Progress in Neuro-Psychopharmacology and Biological Psychiatry, 28*, 849–863.

Kalb, C. (1998, April 27). When drugs do harm. *Newsweek, 131*, 8.

Kalesan, B., Stine, J., & Alberg, A. J. (2006). The joint influence of parental modeling and positive parental concern on cigarette smoking in middle and high school students. *Journal of School Health, 76*, 402–407.

Kalichman, S. C., Eaton, L., Cain, D., Cherry, C., Fuhrel, A., Kaufman, M., et al. (2007). Changes in HIV treatment beliefs and sexual risk behaviors among gay and bisexual men, 1997–2005. *Health Psychology, 26*, 650–656.

Kalman, D., Morissette, S. B., & George, T. P. (2005). Co-morbidity of smoking in patients with psychiatric and substance use disorders. *American Journal of Addictions, 14*, 106–123.

Kamarck, T. W., Muldoon, M. F., Shiffman, S. S., & Sutton-Tyrrell, K. (2007). Experiences of demand and control during daily life are predictors of carotid atherosclerotic progression among healthy men. *Health Psychology, 26*, 324–332.

Kambouropoulos, N. (2003). The validity of the tension-reduction hypothesis in alcohol cue-reactivity research. *Australian Journal of Psychology, 55*(Suppl.), 6.

Kamer, A. R., Craig, R. G., Dasanayke, A. P., Brys, M., Glodzik-Sobanska, L, & de Leon, M. J. (2008). Inflammation and Alzheimer's disease: Possible role of periodontal diseases. *Alzheimer's and Dementia, 4*, 242–250.

Kamiya, J. (1969). Operant control of the EEG alpha rhythm and some of its reported effects on consciousness. In C. Tart (Ed.), *Altered states of consciousness.* New York: Wiley.

Kaner, E. F. S., Beyer, F., Dickinson, H. O., Pienaar, E., Campbell, F., Schlesinger, C., et al. (2007). Effectiveness of brief alcohol interventions in primary care populations. *Cochrane Database of Systematic Reviews*, Cochrane AN: CD004148.

Kanner, A. D., Coyne, J. C., Schaefer, C., & Lazarus, R. S. (1981). Comparison of two modes of stress measurement: Daily hassles and uplifts versus major life events. *Journal of Behavioral Medicine, 4*, 1–39.

Ka'opua, L. S. I., & Mueller, C. W. (2004). Treatment adherence among Native Hawaiians living with HIV. *Social Work, 49*, 55–62.

Kaplan, R. M., & Bush, J. W. (1982). Health-related quality of life measurement for evaluation research and policy analysis. *Health Psychology, 1*, 61–80.

Kaptchuk, T., Eisenberg, D., & Komaroff, A. (2002). Pondering the placebo effect. *Newsweek, 140* (23), 71, 73.

Kaptchuk, T. J., & Miller, F. G. (2005). What is the best and most ethical model for the relationship between mainstream and alternative medicine: Opposition, integration, or pluralism? *Academic Medicine, 80*, 286–290.

Karam, E., Kypri, K., & Salamoun, M. (2007). Alcohol use among college students: An international perspective. *Current Opinion in Psychiatry, 20*, 213–221.

Karani, R., McLaughlin, M. A., & Cassel, C. K. (2001). Exercise in the healthy older adult. *American Journal of Geriatric Cardiology, 10*, 269–273.

Karavidas, M. K., Tsai, P.-S., Yucha, C., McGrady, A., & Lehrer, P. M. (2006). Thermal biofeedback for primary Raynaud's phenomenon: A review of the literature. *Applied Psychophysiology and Biofeedback, 31*, 203–216.

Karl, A., Mühlnickel, W., Kurth, R., & Flor, H. (2004). Neuroelectric source imaging of steady-state movement-related cortical potentials in human upper extremity amputees with and without phantom limb pain. *Pain, 110*, 90–102.

Karlamangla, A. S., Singer, B. H., Williams, D. R., Schwartz, J. E., Matthews, K. A., Kiefe, C. I., et al. (2005). Impact of socioeconomic status on longitudinal accumulation of cardiovascular risk in young adults: The CARDIA Study (USA). *Social Science and Medicine, 60*, 999–1015.

Karoly, P., & Ruehlman, L. S. (2007). Psychosocial aspects of pain-related life task interference: An exploratory analysis in a general population sample. *Pain Medicine, 8*, 563–572.

Kasl, S. V., & Cobb, S. (1966a). Health behavior, illness behavior, and sick role behavior: I. Health and illness behavior. *Archives of Environmental Health, 12*, 246–266.

Kasl, S. V., & Cobb, S. (1966b). Health behavior, illness behavior, and sick role behavior: II. Sick role behavior. *Archives of Environmental Health, 12*, 531–541.

Kaur, S., Cohen, A., Dolor, R., Coffman, C. J., & Bastian, L. A. (2004). The impact of environmental tobacco smoke on women's risk of dying from heart disease: A meta-analysis. *Journal of Women's Health, 13*, 888–897.

Kaushal, N. (2007). Do food stamps cause obesity? Evidence for immigrant experience. *Journal of Health Economics, 26*, 968–991.

Kavookjian, J., Elswick, B. M., & Whetsel, T. (2007). Interventions for being active among individuals with diabetes: A systematic review of the literature. *Diabetes Educator, 33*, 962–988.

Kawachi, I., Daniels, N., & Robinson, D. E. (2005). Health disparities by race and class: Why both matter. *Health Affairs, 24*, 343–352.

Kawada, T. (2004). Difference of body mass index stratified by the period of smoking cessation from a cross-sectional study. *Archives of Medical Research, 35*, 181–184.

Kawamura, N., Kim, Y., & Asukai, N. (2001). Suppression of cellular immunity in men with a past history of post-traumatic stress disorder. *American Journal of Psychiatry, 158*, 484–486.

Kaye, W. (2008). Neurobiology of anorexia and bulimia nervosa. *Physiology and Behavior, 94*, 121–135.

Keane, H. (2003). Anabolic steroids and dependence. *Contemporary Drug Problems, 30*, 541–562.

Keefe, F. J. (1982). Behavioral assessment and treatment of chronic pain: Current status and future directions. *Journal of Consulting and Clinical Psychology, 50*, 896–911.

Keefe, F. J., & Smith, S. J. (2002). The assessment of pain behavior: Implications for applied psychophysiology and future research directions. *Applied Psychophysiology and Biofeedback, 27*, 117–127.

Keefe, F. J., Smith, S. J., Buffington, A. L. H., Gibson, J., Studts, J. L., & Caldwell, D. S. (2002). Recent advances and future directions in the biopsychosocial assessment and treatment of arthritis. *Journal of Consulting and Clinical Psychology, 70*, 640–655.

Keel, P. K., & Klump, K. L. (2003). Are eating disorders culture-bound syndromes? Implications for conceptualizing their etiology. *Psychological Bulletin, 129*, 747–769.

Kehr, B. A. (2004). Computer-enhanced treatment compliance. *Behavioral Health Management, 24*(2), 44–48.

Keith, V., Kronenfeld, J., Rivers, P., & Liang, S. (2005). Assessing the effects of race and ethnicity on use of complementary and alternative therapies in the USA. *Ethnicity and Health, 10*, 19–32.

Keller, A., Hayden, J., Bombardier, C., & van Tulder, M. (2007). Effect sizes of non-surgical treatments of non-specific low-back pain. *European Spine Journal, 16*, 1776–1788.

Kelley, G. A., & Kelley, K. S. (2007). Aerobic exercise and lipids and lipoproteins in children and adolescents: A meta-analysis of randomized controlled trials. *Atherosclerosis, 191*, 447–453.

Kelley, K. W., Bluthé, R.-M., Dantzer, R., Zhou, J.-H., Shen, W.-H., Johnson, R. W., et al. (2003). Cytokine-induced sickness behavior. *Brain, Behavior and Immunity, 17*(Suppl.), 112–118.

Kelly, J. A., & Kalichman, S. C. (2002). Behavioral research in HIV/AIDS primary and secondary prevention: Recent advances and future directions. *Journal of Consulting and Clinical Psychology, 70,* 626–639.

Kelly, J. F. (2003). Self-help for substance-use disorders: History, effectiveness, knowledge gaps, and research opportunities. *Clinical Psychology Review, 23,* 639–664.

Keltner, B., Kelley, F. J., & Smith, D. (2004). Leadership to reduce health disparities. *Nursing Administration Quarterly, 28,* 181–190.

Kemeny, M. E. (2003). The psychobiology of stress. *Current Directions in Psychological Science, 12,* 124–129.

Kemeny, M. E., & Schedlowski, M. (2007). Understanding the interaction between psychosocial stress and immune-related diseases: A stepwise progression. *Brain, Behavior and Immunity, 21,* 1009–1018.

Kendler, K. S., Gatz, M., Gardner, C. O., & Pedersen, N. L. (2007). Clinical indices of familial depression in the Swedish Twin Registry. *Acta Psychiatrica Scandinavica, 115,* 214–220.

Kenntner-Mabiala, R., Weyers, P., & Pauli, P. (2007). Independent effects of emotion and attention on sensory and affective pain perception. *Cognition and Emotion, 21,* 1615–1629.

Keogh, E., Bond, F. W., & Flaxman, P. E. (2006). Improving academic performance and mental health through a stress management intervention: Outcomes and mediators of change. *Behaviour Research and Therapy, 44,* 339–357.

Kerns, R. D., Turk, D. C., & Rudy, T. E. (1985). The West Haven–Yale Multidimensional Pain Inventory. *Pain, 23,* 345–356.

Kerse, N., Buetow, S., Mainous, A. G., III, Young, G., Coster, G., & Arroll, A. (2004). Physician-patient relationship and medication compliance: A primary care investigation. *Annals of Family Medicine, 2,* 455–461.

Kertesz, L. (2003). The numbers behind the news. *Healthplan, 44*(5), 10–14, 16, 18.

Kesaniemi, Y. A, Danforth, E., Jr., Jensen, M. D., Kopelman, P. G., Lefebvre, P., & Reader, B. A. (2001). Dose-response issues concerning physical activity and health: An evidence-based symposium. *Medicine and Science in Sports and Exercise, 33,* S351–S358.

Kesmodel, U., Wisborg, K., Olsen, S. F., Henriksen, T. B., & Secher, N. J. (2002). Moderate alcohol intake during pregnancy and the risk of stillbirth and death in the first year of life. *American Journal of Epidemiology, 155,* 305–312.

Ketonen, M., Pajunen, P., Koukkunen, H., Immonen-Räihä, P., Mustonen, J., Mähönen, M., et al. (2008). Long-term prognosis after coronary artery bypass surgery. *International Journal of Cardiology, 124,* 72–79.

Keys, A., Brozek, J., Henschel, A., Mickelsen, O., & Taylor, H. L. (1950). *The biology of human starvation* (2 vols.). Minneapolis: University of Minnesota Press.

Khalsa, P. S. (2004). Biomechanics of musculoskeletal pain: Dynamics of the neuromatrix. *Journal of Electromyography and Kinesiology, 14,* 109–130.

Kharbanda, R., & MacAllister, R. J. (2005). The atherosclerosis time-line and the role of the endothelium. *Current Medicinal Chemistry—Immunology, Endocrine, and Metabolic Agents, 5,* 47–52.

Khaw, K.-T., Wareham, N., Bingham, S., Luben, R., Welch, A., & Day, N. (2004). Association of hemoglobin A$_{1c}$ with cardiovascular disease and mortality in adults: The European Prospective Investigation into Cancer in Norfolk. *Annals of Internal Medicine, 141,* 413–420.

Kickbusch, I. (2008). Health literacy: An essential skill for the twenty-first century. *Health Education, 108,* 101–104.

Kiecolt-Glaser, J. K. (1999). Stress, personal relationships, and immune function: Health implications. *Brain, Behavior and Immunity, 13,* 61–72.

Kiecolt-Glaser, J. K., Malarkey, W. B., Cacioppo, J. T., & Glaser, R. (1994). Stressful personal relationships: Immune and endocrine function. In R. Glaser & J. K. Kiecolt-Glaser (Eds.), *Handbook of human stress and immunity* (pp. 321–339). San Diego, CA: Academic Press.

Kiecolt-Glaser, J. K., Marucha, P. T., Malarkey, W. B., Mercado, A. M., & Glaser, R. (1995). Slowing of wound healing by psychological stress. *Lancet, 346,* 1194–1196.

Kiecolt-Glaser, J. K., McGuire, L., Robles, T. F., & Glaser, R. (2002). Emotions, morbidity, and mortality: New perspectives from psychoneuroimmunology. *Annual Review of Psychology, 53,* 83–108.

Kiecolt-Glaser, J. K., & Newton, T. L. (2001). Marriage and health: His and hers. *Psychological Bulletin, 127,* 472–503.

Kim, D., Kawachi, I., Hoorn, S. V., Ezzati, M. (2008). Is inequality at the heart of it? Cross-country associations of income inequality with cardiovascular diseases and risk factors. *Social Science and Medicine, 66,* 1719–1732.

Kim, H., Neubert, J. K., Rowan, J. S., Brahim, J. S., Iadarola, M. J., & Dionne, R. A. (2004). Comparison of experimental and acute clinical pain responses in humans as pain phenotypes. *Journal of Pain, 5,* 377–384.

Kimball, C. P. (1981). *The biopsychosocial approach to the patient.* Baltimore: Williams & Wilkins.

King, D., & Pace, L. (2005, April). Sports, steroids, and scandals. *Information Today, 22,* 25–27.

King, J., & Henry, E. (2004, September 4). Bill Clinton awaits heart surgery next week. *CNN Washington Bureau.* Retrieved June 16, 2005, from http://www.cnn.com/2004/ALLPOLITICS/09/03/clinton.tests/

King, K. M., Humen, D. P., Smith, H. L., Phan, C. L., & Teo, K. K. (2001). Psychosocial components of cardiac recovery and rehabilitation attendance. *Heart, 85,* 290–293.

King, L., Saules, K. K., & Irish, J. (2007). Weight concerns and cognitive style: Which carries more "weight" in the prediction of smoking among college women? *Nicotine and Tobacco Research, 9,* 535–543.

King, L. A., & Miner, K. N. (2000). Writing about the perceived benefits of traumatic events: Implications for physical health. *Personality and Social Psychology Bulletin, 26,* 220–230.

King, N., Touyz, S., & Charles, M. (2000). The effect of body dissatisfaction on women's perceptions of female celebrities. *International Journal of Eating Disorders, 27,* 341–346.

King, T. K., Matacin, M., White, K. S., & Marcus, B. H. (2005). A prospective examination of body image and smoking cessation in women. *Body Image, 2,* 19–28.

Kirkwood, G., Rampes, H., Tuffrey, V., Richardson, J., & Pilkington, K. (2005). Yoga for anxiety: A systematic review of the research evidence. *British Journal of Sports Medicine, 39,* 884–891.

Kirsch, I., Moore, T. J., Scoboria, A., & Nicholls, S. S. (2002). The emperor's new drugs: An analysis of antidepressant medication data submitted to the U.S. Food and Drug Administration. *Prevention & Treatment, 5,* Article 23. Available at http://www.journals.apa.org/prevention/volume5/ pre0050023a.html

Kivlinghan, K. T., Granger, D. A., & Booth, A. (2005). Gender differences in testosterone and cortisol response to competition. *Psychoneuroendocrinology, 30,* 58–71.

Klag, S., & Bradley, G. (2004). The role of hardiness in stress and illness: An exploration of the effect of negative affectivity and gender. *British Journal of Health Psychology, 9,* 137–161.

Klatsky, A. L. (2003, February). Drink to your health? *Scientific American, 288,* 75–82.

Klatsky, A. L. (2008). Alcohol, wine, and vascular diseases: An abundance of paradoxes. *American Journal of Physiology: Heart and Circulatory Physiology, 63,* 582–583.

Klatsky, A. L., & Udaltsova, N. (2007). Alcohol drinking and total morality risk. *Annals of Epidemiology, 17*(Suppl.), S63–S67.

Klein, D. A., Bennett, A. S., Schebendach, J., Foltin, R. W., Devlin, M. J., & Walsh, B. T. (2004). Exercise "addiction" in anorexia nervosa: Model development and pilot data. *CNS Spectrums, 9,* 531–537.

Klein, H., Elifson, K. W., & Sterk, C. E. (2003). "At risk" women who think that they have no chance of getting HIV: Self-assessed perceived risks. *Women and Health, 38,* 47–63.

Klein, S., Fontana, L., Young, V. L., Coggan, A. R., Kilo, C., Patterson, B. W., et al. (2004). Absence of an effect of liposuction on insulin action and risk factors for coronary heart disease. *New England Journal of Medicine, 350,* 2549–2557.

Klimenko, E., & Julliard, K. (2007). Communication between CAM mainstream medicine: Delphi panel perspectives. *Complementary Therapies in Clinical Practice, 13,* 46–52.

Klohn, L. S., & Rogers, R. W. (1991). Dimensions of the severity of a health threat: The persuasive effects of visibility, time of onset, and rate of onset on young women's intentions to prevent osteoporosis. *Health Psychology, 10,* 323–329.

Kloner, R. A., & Rezkalla, S. H. (2003). Cocaine and the heart. *New England Journal of Medicine, 348,* 487–488.

Klonoff, E. A., & Landrine, H. (2000). Is skin color a marker for racial discrimination? Explaining the skin color–hypertension relationship. *Journal of Behavioral Medicine, 23,* 329–338.

Kluger, R. (1996). *Ashes to ashes: America's hundred-year cigarette war, the public health and the unabashed triumph of Philip Morris.* New York: Knopf.

Knafl, K. A., & Deatrick, J. A. (2002). The challenge of normalization for families of children with chronic conditions. *Pediatric Nursing, 28,* 49–54.

Knight, K. M., McGowan, L., Dickens, C., & Bundy, C. (2006). A systematic review of motivational interviewing in physical health care settings. *British Journal of Health Psychology, 11,* 319–332.

Knight, S. J., & Emanuel, L. (2007). Processes of adjustment to end-of-life losses: A reintegration model. *Journal of Palliative Medicine, 10,* 1190–1198.

Knutson, K. L., & van Cauter, E. (2008). Associations between sleep loss and increased risk of obesity and diabetes. *Annals of the New York Academy of Sciences, 1129*(Suppl. 1), 287–304.

Knuttgen, H. G. (2007). Strength training and aerobic exercise: Comparison and contrast. *Journal of Strength and Conditioning, 21,* 973–978.

Ko, N.-Y., & Muecke, M. (2005). Reproductive decision-making among HIV-positive couples in Taiwan. *Journal of Nursing Scholarship, 37,* 41–47.

Kobasa, S. C. (1979). Stressful life events, personality, and health: An inquiry into hardiness. *Journal of Personality and Social Psychology, 37,* 1–11.

Kobasa, S. C., & Maddi, S. R. (1977). Existential personality theory. In R. Corsini (Ed.), *Current personality theories* (pp. 242–276). Itasca, IL: Peacock.

Kofman, O. (2002). The role of prenatal stress in the etiology of developmental behavioural disorders. *Neuroscience and Biobehavioral Reviews, 26,* 457–470.

Kohl, H. W., III. (2001). Physical activity and cardiovascular disease: Evidence for a dose response. *Medicine and Science in Sports and Exercise, 33,* S472–S483.

Kohn, L. T., Corrigan, J. M., & Donaldson, M. (Eds.). (1999). *To err is human: Building a safer health system.* Washington, DC: Institute of Medicine.

Köhnke, M. D. (2008). Approach to the genetics of alcoholism: A review based on pathophysiology. *Biochemical Pharmacology, 75,* 160–177.

Komagata, S., & Newton, R. (2003). The effectiveness of tai chi on improving balance in older adults: An evidence-based review. *Journal of Geriatric Physical Therapy, 26*(2), 9–16.

Koopmans, G. T., & Lamers, L. M. (2007). Gender and health care utilization: The role of mental distress and help-seeking propensity. *Social Science & Medicine, 64,* 1216–1230.

Kop, W. J. (2003). The integration of cardiovascular behavioral medicine and psychoneuroimmunology: New developments based on converging research fields. *Brain, Behavior and Immunity, 17,* 233–237.

Kopnisky, K. L., Stoff, D. M., & Rausch, D. M. (2004). Workshop report: The effects of psychological variables on the progression of HIV-1 disease. *Brain, Behavior and Immunity, 18,* 246–261.

Kosok, A. (2006). The moderation management programme in 2004: What type of drinker seeks controlled drinking? *International Journal of Drug Policy, 17,* 295–303.

Koss, M. P. (1990). The women's mental health research agenda: Violence against women. *American Psychologist, 45,* 374–380.

Koss, M. P., Bailey, J. A., Yuan, N. P., Herrara, V. M., & Lichter, E. L. (2003). Depression and PTSD in survivors of male violence: Research and training initiatives to facilitate recovery. *Psychology of Women Quarterly, 27,* 130–142.

Kottow, M. H. (2007). Should research ethics triumph over clinical ethics? *Journal of Evaluation in Clinical Practice, 13,* 695–698.

Kozlowski, L. T., Wilkinson, A., Skinner, W., Kent, C., Franklin, T., & Pope, M. (1989). Comparing tobacco cigarette dependence with other drug dependences. *Journal of the American Medical Association, 261,* 898–901.

Krahn, D. D., Kurth, C. L., Gomberg, E., & Drewnowski, A. (2005). Pathological dieting and alcohol use in college women—A continuum of behaviors. *Eating Behaviors, 6,* 43–52.

Kramer, A. M. (1995). Health care for elderly persons— Myths and realities. *New England Journal of Medicine, 332,* 1027–1029.

Kramsch, D. M., Aspen, A. J., Abramowitz, B. M., Kreimendahl, T., & Hood, W. B., Jr. (1981). Reduction of coronary atherosclerosis by moderate conditioning exercise in monkeys on an atherogenic diet. *New England Journal of Medicine, 305,* 1483–1489.

Krantz, D. S., & McCeney, K. T. (2002). Effects of psychological and social factors on organic disease: A critical assessment of research on coronary heart disease. *Annual Review of Psychology, 53,* 341–369.

Krantz, D. S., Sheps, D. S., Carney, R. M., & Natelson, B. H. (2000). Effects of mental stress in patients with coronary artery disease: Evidence and clinical implications. *Journal of the American Medical Association, 283,* 1800–1802.

Krantz, G., Forsman, M., & Lundberg, U. (2004). Consistency in physiological stress responses and electromyographic activity during induced stress exposure in women and men. *Integrative Physiological and Behavioral Science, 39,* 105–118.

Krarup, L.-H., Truelsen, T., Pedersen, A., Kerke, H., Lindahl, M., Hansen, L., et al. (2007). Level of physical activity in the week preceding an ischemic stroke. *Cerebrovascular Disease, 24,* 296–300.

Krewski, D., Lubin, J. H., Zielinski, J. M., Alavanja, M., Catalan, V. S., Field, R. W., et al. (2006). A combined analysis of North American case-control studies of residential radon and lung cancer. *Journal of Toxicology and Environmental Health, 69,* 533–597.

Krieger, N., Chen, J. T., Waterman, P. D., Rehkopf, D. H., & Subramanian, S. V. (2005). Painting a truer picture of US socioeconomic and racial/ethnic health inequalities: The public health disparities geocoding project. *American Journal of Public Health, 95,* 312–323.

Krisanaprakornkit, T., Krisanaprakornkit, W., Piyavhatkul, N., & Laopaiboon, M. (2006). Meditation therapy for anxiety disorders. *Cochrane Database of Systematic Reviews*, Cochrane AN: CD004998.

Kronish, I. M., Rieckmann, N., Halm, E. A., Shimbo, D., Vorchheimer, D., Haas, D. C., et al. (2006). Persistent depression affects adherence to secondary prevention behaviors after acute coronary syndromes. *Journal of General Internal Medicine, 21,* 1178–1183.

Kruger, J., Galuska, D. A., Serdula, M. K., & Jones, D. A. (2004). Attempting to lose weight: Specific practices among U.S. adults. *American Journal of Preventive Medicine, 26,* 402–406.

Kubetin, S. K. (2001). Weight-loss maintenance requires long-term management. *Family Practice News, 31*(4), 6–7.

Kübler-Ross, E. (1969). *On death and dying.* New York: Macmillan.

Kuepper-Nybelen, J., Rothenbacher, D., & Brenner, H. (2005). Relationship between lifetime alcohol consumption and Helicobacter Pylori infection. *Annals of Epidemiology, 15,* 607–613.

Kung, H. C., Hoyert, D. L., Xu, J. Q., & Murphy, S. L. (2008). Deaths: Final data for 2005. *National Vital Statistics Reports, 56*(10), 1–66.

Kurland, H. (2000). *History of t'ai chi chu'an.* Retrieved May 16, 2008, from http://www.dotaichi.com/Articles/HistoryofTaiChi.htm

Kushi, L., Fee, R. M., Folsom, A. R., Mink, P. J., Anderson, K. E., & Sellers, T. A. (1997). Physical activity and mortality in postmenopausal women. *Journal of the American Medical Association, 227,* 1287–1292.

Kyngäs, H. (2004). Support network of adolescents with chronic disease: Adolescents' perspective. *Nursing and Health Sciences, 6,* 287–293.

Laaksonen, M., Talala, K., Martelin, T., Rahkonen, O., Roos, E., Helakorpi, S., et al. (2008). Health behaviours as explanations for educational level differences in cardiovascular and all-cause mortality: A follow-up of 60,000 men and women over 23 years. *European Journal of Public Health, 18,* 38–43.

Laatikainen, T., Critchley, J., Vartiainen, E., Salomaa, V., Ketonen, M., & Capewell, S. (2005). Explaining the decline in coronary heart disease mortality in Finland between 1982 and 1997. *American Journal of Epidemiology, 162,* 764–773.

Lacey, K., Zaharia, M. D., Griffiths, J., Ravindran, A. V., Merali, Z., & Anisman, H. (2000). A prospective study of neuroendocrine and immune alterations associated with the stress of an oral academic examination among graduate students. *Psychoneuroendocrinology, 25,* 339–356.

Laessle, R. G., Lehrke, S., & Dückers, S. (2007). Laboratory eating behavior in obesity. *Appetite, 49,* 399–404.

Lafferty, W. E., Tyree, P. T., Devlin, S. M., Andersen, M. R., & Diehr, P. K. (2008). Complementary and alternative medicine provider use and expenditures by cancer treatment phase. *American Journal of Managed Care, 14,* 326–334.

Laforge, R. G., Greene, G. W., & Prochaska, J. O. (1994). Psychosocial factors influencing low fruit and vegetable consumption. *Journal of Behavioral Medicine, 17*, 361–374.

Laitinen, M. H., Ngandu, T., Rovio, S., Helkala, E.-L., Uusitalo, U., Viitanen, M., et al. (2006). Fat intake at midlife and risk of dementia and Alzheimer's disease: A population-based study. *Dementia and Geriatric Cognitive Disorders, 22*, 99–107.

Lake, J. (2007). Philosophical problems in medicine and psychiatry, part II. *Integrative Medicine: A Clinician's Journal, 6*(3), 44–47.

Lamptey, P. R. (2002). Reducing heterosexual transmission of HIV in poor countries. *British Medical Journal, 324*, 207–211.

Lancaster, T., Hajek, P., Stead, L. F., West, R., & Jarvis, M. J. (2006). Prevention of relapse after quitting smoking: A systematic review of trials. *Archives of Internal Medicine, 166*, 828–835.

Landrine, H., & Klonoff, E. A. (1996). The Schedule of Racist Events: A measure of racial discrimination and a study of its negative physical and mental health consequences. *Journal of Black Psychology, 22*, 144–168.

Lane, S. D., Cherek, D. R., Tcheremissine, O. V., Lieving, L. M., & Pietras, C. J. (2005). Acute marijuana effects on human risk taking. *Neuropsychopharmacology, 30*, 800–809.

Lang, E. V., Benotsch, E. G., Fick, L. J., Lutgendorf, S., Berbaum, M. L., Berbaum, K. S., et al. (2000). Adjunctive non-pharmacological analgesia for invasive medical procedures: A randomised trial. *Lancet, 355*, 1486–1490.

Lang, F. R., Baltes, P. B., & Wagner, G. G. (2007). Desired lifetime and end-of-life desires across adulthood from 20 to 90: A dual-source information model. *Journals of Gerontology Series B: Psychological Sciences and Social Sciences, 62B*, 268–276.

Langa, K. M., Foster, N. L., & Larson, E. B. (2004). Mixed dementia: Emerging concepts and therapeutic implications. *Journal of the American Medical Association, 292*, 2901–2908.

Langer, E. J., & Rodin, J. (1976). The effects of choice and enhanced personal responsibility for the aged: A field experiment in an institutional setting. *Journal of Personality and Social Psychology, 34*, 191–198.

López-Moreno, J. A., González-Cuevas, G., Moreno, G., & Navarro, M. (2008). The pharmacology of the endocannabinoid system: Functional structural interactions with other neurotransmitter systems and their repercussions in behavioral addiction. *Addiction Biology, 13*, 160–187.

Largo-Wight, E., Peterson, P. M., & Chen, W. W. (2005). Perceived problem solving, stress, and health among college students. *American Journal of Health Behavior, 29*, 360–370.

Larun, L., Nordheim, L. V., Ekeland, E., Hagen, K. B., & Heian, F. (2006). Exercise in prevention and treatment of anxiety and depression among children and young people. *Cochrane Database of Systematic Reviews*, Cochrane AN: CD004691.

Lash, S. J., Stephens, R. S., Burden, J. L., Grambow, S. C., DeMarce, J. M., Jones, M. E., et al. (2007). Contracting, prompting, and reinforcing substance use disorder continuing care: A randomized clinical trial. *Psychology of Addictive Behaviors, 21*, 387–397.

Lasser, K. E., Himmelstein, D. U., & Woolhandler, S. (2006). Access to care, health status, and health disparities in the United States and Canada: Results of a cross-national population-based survey. *American Journal of Public Health, 96*, 1300–1307.

Latkin, C. A., & Knowlton, A. R. (2005). Micro-social structural approaches to HIV prevention: A social ecological perspective. *AIDS Care, 17*(Suppl. 1), 102–113.

La Torre, G., Chiaradia, G., & Ricciardi, G. (2005). School-based smoking prevention in children and adolescents: Review of the scientific literature. *Journal of Public Health, 13*, 285–290.

Latzer, Y., Tzischinsky, O., & Roer, S. (2007). Sleep-wake cycles in obese children with and without binge eating episodes. *Appetite, 49*, 306.

Laucht, M., Becker, K., Frank, J., Schmidt, M. H., Esser, G., Treutlein, J., et al. (2008). Genetic variation in dopamine pathways differentially associated with smoking progression in adolescence. *Journal of the American Academy of Child and Adolescent Psychiatry, 47*, 673–681.

LaVeist, T. A., Bowie, J. V., & Cooley-Quille, M. (2000). Minority health status in adulthood: The middle years of life. *Health Care Financing Review, 21*(4), 9–21.

Lavie, C. J., & Milani, R. V. (2005). Prevalence of hostility in young coronary artery disease patients and effects of cardiac rehabilitation and exercise training. *Mayo Clinic Proceedings, 80*, 335–342.

Lawton, J., Ahmad, N., Peel, E., & Hallowell, N. (2007). Contextualising accounts of illness: Notions of responsibility and blame in white and South Asian respondents' accounts of diabetes causation. *Sociology of Health and Illness, 29*, 891–906.

Lazarou, J., Pomeranz, B. H., & Corey, P. N. (1998). Incidence of adverse drug reactions in hospitalized patients: A meta-analysis of prospective studies. *Journal of the American Medical Association, 278*, 1200–1205.

Lazarus, R. S. (1984). Puzzles in the study of daily hassles. *Journal of Behavioral Medicine, 7*, 375–389.

Lazarus, R. S. (1993). From psychological stress to the emotions: A history of changing outlooks. *Annual Review of Psychology, 44*, 1–21.

Lazarus, R. S. (2000). Toward better research on stress and coping. *American Psychologist, 55*, 665–673.

Lazarus, R. S., & Cohen, J. (1977). Environmental stress. In I. Altman & J. Wohlwill (Eds.), *Human behavior and environment: Advances in theory and research* (Vol. 2, pp. 89–127). New York: Plenum Press.

Lazarus, R. S., & DeLongis, A. (1983). Psychological stress and coping in aging. *American Psychologist, 38*, 245–254.

Lazarus, R. S., DeLongis, A., Folkman, S., & Gruen, R. (1985). Stress and adaptational outcomes. *American Psychologist, 40*, 770–779.

Lazarus, R. S., & Folkman, S. (1984). *Stress, appraisal, and coping.* New York: Springer.

Leape, L. L., & Berwick, D. M. (2005). Five years after *To Err Is Human:* What have we learned? *Journal of the American Medical Association, 293,* 2384–2390.

Lebovits, A. (2007). Cognitive-behavioral approaches to chronic pain. *Primary Psychiatry, 14*(9), 48–50, 51–54.

Lee, I.-M., & Paffenbarger, R. S., Jr. (1998). Life is sweet: Candy consumption and longevity. *British Medical Journal, 317,* 1683–1684.

Lee, I.-M., & Skerrett, P. J. (2001). Physical activity and all-cause mortality. What is the dose-response relation? *Medicine and Science in Sports and Exercise, 33,* S459–S471.

Lee, L. M., Karon, J. M., Selik, R., Neal, J. J., & Fleming, P. L. (2001). Survival after AIDS diagnosis in adolescents and adults during the treatment era, United States, 1984–1997. *Journal of the American Medical Association, 285,* 1308–1315.

Lee, M. S., Kim, M. K., & Ryu, H. (2005). Qi-training (qigong) enhanced immune functions: What is the underlying mechanism? *International Journal of Neuroscience, 115,* 1099–1104.

Lee, M. S., Pittler, M. H., & Ernst, E. (2007). External qigong for pain conditions: A systematic review of randomized clinical trials. *Journal of Pain, 8,* 827–831.

Lee, M. S., Pittler, M. H., Shin, B.-C., & Ernst, E. (2008). Tai chi for osteoporosis: A systematic review. *Osteoporosis International, 19,* 139–146.

Lee, S. H., Akuete, K., Fulton, J., Chelmow, D., Chung, M. A., & Cady, B. (2003). An increased risk of breast cancer after delayed first parity. *American Journal of Surgery, 186,* 409–412.

Leeuw, M., Goossens, M. E. J. B., Linton, S. J., Crombez, G., Boersma, K., & Vlaeyen, J. W. S. (2007). The fear-avoidance model of musculoskeletal pain: Current state of scientific evidence. *Journal of Behavioral Medicine, 30,* 77–94.

Lenssinck, M.-L. B., Damen, L., Verhagen, A. P., Berger, M. Y., Passchier, J., & Koes, B. W. (2004). The effectiveness of physiotherapy and manipulation in patients with tension-type headache: A systematic review. *Pain, 112,* 381–388.

Leo, R. J., & Ligot, J. S. A., Jr. (2007). A systematic review of randomized controlled trials of acupuncture in the treatment of depression. *Journal of Affective Disorders, 97,* 13–22.

Leon, A. S., & Sanchez, O. A. (2001). Response of blood lipids to exercise training alone or combined with dietary intervention. *Medicine and Science in Sports and Exercise, 33,* S502–S515.

Lepore, S. J., Fernandez-Berrocal, P., Ragan, J., & Ramos, N. (2004). It's not that bad: Social challenges to emotional disclosure enhance adjustment to stress. *Anxiety, Stress and Coping, 17,* 341–361.

Lepore, S. J., Revenson, T. A., Weinberger, S. L., Weston, P., Frisina, P. G., Robertson, R., et al. (2006). Effects of social stressors on cardiovascular reactivity in black and white women. *Annals of Behavioral Medicine, 31,* 120–127.

Lestideau, O. T., & Lavallee, L. F. (2007). Structured writing about current stressors: The benefits of developing plans. *Psychology and Health, 22,* 659–676.

Levenson, J. L., & Schneider, R. K. (2007). Infectious diseases. In J. L. Levenson (Ed.), *Essentials of psychosomatic medicine* (pp. 181–204). Washington, DC: American Psychiatric Publishing.

Levenson, R. W., Sher, K. J., Grossman, L. M., Newman, J., & Newlin, D. B. (1980). Alcohol and stress response dampening: Pharmacological effects, expectancy, and tension reduction. *Journal of Abnormal Psychology, 89,* 528–538.

Levenstein, S. (2000). The very model of a modern etiology: A biopsychosocial view of peptic ulcer. *Psychosomatic Medicine, 62,* 176–185.

Leventhal, H., & Avis, N. (1976). Pleasure, addiction, and habit: Factors in verbal report or factors in smoking behavior? *Journal of Abnormal Psychology, 85,* 478–488.

Leventhal, H., Leventhal, E. A., & Cameron, L. (2001). Representations, procedures, and affect in illness self-regulation: A perceptual-cognitive model. In A. Baum, T. A. Revenson, & J. E. Singer (Eds.), *Handbook of health psychology* (pp. 19–47). Mahwah, NJ: Erlbaum.

Levi, L. (1974). Psychosocial stress and disease: A conceptual model. In E. K. E. Gunderson & R. H. Rahe (Eds.), *Life stress and illness* (pp. 8–33). Springfield, IL: Thomas.

Levin, B. E. (2005). Factors promoting and ameliorating the development of obesity. *Physiology and Behavior, 86,* 633–639.

Levin, T., & Kissane, D. W. (2006). Psychooncology—The state of its development in 2006. *European Journal of Psychiatry, 20,* 183–197.

Levy, D., & Brink, S. (2005). *A change of heart: How the people of Framingham, Massachusetts, helped unravel the mysteries of cardiovascular disease.* New York: Knopf.

Lewis, M., & Johnson, M. I. (2006). The clinical effectiveness of therapeutic massage for muscoloskeletal pain: A systematic review. *Physiotherapy, 92,* 146–158.

Lewis, M. A., Hove, M. C., Whiteside, U., Lee, C. M., Kirkeby, B. S., Oster-Aaland, L., et al. (2008). Fitting in and feeling fine: Conformity and coping motives as mediators of the relationship between social anxiety and problematic drinking. *Psychology of Addictive Behaviors, 22,* 58–67.

Ley, P. (1997). Compliance among patients. In A. Baum, S. Newman, J. Weinman, R. West, & C. McManus (Eds.), *Cambridge handbook of psychology, health and medicine* (pp. 281–284). Cambridge, UK: Cambridge University Press.

Li, M. D., Ma, J. Z., & Beuten, J. (2004). Progress in searching for susceptibility loci and genes for smoking-related behaviour. *Clinical Genetics, 66,* 382–392.

Li, Q.-Z., Li, P., Garcia, G. E., Johnson, R. J., & Feng, L. (2005). Genomic profiling of neutrophil transcripts in Asian qigong practitioners: A pilot study in gene regulation by mind-body interaction. *Journal of Alternative and Complementary Medicine, 11*, 29–39.

Li, T.-K., Hewitt, B. G., & Grant, B. F. (2007). The alcohol dependence syndrome, 30 years later: A commentary. *Addiction, 102*, 1522–1530.

Lichtenstein, B. (2005). Domestic violence, sexual ownership, and HIV risk in women in the American deep south. *Social Science and Medicine, 60*, 701–715.

Lieberman, M. A., & Goldstein, B. A. (2006). Not all negative emotions are equal: The role of emotional expression in online support groups for women with breast cancer. *Psycho-Oncology, 15*, 160–168.

Ligier, S., & Sternberg, E. M. (2001). The neuroendocrine system and rheumatoid arthritis: Focus on the hypothalamo-pituitary-adrenal axis. In R. Ader, D. L. Felten, & N. Cohen (Eds.), *Psychoneuroimmunology* (3rd ed., Vol. 2, pp. 449–469). San Diego, CA: Academic Press.

Lilienfeld, A. M., & Lilienfeld, D. E. (1980). *Foundations of epidemiology* (2nd ed.). New York: Oxford University Press.

Lillie-Blanton, M., Maddox, T. M., Rushing, O., & Mensah, G. A. (2004). Disparities in cardiac care: Rising to the challenge of *Healthy People 2010. Journal of the American College of Cardiology, 44*, 503–508.

Lincoln, K. D., Chatters, L. M., & Taylor, R. J. (2003). Psychological distress among Black and White Americans: Differential effects of social support, negative interaction and personal control. *Journal of Health and Social Behavior, 44*, 390–407.

Linde, K., Witt, C. M., Streng, A., Weidenhammer, W., Wagenfeil, S., Brinkhaus, B., et al. (2007). The impact of patient expectations on outcomes in four randomized controlled trials of acupuncture in patients with chronic pain. *Pain, 128*, 264–271.

Linden, W. (2000). Psychological treatments in cardiac rehabilitation: Review of rationales and outcomes. *Journal of Psychosomatic Research, 48*, 443–454.

Lindsay, J., Sykes, E., McDowell, I., Verreault, R., & Laurin, D. (2004). More than epidemiology of Alzheimer's disease: Contributions of the Canadian Study of Health and Aging. *Canadian Journal of Psychiatry, 49*, 83–91.

Lindstrom, H. A., Fritsch, T., Petot, G., Smyth, K. A., Chen, C. H., Debanne, S. M., et al. (2005). The relationship between television viewing in midlife and the development of Alzheimer's disease in a case-control study. *Brain and Cognition, 58*, 157–165.

Ling, D., Niu, T., Feng, Y., Xing, H., & Xu, X. (2004). Association between polymorphism of the dopamine transporter gene and early smoking onset: An interaction risk on nicotine dependence. *Journal of Human Genetics, 49*, 35–39.

Lints-Martindale, A. C., Hadjistavropoulos, T., Barber, B., & Gibson, S. J. (2007). A psychophysical investigation of the Facial Action Coding System as an index of pain variability among older adults with and without Alzheimer's disease. *Pain Medicine, 8*, 678–689.

Litz, B. T., Williams, L., Wang, J., Bryant, R., & Engel, C. C. (2004). A therapist-assisted Internet self-help program for traumatic stress. *Professional Psychology: Research and Practice, 35*, 628–634.

Liu, H., Golin, C. E., Miller, L. G., Hays, R. D., Beck, C. K., Sanandji, S., et al. (2001). A comparison study of multiple measures of adherence to HIV protease inhibitors. *Annals of Internal Medicine, 134*, 968–977.

Livermore, M. M., & Powers, R. S. (2006). Unfulfilled plans and financial stress: Unwed mothers and unemployment. *Journal of Human Behavior in the Social Environment, 13*, 1–17.

Livneh, H., & Antonak, R. F. (2005). Psychosocial adaptation to chronic illness and disability: A primer for counselors. *Journal of Counseling and Development, 83*, 12–20.

Livneh, H., Lott, S. M., & Antonak, R. F. (2004). Patterns of psychosocial adaptation to chronic illness and disability: A cluster analytic approach, *Psychology, Health and Medicine, 9*, 411–430.

Ljungberg, J. K., & Neely, G. (2007). Stress, subjective experience and cognitive performance during exposure to noise and vibration. *Journal of Environmental Psychology, 27*, 44–54.

Lloyd-Williams, M., Dogra, N., & Petersen, S. (2004). First year medical students' attitudes toward patients with life-limiting illness: Does age make a difference? *Palliative Medicine, 18*, 137–138.

Locher, J. L., Yoels, W. C., Maurer, D., & Van Ells, J. (2005). Comfort foods: An exploratory journey into the social and emotional significance of food. *Food and Foodways: History and Culture of Human Nourishment, 13*, 273–297.

Lock, K., Pomerleau, J., Causer, L., Altmann, D. R., & McKee, M. (2005). The global burden of disease attributable to low consumption of fruit and vegetables: Implications for the global strategy on diet. *Bulletin of the World Health Organization, 83*, 100–108.

Locke, J., & le Grange, D. (2005). Family-based treatment of eating disorders. *International Journal of Eating Disorders, 37*, 64–67.

Locke, J., le Grange, D., Agras, W. S., & Dare, C. (2001). *Treatment manual for anorexia nervosa: A family-based approach.* New York: Guilford Press.

Loftus, M. (1995). The other side of fame. *Psychology Today, 28*(3), 48–53, 70, 72, 74, 76, 78, 80–81.

Logan, D. E., & Rose, J. B. (2004). Gender differences in post-operative pain and patient controlled analgesia use among adolescent surgical patients. *Pain, 109*, 481–487.

Lohaus, A., & Klein-Hessling, J. (2003). Relaxation in children: Effects of extended and intensified training. *Psychology and Health, 18*, 237–249.

Lotufo, P. A., Gaziano, J. M., Chae, C. U., Ajani, U. A., Moreno-John, G., Buring, J. E., et al. (2001). Diabetes and all-cause and coronary heart disease mortality among US male physicians. *Archives of Internal Medicine, 161*, 242–247.

Lowes, L., Gregory, J. W., & Lyne, P. (2005). Newly diagnosed childhood diabetes: A psychosocial transition for parents? *Journal of Advanced Nursing, 50*, 253–261.

Lowman, C., Hunt, W. A., Litten, R. Z., & Drummond, D. C. (2000). Research perspectives on alcohol craving: An overview. *Addiction, 95*(Suppl. 2), 45–54.

Lowry, R., Lee, S. M., Galuska, D. A., Fulton, J. E., Barrios, L. C., & Kann, L. (2007). Physical activity-related injury and body mass index among US high school students. *Journal of Physical Activity and Health, 4,* 325–342.

Lucas, A. E. M., Smeenk, F. W. J. M., Smeele, I. J., van Schayck, C. P. (2008). Overtreatment with inhaled corti-costeroids and diagnostic problems in primary care patients, an exploratory study. *Family Practice, 25,* 86–91.

Ludwig, D. S., & Ebbeling, C. B. (2001). Type 2 diabetes mellitus in children: Primary care and public health considerations. *Journal of the American Medical Association, 286,* 1427–1430.

Lukoschek, P. (2003). African Americans' beliefs and attitudes regarding hypertension and its treatment: A qualitative study. *Journal of Health Care for the Poor and Underserved, 14,* 566–587.

Luo, X. (2004). Estimates and patterns of direct health care expenditures among individuals with back pain in the United States. *Spine, 29,* 79–86.

Lustman, P. J., & Clouse, R. E. (2005). Depression in diabetic patients: The relationship between mood and glycemic control. *Journal of Diabetes and Its Complications, 19,* 113–122.

Luthar, S. S., & Latendresse, S. J. (2005). Children of the affluent: Challenges to well-being. *Current Directions in Psychological Science, 14,* 49–53.

Lutz, R. W., Silbret, M., & Olshan, W. (1983). Treatment outcome and compliance with therapeutic regimens: Long-term follow-up of a multidisciplinary pain program. *Pain, 17,* 301–308.

Lynch, H. T., Deters, C. A., Snyder, C. L., Lynch, J. F., Villeneuve, P., Silberstein, J., et al. (2005). BRCA1 and pancreatic cancer: Pedigree findings and their causal relationships. *Cancer Genetics and Cytogenetics, 158,* 119–125.

MacDonald, T. K., Fong, G. T., Zanna, M. P., & Martineau, A. M. (2000). Alcohol myopia and condom use: Can alcohol intoxication be associated with more prudent behavior? *Journal of Personality and Social Psychology, 78,* 605–619.

MacDonald, T. K., MacDonald, G., Zanna, M. P., & Fong, G. T. (2000). Alcohol, sexual arousal, and intentions to use condoms in young men: Applying alcohol myopia theory to risky sexual behavior. *Health Psychology, 19,* 290–298.

MacDougall, J. M., Dembroski, T. M., Dimsdale, J. E., & Hackett, T. P. (1985). Components of Type A, hostility, and anger-in: Further relationships to angiographic findings. *Health Psychology, 4,* 137–142.

Macedo, A., Baños, J.-E., & Farré, M. (2008). Placebo response in the prophylaxis of migraine: A meta-analysis. *European Journal of Pain, 12,* 68–75.

Maciejewski, P. K., Zhang, B., Block, S. D., & Prigerson, H. G. (2007). An empirical examination of the stage theory of grief. *Journal of the American Medical Association, 297,* 716–723.

Mackay, J., & Mensah, G. (2004). *The atlas of heart disease and stroke.* Geneva: World Health Organization and Centers for Disease Control and Prevention.

Mackellar, D. A., Valleroy, L. A., Secura, G. M., Behel, S., Bingham, T., Celentano, D. D., et al. (2007). Perceptions of lifetime risk and actual risk for acquiring HIV among young men who have sex with men. *AIDS and Behavior, 11,* 263–270.

Mackenbach, J. P., Stirbu, I., Roskam, J.-A. R. Schaap, M. M., Menvielle, G., Leinsalu, M., et al. (2008). Socioeconomic inequalities in health in 22 European countries. *New England Journal of Medicine, 358,* 2468–2481.

Macrodimitris, S. D., & Endler, N. S. (2001). Coping, control, and adjustment in Type 2 diabetes. *Health Psychology, 20,* 208–216.

Maddi, S. R. (2005). On hardiness and other pathways to resilience. *American Psychologist, 60,* 261–262.

Maenthaisong, R., Chaiyakunapruk, N., Niruntraporn, S., & Kongkaew, C. (2007). The efficacy of aloe vera used for burn wound healing: A systematic review. *Burns, 33,* 713–718.

Magura, S. (2007). The relationship between substance user treatment and 12-step fellowships: Current knowledge and research questions. *Substance Use and Misuse, 42,* 343–360.

Mahar, M. (2006). *Money-driven medicine: The real reason health care costs so much.* New York: HarperCollins.

Maier, S. F. (2003). Bi-directional immune-brain communication: Implications for understanding stress, pain, and cognition. *Brain, Behavior and Immunity, 17,* 269–285.

Maier, S. F., & Watkins, L. R. (2003). Immune-to-central nervous system communication and its role in modulating pain and cognition: Implications for cancer and cancer treatment. *Brain, Behavior and Immunity, 17,* 125–131.

Maizels, M., & McCarberg, B. (2005). Antidepressants and antiepileptic drugs for chronic non-cancer pain. *American Family Physician, 71,* 483–490.

Major, B., & O'Brien, L. T. (2005). The psychology of stigma. *Annual Review of Psychology, 56,* 393–421.

Malecka-Tendera, E., & Mazur, A. (2006). Childhood obesity: A pandemic of the twenty-first century. *International Journal of Obesity, 30*(Suppl. 2), S1–S3.

Mandayam, S. (2004). Epidemiology of alcoholic liver disease. *Seminars in Liver Disease, 24,* 217–232.

Mangels, A. R., Messina, V., & Melina, V. (2003). Vegetarian diets. *Journal of the American Dietetic Association, 103,* 748–765.

Manheimer, E., White, A., Berman, B., Forys, K., & Ernst, E. (2005). Meta-analysis: Acupuncture for low back pain. *Annals of Internal Medicine, 142,* 651–663.

Manier, D., & Olivares, A. (2005). Who benefits from expressive writing? Moderator variables affecting outcomes of emotional disclosure interventions. *Counseling and Clinical Psychology Journal, 2,* 15–28.

Manimala, M. R., Blount, R. L., & Cohen, L. L. (2000). The effects of parental reassurance versus distraction on child distress and coping during immunizations. *Children's Health Care, 29*, 161–177.

Mann, K. (2004). Pharmacotherapy of alcohol dependence: A review of the clinical data. *CNS Drugs, 18*, 485–504.

Manne, S. L., & Andrykowski, M. A. (2006). Are psychological interventions effective and accepted by cancer patients? II. Using empirically supported therapy guidelines to decide. *Annals of Behavioral Medicine, 32*, 98–103.

Mannino, D. M., Moorman, J. E., Kingsley, B., Rose, D., & Repace, J. (2001). Health effects related to environmental tobacco smoke exposure in children in the United States: Data from the Third National Health and Nutrition Examination Survey. *Archives of Pediatrics and Adolescent Medicine, 155*, 36–41.

Manor, O., Eisenbach, Z., Friedlander, Y., & Kark, J. D. (2004). Educational differentials in mortality from cardiovascular disease among men and women: The Israel Longitudinal Mortality Study. *Annals of Epidemiology, 14*, 453–460.

Manson, J. E., Skerrett, P. J., Greenland, P., & VanItallie, T. B. (2004). The escalating pandemics of obesity and sedentary lifestyle: A call to action for clinicians. *Archives of Internal Medicine, 164*, 249–258.

Mantell, J. E., Stein, Z. A., & Susser, I. (2008). Women in the time of AIDS: Barriers, bargains, and benefits. *AIDS Education and Prevention, 20*, 91–106.

Manzoni, G. C., & Torelli, P. (2002). Epidemiology of migraine. *Journal of Headache & Pain, 4*, S18–S22.

Marcus, D. A. (2001). Gender differences in treatment-seeking chronic headache sufferers. *Headache, 41*, 698–703.

Mårdby, A.-C., Åkerlind, I., & Jörgensen, T. (2007). Beliefs about medicines and self-reported adherence among pharmacy clients. *Patient Education and Counseling, 69*, 158–164.

Marlatt, G. A., Demming, B., & Reid, J. (1973). Loss of control drinking in alcoholics: An experimental analogue. *Journal of Abnormal Psychology, 81*, 233–241.

Marlatt, G. A., & Gordon, J. R. (1980). Determinants of relapse: Implication for the maintenance of behavior change. In P. O. Davidson & S. M. Davidson (Eds.), *Behavioral medicine: Changing health lifestyles* (pp. 410–452). New York: Brunner/Mazel.

Marlatt, G. A., & Rohsenow, D. J. (1980). Cognitive processes in alcohol use: Expectancy and the balanced placebo design. In N. Mello (Ed.), *Advances in substance abuse: Behavioral and biological research*. Greenwich, CT: JAI Press.

Marlowe, N. (1998). Stressful events, appraisal, coping and recurrent headache. *Journal of Clinical Psychology, 54*, 247–256.

Marquié, L., Raufaste, E., Lauque, D., Mariné, C., Ecoiffier, M., & Sorum, P. (2003). Pain rating by patients and physicians: Evidence of systematic miscalibration. *Pain, 102*, 289–296.

Marshall, B. J. (1995). Helicobacter pylori: The etiologic agent for peptic ulcers. *Journal of the American Medical Association, 274*, 1064–1066.

Marsland, A. L., Bachen, E. A., Cohen, S., & Manuck, S. B. (2001). Stress, immunity, and susceptibility to infectious disease. In A. Baum, T. A. Revenson, & J. E. Singer (Eds.), *Handbook of health psychology* (pp. 683–695). Mahwah, NJ: Erlbaum.

Marsland, A. L., Bachen, E. A., Cohen, S., Rabin, B., & Manuck, S. B. (2002). Stress, immune reactivity and susceptibility to infectious disease. *Physiology and Behavior, 77*, 711–716.

Martikainen, P., Valkonen, T., & Martelin, T. (2001). Change in male and female life expectancy by social class: Decomposition by age and cause of death in Finland 1971–95. *Journal of Epidemiology and Community Health, 55*, 494–499.

Martin, C. S., Fillmore, M. T., Chung, T., Easdon, C. M., & Miczek, K. A. (2006). Multidisciplinary perspectives on impaired control over substance use. *Alcoholism: Clinical and Experimental Research, 30*, 265–271.

Martin, P. D., & Brantley, P. J. (2004). Stress, coping, and social support in health and behavior. In J. M. Raczynsky & L. C. Leviton (Eds.), *Handbook of clinical health psychology* (Vol. 2, pp. 233–267). Washington, DC: American Psychological Association.

Martin, P. R., Forsyth, M. R., & Reece, J. (2007). Cognitive-behavioral therapy versus temporal pulse amplitude biofeedback training for recurrent headache. *Behavior Therapy, 38*, 350–363.

Martin, P. R., & Petry, N. M. (2005). Are non-substance-related addictions really addictions? *American Journal on Addictions, 14*, 1–3.

Martin, R., & Lemos, K. (2002). From heart attacks to melanoma: Do common sense models of somatization influence symptoms interpretation for female victims? *Health Psychology, 21*, 25–32.

Martin, R., & Leventhal, H. (2004). Symptom perception and health care–seeking behavior. In J. M. Raczynski & L. C. Leviton (Eds.), *Handbook of clinical health psychology* (Vol. 2, pp. 299–328). Washington, DC: American Psychological Association.

Martin, S. E. (2001). The links between alcohol, crime and the criminal justice system: Explanations, evidence and interventions. *American Journal on Addictions, 10*, 136–158.

Martindale, D. (2001, May 26). Needlework: Whether it's controlling the flow of vital energy or releasing painkilling chemicals, acupuncture seems plausible enough. But does it really work? *New Scientist, 170*, 42–45.

Martinez, F. D. (2001). The coming-of-age of the hygiene hypothesis. *Respiratory Research, 2*, 129–132.

Martins, I. J., Hone, E., Foster, J. K., Sünram-Lea, S. I., Gnjec, A., Fuller, S. J. et al. (2006). Apolipoprotein E, cholesterol metabolism, diabetes, and the convergence of risk factors for Alzheimer's disease and cardiovascular disease. *Molecular Psychiatry, 11*, 721–736.

Martinsen, E. W. (2008). Exercise and depression. *International Journal of Sport and Exercise Psychology, 3*(Special Issue), 469–483.

Martire, L. M., Lustig, A. P., Schulz, R., Miller, G. E., & Helgeson, V. S. (2004). Is it beneficial to involve a family member? A meta-analysis of psychosocial intervention for chronic illness. *Health Psychology, 23,* 599–611.

Martire, L. M., & Schulz, R. (2007). Involving family in psychosocial interventions for chronic illness. *Current Directions in Psychological Science, 16,* 90–94.

Mary-Kate Olsen reportedly suffers anorexia relapse. (2004, October 19). MSNBC Entertainment. Retrieved December 15, 2008, from http://www.msnbc.msn.com/id/6282050/

Mashegoane, S., Moalusi, K. P., Ngoepe, M. A., & Peltzer, K. (2004). The prediction of condom use intention among South African University students. *Psychological Reports, 95,* 407–417.

Mason, J. W. (1971). A reevaluation of the concept of "non-specificity" in stress theory. *Journal of Psychiatric Research, 8,* 323–333.

Mason, J. W. (1975). A historical view of the stress field. Pt. 2. *Journal of Human Stress, 1,* 22–36.

Mason, P. (2005). Deconstructing endogenous pain modulation. *Journal of Neurophysiology, 94,* 1659–1663.

Masters, K. S., & Spielmans, G. I. (2007). Prayer and health: Review, meta-analysis, and research agenda. *Journal of Behavioral Medicine, 30,* 29–338.

Masters, K. S., Spielmans, G. I., & Goodson, J. T. (2005, August). *Meta-analytic review of distant intercessory prayer studies.* Paper presented at the 113th convention of the American Psychological Association, Washington, DC.

Masur, F. T., III. (1981). Adherence to health care regimens. In C. K. Prokop & L. A. Bradley (Eds.), *Medical psychology: Contributions to behavioral medicine.* New York: Academic Press.

Matarazzo, J. D. (1987). Postdoctoral education and training of service providers in health psychology. In G. C. Stone, S. M. Weiss, J. D. Matarazzo, N. E. Miller, J. Rodin, C. D. Belar, et al. (Eds.), *Health psychology: A discipline and a profession* (pp. 371–388). Chicago: University of Chicago Press.

Matarazzo, J. D. (1994). Health and behavior: The coming together of science and practice in psychology and medicine after a century of benign neglect. *Journal of Clinical Psychology in Medical Settings, 1,* 7–39.

Mathers, M. I., Salomon, J. A., Tandon, A., Chatterji, S., Ustün, B., & Murray, C. J. L. (2004). Global patterns of healthy life expectancy in the year 2002. *BMC Public Health, 4,* record 66. Retrieved August 9, 2005, from http://www.biomedcentral.com/1471-2458/4/66

Matthews, K. (2005). Former president to have scar tissue removed. *Associated Press.* Retrieved June 16, 2005, from http://www.greatdreams.com/political/clinton-heart.htm

Matthews, K. A. (2005). Psychological perspectives on the development of heart disease. *American Psychologist, 60,* 783–796.

Matthews, K. A., Kuller, L. H., Chang, Y., & Edmundowicz, D. (2007). Premenopausal risk factors for coronary and aortic calcification: A 20-year follow-up in the healthy women study. *Preventive Medicine, 45,* 302–308.

Matthews, R. J., Jagger, C., & Hancock, R. M. (2006). Does socio-economic advantage lead to a longer, healthier old age? *Social Science and Medicine, 62,* 2489–2499.

Matthies, E., Hoeger, R., & Guski, R. (2000). Living on polluted soil: Determinants of stress symptoms. *Environment and Behavior, 32,* 270–286.

Matud, M. P. (2004). Gender differences in stress and coping styles. *Personality and Individual Differences, 37,* 1401–1415.

Mausbach, B. T., Coon, D. W., Depp, C., Rabinowitz, Y. G., Wilson-Arias, E., Kraemer, H. C., et al. (2004). Ethnicity and time to institutionalization of dementia patients: A comparison of Latina and Caucasian female family caregivers. *Journal of the American Geriatrics Society, 52,* 1077–1084.

May, P. A., & Gossage, J. P. (2001). Estimating the prevalence of fetal alcohol syndrome: A summary. *Alcohol Research and Health, 25,* 159–167.

Mayeaux, R. (2003). Epidemiology of neurogeneration. *Annual Review of Neuroscience, 26,* 81–104.

Mayfield, D. (1976). Alcoholism, alcohol intoxication, and assaultive behavior. *Diseases of the Nervous System, 37,* 228–291.

Maynard, L. M., Serdula, M. K., Galuska, D. A., Gillespie, C., & Mokdad, A. H. (2006). Secular trends in desired weight of adults. *International Journal of Obesity, 30,* 1375–1381.

Mayo Clinic Staff. (2008). *Vegetarian diet: How to get the best nutrition.* Retrieved May 5, 2008, from http://www.mayoclinic.com/print/vegetarian-diet/HQ01596/METHOD=print

Mayo-Smith, M. F., Beecher, L. H., Fischer, T. L., Gorelick, D. A., Guillaunce, J. L., Hill, A., et al. (2004). Management of alcohol withdrawal delirium: An evidence-based practice guideline. *Archives of Internal Medicine, 164,* 1405–1412.

McBride, C. M., Curry, S. J., Grothaus, L. C., Nelson, J. C., Lando, H., & Pirie, P. L. (1998). Partner smoking status and pregnant smoker's perceptions of support for the likelihood of smoking cessation. *Health Psychology, 17,* 63–69.

McCabe, M. P., & Ricciardelli, L. A. (2003). Body image and strategies to lose weight and increase muscle among boys and girls. *Health Psychology, 22,* 39–46.

McCaffrey, A. M., Eisenberg, D. M., Legedza, A. T. R., Davis, R. B., & Phillips, R. S. (2004). Prayer for health concerns: Results of a national survey on prevalence and patterns of use. *Archives of Internal Medicine, 164,* 858–862.

McCallie, M. S., Blum, C. M., & Hood, C. J. (2006). Progressive muscle relaxation. *Journal of Human Behavior in the Social Environment, 13,* 51–66.

McClenahan, C., Shevlin, M., Adamson, G., Bennett, C., & O'Neil, B. (2007). Testicular self-examination: A test of the health belief model and the theory of planned behaviour. *Health Education Research, 22*, 272–284.

McColl, K. E. L., Watabe, H., & Derakhshan, M. H. (2007). Sporadic gastric cancer: A complex interaction of genetic and environmental risk factors. *American Journal of Gastroenterology, 102*, 1893–1895.

McCollum, S. (2003). Living with HIV. *Scholastic Choices, 18*, 6–9.

McCrae, R. R., & Costa, P. T., Jr. (2003). *Personality in adulthood: A five-factor theory perspective* (2nd ed.). New York: Guilford Press.

McCullough, M. E., Hoyt, W. T., Larson, D. S., Koenig, H. G., & Thoresen, C. (2000). Religious involvement and mortality: A meta-analytic review. *Health Psychology, 19*, 211–222.

McDaniel, S. H., Belar, C. D., Schroeder, C., Hargrove, D. S., & Freeman, E. L. (2002). A training curriculum for professional psychologists in primary care. *Professional Psychology: Research and Practice, 33*, 65–72.

McDaniel, S. H., & le Roux, P. (2007). An overview of primary care family psychology. *Journal of Clinical Psychology in Medical Settings, 14*, 23–32.

McEwen, A., West, R., & McRobbie, H. (2008). Motives for smoking and their correlates in clients attending Stop Smoking treatment services. *Nicotine and Tobacco Research, 10*, 843–850.

McEwen, B. S. (2005). Stressed or stressed out: What is the difference? *Journal of Psychiatry and Neuroscience, 30*, 315–318.

McGee, D. L. (2005). Body mass index and mortality: A meta-analysis based on person-level data from twenty-six observational studies. *Annals of Epidemiology, 15*, 87–97.

McGilley, B. M., & Pryor, T. L. (1998). Assessment and treatment of bulimia nervosa. *American Family Physician, 57*, 2743–2750.

McGuire, B. E., & Shores, E. A. (2001). Simulated pain on the Symptom Checklist 90–Revised. *Journal of Clinical Psychology, 57*, 1589–1596.

McHorney, C. A., Schousboe, J. T., Cline, R. R., & Weiss, T. W. (2007). The impact of osteoporosis medication beliefs and side-effect experiences on non-adherence to oral bisphosphonates. *Current Medical Research and Opinion, 23*, 3137–3152.

McHugh, M. D. (2007). Readiness for change and short-term outcomes of female adolescents in residential treatment for anorexia nervosa. *International Journal of Eating Disorders, 40*, 602–612.

McKay, D., & Schare, M. L. (1999). The effects of alcohol and alcohol expectancies on subjective reports and physiological reactivity: A meta-analysis. *Addictive Behaviors, 24*, 633–647.

McKechnie, R., Macleod, R., & Keeling, S. (2007). Facing uncertainty: The lived experience of palliative care. *Palliative and Supportive Care, 5*, 367–376.

McKenzie, K. (2003). Racism and health. *British Medical Journal, 326*, 65–66.

McLean, S., Skirboll, L. R., & Pert, C. B. (1985). Comparison of substance P and enkephalin distribution in rat brain: An overview using radioimmunocytochemistry. *Neuroscience, 14*, 837–852.

McLellan, A. T., Lewis, D. C., O'Brien, C. P., & Kleber, H. D. (2000). Drug dependence, a chronic medical illness: Implications for treatment, insurance, and outcomes. *Journal of the American Medical Association, 284*, 1689–1695.

McNally, R. J. (2003). Progress and controversy in the study of posttraumatic stress disorder. *Annual Review of Psychology, 54*, 229–252.

McRae, C., Cherin, E., Tamazaki, T. G., Diem, G., Vo, A. H., Russell, D., et al. (2004). Effects of perceived treatment on quality of life and medical outcomes in a double-blind placebo surgery trial. *Archives of General Psychiatry, 61*, 412–420.

McWilliams, L. A., Goodwin, R. D., & Cox, B. J. (2004). Depression and anxiety associated with three pain conditions: Results from a nationally representative sample. *Pain, 111*, 77–83.

Mechanic, D. (1978). *Medical sociology* (2nd ed.). New York: Free Press.

Meichenbaum, D. (2007). Stress inoculation training: A preventative and treatment approach. In P. M. Lehrer, R. L. Woolfolk, & W. E. Sime (Eds.), *Principles and practices of stress management* (3rd ed., pp. 497–517). New York: Guilford Press.

Meichenbaum, D., & Cameron, R. (1983). Stress inoculation training: Toward a general paradigm for training coping skills. In D. Meichenbaum & M. E. Jaremko (Eds.), *Stress reduction and prevention* (pp. 115–154). New York: Plenum Press.

Meichenbaum, D., & Turk, D. C. (1976). The cognitive-behavioral management of anxiety, anger and pain. In P. O. Davidson (Ed.), *The behavioral management of anxiety, depression, and pain*. New York: Brunner/Mazel.

Melamed, B. G., Kaplan, B., & Fogel, J. (2001). Childhood health issues across the life span. In A. Baum, T. A. Revenson, & J. E. Singer (Eds.), *Handbook of health psychology* (pp. 449–457). Mahwah, NJ: Erlbaum.

Melnyk, B. M., Small, L., Morrison-Breedy, D., Strasser, A., Spath, L., Kreipe, R., et al. (2007). The COPE Healthy Lifestyles TEEN program: Feasibility, preliminary efficacy, and lessons learned from an after school group intervention with overweight adolescents. *Journal of Pediatric Health Care, 21*, 315–322.

Melzack, R. (1973). *The puzzle of pain*. New York: Basic Books.

Melzack, R. (1975). The McGill Pain Questionnaire: Major properties and scoring methods. *Pain, 1*, 277–299.

Melzack, R. (1987). The short-form McGill Pain Questionnaire. *Pain, 30*, 191–197.

Melzack, R. (1992, April). Phantom limbs. *Scientific American, 266*, 120–126.

Melzack, R. (1993). Pain: Past, present and future. *Canadian Journal of Experimental Psychology, 47*, 615–629.

Melzack, R. (2005). Evolution of the neuromatrix theory of pain. *Pain Practice, 5*, 85–94.

Melzack, R., & Katz, J. (2001). The McGill Pain Questionnaire: Appraisal and current status. In D. C. Turk & R. Melzack (Eds.), *Handbook of pain assessment* (2nd ed., pp. 35–52). New York: Guilford Press.

Melzack, R., & Wall, P. D. (1965). Pain mechanisms: A new theory. *Science, 150*, 971–979.

Melzack, R., & Wall, P. D. (1982). *The challenge of pain.* New York: Basic Books.

Melzack, R., & Wall, P. D. (1988). *The challenge of pain* (Rev. ed.). London: Penguin.

Menckeberg, T. T., Bouvy, M. L., Bracke, M., Kaptein, A. A., Leufkens, H. G., Raaijmakers, J. A. M., et al. (2008). Beliefs about medicines predict refill adherence to inhaled corticosteroids. *Journal of Psychosomatic Research, 64*, 47–54.

Mercer, J. G. J., & Archer, Z. A. (2008). Putting the diet back into diet-induced obesity: Diet-induced hypothalamic gene expression. *European Journal of Pharmacology, 585*, 31–37.

Mercken, L., Candel, M., Willems, P., & de Vries, H. (2007). Disentangling social selection and social influence effects on adolescent smoking: The importance of reciprocity in friendships. *Addiction, 102*, 1483–1492.

Merritt, M. M., Bennett, G. G., Williams, R. B., Sollers, J. J., III, & Thayer, J. F. (2004). Low educational attainment, John Henryism, and cardiovascular reactivity to and recovery from personally relevant stress. *Psychosomatic Medicine, 66*, 49–55.

Metro. (2007, February 19). *Gwyneth reveals cancer curse.* Retrieved June 12, 2008, from http://www.metro.co.uk/fame/article.html?in_article_id=37928&in_page_id=7&in_a_source=

Metropolitan Life Foundation. (1983). Metropolitan height and weight tables. *Statistical Bulletin, 64*(1), 2–9.

Metropolitan Life Insurance Company. (1959). New weight standards for men and women. *Statistical Bulletin, 40*, 1.

Meyer, D., Leventhal, H., & Gutman, M. (1985). Commonsense models of illness: The example of hypertension. *Health Psychology, 4*, 115–135.

Michael, K. C., Torres, A., & Seemann, E. A. (2007). Adolescents' health habits, coping styles and self-concept are predicted by exposure to interparental conflict. *Journal of Divorce and Remarriage, 48*, 155–174.

Michaud, D. S. (2007). Chronic inflammation and bladder cancer. *Urologic Oncology, 25*, 260–268.

Michie, S., O'Connor, D., Bath, J., Giles, M., & Earll, L. (2005). Cardiac rehabilitation: The psychological changes that predict health outcome and healthy behaviour. *Psychology, Health and Medicine, 10*, 88–95.

Milam, J. E. (2004). Posttraumatic growth among HIV/AIDS patients. *Journal of Applied Social Psychology, 34*, 2353–2376.

Miles, L. (2007). Physical activity and the prevention of cancer: A review of recent findings. *Nutrition Bulletin, 32*, 250–282.

Miligi, L., Costantini, A. S., Veraldi, A., Benvenuti, A., & Vineis, P. (2006). Cancer and pesticides. *Annals of the New York Academy of Sciences, 1076*, 366–377.

Millen, J. A., & Bray, S. R. (2008). Self-efficacy and adherence to exercise during and as a follow-up to cardiac rehabilitation. *Journal of Applied Social Psychology, 38*, 2072–2087.

Miller, D. B., & Townsend, A. (2005). Urban hassles as chronic stressors and adolescent mental health: The Urban Hassles Index. *Brief Treatment and Crisis Intervention, 5*, 85–94.

Miller, F. G., & Wager, T. (2004). Painful deception. *Science, 304*, 1109–1111.

Miller, G. E., & Blackwell, E. (2006). Turning up the heat: Inflammation as a mechanism linking chronic stress, depression, and heart disease. *Current Directions in Psychological Science, 15*, 269–272.

Miller, G. E., & Cohen, S. (2001). Psychological interventions and the immune system: A meta-analytic review and critique. *Health Psychology, 20*, 47–63.

Miller, L. G., Liu, H., Hays, R. D., Golin, C. E., Beck, C. K., Asch, S. M., et al. (2002). How well do clinicians estimate patients' adherence to combination antiretroviral therapy? *Journal of General Internal Medicine, 17*, 1–11.

Miller, M., Hemenway, D., & Rimm, E. (2000). Cigarettes and suicide: A prospective study of 50,000 men. *American Journal of Public Health, 90*, 768–773.

Miller, N. E. (1969). Learning of visceral and glandular responses. *Science, 163*, 434–445.

Miller, V. A., & Drotar, D. (2003). Discrepancies between mother and adolescent perceptions of diabetes-related decision-making autonomy and their relationship to diabetes-related conflict and adherence to treatment. *Journal of Pediatric Psychology, 28*, 265–274.

Miller, W. R., & Rollnick, S. (2002). *Motivational interviewing: Preparing people for change* (2nd ed.). New York: Guilford Press.

Miller, W. R., Walters, S. T., & Bennett, M. E. (2001). How effective is alcoholism treatment in the United States? *Journal of Studies on Alcohol, 62*, 211–220.

Miller, W. R., Wilbourne, P. L., & Hettema, J. E. (2003). What works? A summary of alcohol treatment outcome research. In R. K. Hester & W. R. Miller (Eds.), *Handbook of alcoholism treatment approaches: Effective alternatives* (3rd ed., pp. 13–63). Boston: Allyn and Bacon.

Milling, L. S., Kirsch, I., Allen, G. J., & Reutenauer, E. L. (2005). The effects of hypnotic and nonhypnotic imaginative suggestion on pain. *Annals of Behavioral Medicine, 29*, 116–127.

Milling, L. S., Levine, M. R., & Meunier, S. A. (2003). Hypnotic enhancement of cognitive-behavioral interventions for pain: An analogue treatment study. *Health Psychology, 22*, 406–413.

Mills, N., Allen, J., & Morgan, S. C. (2000). Does tai chi/qi gong help patients with multiple sclerosis? *Journal of Bodywork and Movement Therapies, 4*, 39–48.

Milton, B., Cook, P. A., Dugdill, L., Porcellato, L., Springett, J., & Woods, S. E. (2004). Why do primary school children smoke? A longitudinal analysis of predictors of smoking uptake during pre-adolescence. *Public Health, 118*, 247–255.

Mitchell, J. E., & Selders, A. (2005). Recent treatment research in bulimia nervosa. *Eating Disorders Review, 16*(1), 1–3.

Mitchell, M., Johnston, L., & Keppell, M. (2004). Preparing children and their families for hospitalization: A review of the literature. *Paediatric and Child Health Nursing, 7*(2), 5–15.

Mitchell, W. (2001). Neurological and developmental effects of HIV and AIDS in children and adolescents. *Mental Retardation and Developmental Disabilities Research Reviews, 7,* 211–216.

Miyazaki, T., Ishikawa, T., Iimori, H., Miki, A., Wenner, M., Fukunishi, I., et al. (2003). Relationship between perceived social support and immune function. *Stress and Health, 19,* 3–7.

Moen, P., & Yu, Y. (2000). Effective work/life strategies: Working couples, work conditions, gender, and life quality. *Social Problems, 47,* 291–326.

Moerman, D. (2003). Doctors and patients: The role of clinicians in the placebo effect. *Advances, 19*(1), 14–22.

Moerman, D., & Jonas, W. B. (2002). Deconstructing the placebo effect and finding the meaning response. *Annals of Internal Medicine, 136,* 471–476.

Molimard, M., & Le Gros, V. (2008). Impact of patient-related factors on asthma control. *Journal of Asthma, 45,* 109–113.

Monahan, J. L., & Lannutti, P. J. (2000). Alcohol as social lubricant. *Human Communication Research, 26,* 175–202.

Mongan, J. J., Ferris, T. G., & Lee, T. H. (2008). Options for slowing the growth of health care costs. *New England Journal of Medicine, 358,* 1509–1514.

Monroe, S. M., & Harkness, K. L. (2005). Life stress, the "kindling" hypothesis, and the recurrence of depression: Considerations from a life stress perspective. *Psychological Review, 112,* 417–445.

Monteleone, P., DiLieto, A., Castaldo, E., & Maj, M. (2004). Leptin functioning in eating disorders. *CNS Spectrums, 9,* 523–529.

Montgomery, G. H., DuHamel, K. N., & Redd, W. H. (2000). A meta-analysis of hypnotically induced analgesia: How effective is hypnosis? *International Journal of Clinical and Experimental Hypnosis, 48,* 138–153.

Montgomery, G. H., Erblich, J., DiLorenzo, T., & Bovbjerg, D. H. (2003). Family and friends with disease: Their impact on perceived risk. *Preventive Medicine, 37,* 242–249.

Montpetit, M. A., & Bergeman, C. S. (2007). Dimensions of control: Mediational analyses of the stress-health relationship. *Personality and Individual Differences, 43,* 2237–2248.

Moore, J. (2004). The puzzling origins of AIDS. *American Scientist, 92,* 540–547.

Moore, L. L., Visioni, A. J., Qureshi, M. M., Bradlee, M. L., Ellison, R. C., & D'Agostino, R. (2005). Weight loss in overweight adults and the long-term risk of hypertension: The Framingham Study. *Archives of Internal Medicine, 165,* 1298–1303.

Moore, S., Sikora, P., Grunberg, L., & Greenberg, E. (2007). Expanding the tension-reduction model of work stess and alcohol use: Comparison of managerial and non-managerial men and women. *Journal of Management Studies, 44,* 261–283.

Moos, R. H., & Schaefer, J. A. (1984). The crisis of physical illness: An overview and conceptual analysis. In R. H. Moos (Ed.), *Coping with physical illness: Vol. 2. New perspectives* (pp. 3–25). New York: Plenum Press.

Moran, W. R. (2002, January 31). Jackie Joyner-Kersee races against asthma. *USA Today Health.* Retrieved July 7, 2005, from http://www.usatoday.com/news/health/spotlight/2002/01/31/spotlight-kersee.htm

Mørch, L. S., Johansen, D., Løkkegaard, E., Hundrup, Y. A., & Grønbæk, M. (2008). Drinking pattern and mortality in Danish nurses. *European Journal of Clinical Nutrition, 62,* 817–822.

Morgan, W. P. (1979, February). Negative addiction in runners. *The Physician and Sportsmedicine, 7,* 56–63, 67–70.

Morgan, W. P. (1981). Psychological benefits of physical activity. In F. J. Nagle & H. J. Montoye (Eds.), *Exercise in health and disease.* Springfield, IL: Thomas.

Morgan, W. P. (2001). Prescription of physical activity: A paradigm shift. *Quest, 53,* 366–382.

Morillo, L. E., Alarcon, F., Aranaga, N., Aulet, S., Chapman, E., Conterno, L., et al. (2005). Prevalence of migraine in Latin America. *Headache, 45,* 106–117.

Morley, S., de C. Williams, A. C., & Black, S. (2002). A confirmatory factor analysis of the Beck Depression Inventory in chronic pain. *Pain, 99,* 289–298.

Morris, J. C., Storandt, M., Miller, J. P., McKeel, D. W., Price, J. L., Rubin, E. H., et al. (2001). Mild cognitive impairement represents early-stage Alzheimer disease. *Archives of Neurology, 58,* 397–405.

Morris, J. N., Heady, J. A., Raffle, P. A. B., Roberts, C. G., & Parks, J. W. (1953). Coronary heart disease and physical activity of work. *Lancet, 2,* 1053–1057, 1111–1120.

Morrison, C. D. (2008). Leptin resistance and the response to positive energy balance. *Physiology and Behavior, 94,* 660–663.

Morton, J. (2005). Ecstasy: Pharmacology and neurotoxicity. *Current Opinion in Pharmacology, 5,* 79–86.

Morton, S. (2004, November 1). Rare disease makes girl unable to feel pain. Retrieved February 14, 2005, from http://www.msnbc.msn.com/id/6379795/

Moseley, J. B., O'Malley, K. P., Petersen, N. J., Menke, T. J., Brody, B. A., Kuykendall, D. H., et al. (2002). A controlled trial of arthroscopic surgery for osteoarthritis of the knee. *New England Journal of Medicine, 347,* 81–88.

Moskowitz, J. T (2003). Positive affect predicts lower risk of AIDS mortality. *Psychosomatic Medicine, 65,* 620–626.

Moskowitz, J. T., & Wrubel, J. (2005). Coping with HIV as a chronic illness: A longitudinal analysis of illness appraisals. *Psychology and Health, 20,* 509–531.

Mosquera, J. (2008)). Integrative medicine: History, overview, and applications to pain management. In J. F. Audette & A. Bailey (Eds.), *Integrative pain* medicine: The science and practice of complementary and alternative medicine in pain management (pp. 547–570). Totowa, NJ: Humana Press.

Motivala, S. J., & Irwin, M. R. (2007). Sleep and immunity: Cytokine pathways linking sleep and health outcomes. *Current Directions in Psychological Science, 16*, 21–25.

Moyer, C. A., Rounds, J., & Hannum, J. W. (2004). Meta-analysis of massage therapy research. *Psychological Bulletin, 130*, 3–18.

Mozaffarian, D., Longstreth, W. T., Lemaitre, R. N., Manolio, T. A., Kuller, L. H., Burke, G. L., et al. (2005). Fish consumption and stroke risk in elderly individuals: The Cardiovascular Health Study. *Archives of Internal Medicine, 165*, 200–206.

Mukamal, K. J., Conigrave, K. M., Mittleman, M. A., Camargo, C. A., Jr., Stampfer, M. J., Willett, W. C., et al. (2003). Roles of drinking pattern and type of alcohol consumed in coronary heart disease in men. *New England Journal of Medicine, 348*, 109–118.

Mukamal, K. J., Jensen, M. K., Grønbaek, M., Stampfer, M. J., Manson, J. E., Pischon, T., et al. (2005). Drinking frequency, mediating biomarkers, and risk of myocardial infarction in women and men. *Circulation, 112*, 1406–1413.

Mulder, C. L., van Griensven, G. J. P., Sandfort, T. G. M., de Vroome, E. M. M., & Antoni, M. H. (1999). Avoidance as a predictor of the biological course of HIV infection over a 7-year period in gay men. *Health Psychology, 18*, 107–113.

Mullen, J. (2004). Investigating factors that influence individual safety behavior at work. *Journal of Safety Research, 35*, 275–285.

Munaf, M. R., & Johnstone, E. C. (2008). Genes and cigarette smoking. *Addiction, 103*, 893–904.

Murphy, J. K., Stoney, C. M., Alpert, B. S., & Walker, S. S. (1995). Gender and ethnicity in children's cardiovascular reactivity: 7 years of study. *Health Psychology, 14*, 48–55.

Murphy, M. H., Nevill, A. M., Murtagh, E. M., & Holder, R. L. (2007). The effect of walking on fitness, fatness and resting blood pressure: A meta-analysis of randomized, controlled trials. *Preventive Medicine, 44*, 377–385.

Murray, J. A. (2001). Loss as a universal concept: A review of the literature to identify common aspects of loss in diverse situations. *Journal of Loss and Trauma, 6*, 219–231.

Murray, R. P., Connett, J. E., Tyas, S. L., Bond, R., Ekuma, O., Silversides, C. K., et al. (2002). Alcohol volume, drinking pattern, and cardiovascular disease morbidity and mortality: Is there a U-shaped function? *American Journal of Epidemiology, 155*, 242–248.

Murtaugh, M. A. (2004). Meat consumption and the risk of colon and rectal cancers. *Clinical Nutrition, 13*, 61–64.

Must, A., Spadano, J., Coakley, E. H., Field, A. E., Colditz, G., & Dietz, W. H. (1999). The disease burden associated with overweight and obesity. *Journal of the American Medical Association, 282*, 1523–1529.

Mustard, T. R., & Harris, A. V. E. (1989). Problems in understanding prescription labels. *Perceptual and Motor Skills, 69*, 291–299.

Muthen, B. O., & Muthen, L. K. (2000). The development of heavy drinking and alcohol-related problems from ages 18 to 37 in a U.S. national sample. *Journal of Studies on Alcohol, 61*, 290–300.

Myers, J. (2000). Physical activity and cardiovascular disease. *IDEA Health and Fitness Source, 18*, 38–45.

Myers, S. B., Bensoussan, A., O'Connor, J., Paul-Brent, P.-A., Baker, D., Wohlmuth, et al. (2006). A review of reviews of the benefits of naturopathy and Western herbal medicine. In V. Lin et al. (Eds.), *The practice and regulatory requirements of naturopathy and Western herbal medicine* (pp. 68–96). Bundoora, Victoria: School of Public Health, La Trobe University.

Myers, T. C., Wonderlich, S. A., Crosby, R., Mitchell, J. E., Steffen, K. J., Smyth, J., et al. (2006). Is multi-impulsive bulimia a distinct type of bulimia nervosa: Psychopathology and EMA findings. *International Journal of Eating Disorders, 39*, 655–661.

Naimi, T. S., Brown, D. W., Brewer, R. D., Giles, W. H., Mensah, G., Serdula, M. K., et al. (2005). Cardiovascular risk factors and confounders among nondrinking and moderate-drinking U.S. adults. *American Journal of Preventive Medicine, 28*, 369–373.

Napadow, V., Kettner, N., Liu, J., Li, M., Kwong, K. K., Vangel, M., et al. (2007). Hypothalamus and amygdala response to acupuncture stimuli in carpal tunnel syndrome. *Pain, 130*, 254–266.

Naparstek, B. (2007). Guided imagery: A best practice for pregnancy and childbirth. *Journal of Childbirth Education, 22*, 4–8.

Nash, J. M., Park, E. R., Walker, B. B., Gordon, N., & Nicholson, R. A. (2004). Cognitive-behavioral group treatment for disabling headache. *Pain Medicine, 5*, 178–186.

Nash, J. M., & Thebarge, R. W. (2006). Understanding psychological stress, its biological processes, and impact on primary headache. *Headache, 46*, 1377–1386.

Nassiri, M. (2005). The effects of regular relaxation on perceived stress in a group of London primary education teachers. *European Journal of Clinical Hypnosis, 6*, 21–29.

National Association for Sport and Physical Education (NASPE). (2002). *Guidelines for infants and toddlers.* Retrieved August 5, 2002, from www.aahperd.org/naspe/template.cfm?template=toddlers.html

National Center for Complementary and Alternative Medicine (NCCAM). (2002). *What is complementary and alternative medicine?* NCCAM Publication No. D156. Retrieved June 3, 2005, from http://nccam.nih.gov/health/whatiscam/

National Center for Complementary and Alternative Medicine (NCCAM). (2004a). *Manipulative and body-based practices: An overview.* NCCAM Publication No. D238. Retrieved June 3, 2005, from http://nccam.nih.gov/health/backgrounds/manipulative.htm

National Center for Complementary and Alternative Medicine (NCCAM). (2004b). *Mind–body medicine.* Bethesda, MD: Author.

National Center for Complementary and Alternative Medicine (NCCAM). (2004c). *Questions and answers about homeopathy.* Bethesda, MD: Author.

National Center for Complementary and Alternative Medicine (NCCAM). (2004d). *Whole medical systems: An overview.* Bethesda, MD: Author.

National Center for Complementary and Alternative Medicine (NCCAM). (2005). *What is Ayurvedic medicine?* Bethesda, MD: Author.

National Center for Complementary and Alternative Medicine (NCCAM). (2006a). *Massage therapy as CAM.* Bethesda, MD: Author.

National Center for Complementary and Alternative Medicine (NCCAM). (2006b). *Meditation for health purposes.* Bethesda, MD: Author.

National Center for Complementary and Alternative Medicine (NCCAM). (2006c). *Paying for CAM treatment.* Bethesda, MD: Author.

National Center for Complementary and Alternative Medicine (NCCAM). (2006d). *Tai chi for health purposes.* Bethesda, MD: Author.

National Center for Complementary and Alternative Medicine (NCCAM). (2007a). *Biologically based practices: An overview.* Bethesda, MD: Author.

National Center for Complementary and Alternative Medicine (NCCAM). (2007b). *Energy medicine: An overview.* Bethesda, MD: Author.

National Center for Complementary and Alternative Medicine (NCCAM). (2007c). *An introduction to acupuncture.* Bethesda, MD: Author.

National Center for Complementary and Alternative Medicine (NCCAM). (2007d). *An introduction to chiropractic.* Bethesda, MD: Author.

National Center for Complementary and Alternative Medicine (NCCAM). (2007e). *An introduction to naturopathy.* Bethesda, MD: Author.

National Center for Health Statistics (NCHS). (2007). *Health, United States, 2007.* Hyattsville, MD: U.S. Government Printing Office.

National Research Council. (2003). *The polygraph and lie detection.* Washington, DC: National Academies Press. Retrieved August 7, 2004, from http://www.nap.edu/execsumm/0309084369.html

National Task Force on the Prevention and Treatment of Obesity. (2000). Overweight, obesity, and health risk. *Archives of Internal Medicine, 160,* 898–904.

Nayak, M. B., & Kaskutas, L. A. (2004). Risky drinking and alcohol use patterns in a national sample of women of childbearing age. *Addiction, 99,* 1393–1402.

Naylor, R. T., & Marshall, J. (2007). Autogenic training: A key component in holistic medical practice. *Journal of Holistic Healthcare, 4,* 14–19.

Nedrow, A. R., Istvan, J., Haas, M., Barrett, R., Salveson, C., Moore, G., Hammerschlag, R., et al. (2007). Implications for education in complementary and alternative

medicine: A survey of entry attitudes in students at five health professional schools. *Journal of Alternative and Complementary Medicine, 13,* 381–386.

Nelson, H. D., Nevitt, M. C., Scott, J. C., Stone, K. L., & Cummings, S. R. (1994). Smoking, alcohol, and neuromuscular and physical functioning of older women. *Journal of the American Medical Association, 272,* 1825–1831.

Nelson, L. D., & Morrison, E. L. (2005). The symptoms of resource scarcity: Judgments of food and finances influence preferences for potential partners. *Psychological Science, 16,* 167–173.

Nelson, R. (2003). Decade of pain control and research gets into gear in USA. *Lancet, 362,* 1129.

Nemeroff, C. J. (1995). Magical thinking about illness virulence: Conceptions of germs from "safe" versus "dangerous" others. *Health Psychology, 14,* 147–151.

Nestler, E. J., & Malenka, R. C. (2004, March). The addicted brain. *Scientific American, 290,* 78–85.

Nestoriuc, Y., & Martin, A. (2007). Efficacy of biofeedback for migraine: A meta-analysis. *Pain, 128,* 111–127.

Netz, Y., Wu, M.-J., Becker, B. J., & Tenenbaum, G. (2005). Physical activity and psychological well-being in advanced age: A meta-analysis of intervention studies. *Psychology and Aging, 20,* 272–284.

Neumark-Sztainer, D. R., Wall, M. M., Haines, J. I., Story, M. T., Sherwood, N. E. & van den Berg, P. A. (2007). Shared risk and protective factors for overweight and disordered eating in adolescents. *American Journal of Preventive Medicine, 33,* 359–369.

Neumark-Sztainer, D. R., Wall, M. M., Story, M., & Perry, C. L. (2003). Correlates of unhealthy weight-control behaviors among adolescents: Implications for prevention programs. *Health Psychology, 22,* 88–98.

Ng, J. Y. Y., & Tam, S. F. (2000). Effects of exercise-based cardiac rehabilitation on mobility and self-esteem after cardiac surgery. *Perceptual and Motor Skills, 91,* 107–114.

Ng, M. K. C. (2007). New perspectives on Mars and Venus: Unravelling the role of androgens in gender differences in cardiovascular biology and disease. *Heart, Lung and Circulation, 16,* 185–192.

Nicassio, P. M., Meyerowitz, B. E., & Kerns, R. D. (2004). The future of health psychology interventions. *Health Psychology, 23,* 132–137.

Nicoll, R. A., & Alger, B. E. (2004, December). The brain's own marijuana. *Scientific American, 291,* 68–75.

Nied, R. J., & Franklin, B. (2002). Promoting and prescribing exercise for the elderly. *American Family Physician, 65,* 419–426, 427–428.

Nielsen, T. S., & Hansen, K. B. (2007). Do green areas affect health? Results from a Danish survey of the use of green areas and health indicators. *Health and Place, 13,* 839–850.

Nikendei, C., Weisbrod, M., Schild, S., Bender, S., Walther, S., Herzog, W. (2008). Anorexia nervosa: Selective processing of food-related word and pictoral stimuli in recognition and free recall tests. *International Journal of Eating Disorders, 41,* 439–447.

Nikiforov, S. V., & Mamaev, V. B. (1998). The development of sex differences in cardiovascular disease mortality: A historical perspective. *American Journal of Public Health, 88,* 1345–1353.

Nivision, M. E., & Endresen, I. M. (1993). An analysis of relationships among environmental noise, annoyance and sensitivity to noise, and the consequences for health and sleep. *Journal of Behavior Medicine, 16,* 257–276.

Nordström, A., Karlsson, C., Nyquist, F., Olsson, T., Nordström, P., & Karlsson, M. (2005). Bone loss and fracture risk after reduced physical activity. *Journal of Bone and Mineral Research, 20,* 202–207.

Nordstrom, B. L., Kinnunen. T., Utman, C. H., Krall, E. A., Vokanas, P. S., & Garvey, A. J. (2000). Predictors of continued smoking over 25 years of follow-up in the Normative Aging Study. *American Journal of Public Health, 90,* 404–406.

Nori Janosz, K. E., Koenig Berris, K. A., Leff, C., Miller, W. M., Yanez, J., Myers, S., et al. (2008). Clinical resolution of Type 2 diabetes with reduction in body mass index using meal replacement based weight loss. *Vascular Disease Prevention, 5,* 17–23.

Norris, F. H., Byrne, C. M., Diaz, E., & Kaniasty, K. (2001). *The range, magnitude, and duration of effects of natural and human-caused disasters: A review of the empirical literature.* Boston: National Center for PTSD.

North, C. S., Nixon, S. J., Shariat, S., Mallonee, S., McMillen, J. C., Spitznagel, E. L., et al. (1999). Psychiatric disorders among survivors of the Oklahoma City bombing. *Journal of the American Medical Association, 282,* 755–762.

Novack, D. H., Cameron, O., Epel, E., Ader, R., Waldstein, S. R., Levenstein, S., et al. (2007). Psychosomatic medicine: The scientific foundation of the biopsychosocial model. *Academic Psychiatry, 31,* 388–401.

Novins, D. K., Beals, J., Moore, L. A., Spicer, P., & Manson, S. M. (2004). Use of biomedical services and traditional healing options among American Indians: Sociodemographic correlates, spirituality, and ethnic identity. *Medical Care, 42,* 670–679.

O'Brien, K. M., & LeBow, M. D. (2007). Reducing maladaptive weight management practices: Developing a psychoeducational intervention program. *Eating Behaviors, 8,* 195–210.

O'Cleirigh, C., Ironson, G., Weiss, A., & Costa, P. T., Jr. (2007). Conscientiousness predicts disease progression (CD4 number and viral load) in people living with HIV. *Health Psychology, 26,* 473–480.

O'Connor, D. B., & Shimizu, M. (2002). Sense of personal control, stress and coping style: A cross-cultural study. *Stress and Health: Journal of the International Society for the Investigation of Stress, 18,* 173–183.

O'Connor, R. J., McNeill, A., Borland, R., Hammond, D., King, B., Boudreau, C., et al. (2007). Smokers' beliefs about the relative safety of other tobacco products: Findings from the ITC collaboration. *Nicotine and Tobacco Research, 9,* 1033–1042.

Ogden, J. (2003). Some problems with social cognition models: A pragmatic and conceptual analysis. *Health Psychology, 22,* 424–428.

Ogedegbe, G., Schoenthaler, A., & Fernandez, S. (2007). Appointment-keeping behavior is not related to medication adherence in hypertensive African Americans. *Journal of General Internal Medicine, 22,* 1176–1179.

Oguma, Y., Sesso, H. D., Paffenbarger, R. S., Jr., & Lee, I.-M. (2002). Physical activity and all cause mortality in women: A review of the evidence. *British Journal of Sports Medicine, 36,* 162–172.

Oh, Y.-M., Kim, Y. S., Yoo, S. H., Kim, S. K., & Kim, D. S. (2004). Association between stress and asthma symptoms: A population-based study. *Respirology, 9,* 363–368.

O'Hara, P., Connett, J. E., Wee, W. W., Nides, M., Murray, R., & Wise, R. (1998). Early and late weight gain following smoking cessation in the Lung Health Study. *American Journal of Epidemiology, 148,* 821–830.

O'Hare, P. (2007). Merseyside, the first harm reduction conferences, and the early history of harm reduction. *International Journal of Drug Policy, 18,* 141–144.

Okada, S., Hori, N., Kimoto, K., Onozuka, M., Sato, S., & Sasaguri, K. (2007). Effects of biting on elevation of blood pressure and other physiological responses to stress in rats: Biting may reduce allostatic load. *Brain Research, 1185,* 189–194.

Okuda, M., & Nakazawa, T. (2004). *Helicobacter pylori* infection in childhood. *Journal of Gastroenterology, 39,* 809–810.

Oldenburg, R. A., Meijers-Heijboer, H., Cornelisse, C. J., & Devilee, P. (2007). Genetic susceptibility for breast cancer: How many more genes to be found? *Critical Reviews in Oncology/Hematology, 63,* 125–149.

Olesen, J. (1988). Classification and diagnostic criteria for headache disorders, cranial neuralgias, and facial pain: Headache Classification Committee of the International Headache Society [Special issue]. *Cephalalgia, 8*(Suppl. 7).

Olivardia, R., Pope, H. G., & Phillips, K. A. (2000). *The Adonis complex: The secret crisis of male body obsession.* New York: Free Press.

Olsen, R., & Sutton, J. (1998). More hassle, more alone: Adolescents with diabetes and the role of formal and informal support. *Child Care, Health and Development, 24,* 31–39.

Olsen treated for eating disorder. (2004, June 23). *CBS News.* Retrieved July 18, 2005, from http://www.cbsnews.com/stories/2004/06/22/earlyshow/leisure/celebspot/main625389.shtml

Olver, I. N., Taylor, A. E., & Whitford, H. S. (2005). Relationships between patients' pre-treatment expectations of toxicities and post chemotherapy experiences. *Psycho-Oncology, 14,* 25–33.

Oman, D., & Thoresen, C. E. (2002). "Does religion cause health?" Differing interpretations and diverse meanings. *Journal of Health Psychology, 7,* 365–380.

Oman, R. F., & King, A. C. (2000). The effect of life events and exercise program on the adoption and maintenance of exercise behavior. *Health Psychology, 19*, 605–612.

Ondeck, D. M. (2003). Impact of culture on pain. *Home Health Care Management and Practice, 15*, 255–257.

Operario, D., Adler, N. E., & Williams, D. R. (2004). Subjective social status: Reliability and predictive utility for global health. *Psychology and Health, 19*, 237–246.

Orford, J., Krishnan, M., Balaam, M., Everitt, M., & van der Graaf, K. (2004). University student drinking: The role of motivational and social factors. *Drugs: Education, Prevention and Policy, 11*, 407–421.

Ornish, D., Brown, S. E., Scherwitz, L. W., Billings, J. H., Armstrong, W. T., Ports, T., et al. (1990). Can lifestyle changes reverse coronary heart disease? The Lifestyle Heart Trial. *Lancet, 336*, 129–133.

Ornish, D., Scherwitz, L. W., Billings, J. H., Gould, L., Merritt, T. A., Sparler, S., et al. (1998). Intensive lifestyle changes for reversal of coronary heart disease. *Journal of the American Medical Association, 280*, 2001–2007.

Orth-Gomér, K., Wamala, S. P., Horsten, M., Schenck-Gustafsson, K., Scheiderman, N., & Mittleman, M. A. (2000). Marital stress worsens prognosis in women with coronary heart disease: The Stockholm Female Coronary Risk Study. *Journal of the American Medical Association, 284*, 3008–3014.

Ortner, C. N. M., MacDonald, T. K., & Olmstead, M. C. (2003). Alcohol intoxication reduces impulsivity in the delay-discounting paradigm. *Alcohol & Alcoholism, 38*, 151–156.

Osborn, J. W. (2005). Hypothesis: Set-points and long-term control of arterial pressure: A theoretical argument for a long-term arterial pressure control system in the brain rather than the kidney. *Clinical and Experimental Pharmacology and Physiology, 32*, 384–393.

Osborn, R. L., Demoncada, A. C., & Feuerstein, M. (2006). Psychosocial interventions for depression, anxiety, and quality of life in cancer survivors: Meta-analyses. *International Journal of Psychiatry in Medicine, 36*, 13–34.

Osler, M., & Prescott, E. (2003). Educational level as a contextual and proximate determinant of all cause mortality in Danish adults. *Journal of Epidemiology and Community Health, 57*, 266–269.

Ostelo, R. W. J. G., van Tulder, M. W., Vlaeyen, J. W. S., Linton, S. J., Morley, S. J., & Assendelft, W. J. J. (2007). Behavioural treatment for chronic low-back pain. *Cochrane Database of Systematic Reviews*, Cochrane AN: CD002014.

Otchet, F. (1998, Fall). A week in the life of a health psychologist in Canada. *The Health Psychologist, 20*(4), 4–5.

Øystein, K. (2008). A broader perspective on education and mortality: Are we influenced by other people's education? *Social Science and Medicine, 66*, 620–636.

Ozer, E. J. (2005). The impact of violence on urban adolescents: Longitudinal effects of perceived school connection and family support. *Journal of Adolescent Research, 20*, 167–192.

Ozer, E. J., Best, S, R., Lipsey, T. L., & Weiss, D. S. (2003). Predictors of posttraumatic stress disorder and symptoms in adults: A meta-analysis. *Psychological Bulletin, 129*, 52–73.

Paasche-Orlow, M. K., Parker, R. M., Gazmararian, J. A., Nielsen-Bohlman, L. T., & Rudd, R. R. (2005). The prevalence of limited health literacy. *Journal of General Internal Medicine, 20*, 175–184.

Packard, E. (2007). Postgrad growth area: Primary-care psychology. *gradPSYCH, 5*(3), 14–17.

Paffenbarger, R. S., Jr., Gima, A. S., Laughlin, M. E., & Black, R. A. (1971). Characteristics of longshoremen related to fatal coronary heart disease and stroke. *American Journal of Public Health, 61*, 1362–1370.

Paffenbarger, R. S., Jr., Laughlin, M. E., Gima, A. S., & Black, R. A. (1970). Work activity of longshoremen as related to death from coronary heart disease and stroke. *New England Journal of Medicine, 282*, 1109–1114.

Paffenbarger, R. S., Jr., Wing, A. L., & Hyde, R. T. (1978). Physical activity as an index of heart attack risk in college alumni. *American Journal of Epidemiology, 108*, 161–175.

Palm, J. (2004). The nature of and responsibility of alcohol and drug problems: Views among treatment staff. *Addiction Research and Theory, 12*, 413–431.

Palmer, R. F., Katerndahl, D., & Morgan-Kidd, J. (2004). A randomized trial of the effects of remote intercessory prayer: Interactions with personal beliefs on problem-specific outcomes and functional status. *Journal of Alternative and Complementary Medicine, 10*, 438–448.

Palombaro, K. M. (2005). Effects of walking-only interventions on bone mineral density at various skeletal sites: A meta-analysis. *Journal of Geriatric Physical Therapy, 28*(3), 102–107.

Pambianco, G., Costacou, T., & Orchard, T. (2007). The determination of cardiovascular risk factor profiles in Type 1 diabetes. *Diabetes, 56*(Suppl. 1), A176–A177.

Papadaki, A., Hondros, G., Scott, J. A., & Kapsokefalou, M. (2007). Eating habits of university students living at, or away from home in Greece. *Appetite, 49*, 169–176.

Papas, R. K., Belar, C. D., & Rozensky, R. H. (2004). The practice of clinical health psychology: Professional issues. In R. G. Frank, A. Baum, & J. L. Wallander (Eds.), *Handbook of clinical health psychology* (Vol. 3, pp. 293–319). Washington, DC: American Psychological Association.

Parchman, M. L., Noel, P. H., & Lee, S. (2005). Primary care attributes, health care system hassles, and chronic illness. *Medical Care, 43*, 1123–1129.

Park, A., Sher, K. J., & Krull, J. L. (2008). Risky drinking in college changes as fraternity/sorority affiliation changes: A person-environment perspective. *Psychology of Addictive Behaviors, 22*, 219–229.

Park, C. L., & Adler, N. E. (2003). Coping style as a predictor of health and well-being across the first year of medical school. *Health Psychology, 22*, 627–631.

Park, J. (2005). Use of alternative health care. *Health Reports, 16*(2), 39–42.

Parker, C. S., Zhen, C., Price, M., Gross, R., Metlay, J. P., Christie, J. D., et al. (2007). Adherence to warfarin assessed by electronic pill caps, clinician assessment, and patient reports: Results from the IN-RANGE study. *Journal of General Internal Medicine, 22,* 1254–1259.

Parker, R. M., Schaller, J., & Hansmann, S. (2003). Catastrophe, chaos, and complexity models and psychosocial adjustment to disability. *Rehabilitation Counseling Bulletin, 46,* 234–241.

Parrott, D. J., & Zeichner, A. (2002). Effects of alcohol and trait anger on physical aggression in men. *Journal of Studies on Alcohol, 63,* 196–204.

Patel, S. R., Ayas, N. T., Malhotra, M. R., White, D. P., Schemhammer, E. S., Speizer, F. E., et al. (2004). A prospective study of sleep duration and mortality risk in women. *Sleep, 27,* 440–444.

Patterson, D. R., & Jensen, M. P. (2003). Hypnosis and clinical pain. *Psychological Bulletin, 129,* 495–521.

Paul, G., Elam, B., & Verhulst, S. J. (2007). A longitudinal study of students' perceptions of using deep breathing meditation to reduce testing stresses. *Teaching and Learning in Medicine, 19,* 287–292.

Paull, T. T., Cortez, D., Bowers, B., Elledge, S. J., & Gellert, M. (2001). Direct DNA binding by BRCA 1. *Proceedings of the National Academy of Sciences of the United States of America, 98,* 6086–6091.

Pauly, M. V., & Pagán, J. A. (2007). Spillovers and vulnerability: The case of community uninsurance. *Health Affairs, 26,* 1304–1314.

Paun, O., Farran, C. J., Perraud, S., & Loukissa, D. A. (2004). Successful caregiving of persons with Alzheimer's disease. *Alzheimer's Care Quarterly, 5,* 241–251.

Pavlik, V. N., Doody, R. S., Massman, P. J., & Chan, W. (2006). Influence of premorbid IQ and education on progression of Alzheimer's disease. *Dementia and Geriatric Cognitive Disorders, 22,* 367–377.

Pavlin, D. J., Sullivan, M. J. L., Freund, P. R., & Roesen, K. (2005). Catastrophizing: A risk factor for postsurgical pain. *Clinical Journal of Pain, 21,* 83–90.

Paxton, R. J., Valois, R. F., & Drane, J. W. (2004). Correlates of body mass index, weight goals, and weight-management practices among adolescents. *Journal of School Health, 74,* 136–143.

Peay, M. Y., & Peay, E. R. (1998). The evaluation of medical symptoms by patients and doctors. *Journal of Behavioral Medicine, 21,* 57–81.

Peek, M. W., Cargill, A., & Huang, E. S. (2007). Diabetes health disparities: A systematic review of health care interventions. *Medical Care Research and Review, 64*(Suppl.), 101S–156S.

Peele, S. (2002, August 1). Harm reduction in clinical practice. *Counselor: The Magazine for Addiction Professionals,* 28–32.

Peila, R., Rodriguez, B. L., & Launer, L. J. (2002). Type 2 diabetes, APOE gene, and the risk for dementia and related pathologies. *Diabetes, 51,* 1256–1262.

Pelletier, K. R. (2002). Mind as healer, mind as slayer: Mind-body medicine comes of age. *Advances in Mind-Body Medicine, 18,* 4–15.

Penley, J. A., Tomaka, J., & Wiebe, J. S. (2002). The association of coping to physical and psychological health outcomes: A meta-analytic review. *Journal of Behavioral Medicine, 25,* 551–603.

Pennebaker, J. W., Barger, S. D., & Tiebout, J. (1989). Disclosure of traumas and health among Holocaust survivors. *Psychosomatic Medicine, 51,* 577–589.

Pennebaker, J. W., Colder, M., & Sharp, L. K. (1990). Accelerating the coping process. *Journal of Personality and Social Psychology, 58,* 528–537.

Pennebaker, J. W., & Graybeal, A. (2001). Patterns of natural language use: Disclosure, personality, and social integration. *Current Directions in Psychological Science, 10,* 90–93.

Pentz, M. A., Mares, D., Schinke, S., & Rohrbach, L. A. (2004). Political science, public policy, and drug use prevention. *Substance Use and Misuse, 39,* 1821–1865.

Penza-Clyve, S. M., Mansell, C., & McQuaid, E. L. (2004). Why don't children take their asthma medications? A qualitative analysis of children's perspectives on adherence. *Journal of Asthma, 41,* 189–197.

Penzien, D. B., Rains, J. C., & Andrasik, F. (2002). Behavioral management of recurrent headache: Three decades of experience and empiricism. *Applied Psychophysiology and Biofeedback, 27,* 163–181.

Pereira, M. A., Kartashov, A. I., Ebbeling, C. B., Van Horn, L., Slattery, M. L., Jacobs, D. R., Jr., et al. (2005). Fast-food habits, weight gain, and insulin resistance (the CARDIA study): 15-year prospective analysis. *Lancet, 365,* 36–42.

Peres, M. F. P., Mercante, J. P. P., Tanuri, F. C., & Nunes, M. (2006). Chronic migraine prevention with topiramate. *Journal of Headache and Pain, 7,* 185–187.

Peretti-Watel, P., Constance, J., Guilbert, P., Gautier, A., Beck, F., & Moatti, J.-P. (2007). Smoking too few cigarettes to be at risk? Smokers' perceptions of risk and risk denial, a French survey. *Tobacco Control, 16,* 351–356.

Permutt, M. A., Wasson, J., & Cox, N. (2005). Genetic epidemiology of diabetes. *Journal of Clinical Investigation, 115,* 1431–1439.

Perram, S. W. (2006). The results of 47 clinical studies examined in a 30-year period. *American Chiropractor, 28,* 42–44.

Pert, C. B., & Snyder, S. H. (1973). Opiate receptor: Demonstration in nervous tissue. *Science, 179,* 1011–1014.

Pettman, E. (2007). A history of manipulative therapy. *Journal of Manual and Manipulative Therapy, 15,* 165–174.

Phares, V., Steinberg, A. R., & Thompson, J. K. (2004). Gender differences in peer and parental influences: Body image disturbance, self-worth, and psychological functioning in preadolescent children. *Journal of Youth and Adolescence, 33,* 421–429.

Phillips, J. G., & Ogeil, R. P. (2007). Alcohol consumption and computer blackjack. *Journal of General Psychology, 134,* 333–353.

Phipps, E., Braitman, L. E., Stites, S., & Leighton, J. C. (2008). Quality of life and symptom attribution in long-term colon cancer survivors. *Journal of Evaluation in Clinical Practice, 14,* 254–258.

Pho, L., Grossman, D., & Leachman, S. A. (2006). Melanoma genetics: A review of genetic factors and clinical phenotypes in familial melanoma. *Current Opinion in Oncology, 18,* 173–179.

Pickup, J. C., & Renard, E. (2008). Long-acting insulin analogs versus insulin pump therapy for the treatment of Type 1 and Type 2 diabetes. *Diabetes Care, 31*(Suppl.), S140–S145.

Pierce, J. P. (2005). Influence of movie stars on the initiation of adolescent smoking. *Pediatric Dentistry, 27,* 149.

Pierce, J. P., Choi, W. S., Gilpin, E. A., Farkas, A. J., & Berry, C. C. (1998). Tobacco industry promotion of cigarettes and adolescent smoking. *Journal of the American Medical Association, 279,* 511–515.

Pierce, J. P., Distefan, J. M., Kaplan, R. M., & Gilpin, E. A. (2005). The role of curiosity in smoking initiation. *Addictive Behaviors, 30,* 685–696.

Piette, J. D., Heisler, M., Horne, R., & Caleb Alexander, G. (2006). A conceptually based approach to understanding chronically ill patients' responses to medication cost pressures. *Social Science and Medicine, 62,* 846–857.

Pike, K. M., Timothy, B., Vitousek, K., Wilson, G. T., & Bauer, J. (2003). Cognitive behavior therapy in posthospitalization treatment of anorexia nervosa. *American Journal of Psychiatry, 160,* 2046–2049.

Pilkington, K. (2007). Searching for CAM evidence: An evaluation of therapy-specific search strategies. *Journal of Alternative and Complementary Medicine, 13,* 451–460.

Pilote, L., Dasgupta, K., Guru, V., Humphries, K. H., McGrath, J., Norris, C., et al. (2007). A comprehensive view of sex-specific issues related to cardiovascular disease. *Canadian Medical Association Journal, 176*(6), S1–S44.

Pimlott-Kubiak, S., & Cortina, L. M. (2003). Gender, victimization, and outcomes: Reconceptualizing risk. *Journal of Consulting and Clinical Psychology, 71,* 528–539.

Pinel, J. P. J. (2009). *Biopsychology* (7th ed.). Boston: Allyn and Bacon.

Pinel, J. P. J., Assanand, S., & Lehman, D. R. (2000). Hunger, eating, and ill health. *American Psychologist, 55,* 1105–1116.

Pingitore, D., Scheffler, R., Haley, M., Seniell, T., & Schwalm, D. (2001). Professional psychology in a new era: Practice-based evidence from California. *Professional Psychology, Research and Practice, 32,* 585–596.

Piotrowski, C. (1998). Assessment of pain: A survey of practicing clinicians. *Perceptual and Motor Skills, 86,* 181–182.

Piotrowski, C. (2007). Review of the psychological literature on assessment instruments used with pain patients. *North American Journal of Psychology, 9,* 303–306.

Pisinger, C., & Godtfredsen, N. S. (2007). Is there a health benefit of reduced tobacco consumption? A systematic review. *Nicotine and Tobacco Research, 9,* 631–646.

Pisinger, C., & Jorgensen, T. (2007). Weight concerns and smoking in a general population: The Inter99 study. *Preventive Medicine, 44,* 283–289.

Pi-Sunyer, F. X. (2004). The epidemiology of central fat distribution in relation to disease. *Nutrition Reviews, 62,* 120–126.

Pittler, M. H., & Ernst, E. (2008). Is acupuncture an effective treatment for knee osteoarthritis? *Nature Clinical Practice Rheumatology, 4,* 124–125.

Plasqui, G., & Westerterp, K. R. (2007). Physical activity and insulin resistance. *Current Nutrition and Food Science, 3,* 157–160.

Plaut, S. M., & Friedman, S. B. (1981). Psychosocial factors in infectious disease. In R. Ader (Ed.), *Psychoneuroimmunology* (pp. 3–30). New York: Academic Press.

Player, M. S., King, D. E., Mainous, A. G., III, & Geesey, M. E. (2007). Psychosocial factors and progression from prehypertension to hypertension or coronary heart disease. *Annals of Family Medicine, 5,* 403–411.

Pole, N., Best, S. R., Metzler, T., & Marmar, C. R. (2005). Why are Hispanics at greater risk for PTSD? *Cultural Diversity and Mental Health, 11,* 144–161.

Polgar, S., & Ng, J. (2005). Ethics, methodology and the use of placebo controls in surgical trials. *Brain Research Bulletin, 67,* 290–297.

Polich, J. M., Armor, D. J., & Braiker, H. B. (1980). *The course of alcoholism: Four years after treatment.* Santa Monica, CA: Rand.

Polivy, J., Coelho, J., Hargreaves, D., Fleming, A., & Herman, C. P. (2007). The effects of external cues on eating and body weight: Another look at obese humans and rats. *Appetite, 49,* 321.

Polivy, J., & Herman, C. P. (2000). The false-hope syndrome: Unfulfilled expectations of self-change. *Current Directions in Psychological Science, 9,* 128–131.

Polivy, J., & Herman, C. P. (2002). Causes of eating disorders. *Annual Review of Psychology, 53,* 187–214.

Polivy, J., & Herman, C. P. (2004). Sociocultural idealization of thin female body shapes: An introduction to the special issues on body image and eating disorders. *Journal of Social and Clinical Psychology, 23,* 1–6.

Pollard, L. J., & Bates, L. W. (2004). Religion and perceived stress among undergraduates during fall 2000 final examinations. *Psychological Reports, 95,* 999–1006.

Pollock, M. L., Wilmore, J. H., & Fox, S. M., III. (1978). *Health and fitness through physical activity.* New York: Wiley.

Pomerleau, O. F., & Kardia, S. L. R. (1999). Introduction to the features section: Genetic research on smoking. *Health Psychology, 18,* 3–6.

Pool, G. J., Schwegler, A. Fl., Theodore, B. R., & Fuchs, P. N. (2007). Role of gender norms and group identification on hypothetical and experimental pain tolerance. *Pain, 129,* 122–129.

Poole, H., Branwell, R., & Murphy, P. (2006). Factor structure of the Beck Depression Inventory-II in patients with chronic pain. *Clinical Journal of Pain, 22,* 790–798.

Pope, S. K., Shue, V. M., & Beck, C. (2003). Will a healthy lifestyle help prevent Alzheimer's disease? *Annual Review of Public Health, 24,* 111–132.

Popham, R. E. (1978). The social history of the tavern. In Y. Israel, F. B. Glaser, H. Kalant, R. E. Popham, W. Schmidt, & R. G. Smart (Eds.), *Research advances in alcohol and drug problems* (Vol. 2, pp. 225–302). New York: Plenum Press.

Porter, J., & Jick, H. (1980). Addiction rate in patients treated with narcotics. *New England Journal of Medicine, 302,* 123.

Poss, J. E. (2000). Developing a new model for cross-cultural research: Synthesizing the health belief model and the theory of reasoned action. *Advances in Nursing Science, 23,* 1–15.

Poston, W. S. C., Taylor, J. E., Hoffman, K. M., Peterson, A. L., Lando, H. A., Shelton, S., et al. (2008). Smoking and deployment: Perspectives of junior enlisted U.S. Air Force and U.S. Army personnel and their supervisors. *Military Medicine, 173,* 441–447.

Pouchot, J., Le Parc, J.-M., Queffelec, L., Sichère, P., & Flinois, A. (2007). Perceptions in 7700 patients with rheumatoid arthritis compared to their families and physicians. *Joint Bone Spine, 74,* 622–626.

Pouletty, P. (2002). Opinion: Drug addictions: Towards socially accepted and medically treatable diseases. *Nature Reviews Drug Discovery, 1,* 731–736.

Poupard, V. (2007, July 2). *World Health Organization: One billion dead from smoking by century's end.* Retrieved June 3, 2008, from http://www.associatedcontent.com/article/299996/world_health_organization_one_billion.html?cat=5

"Practical Nurse." (2008). Hereditary breast cancer risk overestimated. *Practical Nurse, 35*(9), 9.

Prapavessis, H., Cameron, L., Baldi, J. C., Robinson, S., Borries, K., Harper, T., et al. (2007). The effects of exercise and nicotine replacement therapy on smoking rates in women. *Addictive Behaviors, 32,* 1416–1432.

Preuss, U. W., Schultz, G., Wong, W. M., Watzke, A. B., Barnow, S., & Zimmerman, J. (2004). Current perspectives in genetics and genomics of alcohol dependence. *Current Genomics, 5,* 601–612.

Preventing fatal medical errors. (1999, December 1). *New York Times,* p. A22.

Prince, M. (2004). Care arrangements for people with dementia in developing countries. *International Journal of Geriatric Psychiatry, 19,* 170–177.

Prochaska, J. O., DiClemente, C. C., & Norcross, J. C. (1992). In search of how people change: Applications to addictive behaviors. *American Psychologist, 47,* 1102–1114.

Prochaska, J. O., Norcross, J. C., & DiClemente, C. C. (1994). *Changing for good.* New York: Avon Books.

Psaty, B. M., Anderson, M., Kronmal, R. A., Tracy, R. P., Orchard, T., Fried, L. P., et al. (2004). The association between lipid levels and the risks of incident myocardial infarction, stroke, and total mortality: The Cardiovascular Health Study. *Journal of the American Geriatrics Society, 52,* 1639–1647.

Purslow, L. R., Sandhu, M. S., Forouhi, N., Young, E. H., Luben, R. N., Welch, A. A., et al. (2008). Energy intake at breakfast and weight change: Prospective study of 6,764 middle-aged men and women. *American Journal of Epidemiology, 167,* 188.

Puska, P. (2002). Nutrition and global prevention on non-communicable diseases. *Asia Pacific Journal of Clinical Nutrition, 11*(Suppl. 9), S755–S758.

Puska, P., Vartiainen, E., Tuomilehto, J., Salomaa, V., & Nissinen, A. (1998). Changes in premature death in Finland: Successful long-term prevention of cardiovascular diseases. *Bulletin of the World Health Organization, 76,* 419–425.

Quartana, P. J., Laubmeier, K. K., & Zakowski, S. G. (2006). Psychological adjustment following diagnosis and treatment of cancer: An examination of the moderating role of positive and negative emotional expressivity. *Journal of Behavioral Medicine, 29,* 487–498.

Quinn, J. F., Bodenhamer-Davis, E., & Koch, D. S. (2004). Ideology and the stagnation of AODA treatment modalities in America. *Deviant Behavior, 25,* 109–131.

Quinn, J. R. (2005). Delay in seeking care for symptoms of acute myocardial infarction: Applying a theoretical model. *Research in Nursing and Health, 28,* 283–294.

Quist, M., Rorth, M., Zacho, M., Andersen, C., Moeller, T., Midtgaard, J., et al. (2006). High-intensity resistance and cardiovascular training improve physical capacity in cancer patients undergoing chemotherapy. *Scandinavian Journal of Medicine and Science in Sports, 16,* 349–357.

Qureshi, A. A., Laden, F., Colditz, G. A., & Hunter, D. J. (2008). Geographic variation and risk of skin cancer in US women. *Archives of Internal Medicine, 168,* 501–507.

Rabin, C., Leventhal, H., & Goodin, S. (2004). Conceptualization of disease timeline predicts posttreatment distress in breast cancer patients. *Health Psychology, 23,* 407–412.

Rahim-Williams, F. B., Riley, J. L., III, Herrera, D., Campbell, C. M., Hastie, B. A., & Fillingim, R. B. (2007). Ethnic identity predicts experimental pain sensitivity in African Americans and Hispanics. *Pain, 129,* 177–184.

Rainville, P., & Price, D. D. (2003). Hypnosis phenomenology and the neurobiology of consciousness. *International Journal of Clinical and Experimental Hypnosis, 51*(Special Issue, Pt. 1), 105–129.

Rainwater, D. L., Mitchell, B. D., Gomuzzie, A. G., Vandeberg, J. L., Stein, M. P., & MacCluer, J. W. (2000). Associations among 5-year changes in weight, physical activity, and cardiovascular disease risk factors in Mexican Americans. *American Journal of Epidemiology, 152,* 974–982.

Ramsay, S., Ebrahim, S., Whincup, P., Papacosta, O., Morris, R., Lennon, L., et al. (2008). Social engagement and the risk of cardiovascular disease mortality: Results of a prospective population-based study of older men. *Annals of Epidemiology, 18,* 476–483.

Rapoff, M. A. (2003). Pediatric measures of pain: The Pain Behavior Observation Method, Pain Coping Questionnaire (PCQ), and Pediatric Pain Questionnaire (PPQ). *Arthritis and Rheumatism: Arthritis Care and Research, 49*(5, Suppl.), S90–S91.

Rashidi, A., Mohammadpour-Ahranjani, B., Vafa, M. R., & Karandish, M. (2005). Prevalence of obesity in Iran. *Obesity Reviews, 6,* 191–192.

Raum, E., Rothenbacher, D., Ziegler, H., & Brenner, H. (2007). Heavy physical activity: Risk or protective factor for cardiovascular disease? A life course perspective. *Annals of Epidemiology, 17,* 417–424.

Raymond, J., Pierce, E., Smith, S., Wagner, J. P., Gordon-Thomas, J., & Wirzbicki, A. (2001, April 9). Playing with pain killers. *Newsweek,* 44–47.

Raynor, H. A., & Epstein, L. H. (2001). Dietary variety: Energy regulation and obesity. *Psychological Bulletin, 127,* 325–341.

Rayworth, B. B. (2004). Childhood abuse and risk of eating disorders in women. *Epidemiology, 15,* 271–278.

Read, J. P., Wood, M. D., & Capone, J. C. (2005). A prospective investigation of relations between social influences and alcohol involvement during the transition into college. *Journal of Studies on Alcohol, 66,* 23–34.

Reader, D. M. (2007). Medical nutrition therapy and lifestyle interventions. *Diabetes Care, 30*(Suppl. 2), S188–S193.

Reagan, N. (2000). *I love you Ronnie: The letters of Ronald Reagan to Nancy Reagan.* New York: Random House.

Reed, G. M., & Scheldeman, L. (2004). News. *European Psychologist, 9,* 184–187.

Reeves, J. L., II, Graff-Radford, S. B., & Shipman, D. (2004). The effects of transcutaneous electrical nerve stimulation on experimental pain and sympathetic nervous system response. *Pain Medicine, 5,* 150–161.

Regoeczi, W. C. (2003). When context matters: A multilevel analysis of household and neighbourhood crowding on aggression and withdrawal. *Journal of Environmental Psychology, 23,* 457–470.

Rehm, J., Room, R., Monteiro, M., Gmel, G., Graham, K., Rehn, N., et al. (2003). Alcohol as a risk factor for global burden of disease. *European Addiction Research, 9,* 157–164.

Reich, A., Müller, G., Gelbrich, G., Deutscher, K., Gödicke, R., & Kiess, W. (2003). Obesity and blood pressure—Results from the examination of 2365 schoolchildren in Germany. *International Journal of Obesity, 27,* 1459–1464.

Reiche, E. M. V., Nunes, S. O. V., & Morimoto, H. K. (2004). Stress, depression, the immune system, and cancer. *Lancet Oncology, 5,* 617–625.

Reid, C. M., Gooberman-Hill, R., & Hanks, G. W. (2008). Opioid analgesics for cancer pain: Symptom control for the living or comfort for the dying? A qualitative study to investigate the factors influencing the decision to accept morphine for pain caused by cancer. *Annals of Oncology, 19,* 44.

Reilly, T., & Woo, G. (2004). Social support and maintenance of safer sex practices among people living with HIV/AIDS. *Health and Social Work, 29,* 97–105.

Reitz, C., Tang, M. X., Manly, J., Schupf, N., Mayeaux, R., & Luchsinger, J. A. (2008). Plasma lipid levels in the elderly are not associated with the risk of mild cognitive impairment. *Dementia and Geriatric Cognitive Disorders, 25,* 232–237.

Rentz, C., Krikorian, R., & Keys, M. (2005). Grief and mourning from the perspective of the person with a dementing illness: Beginning the dialogue. *Omega: Journal of Death and Dying, 50,* 165–179.

Renz, H., Blümer, N., Virna, S., Sel, S., & Garn, H. (2006). The immunological basis of the hygiene hypothesis. *Chemical Immunology and Allergy, 91,* 30–48.

Research and Policy Committee. (2002). *A new vision for healthcare: A leadership role for business.* New York: Committee for Economic Development.

Resnicow, K., DiIorio, C., Soet, J. E., Borrelli, B., Hecht, J., & Ernst, D. (2002). Motivational interviewing in health promotion: It sounds like something is changing. *Health Psychology, 21,* 444–451.

Resnicow, K., Jackson, A., Wang, T., Aniridya, K. D., McCarty, F., Dudley, W. N., et al. (2001). A motivational interviewing intervention to increase fruit and vegetable intake through Black churches: Results of the Eat for Life trial. *American Journal of Public Health, 91,* 1686–1693.

Resnik, D. B. (2008). Randomized controlled trials in environmental health research: Ethical issues. *Journal of Environmental Health, 70,* 28–30.

Rethorst, C. D., Wipfli, B. M., & Landers, D. M. (2007). The effect of exercise on depression: Examining clinical significance. *Journal of Sport and Exercise Psychology, 29*(Suppl.), S198.

Reuben, A. (2008). Alcohol and the liver. *Current Opinion in Gastroenterology, 24,* 328–338.

Rhee, Y., Taitel, M. S., Walker, D. R., & Lau, D. T. (2007). Narcotic drug use among patients with lower back pain in employer health plans: A retrospective analysis of risk factors and health care services. *Clinical Therapeutics, 29*(Suppl. 1), 2603–2612.

Riazi, A., Pickup, J., & Bradley, C. (2004). Daily stress and glycaemic control in Type 1 diabetes: Individual differences in magnitude, direction, and timing of stress-reactivity. *Diabetes Research and Clinical Practice, 66,* 237–244.

Ricciardelli, L. A., McCabe, M. P., Williams, R. J., & Thompson, J. K. (2007). The role of ethnicity and culture in body image and disordered eating among males. *Clinical Psychology Review, 27,* 582–606.

Rice, D. P., & Fineman, N. (2004). Economic implications of increased longevity in the United States. *Annual Review of Public Health, 25,* 457–473.

Richardson, J., Smith, J. E., McCall, G., Richardson, A., Pilkington, K., & Kirsch, I. (2007). Hypnosis for nausea and vomiting in cancer chemotherapy: A systematic review of the research evidence. *European Journal of Cancer Care, 16,* 402–412.

Richardson, K. M., & Rothstein, H. R. (2008). Effects of occupational stress management intervention programs: A meta-analysis. *Journal of Occupational Health Psychology, 13,* 69–93.

Richman, J. A., Cloninger, L., & Rospenda, K. M. (2008). Macrolevel stressors, terrorism, and mental health outcomes: Broadening the stress paradigm. *American Journal of Public Health, 98*, 323–329.

Rietveld, S., & Koomen, J. M. (2002). A complex system perspective on medication compliance: Information for healthcare providers. *Disease Management and Health Outcomes, 10*, 621–630.

Riley, J. L., III, Wade, J. B., Myers, C. D., Sheffield, D., Papas, R. K., & Price, D. D. (2002). Racial/ethnic differences in the experience of chronic pain. *Pain, 100*, 291–298.

Rimm, E. B., & Moats, C. (2007). Alcohol and coronary heart disease: Drinking patterns and mediators of effect. *Annals of Epidemiology, 17*(Suppl.), S3–S7.

Rimm, E. B., Williams, P., Fosher, K., Criqui, M., & Stampfer, M. J. (1999). Moderate alcohol intake and lower risk of coronary heart disease: Meta-analysis of effects on lipids and haemostatic factors. *British Medical Journal, 319*, 1523–1528.

Ringström, G., Abrahamsson, H., Strid, H., & Simrén, M. (2007). Why do subjects with irritable bowel syndrome seek health care for their symptoms? *Scandinavian Journal of Gastroenterology, 42*, 1194–1203.

Rissanen, A., Hakala, P., Lissner, L., Mattlar, C.-E., Koskenvuo, M., & Rönnemaa, T. (2002). Acquired preference especially for dietary fat and obesity: A study of weight-discordant monozygotic twin pairs. *International Journal of Obesity and Related Metabolic Disorders, 26*, 973–977.

Ritter, A., & Cameron, J. (2006). A review of the efficacy and effectiveness of harm reduction strategies for alcohol, tobacco and illicit drugs. *Drug and Alcohol Review, 25*, 611–624.

Roberts, S. O. (2002). A strong start: Strength and resistance training guidelines for children and adolescents. *American Fitness, 20*(1), 34–38.

Roberts, W. O. (2007). Heat and cold: What does the environment do to marathon injury? *Sports Medicine, 37*, 400–403.

Robine, J.-M., Jagger, C., Mathers, C. D., Crimmins, E. M., & Suzman, R. M. (2003). *Determining health expectancies.* Chichester, UK: Wiley.

Robine, J.-M., & Ritchie, K. (1991). Healthy life expectancy: Evaluation of global indicator of change in population health. *British Medical Journal, 302*, 457–460.

Robins, L. N. (1995). The natural history of substance use as a guide to setting drug policy. *American Journal of Public Health, 85*, 12–13.

Robinson, L., Clare, L., & Evans, K. (2005). Making sense of dementia and adjusting to loss: Psychological reactions to a diagnosis of dementia in couples. *Aging and Mental Health, 9*, 337–347.

Robinson, M. E., Gagnon, C. M., Dannecker, E. A., Brown, J. L., Jump, R. L., & Price, D. D. (2003). Sex differences in common pain events: Expectations and anchors. *Journal of Pain, 4*, 40–45.

Robinson-Whelen, S., Tada, Y., MacCallum, R. C., McGuire, L., & Kiecolt-Glaser, J. K. (2001). Long-term caregiving: What happens when it ends? *Journal of Abnormal Psychology, 110*, 573–584.

Robles, T. F., Glaser, R., & Kiecolt-Glaser, J. K. (2005). Out of balance: A new look at chronic stress, depression, and immunity. *Current Directions in Psychological Science, 14*, 111–115.

Rock, V. J., Malarcher, A., Kahende, J. W., Asman, K., Husten, C., & Caraballo, R. (2007). Cigarette smoking among adults—United States, 2006. *Morbidity and Mortality Weekly Reports, 56*, 1157–1161.

Rockhill, B., Willett, W. C., Manson, J. E., Leitzmann, M. F., Stampfer, M. J., Hunter, D. J., et al. (2001). Physical activity and mortality: A prospective study among women. *American Journal of Public Health, 91*, 578–583.

Röder, C. H., Michal, M., Overbeck, G., van de Ven, V. G., & Linden, D. E. J. (2007). Pain response in depersonalization: A functional imaging study using hypnosis in health subjects. *Psychotherapy and Psychosomatics, 76*, 115–121.

Rodin, J., & Langer, E. J. (1977). Long-term effects of a control-relevant intervention with the institutionalized aged. *Journal of Personality and Social Psychology, 35*, 897–902.

Rodin, J., Silberstein, L., & Striegel-Moore, R. (1985). Women and weight: A normative discontent. In T. B. Sonderegger (Ed.), *Psychology and gender* (pp. 267–307). Lincoln: University of Nebraska Press.

Rodu, B., & Cole, P. (2007). Declining mortality from smoking in the United States. *Nicotine and Tobacco Research, 9*, 781–784.

Roe, S., & Becker, J. (2005). Drug prevention with vulnerable young people: A review. *Drugs: Education, Prevention and Policy, 12*, 85–99.

Roelofs, J., Boissevain, M. D., Peters, M. L., de Jong, J. R., & Vlaeyen, J. W. S. (2002). Psychological treatments for chronic low back pain: Past, present, and beyond. *Pain Reviews, 9*, 29–40.

Roesch, S. C., Dunkel-Schetter, C., Woo, G., & Hobel, C. J. (2004). Modeling the types and timing of stress in pregnancy. *Anxiety, Stress and Coping, 17*, 87–102.

Roesch, S. L., Adams, L., Hines, A., Palmores, A., Vyas, P., Tran, C., et al. (2005). Coping with prostate cancer: A meta-analytic review. *Journal of Behavioral Medicine, 28*, 281–293.

Rogers, C. J., Colbert, L. H., Greiner, J. W., Perkins, S. N., & Hursting, S. D. (2008). Physical activity and cancer prevention: Pathways and targets for intervention. *Sports Medicine, 38*, 271–296.

Rollins, S. Z., & Garrison, M. E. B. (2002). The Family Daily Hassles Inventory: A preliminary investigation of reliability and validity. *Family and Consumer Sciences Research Journal, 31*, 135–154.

Ronan, G. F., Dreer, L. W., Dollard, K. M., & Ronan, D. W. (2004). Violent couples: Coping and communication skills. *Journal of Family Violence, 19*, 131–137.

Room, R., & Day, N. (1974). Alcohol and mortality. In M. Keller (Ed.), *Second special report to the U.S. Congress: Alcohol and health.* Washington, DC: U.S. Government Printing Office.

Rosal, M. C., Olendzki, B., Reed, G. W., Gumieniak, O., Scavron, J., & Ockene, I. (2005). Diabetes self-management among low-income Spanish-speaking patients: A pilot study. *Annals of Behavioral Medicine, 29*, 225–235.

Rosario, M., Salzinger, S., Feldman, R. S., & Ng-Mak, D. S. (2008). The roles of social support and coping. *American Journal of Community Psychology, 41*, 43–62.

Rosen, C. S. (2000). Is the sequencing of change processes by stage consistent across health problems? A meta-analysis. *Health Psychology, 19*, 593–604.

Rosenberg, E., Leanza, Y., & Seller, R. (2007). Doctor-patient communication in primary care with an interpreter: Physician perceptions of professional and family interpreters. *Patient Education and Counseling, 67*, 286–292.

Rosenberg, H., & Melville, J. (2005). Controlled drinking and controlled drug use as outcome goals in British treatment services. *Addiction Research and Theory, 13*, 85–92.

Rosenberg, N. L., Grigsby, J., Dreisbach, J., Busenbark, D., & Grigsby, P. (2002). Neuropsychologic impairment and MRI abnormalities associated with chronic solvent abuse. *Journal of Toxicology: Clinical Toxicology, 40*, 21–34.

Rosenberg, S. D., Lu, W., Mueser, K. T., Jankowski, M. K., & Cournos, F. (2007). Correlates of adverse childhood events among adults with schizophrenia spectrum disorders. *Psychiatric Services, 58*, 245–253.

Rosenblatt, K. A., Wicklund, K. G., & Stanford, J. L. (2000). Sexual factors and the risk of prostate cancer. *American Journal of Epidemiology, 152*, 1152–1158.

Rosengren, A., Hawken, S., Ounpuu, S., Sliwa, K., Zubaid, M., Almahmeed, W. A., et al. (2004). Association of psychosocial risk factors with risk of acute myocardial infarction in 11119 cases and 13648 controls from 52 countries (the INTERHEART study): Case-control study. *Lancet, 364*, 953–962.

Rosenman, R. H., Brand, R. J., Jenkins, C. D., Friedman, M., Straus, R., & Wurm, M. (1975). Coronary heart disease in the Western Collaborative Group Study: Final follow-up of 8 1/2 years. *Journal of the American Medical Association, 233*, 872–877.

Rosier, E. M., Iadarola, M. J., & Coghill, R. C. (2002). Reproducibility of pain measurement and pain perception. *Pain, 98*, 205–216.

Ross, L., Kohier, C. L., Grimley, D. M., & Anderson-Lewis, C. (2007). The theory of reasoned action and intention to seek cancer information. *American Journal of Health Behavior, 31*, 123–134.

Ross, M. J., & Berger, R. S. (1996). Effects of stress inoculation training on athletes' postsurgical pain and rehabilitation after orthopedic injury. *Journal of Consulting and Clinical Psychology, 64*, 406–410.

Rössler, W., Lauber, C., Angst, J., Haker, H., Gamma, A., Eich, D., et al. (2007). The use of complementary and alternative medicine in the general population: Results from a longitudinal community study. *Psychological Medicine, 37*, 73–84.

Rossow, I., Grøholt, B., & Wichstrøm, L. (2005). Intoxicants and suicidal behaviour among adolescents: Changes in levels and associations from 1992 to 2002. *Addiction, 100*, 79–88.

Roter, D. L., & Hall, J. A. (2004). Physician gender and patient-centered communication: A critical review of empirical research. *Annual Review of Public Health, 25*, 497–519.

Rotskoff, L. (2002). *Love on the rocks: Men, women, and alcohol in post–World War II America.* Chapel Hill: University of North Carolina Press.

Rotter, J. B. (1966). Generalized expectancies for internal versus external control of reinforcement. *Psychological Monographs, 80*(Whole No. 609).

Rouse, B. A. (Ed.). (1998). *Substance abuse and mental health statistics source book.* Rockville, MD: Department of Health and Human Services, Substance Abuse and Mental Health Services Administration.

Rozanski, A., Blumenthal, J. A., Davidson, K. W., Saab, P. G., & Kubzansky, L. (2005). The epidemiology, pathophysiology, and management of psychosocial risk factors in cardiac practice: The emerging field of behavioral cardiology. *Journal of the American College of Cardiology, 45*, 637–651.

Rozin, P. (1999). Food is fundamental, fun, frightening, and far-reaching. *Social Research, 66*, 9–30.

Rozin, P., Kabnick, K., Pete, E., Fischler, C., & Shields, C. (2003). The ecology of eating. *Psychological Science, 14*, 450–454.

Rubak, S., Sanboek, A., Lauritzen, T., & Christensen, B. (2005). Motivational interviewing: A systematic review and meta-analysis. *British Journal of General Practice, 55*, 305–312.

Rubenstein, S., & Caballero, B. (2000). Is Miss America an undernourished role model? *Journal of the American Medical Association, 283*, 1569.

Rucker, D., Padawal, J., Li, S. K., Curioni, C., & Lau, D. C. W. (2007). Long term pharmacotherapy for obesity and overweight: Updated meta-analysis. *British Medical Journal, 335*, 1194–1199.

Rudd, R. E. (2007). Health literacy skills of U.S. adults. *American Journal of Health Behavior, 31*, S8–S18.

Ruitenberg, A., van Swieten, J. C., Wittman, J. C. M., Mehta, K. M., van Duijn, C. M., Hofman, A., et al. (2002). Alcohol consumption and the risk of dementia: The Rotterdam study. *Lancet, 359*, 281–286.

Rutledge, P. C., Park, A., & Sher, K. J. (2008). 21st birthday drinking: Extremely extreme. *Journal of Consulting and Clinical Psychology, 76*, 511–516.

Rutten, G. (2005). Diabetes patient education: Time for a new era. *Diabetic Medicine, 22*, 671–673.

Ryan, C. J., & Zerwic, J. J. (2003). Perceptions of symptoms of myocardial infarction related to health care seeking behaviors in the elderly. *Journal of Cardiovascular Nursing, 18*, 184–196.

Ryan, M. P. (2008). The antidepressant effects of physical activity: Mediting self-esteem and self-efficacy mechanisms. *Psychology and Health, 23*, 279–307.

Sääkslahti, A., Numminen, P., Varstala, V., Helenius, H., Tammi, A., Viikari, J., et al. (2004). Physical activity as a preventive measure for coronary heart disease risk factors in early childhood. *Scandinavian Journal of Medicine and Science in Sports, 14,* 143–149.

Sabia, S., Marmot, M., Dufouil, C., & Singh-Manoux, A. (2008). Smoking history and cognitive function in middle age from the Whitehall II study. *Archives of Internal Medicine, 168,* 1165–1173.

Sacco, R. L., Benson, R. T., Kargman, D. E., Boden-Albala, B., Tuck, C., Lin, I-F., et al. (2001). High-density lipoprotein cholesterol and ischemic stroke in the elderly: The Northern Manhattan Stroke Study. *Journal of the American Medical Association, 285,* 2729–2735.

Sachdev, P., Mondraty, N., Wen, W., & Gulliford, K. (2008). Brains of anorexia nervosa patients process self-images differently from non-self-images: An fMRI study. *Neuropsychologia, 46,* 2161–2168.

Sackett, D. L., & Snow, J. C. (1979). The magnitude of compliance and noncompliance. In R. B. Haynes, D. W. Taylor, & D. L. Sackett (Eds.), *Compliance in health care* (pp. 11–22). Baltimore: Johns Hopkins University Press.

Sahloff, E. G. (2005). Current issues in the development of a vaccine to prevent human immunodeficiency virus. *Pharmacotherapy, 25,* 741–747.

Samuelson, M., Carmody, J., Kabat-Zinn, J., & Bratt, M. A. (2007). Mindfulness-based stress reduction in Massachusetts correctional facilities. *Prison Journal, 87,* 254–268.

Sánchez del Rio, M., & Alvarez Linera, J. (2004). Functional neuroimaging of headaches. *Lancet Neurology, 3,* 645–651.

Sancier, K. M., & Holman, D. (2004). Commentary: Multifaceted health benefits of medical *Qigong. Journal of Alternative and Complementary Medicine, 10,* 163–165.

Sanders, S. (2005). Is the glass half empty or half full? Reflections on strain and gain in caregivers of individuals with Alzheimer's disease. *Social Work in Health Care, 40*(3), 57–73.

Sanders, S. H. (2006). Behavioral conceptualization and treatment for chronic pain. *Behavior Analyst Today, 7,* 253–261.

Sapolsky, R. M. (1998). *Why zebras don't get ulcers: An updated guide to stress, stress-related diseases, and coping.* New York: Freeman.

Sapolsky, R. M. (2004). Social status and health in humans and other animals. *Annual Review of Anthropology, 33,* 393–418.

Sasaki, M., & Yamasaki, K. (2007). Stress coping and the adjustment process among university freshmen. *Counselling Psychology Quarterly, 20,* 51–67.

Sattin, R. W., Easley, K. A., Wolf, S. L., Chen, Y., & Kutner, M. H. (2005). Reduction in fear of falling through intense tai chi exercise training in older, transitionally frail adults. *Journal of the American Geriatrics Society, 53,* 1168–1178.

Sattler, G. (2005). Advances in liposuction and fat transfer. *Dermatology Nursing, 17,* 133–139.

Saunders, T., Driskell, J. E., Johnston, J. H., & Sales, E. (1996). The effects of stress inoculation training on anxiety and performance. *Journal of Occupational Health Psychology, 1,* 170–186.

Sayette, M. A., Kirchner, T. R., Moreland, R. L., Levine, J. M., & Travis, T. (2004). Effects of alcohol on risk-seeking behavior: A group-level analysis. *Psychology of Addictive Behaviors, 18,* 190–193.

Scarpa, A., Haden, S. C., & Hurley, J. (2006). Community violence victimization and symptoms of posttraumatic stress disorder: The moderating effects of coping and social support. *Journal of Interpersonal Violence, 21,* 446–469.

Scarscelli, D. (2006). Drug addiction between deviance and normality: A study of spontaneous and assisted remission. *Contemporary Drug Problems, 33,* 237–274.

Schachter, S. (1980). Urinary pH and the psychology of nicotine addiction. In P. O. Davidson & S. M. Davidson (Eds.), *Behavioral medicine: Changing health lifestyles* (pp. 70–93). New York: Brunner/Mazel.

Schachter, S. (1982). Recidivism and self-cure of smoking and obesity. *American Psychologist, 37,* 436–444.

Schaffer, M., Jeglic, E. L., & Stanley, B. (2008). The relationship between suicidal behavior, ideation, and binge drinking among college students. *Archives of Suicide Research, 12,* 124–132.

Schell, L. M., & Denham, M. (2003). Environmental pollution in urban environments and human biology. *Annual Review of Anthropology, 32,* 111–134.

Schenker, S. (2001, September). The truth about fad diets. *Student BMJ,* 318–319.

Schindler, L., Kerrigan, D, & Kelly, J. (2002). *Understanding the immune system.* Retrieved January 29, 2002, from newscenter.cancer.gov/sciencebehind/immune

Schlebuisch, L. (2004). The development of a stress symptom checklist. *South African Journal of Psychology, 34,* 327–346.

Schlenger, W. E., Caddell, J. M., Ebert, L., Jordan, B. K., Rourke, K. M., Wilson, D., et al. (2002). Psychological reactions to terrorist attacks: Findings from the National Study of Americans' Reactions to September 11. *Journal of the American Medical Association, 288,* 581–588.

Schlicht, W., Kanning, M., & Bös, K. (2007). Psychosocial interventions to influence physical inactivity as a risk factor: Theoretical models and practical evidence. In J. Dordan, B. Bardé, & A. M. Zieher (Eds.), *Contributions toward evidence-based psychocardiology: A systematic review of the literature* (pp. 107–123). Washington, DC: American Psychological Association.

Schmaltz, H. N., Southern, D., Ghali, W. A., Jelinski, S. F., Parsons, G. A., King, K., et al. (2007). Living alone, patient sex and mortality after acute myocardial infarction. *Journal of General Internal Medicine, 22,* 572–578.

Schneider, E. C., Zaslavsky, A. M., & Epstein, A. M. (2002). Racial disparities in the quality of care for enrollees in Medicare managed care. *Journal of the American Medical Association, 287,* 1288–1294.

Schneiderman, N., Saab, P. G., Carney, R. M., Raczynski, J. M., Cowan, M. J., Berkman, L. F., et al. (2004). Psychosocial treatment within sex by ethnicity subgroups in the Enhancing Recovery in Coronary Heart Disease clinical trial. *Psychosomatic Medicine, 66*, 475–483.

Schnittker, J. (2004). Education and the changing shape of the income gradient in health. *Journal of Health and Social Behavior, 45*, 286–305.

Schnittker, J. (2007). Working more and feeling better: Women's health, employment, and family life. *American Sociological Review, 72*, 221–238.

Schnoll, R. A., Patterson, F., & Lerman, C. (2007). Treating tobacco dependence in women. *Journal of Women's Health, 16*, 1211–1218.

Schoenbaum, M. (1997). Do smokers understand the mortality effects of smoking? Evidence from the Health Retirement Survey. *American Journal of Public Health, 87*, 755–759.

Schofield, W. (1969). The role of psychology in the delivery of health services. *American Psychologist, 24*, 568–584.

Scholey, A. B., Robertson, B., Haskell, C. F., Milne, A. L., & Kennedy, D. O. (2008). Effects of chewing gum on subjective and physiological stress responses. *Appetite, 50*, 565.

Schousboe, K., Visscher, P. M., Erbas, B., Kyvik, K. O., Hopper, J. L., Henriksen, J. E., et al. (2004). Twin study of genetic and environmental influences on adult body size, shape, and composition. *International Journal of Obesity, 28*, 39–48.

Schrijvers, C. T., Stronks, K., van de Mheen, H. D., & Mackenbach, J. P. (1999). Explaining educational differences in mortality: The role of behavioral and material factors. *American Journal of Public Health, 89*, 535–540.

Schroeder, K., Fahey, T., & Ebrahim, S. (2007). Interventions for improving adherence to treatment in patients with high blood pressure in ambulatory settings. *Cochrane Database of Systematic Reviews*, Cochrane AN: CD004804.

Schroeder, K. E. E. (2004). Coping competence as predictor and moderator of depression among chronic disease patients. *Journal of Behavioral Medicine, 27*, 123–145.

Schroevers, M., Ranchor, A. V., & Sanderman, R. (2006). Adjustment to cancer in the 8 years following diagnosis: A longitudinal study comparing cancer survivors with healthy individuals. *Social Science and Medicine, 63*, 598–610.

Schuckit, M. A. (2000). Keep it simple. *Journal of Studies on Alcohol, 61*, 781–782.

Schulz, R., & Aderman, D. (1974). Clinical research and the stages of dying. *Omega: Journal of Death and Dying, 5*, 137–143.

Schulze, A., & Mons, U. (2006). The evolution of educational inequalities in smoking: A changing relationship and a cross-over effect among German birth cohorts of 1921–70. *Addiction, 101*, 1051–1056.

Schupf, N., Costa, R., Luchsinger, J., Tang, M., Lee, J. H., & Mayeaux, R. (2005). Relationship between plasma lipids and all-cause mortality in nondemented elderly. *Journal of the American Geriatrics Society, 53*, 219–226.

Schuster, M. A., Stein, B. D., Jaycox, L. H., Collins, R. L., Marshall, G. N., Elliott, M. N., et al. (2001). A national survey of stress reactions after the September 11, 2001, terrorist attacks. *New England Journal of Medicine, 345*, 1507–1512.

Schwartz, B. S., Stewart, W. F., Simon, D., & Lipton, R. B. (1998). Epidemiology of tension-type headache. *Journal of the American Medical Association, 279*, 381–383.

Schwartz, G. E., & Weiss, S. M. (1978). Behavioral medicine revisited: An amended definition. *Journal of Behavioral Medicine, 1*, 249–251.

Schwarzer, R., Luszczynska, A., Ziegelmann, J. P., Scholz, U., & Lippke, S. (2008). Social-cognitive predictors of physical exercise adherence: Three longitudinal studies in rehabilitation. *Health Psychology, 27*(Suppl.), S54–S63.

Sclafani, A. (2001). Psychobiology of food preferences. *International Journal of Obesity, 25*(Suppl. 5), S13–S16.

Sclafani, A., & Springer, D. (1976). Dietary obesity in adult rats: Similarities to hypothalamic and human obesity. *Physiology and Behavior, 17*, 461–471.

Scott, D. J., Stohler, C. S., Egnatuk, C. M., Wang, H., Koeppe, R. A., & Zubieta, J.-K. (2008). Placebo and nocebo effects are defined by opposite opioid and dopaminergic responses. *Archives of General Psychiatry, 65*, 220–231.

Scully, J. A., Tosi, H., & Banning, K. (2000). Life events checklists: Revisiting the Social Readjustment Rating Scale after 30 years. *Educational and Psychological Measurement, 60*, 864–876.

Searle, A., & Bennett, P. (2001). Psychological factors and inflammatory bowel disease: A review of a decade of literature. *Psychology and Health Medicine, 6*, 121–135.

Searle, A., Norman, P., Thompson, R., & Vedhara, K. (2007). A prospective examination of illness beliefs and coping in patients with Type 2 diabetes. *British Journal of Health Psychology, 12*, 621–638.

Sears, S. R., & Stanton, A. L. (2001). Expectancy-value constructs and expectancy violation as predictors of exercise adherence in previously sedentary women. *Health Psychology, 20*, 326–333.

Sebre, S., Sprugevica, I., Novotni, A., Bonevski, D., Pakal-niskiene, V., Popescu, D., et al. (2004). Cross-cultural comparisons of child-reported emotional and physical abuse: Rates, risk factors and psychosocial symptoms. *Child Abuse and Neglect, 28*, 113–127.

Secker-Walker, R. H., Flynn, B. S., Solomon, L. J., Skelly, J. M., Dorwaldt, A. L., & Ashikaga, T. (2000). Helping women quit smoking: Results of a community intervention program. *American Journal of Public Health, 90*, 940–946.

Segall, A. (1997). Sick role concepts and health behavior. In D. S. Gochman (Ed.), *Handbook of health behavior research: Vol.1. Personal and social determinants* (pp. 289–301). New York: Plenum Press.

Segerstrom, S. C. (2005). Optimism and immunity: Do positive thoughts always lead to positive effects? *Brain, Behavior, and Immunity, 19*, 195–200.

Segerstrom, S. C. (2007). Stress, energy, and immunity: An ecological view. *Current Directions in Psychological Science, 16*, 326–330.

Segerstrom, S. C., & Miller, G. E. (2004). Psychological stress and the human immune system: A meta-analytic study of 30 years of inquiry. *Psychological Bulletin, 130*, 601–630.

Seifert, T. (2005). Anthropomorphic characteristics of center-fold models: Trends toward slender figures over time. *Journal of Eating Disorders, 37*, 271–274.

Seitz, H. K., & Maurer, B. (2007). The relationship between alcohol metabolism, estrogen levels, and breast cancer risk. *Alcohol Research and Health, 30*, 42–43.

Seligman, M. E. P., & Csikszentmihalyi, M. (2000). Positive psychology. *American Psychologist, 55*, 5–14.

Selkoe, D. J. (2007). Developing preventive therapies for chronic diseases: Lessons learned from Alzheimer's disease. *Nutrition Reviews, 65*(Suppl.), S239–S243.

Selye, H. (1956). *The stress of life.* New York: McGraw-Hill.

Selye, H. (1976). *Stress in health and disease.* Reading, MA: Butterworths.

Selye, H. (1982). History and present status of the stress concept. In L. Goldberger & S. Breznitz (Eds.), *Handbook of stress: Theoretical and clinical aspects* (pp. 7–17). New York: Free Press.

Seow, D., & Gauthier, S. (2007). Pharmacotherapy of Alzheimer disease. *Canadian Journal of Psychiatry, 52*, 620–629.

Sepa, A., Wahlberg, J., Vaarala, O., Frodi, A., & Ludvigsson, J. (2005). Psychological stress may induce diabetes-related autoimmunity in infancy. *Diabetes Care, 28*, 290–295.

Sepulveda, M.-J., Bodenheimer, T., & Grundy, P. (2008). Primary care: Can it solve employers' health care dilemma? *Health Affairs, 27*, 151–158.

Severson, H. H., Forrester, K. K., & Biglan, A. (2007). Use of smokeless tobacco is a risk factor for cigarette smoking. *Nicotine and Tobacco Research, 9*, 1331–1337.

Shai, I., Schwarzfuchs, D., Henkin, Y., Shahar, D. R., Witkow, S., Greenberg, I., et al. (2008). Weight loss with a low-carbohydrate, Mediterranean, or low-fat diet. *New England Journal of Medicine, 359*, 229–241.

Shankar, A., Conner, M., & Bodnasky, H. J. (2007). Can the theory of planned behaviour predict maintenance of a frequently a repeated behaviour? *Health and Medicine, 12*, 213–224.

Shaper, A. G., Wannamethee, S. G., & Walker, M. (2003). Pipe and cigar smoking and major cardiovascular events, cancer incidence and all-cause mortality in middle-aged British men. *International Journal of Epidemiology, 32*, 802–808.

Shapiro, A. K. (1970). Placebo effects in psychotherapy and psychoanalysis. *Journal of Clinical Pharmacology, 10*, 73–78.

Shapiro, D., Cook, I. A., Davydov, D. M., Ottaviani, C., Leuchter, A. F., & Abrams, M. (2007). Yoga is a complementary treatment of depression: Effects of traits and moods on treatment outcome. *Evidence-Based Complementary and Alternative Medicine, 4*, 493–502.

Sharp, K., & Thombs, D. L. (2003). A cluster analytic study of osteoprotective behavior in undergraduates. *American Journal of Health Behavior, 27*, 364–372.

Sharpe, L., Sensky, T., Timberlake, N., Ryan, B., Brewin, C. R., & Allard, S. (2001). A blind, randomized controlled trial of cognitive-behavioral intervention for patients with recent onset rheumatoid arthritis: Preventing psychological and physical mobility. *Pain, 89*, 275–283.

Sharpley, C. F., Tanti, A., Stone, J. M., & Lothian, P. J. (2004). The effects of Live Events Inventory. *Counselling Psychology Quarterly, 17*, 45–52.

Shavelson, L. (2001). *Hooked: Five addicts challenge our misguided drug rehab system.* New York: New Press.

Sheehy, R., & Horan, J. J. (2004). Effects of stress inoculation training for 1st-year law students. *International Journal of Stress Management, 11*, 41–55.

Sheese, B. E., Brown, E. L., & Graziano, W. G. (2004). Emotional expression in cyberspace: Searching for moderators of the Pennebaker disclosure effect via e-mail. *Health Psychology, 23*, 457–464.

Sheffer, C. E,, Deisinger, J. A., Cassisi, J. E., & Lofland, K. (2007). A revised taxonomy of patients with chronic pain. *Pain Medicine, 8*, 312–325.

Shell, E. R. (2000, May). Does civilization cause asthma? *Atlantic Monthly, 285*, 90–92, 94, 96–98, 100.

Shen, B.-J., Avivi, Y. E., Todaro, J. F., Spiro, A., Laurenceau, J.-P., Ward, K. D., et al. (2008). Anxiety characteristics independently and prospectively predict myocardial infarction in men: The unique contribution of anxiety among psychologic factors. *Journal of the American College of Cardiology, 51*, 113–119.

Shen, B.-J., Stroud, L. R., & Niaura, R. (2004). Ethnic differences in cardiovascular responses to laboratory stress: A comparison between Asian and White Americans. *International Journal of Behavioral Medicine, 11*, 181–186.

Shen, Z., Chen, J., Sun, S., Yu, B., Chen, Z., Yang, J., et al. (2003). Psychosocial factors and immunity of patients with generalized anxiety disorder. *Chinese Mental Health Journal, 17*, 397–400.

Sheps, D. S. (2007). Psychological stress and myocardial ischemia: Understanding the link and implications. *Psychosomatic Medicine, 69*, 491–492.

Sher, K. J. (1987). Stress response dampening. In H. T. Blane & K. E. Leonard (Eds.), *Psychological theories of drinking and alcoholism* (pp. 227–271). New York: Guilford Press.

Sher, K. J., & Levenson, R. W. (1982). Risk for alcoholism and individual differences in the stress-response-dampening effect of alcohol. *Journal of Abnormal Psychology, 91*, 350–367.

Shernoff, M. (2006). Condomless sex: Gay men, barebacking, and harm reduction. *Social Work, 51*, 106–113.

Sherry, B. (2007). Interventions to prevent or treat obesity in preschool children: A review of evaluated programs. *Nutrition Research Newsletter, 26*, 3–5.

Sherwood, L. (2001). *Human physiology: From cells to systems* (4th ed.). Pacific Grove, CA: Brooks/Cole.

Shi, S., & Klotz, U. (2008). Clinical use and pharmacological properties of selective COX-2 inhibitors. *European Journal of Clinical Pharmacology, 64*, 233–252.

Shields, M. (2004). Stress, health and the benefit of social support. *Health Reports, 15*(1), 9–38.

Shiffman, S., Balabanis, M. H., Paty, J. A., Engberg, J., Gwaltney, C. J., Liu, K. S., et al. (2000). Dynamic effects of self-efficacy on smoking lapse and relapse. *Health Psychology, 19*, 315–323.

Shiffman, S., Brockwell, S. E., Pillitteri, J. L., & Gitchell, J. G. (2008). Use of smoking-cessation treatments in the United States. *American Journal of Preventive Medicine, 34*, 102–111.

Shimabukuro, J., Awata, S., & Matsuoka, H. (2005). Behavioral and psychological symptoms of dementia characteristics of mild Alzheimer patients. *Psychiatry and Clinical Neurosciences, 59*, 274–279.

Shinnick, P. (2006). Qigong: Where did it come from? Where does it fit in science? What are the advances? *Journal of Alternative and Complementary Medicine, 12*, 351–353.

Shmueli, A., & Shuval, J. (2007). Are users of complementary and alternative medicine sicker than non-users? *Evidence-Based Complementary and Alternative Medicine, 4*, 251–255.

Siegel, M., & Biener, L. (2000). The impact of an antismoking media campaign on progression to established smoking: Results of a longitudinal youth study. *American Journal of Public Health, 90*, 380–386.

Siegel, M., & Skeer, M. (2003). Exposure to secondhand smoke and excess lung cancer mortality risk among workers in the "5 B's": Bars, bowling alleys, billiard halls, betting establishments, and bingo parlours. *Tobacco Control, 12*, 333–338.

Siegler, B. (2003, August 6–12). Actress Halle Berry battles diabetes. *Miami Times, 80*(48), 4B.

Siegler, I. C., Bastian, L. A., Steffens, D. C., Bosworth, H. B., & Costa, P. T. (2002). Behavioral medicine and aging. *Journal of Consulting and Clinical Psychology, 70*, 843–851.

Siegman, A. W. (1994). From Type A to hostility to anger: Reflections on the history of coronary-prone behavior. In A. W. Siegman & T. W. Smith (Eds.), *Anger, hostility, and the heart* (pp. 1–21). Hillsdale, NJ: Erlbaum.

Siemiatycki, J., Richardson, L., Straif, K., Latreille, B., Lakhani, R., Campbell, S., et al. (2004). Listing occupations carcinogens. *Environmental Health Perspectives, 112*, 1447–1459.

Sigmon, S. T., Stanton, A. L., & Snyder, C. R. (1995). Gender differences in coping: A further test of socialization and role constraint theories. *Sex Roles, 33*, 565–587.

Silagy, C., Lancaster, T., Stead, L., Mant, D., & Fowler, G. (2005). Nicotine replacement therapy for smoking cessation. *Cochrane Library*. Retrieved July 18, 2005, from http://www.cochrane.org/cochrane/revabstr/ab000146.htm

Silberstein, S. D. (2004). Migraine pathophysiology and its clinical implications. *Cephalalgia, 24*(Suppl. 2), 2–7.

Silverman, S. M. (2008). Lindsay Lohan opens up about recent troubles. *People*. Retrieved March 6, 2008, from http://www.people.com/people/article/0,20181019,00.html

Simoni, J. M., Frick, P. A., & Huang, B. (2006). A longitudinal evaluation of a social support model of medication adherence among HIV-positive men and women an antiretroviral therapy. *Health Psychology, 25*, 74–81.

Simonsick, E. M., Guralnik, J. M., Volpato, S., Balfour, J., & Fried, L. P. (2005). Just get out the door! Importance of walking outside the home for maintaining mobility: Findings from the Women's Health and Aging Study. *Journal of the American Geriatrics Society, 53*, 198–203.

SIMpill. (2008). About us. Retrieved Feb. 28, 2008, from http://www.simpill.com/

Simpson, S. H., Eurich, D. T., Majundar, S. R., Padwal, R. S., Tsuyuki, R. T., Varney, J., et al. (2006). A meta-analysis of the association between adherence to drug therapy and mortality. *British Medical Journal, 333*, 15–18.

Sims, E. A. H. (1974). Studies in human hyperphagia. In G. Bray & J. Bethune (Eds.), *Treatment and management of obesity*. New York: Harper & Row.

Sims, E. A. H. (1976). Experimental obesity, dietary-induced thermogenesis, and their clinical implications. *Clinics in Endocrinology and Metabolism, 5*, 377–395.

Sims, E. A. H., Danforth, E., Jr., Horton, E. S., Bray, G. A., Glennon, J. A., & Salans, L. B. (1973). Endocrine and metabolic effects of experimental obesity in man. *Recent Progress in Hormonal Research, 29*, 457–496.

Sims, E. A. H., & Horton, E. S. (1968). Endocrine and metabolic adaptation to obesity and starvation. *American Journal of Clinical Nutrition, 21*, 1455–1470.

Singletary, K. W., & Gapstur, S. M. (2001). Alcohol and breast cancer: Review of epidemiologic and experimental evidence and potential mechanisms. *Journal of the American Medical Association, 286*, 2143–2151.

Sitzer, D. I., Twamley, E. W., & Jeste, D. V. (2006). Cognitive training in Alzheimer's disease: A meta-analysis of the literature. *Acta Psychiatrica Scandinavica, 114*, 75–90.

Sjöström, L., Lindroos, A.-K., Peltonen, M., Torgerson, J., Bouchard, C., Carlsson, B., et al. (2004). Lifestyle, diabetes, and cardiovascular risk factors 10 years after bariatric surgery. *New England Journal of Medicine, 351*, 2683–2693.

Skinner, B. F. (1953). *Science and human behavior*. New York: Macmillan.

Skinner, B. F. (1987). *Upon further reflection*. Englewood Cliffs, NJ: Prentice-Hall.

Skinner, T. C., Hampson, S. E., & Fife-Schaw, C. (2002). Personality, personal model beliefs, and self-care in adolescents and young adults with Type 1 diabetes. *Health Psychology, 21*, 61–70.

Skybo, T., & Ryan-Wenger, N. (2003). Measures of overweight status in school-age children. *Journal of School Nursing, 19*, 172–180.

Slater, J., & Depue, R. A. (1981). The contribution of environmental events and social support to serious suicide attempts in primary depressive disorder. *Journal of Abnormal Psychology, 90*, 275–285.

Slomkowski, C., Rende, R., Novak, S., Lloyd-Richardson, E., & Niaura, R. (2005). Sibling effects on smoking in adolescence: Evidence for social influence from a genetically informative design. *Addiction, 100*, 430–438.

Slugg, R. M., Meyer, R. A., & Campbell, J. N. (2000). Response of cutaneous A- and C-fiber nociceptors in the monkey to controlled-force stimuli. *Journal of Neurophysiology, 83*, 2179–2191.

Small, B. J., Rosnick, C. B., Fratiglioni, L., & Bäckman, L. (2004). Apolipoprotein ε and cognitive performance: A meta-analysis. *Psychology and Aging, 19*, 592–600.

Smedslund, G., & Ringdal, G. I. (2004). Meta-analysis of the effects of psychosocial interventions on survival time in cancer patents. *Journal of Psychosomatic Research, 57*, 123–131.

Smetana, G. W. (2000). The diagnostic value of historical features in primary headache syndromes: A comprehensive review. *Archives of Internal Medicine, 160*, 2729–2740.

Smiles, R. V. (2002). Race matters in health care: Experts say eliminating racial and ethnic health disparities is the civil rights issue of our day. *Black Issues in Higher Education, 19*(7), 22–29.

Smith, D. A., Ness, E. M., Herbert, R., Schechter, C. B., Phillips, R. A., Diamond, J. A., et al. (2005). Abdominal diameter index: A more powerful anthropometric measure for prevalent coronary heart disease risk in adult males. *Diabetes, Obesity and Metabolism, 7*, 370–380.

Smith, D. P., & Bradshaw B. S. (2006). Rethinking the Hispanic paradox: Death rates and life expectancy for US non-Hispanic white and Hispanic populations. *American Journal of Public Health, 96*, 1686–1692.

Smith, J. E., Richardson, J., Hoffman, C., & Pilkington, K. (2005). Mindfulness-based stress reduction as supportive therapy in cancer care: Systematic review. *Journal of Advanced Nursing, 52*, 315–327.

Smith, K. M., & Sahyoun, N. R. (2005). Fish consumption: Recommendations versus advisories, can they be reconciled? *Nutrition Reviews, 63*, 39–46.

Smith, L. A., Roman, A., Dollard, M. F., Winefield, A. H., & Siegrist, J. (2005). Effort-reward imbalance at work: The effects of work stress on anger and cardiovascular disease symptoms in a community sample. *Stress and Health: Journal of the International Society for the Investigation of Stress, 21*, 113–128.

Smith, T. W., & Ruiz, J. M. (2002). Psychosocial influences on the development and course of coronary heart disease: Current status and implications for research and practice. *Journal of Consulting and Clinical Psychology, 70*, 548–568.

Smith, T. W., & Suls, J. (2004). Introduction to the special section on the future of health psychology. *Health Psychology, 23*, 115–118.

Smoking List. (2004). *Christy Turlington.* Retrieved July 19, 2005, from http://smokingsides.com/asfs/T/Turlington.html

Smoot, T. M., Xu, P., Kuppersmith, N. C., Singh, K. P., & Hilserath, P. (2006). Gastric bypass surgery in the United States, 1998–2002. *American Journal of Public Health, 96*, 1187–1189.

Smyth, J. M., Stone, A. A., Hurewitz, A., & Kaell, A. (1999). Effects of writing about stressful experiences on symptom reduction in patients with asthma or rheumatoid arthritis: A randomized trial. *Journal of the American Medical Association, 281*, 1304–1309.

Snyder, J. L., & Bowers, T. G. (2008). The efficacy of acamprosate and naltrexone in the treatment of alcohol dependence: A relative benefits analysis of randomized controlled trials. *American Journal of Drug and Alcohol Abuse, 34*, 449–461.

Snyder, S. H. (1977, March). Opiate receptors and internal opiates. *Scientific American, 236*, 44–56.

Sobel, B. E., & Schneider, D. J. (2005). Cardiovascular complications in diabetes mellitus. *Current Opinion in Pharmacology, 5*, 143–148.

Sobell, L. C., Cunningham, J. A., & Sobell, M. B. (1996). Recovery from alcohol problems with and without treatment: Prevalence in two population surveys. *American Journal of Public Health, 86*, 966–972.

Sola-Vera, J., Sáez, J., Laveda, R., Girona, E., García-Sepulcre, M. F., Cuesta, A., et al. (2008). Factors associated with non-attendance at outpatient endoscopy. *Scandinavian Journal of Gastroenterology, 43*, 202–206.

Solomon, G. F., & Moos, R. H. (1964). Emotions, immunity, and disease: A speculative theoretical integration. *Archives of General Psychiatry, 11*, 657–674.

Song, M.-Y., John, M., & Dobs, A. S. (2007). Clinicians' attitudes and usage of complementary and alternative integrative medicine: A survey at the Johns Hopkins Medical Institute. *Journal of Alternative and Complementary Medicine, 13*, 305–306.

Song, Y.-M., Sung, J., & Kim, J. S. (2000). Which cholesterol level is related to the lowest mortality in a population with low mean cholesterol level: A 6.4-year follow-up study of 482,472 Korean men. *American Journal of Epidemiology, 151*, 739–747.

Sont, W. N., Zielinski, J. M., Ashmore, J. P., Jiang, H., Krewski, D., Fair, M. E., et al. (2001). First analysis of cancer incidence and occupational radiation exposure based on the National Dose Registry of Canada. *American Journal of Epidemiology, 153*, 309–318.

Sørensen, T. I., Rissanen, A., Korkeila, M., & Kaprio, J. (2005). Intention to lose weight, weight changes, and 18-y mortality in overweight individuals without co-morbidities. *PLoS Medicine, 2*, 510–520.

Soriano, C. G. (2004, June 22). Mary-Kate Olsen seeks treatment for eating disorder. *USA Today People.* Retrieved

July 18, 2005, from http://www.usatoday.com/ life/people/2004–06–22–olsen-treatment_x.htm

Sours, J. A. (1980). *Starving to death in a sea of objects: The anorexia nervosa syndrome.* New York: Aronson.

Spiegel, D. (2004). Commentary on "Meta-analysis of the effects of psychosocial interventions on survival time and mortality in cancer patients" by Geir Smedslund and Gerd Inter Ringdal. *Journal of Psychosomatic Research, 57,* 133–135.

Spiegel, D., & Giese-Davis, J. (2003). Depression and cancer: Mechanisms and disease progression. *Biological Psychiatry, 54,* 269–282.

Spiegel, D., Kraemer, H. C., Bloom, J. R., & Gottheil, E. (1989). Effect of psychosocial treatment on survival of patients with metastatic breast cancer. *Lancet, ii,* 888-891.

Spierings, E. L. H., Ranke, A. H., & Honkoop, P. C. (2001). Precipitating and aggravating factors of migraine versus tension-type headache. *Headache, 41,* 554–558.

Spitzer, B. L., Henderson, K. A., & Zivian, M. T. (1999). Gender differences in population versus media body size: A comparison over four decades. *Sex Roles, 40,* 545–566.

Spring, B., Cook, J., Appelhans, B., Maloney, A., Richmond, M., Vaughn, J., et al. (2008). Nicotine effects on affective response in depression-prone smokers. *Psychopharmacology, 196,* 461–471.

Springer, J. F., Sale, E., Kasim, R., Winter, W., Sambrano, S., & Chipungu, S. (2004). Effectiveness of culturally specific approaches to substance abuse prevention: Findings for CSAP's national cross-site evaluation of high risk youth programs. *Journal of Ethnic and Cultural Diversity in Social Work, 13,* 1–23.

Sri Vengadesh, G., Sistla, S. C., & Smile, S. R. (2005). Postoperative pain relief following abdominal operations: A prospective randomised study of comparison of patient controlled analgesia with conventional parental opioids. *Indian Journal of Surgery, 67,* 34–37.

Stacey, P. S., & Sullivan, K. A. (2004). Preliminary investigation of thiamine and alcohol intake in clinical and healthy samples. *Psychological Reports, 94,* 845–848.

Staessen, J. A., Wang, J., Bianchi, G., & Birkenhager, W. H. (2003). Essential hypertension. *Lancet, 361,* 1629–1641.

Stafford, M., Chandola, T., & Marmot, M. (2007). Between fear of crime and mental health and physical functioning. *American Journal of Public Health, 97,* 2076–2081.

Stallworth, J., & Lennon, J. L. (2003). An interview with Dr. Lester Breslow. *American Journal of Public Health, 93,* 1803–1805.

Stamler, J., Elliott, P., Dennis, B., Dyer, A. R., Kesteloot, H., Liu, K., et al. (2003). INTERMAP: Background, aims, design, methods, and descriptive statistics (nondietary). *Journal of Human Hypertension, 17,* 591–608.

Stamler, J., Stamler, R., Neaton, J. D., Wentworth, D., Daviglus, M. L., Garside, D., et al. (1999). Low risk-factor profile and long-term cardiovascular and noncardiovascular mortality and life expectancy: Findings for 5 large cohorts of young adult and middle-aged men and women. *Journal of the American Medical Association, 282,* 2012–2018.

Stampfer, M. J., Hu, F. B., Manson, J. E., Rimm, E. B., & Willett, W. C. (2000). Primary prevention of coronary heart disease in women through diet and lifestyle. *New England Journal of Medicine, 343,* 16–22.

Standridge, J. B., Zylstra, R. G., & Adams, S. M. (2004). Alcohol consumption: An overview of benefits and risks. *Southern Medical Journal, 97,* 664–672.

Stanner, S. A., Hughes, J., Kelly, C. N. M., & Buttriss, J. (2004). A review of the epidemiological evidence for the "antioxidant hypothesis." *Public Health Nutrition, 7,* 407–422.

Stanton, A. L., Revenson, T. A., & Tennen, H. (2007). Health psychology: Psychological adjustment to chronic disease. *Annual Review of Psychology, 58,* 565–592.

Stanton, J. M., Balzer, W. K., Smith, P. C., Parra, L. F., & Ironson, G. (2001). A general measure of work stress: The Stress in General scale. *Educational and Psychological Measurement, 61,* 866–887.

Stapleton, J. A., Sutherland, G., & O'Gara, C. (2007). Association between dopamine transporter genotypes and smoking cessation: A meta-analysis. *Addiction Biology, 12,* 221–226.

Starkstein, S. E., Jorge, R., Mizrahi, R., Adrian, J., & Robinson, R. G. (2007). Insight and danger in Alzheimer's disease. *European Journal of Neurology, 14,* 455–460.

Stason, W., Neff, R., Miettinen, O., & Jick, H. (1976). Alcohol consumption and nonfatal myocardial infarction. *American Journal of Epidemiology, 104,* 603–608.

Staton, L. J., Panda, M., Chen, I., Genao, I., Kurz, J., Pasanen, M., et al. (2007). When race matters: Disagreement in pain perception between patients and their physicians in primary care. *Journal of the National Medical Association, 99,* 532–537.

Stead, L. F., Bergson, G., & Lancaster, T. (2008). Physician advice for smoking cessation. *Cochrane Database of Systematic Reviews,* Cochrane AN: CD000165.

Stead, L. F., Perera, R., Bullen, C., Mant, D., & Lancaster, T. (2008). Nicotine replacement therapy for smoking cessation. *Cochrane Database of Systematic Reviews,* Cochrane AN: CD000146.

Steele, C. (1997). A threat in the air: How stereotypes shape intellectual identity and performance. *American Psychologist, 52,* 613–629.

Steele, C. M., & Josephs, R. A. (1990). Alcohol myopia: Its prized and dangerous effects. *American Psychologist, 45,* 921–933.

Steffen, K. J., Mitchell, J. E., Roerig, J. L., & Lancaster, K. L. (2007). The eating disorders medicine cabinet revisited: A clinician's guide to ipecac and laxatives. *International Journal of Eating Disorders, 40,* 360–368.

Steffens, A. A., Moreira, L. B., Fuchs, S. C., Wiehe, M., Gus, M., & Fuchs, F. D. (2006). Incidence of hypertension by alcohol consumption: Is it modified by race? *Journal of Hypertension, 24,* 1489–1492.

Stein, M. B., Schork, N. J., & Gelernter, J. (2008). Gene-by-environment (serotonin transporter and childhood maltreatment) interaction for anxiety sensitivity, an intermediate phenotype for anxiety disorders. *Neuropsychopharmacology, 33,* 312–319.

Steinbrook, R. (2004). The AIDS epidemic in 2004. *New England Journal of Medicine, 351,* 115–117.

Steptoe, A., Hamer, M., & Chida, Y. (2007). The effects of acute psychological stress on circulating inflammatory factors in humans: A review and meta-analysis. *Brain, Behavior and Immunity, 21,* 901–912.

Steptoe, A., Wardle, J., Bages, N., Sallis, J. F., Sanabria-Ferrand, P.-A., & Sanchez, M. (2004). Drinking and driving in university students: An international study of 23 countries. *Psychology and Health, 19,* 527–540.

Stevens, S. L., Colwell, B., Smith, D. W., Robinson, J., & McMillan, C. (2005). An exploration of self-reported negative affect by adolescence as a reason for smoking: Implications for tobacco prevention and intervention programs. *Preventive Medicine, 41,* 589–596.

Stewart, J. C., Janicki, D. L., & Kamarck, T. W. (2006). Cardiovascular reactivity to and recovery from psychological challenge as predictors of 3-year change in blood pressure. *Health Psychology, 25,* 111–118.

Stewart, K. L. (2004). Pharmacological and behavioral treatments for migraine headaches: A meta-analytic review. *Dissertation Abstracts International: Section B, 65*(3-B), 1535.

Stewart, L. K., Flynn, M. G., Campbell, W. W., Craig, B. A., Robinson, J. P., Timmerman, K. L., et al. (2007). The influence of exercise training on inflammatory cytokines and C-reactive protein. *Medicine and Science in Sports and Exercise, 39,* 1714–1719.

Stewart-Knox, B. J., Sittlington, J., Rugkåsa, J., Harrisson, S., Treacy, M., & Abaunza, P. S. (2005). Smoking and peer groups: Results from a longitudinal qualitative study of young people in Northern Ireland. *British Journal of Social Psychology, 44,* 397–414.

Stewart-Williams, S. (2004). The placebo puzzle: Putting together the pieces. *Health Psychology, 23,* 198–206.

Stice, E., & Bearman, S. K. (2001). Body-image and eating disturbances prospectively predict increases in depressive symptoms in adolescent girls: A growth curve analysis. *Developmental Psychology, 37,* 597–607.

Stice, E., Presnell, K., Groesz, L., & Shaw, H. (2005). Effects of a weight maintenance diet on bulimic symptoms in adolescent girls: An experimental test of the dietary restraint theory. *Health Psychology, 24,* 402–412.

Stice, E., Presnell, K., & Spangler, D. (2002). Risk factors for binge eating onset in adolescent girls: A 2-year prospective investigation. *Health Psychology, 21,* 131–138.

Stice, E., Trost, A., & Chase, A. (2003). Healthy weight control and dissonance-based eating disorder prevention programs: Results from a controlled trial. *International Journal of Eating Disorders, 33,* 10–21.

Stickney, S. R., Black, D. R. (2008). Physical self-perception, body dysmorphic disorder, and smoking behavior. *American Journal of Health Behavior, 32,* 295–304.

Stojanovich, L., & Marisavljevich, D. (2008). Stress as a trigger of autoimmune disease. *Autoimmunity Review, 7,* 209–213.

Stokols, D. (1972). On the distinction between density and crowding: Some implications for future research. *Psychological Review, 79,* 275–277.

Stone, A. A., Reed, B. R., & Neale, J. M. (1987). Changes in daily event frequency precedes episodes of physical symptoms. *Journal of Human Stress, 13,* 70–74.

Stone, G. C. (1987). The scope of health psychology. In G. C. Stone, S. M. Weiss, J. D. Matarazzo, N. E. Miller, J. Rodin, C. D. Belar, et al. (Eds.), *Health psychology: A discipline and a profession* (pp. 27–40). Chicago: University of Chicago Press.

Storr, C. L., Lalongo, N. S., Anthony, J. C., & Breslau, N. (2007). Childhood antecedents of exposure to traumatic events and posttraumatic stress disorder. *American Journal of Psychiatry, 164,* 119–125.

Strandberg, T. E., Strandberg, A., Rantanen, K., Salomaa, V. V., Pitkälä, K., & Miettinen, T. A. (2004). Low cholesterol, mortality, and quality of life in old age during a 39-year follow-up. *Journal of the American College of Cardiology, 44,* 1002–1008.

Strasser, A. A., Lerman, C., Sanborn, P. M., Pickworth, W. B., & Feldman, E. A. (2007). New lower nicotine cigarettes can produce compensatory smoking and increased carbon monoxide exposure. *Drug and Alcohol Dependence, 86,* 294–300.

Straus, M. A. (2008). Dominance and symmetry in partner violence by male and female university students in 32 nations. *Children and Youth Services Review, 30,* 252–275.

Strazdins, L., & Broom, D. H. (2007). The mental health costs and benefits of giving social support. *International Journal of Stress Management, 14,* 370–385.

Streltzer, J. (1997). Pain. In W.-S. Tseng & J. Streltzer (Eds.), *Culture and psychopathology: A guide to clinical assessment* (pp. 87–100). New York: Brunner/Mazel.

Streppel, M. T., Boshuizen, H. C., Ocké, M. C., Kok, F. J., & Kromhout, D. (2007). Mortality and life expectancy in relation to long-term cigarette, cigar and pipe smoking: The Zutphen study. *Tobacco Control, 16,* 107–113.

Striegel-Moore, R. H., Franko, D. L., Thompson, D., Barton, B., Schreiber, G. B., & Daniels, S. R. (2004). Changes in weight and body image over time in women with eating disorders. *International Journal of Eating Disorders, 36,* 315–327.

Strigo, I. A., Duncan, G. H., Boivin, M., & Bushnell, M. C. (2003). Differentiation of visceral and cutaneous pain in the human brain. *Journal of Neurophysiology, 89,* 3294–3303.

Strine, T. W., Mokdad, A. H., Balluz, L. S., Berry, J. T., & Gonzalez, O. (2008). Impact of depression and anxiety on quality of life, health behaviors, and asthma control among adults in the United States with asthma, 2006. *Journal of Asthma, 45,* 123–133.

Stroebe, W., Papies, E. K., & Aarts, H. (2008). From homeostatic to hedonic theories of eating: Self-regulatory failure in food-rich environments. *Applied Psychology: An International Review, 57*(Suppl.), 172–193.

Strong, C. A. (1895). The psychology of pain. *Psychological Review, 2*, 329–347.

Stotts, J., Lohse, B., Patterson, J., Horacek, T., White, A., & Greene, G. (2007). Eating competence in college students nominates a non-dieting approach to weight management. *FASEB Journal, 21*, A301.

Stroebe, W. (2008). *Dieting, overweight, and obesity: Self-regulation in a food-rich environment.* Washington, DC: American Psychological Association.

Stroud, C. B., Davila, J., & Moyer, A. (2008). The relationship between stress and depression in first onsets versus recurrences: A meta-analytic review. *Journal of Abnormal Psychology, 117*, 206–213.

Stuart, R. B. (1967). Behavioral control of overeating. *Behavior Research and Therapy, 5*, 357–365.

Stunkard, A. J., & Allison, K. C. (2003). Binge eating disorder: Disorder or marker? *International Journal of Eating disorders, 34*(Suppl. 1), S107–S116.

Stunkard, A. J., Harris, J. R., Pedersen, N. L., & McClean, G. E. (1990). The body-mass index of twins who have been reared apart. *New England Journal of Medicine, 322*, 1483–1487.

Stunkard, A. J., Sørensen, T. I. A., Hanis, C., Teasdale, T. W., Chakraborty, R., Schull, W. J., et al. (1986). An adoption study of human obesity. *New England Journal of Medicine, 314*, 193, 198.

Stürmer, T., Hasselbach, P., & Amelang, M. (2006). Personality, lifestyle, and risk of cardiovascular disease and cancer: Follow-up of population based cohort. *British Medical Journal, 332*, 1359.

Su, D., Li, L., & Pagán, J. A. (2008). Acculturation and the use of complementary and alternative medicine. *Social Science and Medicine, 66*, 439–453.

Suarez, E. C., Saab, P. G., Llabre, M. M., Kuhn, C. M., & Zimmerman, E. (2004). Ethnicity, gender, and age effects on adrenoceptors and physiological responses to emotional stress. *Psychophysiology, 41*, 450–460.

Substance Abuse and Mental Health Services Administration (SAMHSA). (2007). *Results from the 2006 National Survey on Drug Use and Health: National findings* (Office of Applied Studies NSDUH Series H-32, DHHS Publication No. SMA 07-4293). Rockville, MD: National Clearinghouse for Alcohol and Drug Information.

Sufka, K. J., & Price, D. D. (2002). Gate control theory reconsidered. *Brain & Mind, 3*, 277–290.

Suls, J., & Bunde, J. (2005). Anger, anxiety, and depression as risk factors for cardiovascular disease: The problems and implications of overlapping affective dispositions. *Psychological Bulletin, 131*, 260–300.

Suls, J., & Rothman, A. (2004). Evolution of the biopsychosocial model: Prospects and challenges for health psychology. *Health Psychology, 23*, 119–125.

Sundblad, G. M. B., Saartok, T., & Engström, L.-M. T. (2007). Prevalence and co-occurrence of self-rated pain and perceived health in school-children: Age and gender differences. *European Journal of Pain, 11*, 171–180.

Surtees, P. G., Wainwright, N. W. J., Luben, R., Day, N. E., & Khaw, K.-T. (2005). Prospective cohort study of hostility and the risk of cardiovascular disease mortality. *International Journal of Cardiology, 100*, 155–161.

Surwit, R. S., Van Tilburg, M. A. L., Zucker, N., McCaskill, C. C., Parekh, P., Feinglos, M. N., et al. (2002). Stress management improves long-term glycemic control in Type 2 diabetes. *Diabetes Care, 25*, 30–34.

Susser, M. (1991). What is a cause and how do we know one? A grammar for pragmatic epidemiology. *American Journal of Epidemiology, 133*, 635–648.

Sutton, S., McVey, D., & Glanz, A. (1999). A comparative test of the theory of reasoned action and the theory of planned behavior in the prediction of condom use intentions in a national sample of English young people. *Health Psychology, 18*, 72–81.

Svansdottir, H. B., Snaedal, J. (2006). Music therapy in moderate and severe dementia of Alzheimer's type: A case-control study. *International Psychogeriatrics, 18*, 613–621.

Svetkey, L. P., Stevens, V. J., Brantley, P. J., Appel, L. J., Hollis, J. F., Loria, C. M., et al. (2008). Comparison of strategies for sustaining weight loss. *Journal of the American Medical Association, 299*, 1139–1148.

Swaim, R. C., Perrine, N. E., & Aloise-Young, P. A. (2007). Gender differences in a comparison of two tested etiological models of cigarette smoking among elementary school students. *Journal of Applied Social Psychology, 37*, 1681–1696.

Sweeney, C. T., Fant, R. V., Fagerstrom, K. O., McGovern, F., & Henningfield, J. E. (2001). Combination nicotine replacement therapy for smoking cessation rationale, efficacy and tolerability. *CNS Drugs, 15*, 453–467.

Sypeck, M. F., Gray, J. J., Etu, S. F., Ahrens, A. H., Mosimann, J. E., & Wiseman, C. V. (2006). Cultural representations of thinness in women, redux: Playboy magazine's depiction of beauty from 1979 to 1999. *Body Image, 3*, 229–235.

Syrjala, K. L., & Abrams, J. (1999). Cancer pain. In R. J. Gatchel & D. C. Turk (Eds.), *Psychosocial factors in pain: Critical perspectives* (pp. 301–314). New York: Guilford Press.

Szapary, P. O., Bloedon, L. T., & Foster, B. D. (2003). Physical activity and its effects on lipids. *Current Cardiology Reports, 5*, 488–492.

Szegedi, A., Kohnen, R., Dienel, A., & Kieser, M. (2005). Acute treatment of moderate to severe depression with Hypericum extract WS® 5570 (St. John's Wort): Randomized, controlled, double-blind, non-inferiority trial versus Paroxetine. *British Medical Journal, 330* (7490), 503.

Szekely, C. A., Breitner, J. C., Fitzpatrick, A. L., Rea, T. D., Psalty, B. M., Kuller, L. H., et al. (2008). NSAID use and dementia risk in the Cardiovascular Health Study: Role of APOE and NSAID type. *Neurology, 70*, 17–24.

Tacker, D. H., & Okorodudu, A. O. (2004). Evidence for injurious effect of cocaethylene in human microvascular endothelial cells. *Clinica Chimica Acta, 345*, 69–76.

Takkouche, B., Regueira, C., & Gestal-Otero, J. J. (2001). A cohort study of stress and the common cold. *Epidemiology, 12,* 345–349.

Talbot, M. (2000, January 9). The placebo prescription. *New York Times Magazine,* pp. 34–39, 44, 58–60.

Tam, C. S., Garnett, S. P., Cowell, C. T., Campbell, K., Cabrera, G., & Baur, L. A. (2006). Soft drink consumption and excess weight gain in Australian school students: Results from the Nepean study. *International Journal of Obesity, 30,* 1091–1093.

Tang, B. M. P., Eslick, G. D., Nowson, C., Smith, C., & Bensoussan, A. (2007). Use of calcium or calcium in combination with vitamin D supplementation to prevent fractures and bone loss in people aged 50 years and older: A meta-analysis. *Lancet, 370,* 657–666.

Tanofsky-Kraff, M., Marcus, M. D., Yanovski, S. Z., & Yanovski, J. A. (2008). Loss of control eating disorder in children age 12 years and younger: Proposed research criteria. *Eating Behaviors, 9,* 360–365.

Tardon, A., Lee, W. J., Delgaldo-Rodriques, M., Dosemeci, M., Albanes, D., Hoover, R., et al. (2005). Leisure-time physical activity and lung cancer: A meta-analysis. *Cancer Causes and Control, 16,* 389–397.

Tate, S. R., Brown, S. A., Unrod, M., & Ramo, D. E. (2004). Context of relapse for substance-dependent adults with and without comorbid psychiatric disorders. *Addictive Behaviors, 29,* 1707–1724.

Taylor, D. H., Jr., Hasselblad, V., Henley, S. J., Thun, M. J., & Sloan, F. A. (2002). Benefits of smoking cessation for longevity. *American Journal of Public Health, 92,* 990–996.

Taylor, E. N., Stampfer, M. J., & Curhan, G. C. (2005). Obesity, weight gain, and the risk of kidney stones. *Journal of the American Medical Association, 293,* 455–462.

Taylor, R. S., Brown, A., Ebrahim, S., Jolliffe, J., Noorani, H., Rees, K., et al. (2004). Exercise-based rehabilitation for patients with coronary heart disease: Systematic review and meta-analysis of randomized controlled trials. *American Journal of Medicine, 116,* 682–692.

Taylor, S. E. (2002). *The tending instinct: How nurturing is essential to who we are and how we live.* New York: Times Books, Henry Holt and Company.

Taylor, S. E. (2006). Tend and befriend: Biobehavioral bases of affiliation under stress. *Current Directions in Psychological Science, 15,* 273–277.

Taylor, S. E., Klein, L. C., Lewis, B. P., Gruenewald, T. L., Gurung, R. A. R., & Updegraff, J. A. (2000). Biobehavioral responses to stress in females: Tend-and-befriend, not fight-or-flight. *Psychological Review, 107,* 411–429.

Taylor, S. E., Sherman, D. K., Kim, H. S., Jarcho, J., Takagi, K., & Dunagan, M. S. (2004). Culture and social support: Who seeks it and why? *Journal of Personality and Social Psychology, 87,* 354–362.

Taylor-Piliae, R. E., Haskell, W. L., Waters, C. M., & Froelicher, E. S. (2006). Change in perceived psychosocial status following a 12-week Tai Chi exercise programme. *Journal of Advanced Nursing, 54,* 313–329.

Tedeschi, R. G., & Calhoun, L. G. (2006). Time of change? The spiritual challenges of bereavement and loss. *Omega: Journal of Death and Dying, 53,* 105–116.

Tedeschi, R. G., & Calhoun, L. G. (2008). Beyond the concept of recovery: Growth and the experience of loss. *Death Studies, 32,* 27–39.

Telama, R., Yang, X., Viikari, J., Välimäki, I., Wanne, O., & Raitakari, O. (2005). Physical activity from childhood to adulthood: A 21-year tracking study. *American Journal of Preventive Medicine, 28,* 267–273.

Templeton, D. (2008, April 15). Bill Clinton's heart troubles hard to detect, experts say. *Pittsburg Post-Gazette.* Retrieved June 1, 2008, from http://www.post-gazette.com/pg/08106/873418-114.stm

Terry, A., Szabo, A., & Griffiths, M. D. (2004). The Exercise Addiction Inventory: A new brief screening tool. *Addiction Research and Theory, 12,* 489–499.

Testa, M., Vazile-Tamsen, C., & Livingston, J. A. (2004). The role of victim and perpetrator intoxication on sexual assault outcomes. *Journal of Studies on Alcohol, 65,* 320–329.

Theberge, N. (2008). The integration of chiropractors into healthcare teams: A case study from sport medicine. *Sociology of Health and Illness, 30,* 19–34.

Theis, K. A., Helmick, C. G., & Hootman, J. M. (2007). Arthritis burden and impact are greater among U.S. women than men: Intervention opportunities. *Journal of Women's Health, 16,* 441–453.

Then and now: Magic Johnson. (2005, June 22). *CNN.* Retrieved July 1, 2005, from http://www.cnn.com/2005/US/01/17/cnn25.tan.johnson/

Thomas, J. J., Keel, P. K., & Heatherton, T. E. (2005). Disordered eating attitudes and behaviors in ballet students: Examination of environmental and individual risk factors. *International Journal of Eating Disorders, 38,* 263–268.

Thomas, W., White, C. M., Mah, J., Geisser, M. S., Church, T. R., & Mandel, J. S. (1995). Longitudinal compliance with annual screening for fecal occult blood. *American Journal of Epidemiology, 142,* 176–182.

Thompson, P. D. (2001, January). Exercise rehabilitation for cardiac patients: A beneficial but underused therapy. *The Physician and Sportsmedicine, 29,* 69–75.

Thompson, P. D., Franklin, B. A., Balady, G. J., Blair, S. N., Corrado, D., Domenico, E., III, et al. (2007). Exercise and acute cardiovascular events: Placing the risks into perspective. *Medicine and Science in Sports and Exercise, 39,* 886–897.

Thompson, S. H., & Hammond, K. (2003). Beauty is as beauty does: Body image and self-esteem of pageant contestants. *Eating and Weight Disorders, 8,* 231–237.

Thorburn, A. W. (2005). Prevalence of obesity in Australia. *Obesity Reviews, 6,* 187–189.

Thorn, B., & Saab, P. (2001). Notes from the APS Council of Representatives (CoR) Meeting. *Health Psychologist, 23*(3), 5, 8.

Thorn, B. E., & Kuhajda, M. C. (2006). Group cognitive therapy for chronic pain. *Journal of Clinical Psychology, 62,* 1355–1366.

Thorn, B. E., Pence, L. B., Ward, L. C., Kilgo, G., Clements, K. L., Cross, T. H., et al. (2007). A randomized clinical trial of targeted cognitive behavioral treatment to reduce catastrophizing in chronic headache sufferers. *Journal of Pain, 8*, 938–949.

Thun, M. J., Day-Lally, C. A., Calle, E. E., Flanders, W. D., & Heath, C. W., Jr. (1995). Excess mortality among cigarette smokers: Changes in a 20-year interval. *American Journal of Public Health, 85*, 1223–1230.

Thune, I., Brenn, T., Lund, E., & Gaard, M. (1997). Physical activity and the risk of breast cancer. *New England Journal of Medicine, 336*, 1269–1275.

Thune, I., & Furberg, A. S. (2001). Physical activity and cancer risk: Dose-response and cancer, all sites and site-specific. *Medicine and Science in Sports and Exercise, 33*, S530–S550.

Thuné-Boyle, I. C. V., Myers, L. B., & Newman, S. P. (2006). The role of illness beliefs, treatment beliefs, and perceived severity of symptoms in explaining distress in cancer patients during chemotherapy treatment. *Behavioral Medicine, 32*, 19–29.

Thygesen, L. C., Johansen, C., Keiding, N., Giovannucci, E., & Grønbæk, M. (2008). Effects of sample attrition in a longitudinal study of the association between alcohol intake and all-cause mortality. *Addiction, 103*, 1149–1159.

Tice, D. M., Bratslavsky, E., & Baumeister, R. F. (2001). Emotional distress regulation takes precedence over impulse control: If you feel bad, do it! *Journal of Personality and Social Psychology, 80*, 53–67.

Tobar, D. A. (2005). Overtraining and staleness: The importance of psychological monitoring. *International Journal of Sport and Exercise Psychology, 3*, 455–468.

Tolfrey, K. (2004). Lipid-lipoproteins in children: An exercise dose-response study. *Medicine and Science in Sports and Exercise, 36*, 418–427.

Tolfrey, K., Jones, A. M., & Campbell, I. G. (2000). The effect of aerobic exercise training on the lipid-lipoprotein profile of children and adolescents. *Sports Medicine, 29*, 99–112.

Tolstrup, J. S., Nordestgaard, B. G., Rasmussen, S., Tybjærg-Hansen, & Grønbæk, M. (2008). Alcoholism and alcohol drinking habits predicted from alcohol dehydrogenase genes. *Pharmacogenomics Journal, 8*, 220–227.

Tomar, S. L. (2007). Epidemiologic perspectives on smokeless tobacco marketing and population harm. *American Journal of Preventive Medicine, 33*(6, Suppl.), S387–S397.

Tomar, S. L., & Hatsukami, D. K. (2007). Perceived risk of harm from cigarettes or smokeless tobacco among U.S. high school seniors. *Nicotine and Tobacco Research, 9*, 1191–1196.

Tomfohr, L. M., Martin, T. M., & Miller, G. E. (2008). Symptoms of depression and impaired endothelial function in healthy adolescent women. *Journal of Behavioral Medicine, 31*, 137–143.

Toneatto, T., & Nguyen, L. (2007). Does mindfulness meditation improve anxiety and mood symptoms? A review of the controlled research. *Canadian Journal of Psychiatry, 52*, 260–266.

Torpy, J. M. (2006). Eating fish: Health benefits and risks. *Journal of the American Medical Association, 296*, 1926.

Torstveit, M. K., Rosenvinge, J. H., & Sundgot-Borgen, J. (2008). Prevalence of eating disorders and the predictive power of risk models in female elite athletes: A controlled study. *Scandinavian Journal of Medicine and Science in Sports, 18*, 108–118.

Tousignant-Laflamme, Y., Rainville, P., & Marchand, S. (2005). Establishing a link between heart rate and pain in healthy subjects: A gender effect. *Journal of Pain, 6*, 341–347.

Tovian, S. M. (2004). Health services and health care economics: The health psychology marketplace. *Health Psychology, 23*, 138–141.

Townley, B. (2004, February 2). *Drew Barrymore confirms lesbian past.* Retrieved March 29, 2005, from http://uk.gay.com/headlines/5749

Tractenberg, R. E., Singer, C. M., & Kaye, J. A. (2005). Symptoms of sleep disturbance in persons with Alzheimer's disease and normal elderly. *Journal of Sleep Research, 14*, 177–185.

Traditional Chinese Medicine World Foundation (TCMWF). (2005–2008). What is traditional Chinese medicine? Retrieved April 21, 2008, from http://www.tcmworld.org/what_is_tcm/

Tramer, M. R., Carroll, D., Campbell, F. A., Reynolds, D. J. M., Moore, R. A., & McQuay, H. J. (2001). Cannabinoids for control of chemotherapy induced nausea and vomiting: Quantitative systematic review. *British Medical Journal, 323*, 16–20.

Travis, L. (2001). Training for interdisciplinary healthcare. *Health Psychologist, 23*(1), 4–5.

Treiber, F. A., Davis, H., Musante, L., Raunikar, R. A., Strong. W. G., McCaffrey, F., et al. (1993). Ethnicity, gender, family history of myocardial infarction, and menodynamic responses to laboratory stressors in children. *Health Psychology, 12*, 6–15.

Tremblay, A. (2004). Dietary fat and body weight set point. *Nutrition Reviews, 62*(Suppl.), 75–77.

Tremblay, L., & Frigon, J.-Y. (2004). Biobehavioural and cognitive determinants of adolescent girls' involvement in sexual risk behaviours: A test of three theoretical models. *Canadian Journal of Human Sexuality, 13*, 29–43.

Treur, T., Koperdák, M., Rózsa, S., & Füredi, J. (2005). The impact of physical and sexual abuse on body image in eating disorders. *European Eating Disorders Review, 13*, 106–111.

Troxel, W. M., Matthews, K. A., Bromberger, J. T., & Sutton-Tyrrell, K. (2003). Chronic stress burden, discrimination, and subclinical carotid artery disease in African American and Caucasian women. *Health Psychology, 22*, 300–309.

Troxel, W. M., Matthews, K. A., Gallo, L. C., & Kuller, L. H. (2005). Marital quality and occurrence of the metabolic syndrome in women. *Archives of Internal Medicine, 165*, 1022–1027.

Trunko, M. E., Rockwell, R. E., Curry, E., Runfola, C., & Kaye, W. H. (2007). Management of bulimia nervosa. *Women's Health, 3*, 255–265.

The truth about dieting. (2002, June). *Consumer Reports, 67*(6), 26–31.

Tsai, A. G., & Wadden, T. A. (2005). Systematic review: An evaluation of major commercial weight loss programs in the United States. *Annals of Internal Medicine, 142,* 56–66.

Tsao, J. C. I (2007). Effectiveness of massage therapy for chronic, non-malignant pain: A review. *Evidence-Based Complementary and Alternative Medicine, 4,* 165–179.

Tsao, J. C. I., & Zeltzer, L. K. (2005). Complementary and alternative medicine approaches for pediatric pain: A review of the state-of-the-science. *Evidence-Based Complementary and Alternative Medicine, 2,* 149–159.

Tsiotra, P. C., & Tsigos, C. (2006). Stress, the endoplasmic reticulum, and insulin resistance. In G. P. Chrousos & C. Tsigos (Eds.), *Stress, obesity, and metabolic syndrome* (pp. 63–76). New York: Annals of the New York Academy of Sciences.

Tucker, J. A., Phillips, M. M., Murphy, J. G., & Raczynski, J. M. (2004). Behavioral epidemiology and health psychology. In R. G. Frank, A. Baum, & J. L. Wallander (Eds.), *Handbook of clinical health psychology* (Vol. 3, pp. 435–464). Washington, DC: American Psychological Association.

Tucker, J. S., Orlando, M., & Ellickson, P. L. (2003). Patterns and correlates of binge drinking trajectories form early adolescence to young adulthood. *Health Psychology, 22,* 79–87.

Tucker, O. N., Szomstein, S., & Rosenthal, R. J. (2007). Nutritional consequences of weight loss surgery. *Medical Clinics of North America, 91,* 499–513.

Turk, D. C. (1978). Cognitive behavioral techniques in the management of pain. In J. P. Foreyt & D. P. Rathjen (Eds.), *Cognitive behavior therapy.* New York: Plenum Press.

Turk, D. C. (2001). Physiological and psychological bases of pain. In A. Baum, T. A. Revenson, & J. E. Singer (Eds.), *Handbook of health psychology* (pp. 117–131). Mahwah, NJ: Erlbaum.

Turk, D. C., & McCarberg, B. (2005). Non-pharmacological treatments for chronic pain: A disease management context. *Disease Management and Health Outcomes, 13,* 19–30.

Turk, D. C., & Melzack, R. (2001). The measurement of pain and the assessment of people experiencing pain. In D. C. Turk & R. Melzack (Eds.), *Handbook of pain assessment* (2nd ed., pp. 3–11). New York: Guilford Press.

Turk, D. C., & Rudy, T. E. (1988). Toward an empirically derived taxonomy of chronic pain patients: Integration of psychological assessment data. *Journal of Consulting and Counseling Psychology, 56,* 233–238.

Turner, J., & Kelly, B. (2000). Emotional dimensions of chronic disease. *Western Journal of Medicine, 172,* 124–128.

Turner, J. A., Deyo, R. A., Loeser, J. D., Von Korff, M., & Fordyce, W. E. (1994). The importance of placebo effects in pain treatment and research. *Journal of the American Medical Association, 271,* 1609–1614.

Turner, R. J., & Avison, W. R. (2003). Status variations in stress exposure: Implications for the interpretation of research on race, socioeconomic status, and gender. *Journal of Health and Social Behavior, 44,* 488–505.

Turner, R. J., & Wheaton, B. (1995). Checklist measurement of stressful life events. In S. Cohen, R. C. Kessler, & L. U. Gordon (Eds.), *Measuring stress: A guide for health and social scientists* (pp. 29–58). New York: Oxford University Press.

Turnipseed, D. L. (2003). Hardy personality: A potential link with organizational citizenship behavior. *Psychological Reports, 93,* 529–543.

Turpin, R. S., Simmons, J. B., Lew, J. F., Alexander, C. M., Dupee, M. A., Kavanagh, P., et al. (2004). Improving treatment regimen adherence in coronary heart disease by targeting patient types. *Disease Management and Health Outcomes, 12,* 377–383.

Twardella, D., Loew, M., Rothenbacher, D., Stegmaier, C., Ziegler, H., & Brenner, H. (2006). The impact of body weight on smoking cessation in German adults. *Preventive Medicine, 42,* 109–113.

Twenge, J. M., Liqing, Z., & Im, C. (2004). It's beyond my control: A cross-temporal meta-analysis of increasing externality in locus of control, 1960–2002. *Personality and Social Psychology Review, 8,* 308–319.

Tylka, T. L. (2004). The relation between body dissatisfaction and eating disorder symptomatology: An analysis of moderating variables. *Journal of Counseling Psychology, 51,* 178–191.

UCLA Cousins Center. (2007). *Overview.* Retrieved May 29, 2008, from http://www.cousinspni.org/about_front.html

Ullrich, P. M., Rothrock, N. E., Lutgendorf, S. K., Jochimsen, P. R., & Williams, R. D. (2008). Adjustment and discussion of cancer: A comparison of breast and prostate cancer survivors. *Psychology and Health, 23,* 391–406.

Ulmer, H., Kelleher, C., Diem, G., & Concin, H. (2004). Why Eve is not Adam: Prospective follow-up of 149,650 women and men of cholesterol and other risk factors related to cardiovascular and all-cause mortality. *Journal of Women's Health, 13,* 41–53.

Ulrich, C. (2002). High stress and low income: The environment of poverty. *Human Ecology, 30*(4), 16–18.

UNAIDS. (2007). *AIDS epidemic update, 2007.* Geneva: Joint United Nations Programme on HIV/AIDS.

UNAIDS. (2008). *Toward universal access: Scaling up priority HIV/AIDS interventions in the health sector: A progress report 2008.* Geneva: World Health Organization.

Unger, J. B., Boley Cruz, T., Rohrbach, L. A., Ribisl, K. M., Baezconde-Garbanati, L., Chen, X., et al. (2000). English language use as a risk factor for smoking initiation among Hispanic and Asian American adolescents: Evidence for mediation by tobacco-related beliefs and social norms. *Health Psychology, 19,* 403–410.

Unger, J. B., Reynolds, K., Shakib, S., Spruijt-Metz, D., Sun, P., & Johnson, C. A. (2004). Acculturation, physical activity, and fast-food consumption among Asian-American and Hispanic adolescents. *Journal of Community Health, 29,* 467–481.

U.S. Bureau of the Census (USBC). (1975). *Historical statistics of the United States: Colonial times to 1970: Part 1*. Washington, DC: U.S. Government Printing Office.

U.S. Census Bureau (USCB). (2007). *Statistical abstract of the United States: 2008* (127th edition). Washington, DC: U.S. Government Printing Office.

U.S. Department of Health and Human Services (USDHHS). (1990). *The health benefits of smoking cessation: A report of the Surgeon General* (DHHS Publication No. CDC 90-8416). Washington, DC: U.S. Government Printing Office.

U.S. Department of Health and Human Services (USDHHS). (1991). *Healthy people 2000: National health promotion and disease prevention objectives*. (PHS Publication No. 91-50212). Washington, DC: Author.

U.S. Department of Health and Human Services (USDHHS). (1995). *Healthy People 2000 review, 1994* (DHHS Publication No. PHS 95-1256-1). Washington, DC: U.S. Government Printing Office.

U.S. Department of Health and Human Services (USDHHS). (1996). *Physical activity and health: A report of the Surgeon General*. Atlanta, GA: Centers for Disease Control and Prevention.

U.S. Department of Health and Human Services (USDHHS). (2000). *Healthy People 2010: Understanding and improving health* (2nd ed.). Washington, DC: U.S. Government Printing Office.

U.S. Department of Health and Human Services (USDHHS). (2003). *The seventh report of the Joint National Committee on Prevention, Detection, Evaluation and Treatment of High Blood Pressure* (NIH Publication No. 03–5233). Washington, DC: Author.

U.S. Department of Health and Human Services (USDHHS). (2004). *The health consequences of smoking: A report of the Surgeon General*. Atlanta, GA: Author.

U.S. Department of Health and Human Services (USDHHS). (2006). *The health consequences of involuntary exposure to tobacco smoke: A report of the Surgeon General*. Atlanta, GA: Author.

U.S. Department of Health and Human Services (USDHHS). (2007). *Healthy people 2010 midcourse review*. Retrieved August 5, 2008, from http://www.healthypeople.gov/Data/midcourse/

U.S. Public Health Service (USPHS). (1964). *Smoking and health: Public Health Service report of the Advisory Committee to the Surgeon General of the Public Health Service* (PHS Publication No. 1103). Washington, DC: U.S. Government Printing Office.

Uzunca, K., Birtane, M., Durmus-Altun, G., & Ustun, F. (2005). High bone mineral density in loaded skeletal regions of former professional football (soccer) players: What is the effect of time after career? *British Journal of Sports Medicine, 39*, 154–158.

Vainionpää, A., Korpelainen, R., Leppäluoto, J., & Jämsä, T. (2005). Effects of high-impact exercise on bone mineral density: A randomized controlled trial in premenopausal women. *Osteoporosis International, 16*, 191–197.

van Baal, P. H. M., Polder, J. J., de Wit, G. A., Hoogenveen, R. T., Feenstra, T. L., Bohuizen, H. C., et al. (2008). Lifetime medical costs of obesity: Prevention no cure for increasing health expenditure. *PLoS Medicine, 5*(2), 0242–0249.

van Cauter, E., Holmbäck, U., Knutson, K., Leproult, R., Miller, A., Nedeltcheva, A., et al. (2007). Impact of sleep and sleep loss on neuroendocrine and metabolic function. *Hormone Research, 67*(Suppl. 1), 2–9.

Van den Beuken-van Everdingen, M. H. J., de Rijke, J. M., Kessels, A. G., Schouten, H. C., van Kleef, M., & Patijn, J. (2007). High prevalence of pain in patients with cancer in a large population-based study in The Netherlands. *Pain, 132*, 312–320.

Van Den Buick, J. (2004). The relationship between television fiction and fear of crime: An empirical comparison of three causal explanations. *European Journal of Communication, 19*, 239–248.

Van der Does, A. J., & Van Dyck, R. (1989). Does hypnosis contribute to the care of burn patients? Review of evidence. *General Hospital Psychiatry, 11*, 119–124.

van Hanswijck de Jonge, P., van Furth, E. F., Lacey, J. H., & Waller, G. (2003). The prevalence of DSM-IV personality pathology among individuals with bulimia nervosa, binge eating disorder and obesity. *Psychological Medicine, 33*, 1311–1317.

van Reekum, R., Binns, M., Clarke, D., Chayer, C., Conn, D., & Herrmann, N. (2005). Is late-life depression a predictor of Alzheimer's disease? Results from a historical cohort study. *International Journal of Geriatric Psychiatry, 20*, 80–82.

van Ryn, M., & Burke, J. (2000). The effect of patient race and socio-economic status on physicians' perception of patients. *Social Science and Medicine, 50*, 813–828.

van Zundert, J., & van Kleef, M. (2005). Low back pain: From algorithm to cost-effectiveness? *Pain Practice, 5*, 179–189.

Varady, K. A., & Jones, P. J. H. (2005). Combination diet and exercise interventions for the treatment of dysilpidemia: An effective preliminary strategy to lower cholesterol levels? *Journal of Nutrition, 135*, 1829–1835.

Vastag, B. (2001). Quitting smoking harder for women. *Journal of the American Medical Association, 285*, 2966.

Veldtman, G. R., Matley, S. L., Kendall, L., Quirk, J., Gibbs, J. L., Parsons, J. M., et al. (2001). Illness understanding in children and adolescents with heart disease. *Western Journal of Medicine, 174*, 171–173.

Velicer, W. F., Fava, J. L., Keller, S., Ramelson, H., Friedman, R. H., Gulliver, S. B., et al. (2006). Evaluating nicotine replacement therapy and stage-based therapies in a population-based effectiveness trial. *Journal of Consulting and Clinical Psychology, 74*, 1162–1172.

Velicer, W. F., & Prochaska, J. O. (2008). Stages and non-stage theories of behavior and behavior change: A comment on Schwarzer. *Applied Psychology: An International Review, 57*, 75–83.

Velligan, D. I., Wang, M., Diamond, P., Glahn, D. C., Castillo, D., Bendle, S., et al. (2007). Relationships among subjective and objective measures of adherence to oral antipsychotic medications. *Psychiatric Services, 58,* 1187–1192.

Vemuri, P., Gunter, J. L., Senjem, M. L., Whitwell, J. L., Kantarci, K., Knopman, D. S., et al. (2008). Alzheimer's disease diagnosis in individual subjects using structural MR images: Validation studies. *NeuroImage, 39,* 1186–1197.

Venn, A., & Britton, J. (2007). Exposure to secondhand smoke and biomarkers of cardiovascular disease risk in never-smoking adults. *Circulation, 115,* 900–995.

Verkaik, R., Van Weert, J. C. M., & Francke, A. L. (2005). The effects of psychosocial methods on depressed, aggressive and apathetic behaviors of people with dementia: A systematic review. *International Journal of Geriatric Psychiatry, 20,* 301–314.

Verma, K. B., & Khan, M. I. (2007). Social inhibition, negative affectivity and depression in cancer patients with Type D personality. *Social Science International, 23,* 114–122.

Vermeire, E., Hearnshaw, H., Van Royen, P., & Denekens, J. (2001). Patient adherence to treatment: Three decades of research. A comprehensive review. *Journal of Clinical Pharmacy and Therapeutics, 26,* 331–342.

Vineis, P. (2005). Environmental tobacco smoke and risk of respiratory cancer and chronic obstructive pulmonary disease in former smokers and never smokers in the EPC prospective study. *British Medical Journal, 330,* 277–280.

Virmani, R., Burke, A. P., & Farb, A. (2001). Sudden cardiac death. *Cardiovascular Pathology, 10,* 211–218.

Visser, M. (1999). Food and culture: Interconnections. *Social Research, 66,* 117–132.

Vlachopoulos, C., Rokkas, K., Ioakeimidis, N., & Stefanadis, C. (2007). Inflammation, metabolic syndrome, erectile dysfunction, and coronary artery disease: Common links. *European Urology, 52,* 1590–1600.

Voas, R. B., Roman, T. E., Tippetts, A. S., & Durr-Holden, C. D. M. (2006). Drinking status and fatal crashes: Which drinkers contribute most to the problem? *Journal of Studies on Alcohol, 67,* 722–729.

Vollrath, M. E., Landolt, M. A., Gnehm, H. E., Laimbacher, J., & Sennhauser, F. H. (2007). Child and parental personality are associated with glycaemic control in Type 1 diabetes. *Diabetic Medicine, 24,* 1028–1033.

von Baeyer, C. L., & Spagrud, L. J. (2007). Systematic review of observational (behavioral) measures of pain for children and adolescents aged 3 to 18 years. *Pain, 127,* 140–150.

von Hertzen, L. C., & Haahtela, T. (2004). Asthma and atopy—The price of affluence? *Allergy, 59,* 124–137.

von Känel, R., Hepp, U., Kraemer, B., Traber, R., Keel, M., Mica, L., et al. (2007). Evidence for low-grade systemic proinflammatory activity in patients with posttraumatic stress disorder. *Journal of Psychiatric Research, 41,* 744–752.

Von Korff, M., Barlow, W., Cherkin, D., & Deyo, R. A. (1994). Effects of practice style in managing back pain. *Annals of Internal Medicine, 121,* 187–195.

Voukelatos, A., Cummings, R. G., Lord, S. R., & Rissel, C. (2007). A randomized, controlled trial of tai chi for the prevention of falls: The central Sydney tai chi trial. *Journal of the American Geriatrics Society, 55,* 1195–1191.

Wadden, T. A., Crerand, C. E., & Brock, J. (2005). Behavioral treatment of obesity. *Psychiatric Clinics of North America, 28,* 151–170.

Wager, T. D., Rilling, J. K., Smith, E. E., Sololik, A., Casey, K. L., Davidson, R. J., et al. (2004). Placebo-induced changes in fMRI in the anticipation and experience of pain. *Science, 303,* 1162–1167.

Waite-Jones, J. M., & Madill, A. (2008a). Amplified ambivalence: Having a sibling with juvenile idiopathic arthritis. *Psychology and Health, 23,* 477–492.

Waite-Jones, J. M., & Madill, A. (2008b). Concealed concern: Fathers' experiences of having a child with juvenile idiopathic arthritis. *Psychology and Health, 23,* 585–601.

Walach, H., & Jonas, W. B. (2004). Placebo research: The evidence base for harnessing self-healing capacities. *Journal of Alternative and Complementary Medicine, 10*(Suppl.), S103–S112.

Wald, H. S., Dube, C. E., & Anthony, D. C. (2007). Untangling the Web—The impact of Internet use on health care and the physician-patient relationship. *Patient Education and Counseling, 68,* 218–224.

Walen, H. R., & Lachman, M. E. (2000). Social support and strain from partner, family, and friends: Costs and benefits for men and women in adulthood. *Journal of Social and Personal Relationships, 17,* 5–30.

Walker, A. R. P., Walker, B. F., & Adam, F. (2003). Nutrition, diet, physical activity, smoking, and longevity: From primitive hunter-gatherer to present passive consumer—How far can we go? *Nutrition, 19,* 169–173.

Walker, E. A., Mertz, C. K., Kalten, M. R., & Flynn, J. (2003). Risk perception for developing diabetes. *Diabetes Care, 26,* 2543–2548.

Wall, P. (2000). *Pain: The science of suffering.* New York: Columbia University Press.

Waltenbaugh, A. W., & Zagummy, M. J. (2004). Optimistic bias and perceived control among cigarette smokers. *Journal of Alcohol and Drug Education, 47,* 20–33.

Walter, H., Gutierrez, K., Ramskogler, K., Hertling, I., Dvorak, A., & Lesch, O. M. (2003). Gender-specific differences in alcoholism: Implications for treatment. *Archives of Women's Mental Health, 6,* 253–258.

Walters, G. D. (2000). Spontaneous remission from alcohol, tobacco, and other drug abuse: Seeking quantitative answers to qualitative questions. *American Journal of Drug and Alcohol Abuse, 26,* 443–460.

Walton, K. G., Schneider, R. H., Nidich, S. I., Salerno, J. W., Nordstrom, C. K., & Merz, C. N. B. (2002). Psychosocial stress and cardiovascular disease Part 2: Effectiveness of the Transcendental Meditation program in treatment and prevention. *Behavioral Medicine, 28,* 106–123.

Wamala, S. P., Mittleman, M. A., Horsten, M., Schenck-Gustafsson, K., & Orth-Gomér, K. (2000). Job stress and the occupational gradient in coronary heart disease risk in women: The Stockholm Female Coronary Risk study. *Social Science and Medicine, 51*, 481–489.

Wang, G.-J., Volkow, N. D., Fowler, J. S., Franceschi, D., Wong, C. T., Pappas, N. R., et al. (2003). Alcohol intoxication induces greater reductions in brain metabolism in male than in female subjects. *Alcoholism: Clinical and Experimental Research, 27*, 909–917.

Wang, H.-W., Mittleman, M. A., & Orth-Gomér, K. (2005). Influence of social support on progression of coronary artery disease in women. *Social Science and Medicine, 60*, 599–607.

Wang, H.-X., Leineweber, C., Kirkeeide, R., Svane, B., Schenck-Guftafsson, K., Theorell, T., et al. (2007). Psychosocial stress and atherosclerosis: Family and work stress accelerate progression of coronary disease in women. The Stockholm Female Coronary Angiography Study. *Journal of Internal Medicine, 261*, 245–254.

Wang, J. L., Lesage, A., Schmitz, N., & Drapeau, A. (2008) The relationship between work stress and mental disorders in men and women: Findings from a population-based study. *Journal of Epidemiology and Community Health, 62*, 42–47.

Wang, Y. (2004). Diet, physical activity, childhood obesity and risk of cardiovascular disease. *International Congress Series, 1262*, 176–179.

Wang, Y., Chen, X., Song, Y., Caballero, B., & Cheskin, L. J. (2008). Association between obesity and kidney disease: A systematic review and meta-analysis. *Kidney International, 3*, 19–33.

Wannamethee, S. G., Shaper, A. G., & Lennon, L. (2005). Reasons for intentional weight loss, unintentional weight loss, and mortality in older men. *Archives of Internal Medicine, 165*, 1035–1040.

Warburton, D. E. R., Nicol, C. W., Bredin, S. S. D. (2006). Health benefits of physical activity: The evidence. *Canadian Medical Association Journal, 174*, 801–809.

Wardle, J., & Johnson, F. (2002). Weight and dieting: Examining levels of weight concern in British adults. *International Journal of Obesity, 26*, 1144–1149.

Warner, R., & Griffiths, M. D. (2006). A qualitative thematic analysis of exercise addiction: An exploratory study. *International Journal of Mental Health and Addiction, 4*, 13–26.

Warren, C. W., Jones, N. R., Peruga, A., Chauvin, J., Baptiste, J.-P., de Silva, V. C., et al. (2008). Global youth tobacco surveillance, 2000–2007. *Morbidity and Mortality Weekly Reports, 57*(SS-1), 1–27.

Watanabe, T., Higuchi, K., Tanigawa, T., Tominaga, K., Fujiwara, Y., & Arakawa, T. (2002). Mechanisms of peptic ulcer recurrence: Role of inflammation. *Inflammopharmacology, 10*, 291–302.

Watkins, L. R., Hutchinson, M. R., Ledeboer, A., Wieseler-Frank, J., Milligan, E. D., & Maier, S. F. (2007). Glia as the "bad guys": Implications for improving clinical pain control and the clinical utility of opioids. *Brain, Behavior and Immunity, 21*, 131–146.

Watkins, L. R., & Maier, S. F. (2003). When good pain turns bad. *Current Directions in Psychological Science, 12*, 232–236.

Watkins, L. R., & Maier, S. F. (2005). Immune regulation of central nervous system function: From sickness responses to pathological pain. *Journal of Internal Medicine, 257*, 139–155.

Waye, K. P., Bengtsson, J., Rylander, R., Hucklebridge, F., Evans, P., & Clow, A. (2002). Low frequency noise enhances cortisol among noise sensitive subjects during work performance. *Life Sciences, 70*, 745–758.

Wayne, P. M., Kiel, D. P., Krebs, D. E., Davis, R. B., Savetsky-German, J., Connelly, M., et al. (2007). The effects of tai chi on bone mineral density in postmenopausal women: A systematic review. *Archives of Physical Medicine and Rehabilitation, 88*, 673–680.

Wechsler, H., Lee, J. E., Kuo, M., Seibring, M., Nelson, T. F., & Lee, H. (2002). Trends in college binge drinking during a period of increased prevention efforts: Findings for 4 Harvard School of Public Health College Alcohol Study surveys: 1993–2001. *Journal of American College Health, 50*, 203–217.

Wee, C. C., Rigotti, N. A., Davis, R. B., & Phillips, R. S. (2001). Relationship between smoking and weight control efforts among adults in the United States. *Archives of Internal Medicine, 161*, 546–550.

Weems, C. F., Watts, S. E., Marsee, M. A., Taylor, L. K., Costa, N. M., Cannon, M. F., et al. (2007). The psychological impact of Hurricane Katrina: Contextual differences in psychological symptoms, social support, and discrimination. *Behavior Research and Therapy, 45*, 2295–2306.

Weidner, G. (2000). Why do men get more heart disease than women? An international perspective. *Journal of American College Health, 48*, 291–296.

Weidner, G., & Cain, V. S. (2003). The gender gap in heart disease: Lessons from Eastern Europe. *American Journal of Public Health, 93*, 768–770.

Weil, C. M., Wade, S. L., Bauman, L. J., Lynn, H., Mitchell, H., & Lavigne, J. (1999). The relationship between psychosocial factors and asthma morbidity in inner-city children with asthma. *Pediatrics, 104*, 1274–1280.

Weil, J. M., & Lee, H. H. (2004). Cultural considerations in understanding family violence among Asian American Pacific islander families. *Journal of Community Health Nursing, 21*, 217–227.

Weinberger, A. H., Krishnan-Sarin, S., Mazure, C. M., & McKee, S. A. (2008). Relationship of perceived risks of smoking cessation to symptoms of withdrawal, craving, and depression during short-term smoking abstinence. *Addictive Behaviors, 33*, 960–963.

Weiner, H., & Shapiro, A. P. (2001). *Helicobacter pylori*, immune function, and gastric lesions. In R. Ader, D. L. Felten, & N. Cohen (Eds.), *Psychoneuroimmunology* (3rd ed., Vol. 2, pp. 671–686). San Diego, CA: Academic Press.

Weiner, M. F., Hynan, L. S., Bret, M. E., & White, C., III. (2005). Early behavioral symptoms and course of Alzheimer's disease. *Acta Psychiatrica Scandinavica, 111*, 367–371.

Weingart, S. N., Pagovich, O., Sands, D. Z., Li, J. M., Aronson, M. D., Davis, R. B., et al. (2006). Patient-reported service quality on a medicine unit. *International Journal for Quality in Health Care, 18,* 95–101.

Weingarten, S. R., Henning, J. M., Badamgarav, E., Knight, K., Hasselblad, V., Gano, A., Jr., et al. (2002). Interventions used in disease management programmes for patients with chronic illness—Which ones work? Meta-analysis of published reports. *British Medical Journal, 325,* 925–928.

Weinstein, N. D. (1980). Unrealistic optimism about future life events. *Journal of Personality and Social Psychology, 39,* 806–820.

Weinstein, N. D. (1984). Why it won't happen to me: Perceptions of risk factors and susceptibility. *Health Psychology, 3,* 431–457.

Weinstein, N. D. (1988). The precaution adoption process. *Health Psychology, 7,* 355–386.

Weinstein, N. D. (2000). Perceived probability, perceived severity, and health-protective behavior. *Health Psychology, 19,* 65–74.

Weinstein, N. D. (2001). Smokers' recognition of their vulnerability to harm. In P. Slovic (Ed.), *Smoking: Risk, perception and policy* (pp. 81–96). Thousand Oaks, CA: Sage.

Weinstein, N. D., Lyon, J. E., Sandman, P. M., & Cuite, C. L. (2003). Experimental evidence for stages of health behavior change: The precaution adoption process model applied to home radon testing. In P. Salovey & A. J. Rothman (Eds.), *Social psychology of health* (pp. 249–260). New York: Psychology Press.

Weir, H. K., Thun, M. J., Hankey, B. F., Ries, L. A. G., Howe, H. L., Wingo, P. A., et al. (2003). Annual report to the nation on the status of cancer, 1975–2000, featuring the uses of surveillance data for cancer prevention and control. *Journal of the National Cancer Institute, 95,* 1276–1299.

Weisli, P., Schmid, C., Kerwer, O., Nigg-Koch, C., Klaghofer, R., & Seifert, B. (2005). Acute psychological stress affects glucose concentrations in patients with Type I diabetes following food intake but not in the fasting state. *Diabetes Care, 28,* 1910–1915.

Weiss, J. R., Moysich, K. B., & Swede, H. (2005). Epidemiology of male breast cancer. *Cancer Epidemiology, Biomarkers and Prevention, 14,* 20–26.

Weiss, J. W., Cen, S., Schuster, D. V., Unger, J. B., Johnson, C. A., Mouttapa, M., et al. (2006). Longitudinal effects of pro-tobacco and anti-tobacco messages on adolescent smoking susceptibility. *Nicotine and Tobacco Research, 8,* 455–465.

Weiss, R. (1999, November 30). Medical errors blamed for many deaths; as many as 98,000 a year in US linked to mistakes. *Washington Post,* p. A1.

Weitz, R. (2007). *The sociology of health, illness, and health care: A critical approach* (4th ed.). Belmont, CA: Wadsworth.

Wen, C., Tsai, S. P., Cheng, T. Y., Chan, H., T., Chung, W. S. I., & Chen, C. J. (2005). Excess injury mortality among smokers: A neglected tobacco hazard. *Tobacco Control, 14*(Suppl. 1), 28–32.

Wen, M. (2007). Racial and ethnic differences in general health status and limiting health conditions among American children: Parental reports in the 1999 National Survey of America's Families. *Ethnicity and Health, 12,* 401–422.

Wendel-Vos, G. C., Schuit, A. J., Feskens, E. J., Boshuizen, H. C., Verschuren, W. M., Saris, W. H., et al. (2004). Physical activity and stroke: A meta-analysis of observational data. *International Journal of Epidemiology, 33,* 787–798.

Wennberg, P., Eliasson, M., Hallmans, G., Johansson, L., Boman, K., & Jansson, J.-H. (2007). The risk of myocardial infarction and sudden cardiac death amongst snuff users with or without a previous history of smoking. *Journal of Internal Medicine, 262,* 360–367.

Wenzel, S. E. (2006). Asthma: Defining of the persistent adult phenotypes. *Lancet, 368,* 804–813.

West, S. L., & O'Neal, K. K. (2004). Project D.A.R.E. outcome effectiveness revisited. *American Journal of Public Health, 94,* 1027–1029.

Westerfelt, A. (2004). A qualitative investigation of adherence issues for men who are HIV positive. *Social Work, 49,* 231–239.

Westover, A. N., Nakonezny, P. A., & Haley, R. W. (2008). Acute myocardial infarction in young adults who abuse amphetamines. *Drug and Alcohol Dependence, 96,* 49–56.

Wetter, D. W., Cofta-Gunn, L., Fouladi, R. T., Irvin, J. E., Daza, P., Mazas, C., et al. (2005). Understanding the association among education, employment characteristics, and smoking. *Addictive Behaviors, 30,* 905–914.

White, S., Chen, J., & Atchison, R. (2008). Relationship of preventive health practices and health literacy: A national study. *American Journal of Health Behavior, 32,* 227–242.

White, W. L. (2004). Addiction recovery mutual aid groups: An enduring international phenomenon. *Addiction, 99,* 532–538.

Whitfield, K. E., Weidner, G., Clark, R., & Anderson, N. B. (2002). Sociodemographic diversity in behavioral medicine. *Journal of Consulting and Clinical Psychology, 70,* 463–481.

Wiehe, S. E., Garrison, M. M., Christakis, D. A., Ebel, B. E., & Rivara, F. P. (2005). A systematic review of school-based smoking prevention trials with long-term follow-up. *Journal of Adolescent Health, 36,* 162–169.

Wilbert-Lampen, U., Leistner, D., Greven, S., Pohl, T., Sper, S., Völker, C., et al. (2008). Cardiovascular events during World Cup Soccer. *New England Journal of Medicine, 358,* 475–483.

Wiley, J. A., & Camacho, T. C. (1980). Life-style and future health: Evidence from the Alameda County Study. *Preventive Medicine, 9,* 1–21.

Williams, L. J., Jacka, F. N., Pasco, J. A., Dodd, S., & Berk, M. (2006). Depression and pain: An overview. *Acta Neuropsychiatrica, 18,* 79–87.

Williams, M. T., & Hord, H. G. (2005). The role of dietary factors in cancer prevention: Beyond fruits and vegetables. *Nutrition in Clinical Practice, 20,* 451–459.

Williams, P. G., Holmbeck, G. N., & Greenley, R. N. (2002). Adolescent health psychology. *Journal of Consulting and Clinical Psychology, 70,* 828–842.

Williams, P. T. (2001). Health effects resulting from exercise versus those from body fat loss. *Medicine and Science in Sports and Exercise, 33,* S611–S621.

Williams, R. B., Jr. (1989). *The trusting heart: Great news about Type A behavior.* New York: Times Books.

Williamson, D. A., Thaw, J. M., & Varnado-Sullivan, P. J. (2001). Cost-effectiveness analysis of a hospital-based cognitive-behavioral treatment program for eating disorders. *Behavior Therapy, 32,* 459–470.

Wills, T. A. (1998). Social support. In E. A. Blechman & K. D. Brownell (Eds.), *Behavioral medicine and women: A comprehensive handbook* (pp. 118–128). New York: Guilford Press.

Wills, T. A., Sargent, J. D., Stoolmiller, M., Gibbons, F. X., & Gerrard, M. (2008). Movie smoking exposure and smoking onset: A longitudinal study of meditation processes in a representative sample of U.S. adolescents. *Psychology of Addictive Behaviors, 22,* 269–277.

Wills-Karp, M. (2004). Interleukin-13 in asthma pathogenesis. *Immunological Reviews, 202,* 175–190.

Wilson, B., & McSherry, W. (2006). A study of nurses' inferences of patients' physical pain. *Journal of Clinical Nursing, 15,* 459–468.

Wilson, G. T., Fairburn, C. G., Agras, W. S., Walsh, B. T., & Kraemer, H. (2002). Cognitive-behavioral therapy for bulimia nervosa: Time course and mechanisms of change. *Journal of Consulting and Clinical Psychology, 70,* 267–274.

Wilson, J. F. (2001, October 29). Pain research comes into its own: Molecular biology may provide answers to relief. *The Scientist, 15*(21), 16–17.

Wimberly, S. R., Carver, C. S., Laurenceau, J.-P., Harris, S. D., & Antoni, M. H. (2005). Perceived partner reactions to diagnosis and treatment of breast cancer: Impact on psychosocial and psychosexual adjustment. *Journal of Consulting and Clinical Psychology, 73,* 300–311.

Windle, M., & Windle, R. C. (2001). Depressive symptoms and cigarette smoking among middle adolescents: Prospective associations and intrapersonal and interpersonal influences. *Journal of Consulting and Clinical Psychology, 69,* 215–226.

Wing, R. R., Gorin, A. A., Raynor, H. A., Tate, D. F., Fava, J. L., & Machan, J. (2007). "STOP Regain": Are there negative effects of daily weighing? *Journal of Consulting and Clinical Psychology, 75,* 652–656.

Wing, R. R., & Polley, B. A. (2001). Obesity. In A. Baum, T. A. Revenson, & J. E. Singer (Eds.), *Handbook of health psychology* (pp. 263–279). Mahwah, NJ: Erlbaum.

Wingard, D. L., Berkman, L. F., & Brand, R. J. (1982). A multivariate analysis of health-related practices: A nine-year mortality follow-up of the Alameda County study. *American Journal of Epidemiology, 116,* 765–775.

Winterling, J., Glimelius, B., & Nordin, K. (2008). The importance of expectations on the recovery period after cancer treatment. *Psycho-Oncology, 17,* 190–198.

Wipfli, B. M., Rethorst, C. D., & Landers, D. M. (2008). The anxiolytic effects of exercise: A meta-analysis of randomized trials and dose-response analysis. *Journal of Sport and Exercise Psychology, 30,* 392–410.

Wisborg, K., Kesmodel, U., Henriksen, T. B., Olsen, S. F., & Secher, N. J. (2001). Exposure to tobacco smoke in utero and the risk of stillbirth and death in the first year of life. *American Journal of Epidemiology, 154,* 322–327.

Wise, J. (2000). Largest-ever study shows reduction in cardiovascular mortality. *Bulletin of the World Health Organization, 78,* 562.

Wiseman, C. V., Gray, J. J., Mosimann, J. E., & Ahrens, A. H. (1992). Cultural expectations of thinness in women: An update. *International Journal of Eating Disorders, 11,* 85–89.

Wiseman, C. V., Sunday, S. R., & Becker, A. E. (2005). Impact of the media on adolescent body image. *Child and Adolescent Psychiatric Clinics of North Americs, 14,* 453–471.

Witkiewitz, K., & Marlatt, G. A. (2004). Relapse prevention for alcohol and drug problems. *American Psychologist, 59,* 224–235.

Witt, C. M., Brinkhaus, B., Reinhold, T., & Willich, S. N. (2006). Efficacy, effectiveness, safety and costs of acupuncture for chronic pain—Results of a large research initiative. *Acupuncture in Medicine, 24*(Suppl.), 33–39.

Wolfgang, M. E. (1957). Victim precipitated criminal homicide. *Journal of Criminal Law and Criminology, 48,* 1–11.

Wonderlich, S. A., Crosby, R. D., Joiner, T., Peterson, C. B., Bardone-Cone, A., Klein, M., et al. (2005). Personality subtyping and bulimia nervosa: Psychopathological and genetic correlates. *Psychological Medicine, 35,* 649–657.

Wonderlich, S. A., Wilsnack, R. W., Wilsnack, S. C., & Harris, T. R. (1996). Childhood sexual abuse and bulimic behavior in a nationally representative sample. *American Journal of Public Health, 86,* 1082–1086.

Wood, P. D., Stefanick, M. L., Dreon, D. M., Frey-Hewitt, B., Garay, S. C., Williams, P. T., et al. (1988). Changes in plasma lipids and lipoproteins in overweight men during weight loss through dieting compared with exercise. *New England Journal of Medicine, 319,* 1173–1179.

Woodhouse, A. (2005). Phantom limb sensation. *Clinical and Experimental Pharmacology and Physiology, 32,* 132–134.

Woodside, D. B. (2002). Eating disorders in men: An overview. *Healthy Weight Journal, 16*(4), 52–55.

Woolrich, R. A., Cooper, M. J., & Turner, H. M. (2008). Metacognition in patients with anorexia nervosa, dieting and non-dieting women: A preliminary study. *European Eating Disorders Review, 16,* 11–20.

Woolridge, E., Barton, S., Samuel, J., Osorio, J., Dougherty, A., & Holdcroft, A. (2005). Cannabis use in HIV for pain and other medical symptoms. *Journal of Pain and Symptom Management, 29,* 358–367.

World Cancer Research Fund/American Institute for Cancer Research (WCRF/AICR). (2007). *Food, nutrition, physical activity, and the prevention of cancer: A global perspective.* Washington, DC: AICR.

World Health Organization. (2008a). *The WHO report on the global tobacco epidemic, 2008.* Geneva: Author.

World Health Organization. (2008b). *World health 2008.* Geneva: WHO Press.

World Medical Association. (2004). *Declaration of Helsinki: Ethical principles for medical research involving human subjects.* Retrieved February 7, 2008, from http://www.wma.net/e/policy/b3.htm

Wright, C. E., O'Donnell, K., Brydon, L., Wardle, J., & Steptoe, A. (2007). Family history of cardiovascular disease is associated with cardiovascular responses to stress in healthy young men and women. *International Journal of Psychophysiology, 63,* 275–282.

Wright, R. J., Mitchell, H., Visness, C. M., Cohen, S., Stout, J., Evans, R., et al. (2004). Community violence and asthma morbidity: The Inner-City Asthma Study. *American Journal of Public Health, 94,* 625–632.

Writing Group for the Women's Health Initiative Investigators. (2002). Risks and benefits of estrogen plus progestin in healthy postmenopausal women: Principal results from the Women's Health Initiative randomized controlled trial. *Journal of the American Medical Association, 288,* 321–333.

Wyden, P. (1965). *The overweight society.* New York: Morrow.

Xin, L., Miller, Y. D., & Brown, W. J. (2007). A qualitative review of the role of qigong in the management of diabetes. *Journal of Alternative and Complementary Medicine, 13,* 427–434.

Xue, C. C. L., Zhang, A. L., Lin, V., Da Costa, C., & Story, D. F. (2007). Complementary and alternative medicine use in Australia: A national population-based survey. *Journal of Alternative and Complementary Medicine, 13,* 643–650.

Yager, J. (2008). Binge eating disorder: The search for better treatments. *American Journal of Psychiatry, 165,* 4–6.

Yang, Y., Verkuilen, J., Rosengren, K. S., Mariani, R. A., Reed, M., Grubisich, S. A., et al. (2007). Effects of a taiji and qigong intervention on the antibody response to influenza vaccine in older adults. *American Journal of Chinese Medicine, 35,* 597–607.

Yano, E., Wang, Z.-M., Wang, X.-R., Wang, M.-Z., & Lan, Y.-J. (2001). Cancer mortality among workers exposed to amphibole-free chrysotile, asbestos. *American Journal of Epidemiology, 154,* 538–543.

Yarnold, P. R., Michelson, E. A., Thompson, D. A., & Adams, S. L. (1998). Predicting patient satisfaction: A study of two emergency departments. *Journal of Behavioral Medicine, 21,* 545–563.

Ye, X., Gross, C. R., Schommer, J., Cline, R., & St. Peter, W. L. (2007). Association between copayment and adherence to statin treatment initiated after coronary heart disease hospitalization: A longitudinal, retrospective, cohort study. *Clinical Therapeutics, 29,* 2748–2757.

Yi, H.-Y., Chen, C. M., & Williams, G. D. (2006). *Trends in alcohol-related fatal traffic crashes, United States, 1982–2004* (Alcohol Epidemiologic Data System, Surveillance Report No. 76). Arlington, VA: National Institute of Alcohol Abuse and Alcoholism.

Ylvén, R., Björck-Åkesson, E., & Granlund, M. (2006). Literature review of positive functioning in families with children with a disability. *Journal of Policy and Practice in Intellectual Disabilities, 3,* 253–270.

Yong, H.-H., Borland, R., Hyland, A., & Siahpush, M. (2008). How does a failed quit attempt among regular smokers affect their cigarette consumption? Findings from the International Tobacco Control Four-Country Survey (ITC-4). *Nicotine and Tobacco Research, 10,* 897–905.

You, R. X., Thrift, A. G., McNeil, J. J., Davis, S. M., & Donnan, G. A. (1999). Ischemic stroke risk and passive exposure to spouses' cigarette smoking. *American Journal of Public Health, 89,* 572–575.

Young, K. M., Northern, J. J., Lister, K. M., Drummond, J. A., & O'Brien, W. H. (2007). A meta-analysis of family-behavioral weight-loss treatments for children. *Clinical Psychology Reviews, 27,* 240–249.

Young, L. R., & Nestle, M. (2002). The contribution of expanding portion sizes to the US obesity epidemic. *American Journal of Public Health, 92,* 246–249.

Yu, L., Chiu, C.-H., Lin, Y.-S., Wang, H.-H., & Chen, J.-W. (2007). Testing a model of stress and health using meta-analytic path analysis. *Journal of Nursing Research, 15,* 202–214.

Yu, Z., Nissinen, A., Vartiainen, E., Song, G., Guo, Z., Zheng, G., et al. (2000). Associations between socio-economic status and cardiovascular risk factors in an urban population in China. *Bulletin of the World Health Organization, 78,* 1296–1305.

Yuhas, N., McGowan, B., Fontaine, T., Czech, J., & Gambrell-Jones, J. (2006). Psychosocial interventions for disruptive symptoms of dementia. *Journal of Psychosocial Nursing and Mental Health Services, 44,* 34–42.

Yusuf, S., Hawken, S., Ôunpuu, S., Bautista, L., Franzosi, M. G., Commerford, P., et al. (2005). Obesity and the risk of myocardial infarction in 2700 participants from 52 countries: A case-control study. *Lancet, 366,* 1640–1649.

Yusuf, S., Hawken, S., Ôunpuu, S., Dans, T., Avezum, A., Lanas, F., et al. (2004). Effect of potentially modifiable risk factors associated with myocardial infarction in 52 countries (the INTERHEART study): Case-control study. *Lancet, 364,* 937–952.

Zaarcadoolas, C., Pleasant, A., & Greer, D. S. (2005). Understanding health literacy: An expanded model. *Health Promotion International, 20,* 195–203.

Zack, M., Poulos, C. X., Aramakis, V. B., Khamba, B. K., & MacLeod, C. M. (2007). Effects of drink-stress sequence and gender on alcohol stress response dampening in high and low anxiety sensitive drinkers. *Alcoholism: Clinical and Experimental Research, 31,* 411–422.

Zagorsky, J. L. (2004). The wealth effects of smoking. *Tobacco Control, 13,* 370–374.

Zakhari, S. (2006). Overview: How is alcohol metabolized by the body? *Alcohol Research and Health, 29,* 245–255.

Zakowski, S. G., Ramati, A., Morton, C., & Flanigan, R. (2004). Written emotional disclosure buffers the effects of social constraints on distress among cancer patients. *Health Psychology, 23*, 555–563.

Zautra, A. J. (2003). *Emotions, stress, and health.* New York: Oxford University Press.

Zehnacker, C. H., & Bemis-Dougherty, A. (2007). Effect of weighted exercises on bone mineral density in post menopausal women: A systematic review. *Journal of Geriatric Physical Therapy, 30*, 79–88.

Zelenko, M., Lock, J., Kraemer, H. C., & Steiner, H. (2000). Perinatal complications and child abuse in a poverty sample. *Child Abuse and Neglect, 24*, 939–950.

Zhan, C., & Miller, M. R. (2003). Excess length of stay, charges, and mortality attributable to medical injuries during hospitalization. *Journal of the American Medical Association, 290*, 1868–1874.

Zhang, B., Ferrence, R., Cohen, J., Bondy, S., Ashley, M. J., Rehm, J., et al. (2005). Smoking cessation and lung cancer mortality in a cohort of middle-aged Canadian women. *Annals of Epidemiology, 15*, 302–309.

Zigman, J. M., & Elmquist, J. K. (2003). Minireview: From anorexia to obesity—The yin and yang of body weight control. *Endocrinology, 144*, 1349–1356.

Zijlstra, G. A., Rixt, H., Jolanda, C. M., van Rossum, E., van Eijk, J. T., Yardley, L., et al. (2007). Interventions to reduce fear of falling in community-living older people: A systematic review. *Journal of American Geriatrics Society, 55*, 603–615.

Zimmerman, M. (1983). Methodological issues in the assessment of life events: A review of issues and research. *Clinical Psychology Review, 3*, 339–370.

Zimmerman, R. (2006, November 20). Cell phones provide medication information and reminders. *Wall Street Journal.*

Zimmerman, T., Heinrichs, N., & Baucom, D. H. (2007). "Does one size fit all?" Moderators in psychosocial interventions for breast cancer patients: A meta-analysis. *Annals of Behavioral Medicine, 34*, 225–239.

Zinberg, N. E. (1984). *Drug, set, and setting: The basis for controlled intoxicant use.* New Haven, CT: Yale University Press.

Zoller, H. (2005). Women caught in the multi-causal web: A gendered analysis of *Healthy People 2010. Communication Studies, 56*, 175–192.

Zorrilla, E. P., Luborsky, L., McKay, J. R., Rosenthal, R., Houldin, A., Tax, A., et al. (2001). The relationship of depression and stressors to immunological assays: A meta-analytic review. *Brain, Behavior and Immunity, 15*, 199–226.

Zubin, J., & Spring, B. (1977). Vulnerability: A new view of schizophrenia. *Journal of Abnormal Psychology, 86*, 103–127.

Zyazema, N. Z. (1984). Toward better patient drug compliance and comprehension: A challenge to medical and pharmaceutical services in Zimbabwe. *Social Science and Medicine, 18*, 551–554.

Zywiak, W. H., Stout, R. L., Longabaugh, R., Dyck, I., Connors, G. J., & Maisto, S. A. (2006). Relapse-onset factors in Project MATCH: The relapse questionnaire. *Journal of Substance Abuse Treatment, 31*, 341–345.

Name Index

SUBJECT INDEX

1. **False**—According to most health psychologists, health is more than the absence of disease; it is a positive state of well being. (Chapter 1)

2. **False**—The United States ranks in 14th place in terms of life expectancy. (Chapter 1)

3. **False**—The increase in life expectancy during the 20th century was primarily the result of decreases in infant mortality and improvements in public health. (Chapter 1)

4. **False**—The relationship between stress and disease is less certain than most people imagine. (Chapter 6)

5. **True**—People who maintain close to ideal weight are healthier and live longer than those who are either heavier or thinner. (Chapter 14)

6. **False**—Progress in research comes through the cumulative knowledge from many studies. (Chapter 2)

7. **True**—Smoking is the leading cause of preventable death in the United States. (Chapter 12)

8. **True**—Effective coping strategies allow people to deal with stress. (Chapter 5)

9. **False**—Although smoking contributes to the development of heart disease, more smoking-related cancer deaths occur than smoking-related heart disease deaths. (Chapter 12)

10. **False**—Correlation does not demonstrate a cause-and-effect relationship. (Chapter 2)

11. **False**—High cholesterol levels are related to increased heart disease risk during middle age, but after age 60, that relationship is not strong; low cholesterol becomes more of a risk. (Chapter 9)

12. **True**—Physical activity is another of the health habits that the Alameda County Study showed to be related to better health and longer life. (Chapter 2 & Chapter 15)

13. **False**—Lung cancer is the leading cause of cancer death for both women and men. (Chapter 10)

14. **True**—Not only overweight but also fat distribution poses health risks. (Chapter 14)

15. **True**—Stress affects the immune system, making people more vulnerable to infectious disease. (Chapter 6)

16. **False**—Female college students are more likely to use seat belts than male college students. (Chapter 16)